SMART DENTAL REVISION

Suraj Kumar MDS
Postgraduate Resident
Department of Oral and Maxillofacial Surgery
SGR College, Bangalore
Karnataka, India

JAYPEE The Health Sciences Publisher
New Delhi | London | Philadelphia | Panama

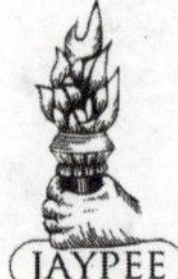

JAYPEE **Jaypee Brothers Medical Publishers (P) Ltd**

Headquarters

Jaypee Brothers Medical Publishers (P) Ltd
4838/24, Ansari Road, Daryaganj
New Delhi 110 002, India
Phone: +91-11-43574357
Fax: +91-11-43574314
Email: jaypee@jaypeebrothers.com

Overseas Offices

J.P. Medical Ltd
83, Victoria Street, London
SW1H 0HW (UK)
Phone: +44-20 3170 8910
Fax: +44 (0)20 3008 6180
Email: info@jpmedpub.com

Jaypee-Highlights Medical Publishers Inc
City of Knowledge, Bld. 237, Clayton
Panama City, Panama
Phone: +1 507-301-0496
Fax: +1 507-301-0499
Email: cservice@jphmedical.com

Jaypee Medical Inc.
The Bourse
111, South Independence Mall East
Suite 835, Philadelphia, PA 19106, USA
Phone: +1 267-519-9789
Email: joe.rusko@jaypeebrothers.com

Jaypee Brothers Medical Publishers (P) Ltd
17/1-B, Babar Road, Block-B, Shaymali
Mohammadpur, Dhaka-1207
Bangladesh
Mobile: +08801912003485
Email: jaypeedhaka@gmail.com

Jaypee Brothers Medical Publishers (P) Ltd
Bhotahity, Kathmandu, Nepal
Phone: +977-9741283608
Email: Kathmandu@jaypeebrothers.com

Website: www.jaypeebrothers.com
Website: www.jaypeedigital.com

Inquiries for bulk sales may be solicited at: jaypee@jaypeebrothers.com

Smart Dental Revision

First Edition: 2015

ISBN 978-93-5152-674-2

Printed at Rajkamal Electric Press, Plot No. 2, Phase-IV, Kundli, Haryana.

Dedicated

to

My Parents

Preface

Firstly I would like to bring to the notice of MDS ASPIRANTS that I have NOT covered the BASICS in this book. You can get it in any MCQs books. Moreover it is even presumed that after passing Degree Course of 4 years, the aspirants will be well-versed with the BASIC knowledge. In this book, I have covered only those points which are FREQUENTLY asked in any competitive MDS entrance examination and which are commonly OVERLOOKED by the aspirants. Moreover I have also discussed the points from which new questions might be asked related to the previous years questions. Also certain CONCEPTS which I had formed during my preparatory period which had commonly baffled me has been put-up in a simple way.

There are also certain TRICKS to remember the important forgettable points which is solely my BRAIN CHILD

I have also tried to represent certain difficult points in diagrammatic/tabular/flow chart format as it is easy to learn.

To sum-up, this book is FULL of competitive CONCEPTS and less of BASICS.

Suraj Kumar

Acknowledgments

- I would like to thank all my teachers who have been a source of inspiration, encouragement and support.
- My special thanks are due to Dr Rashmi Sinha to enrich this book.

Contents

CHAPTER

1 Dental Material, Operative Dentistry and Prosthodontics

Topic

PHYSICAL PROPERTIES

- Glass Transition Temperature:

• It is the temperature at which abrupt increase in COTE occurs indicating increased molecular mobility.
• It is a characteristic of GLASSY structure
• For INLAY wax = 35 ^{0}C (Q)
• For impression compound = 35 to 30 ^{0}C *(AIIMS Nov.10, AIPG 07)*

- Benzold – Bruck effect (PGI 11) vs Metamerism

• BENZOLD – BRUCK effect	• METAMERISM
• Change in color due to change in BRIGHTNESS	• different colour under different LIGHT SOURCE [Q]
• Change in value of hue with change in luminance *(PGI june 11)*	

- Munsell 's system measures and defines color quantitatively *(AIIMS Nov. 10, AIPG 07)*
- **Water contact angle:**

• Hydrophobic = polysulfide (82), addition and condensation polysilicone (has the HIGHEST contact angle value = 98) *(PGI 10)*
• Hydrophilic = polyether, alginate, agar (agar + alginate >>> polyether) These are the only hydrophilic impression materials [Q]

- Poisson's ratio:

$$\frac{\text{Lateral strain}}{\text{Axial strain}} = 0.5 \text{ (for isotropic material at constant volume)}$$

- Stress: It is the Internal [Q] resistance against applied force/load
- Elastic Limit " Maximum stress" > proportional limit
- Permanent distortion occurs when ELASTIC limit is exceede
- Proportional limit = GREATEST stress
- toughness

Toughness of dentine > enamel [Q]
$\alpha = \frac{1}{\text{hardness}}$ $\alpha = \frac{1}{\text{brittleness}}$ ductility e.g tempering of steel [Q]

- Bingham Body behavior:

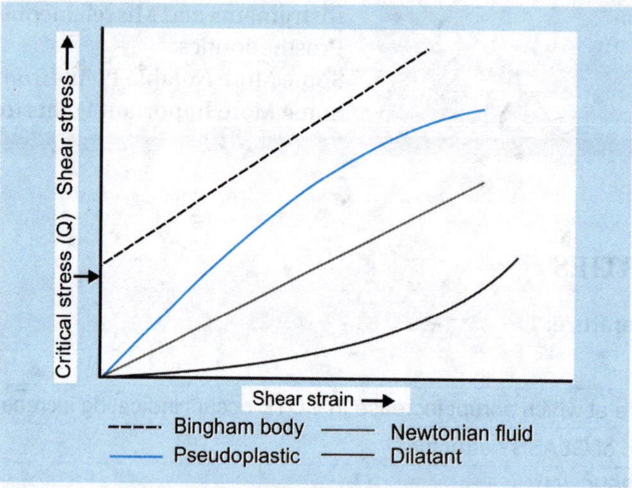

Fig 1.1: Bingham body behavior

- **Concept:** Viscoelastic deformation: applied force produces ELASTIC strain, plastic strain/combination of elastic + plastic strain.
- Plastic deformation: Is irreversible.new permanent shape taken up
- Elastic deformation: Is reversible and will be completely recovered
- Viscoelastic deformation: PARTIAL recovery [Q]. It is a characteristic of POLYMER that behave as elastic solids and viscous liquid.AMALGAM is also viscoelastic.
- THIXOTROPIC fluid → viscosity ↓ses under pressure, e.g APF gel [Q] (compare with pseudoplastic)

- Stress strain graph:

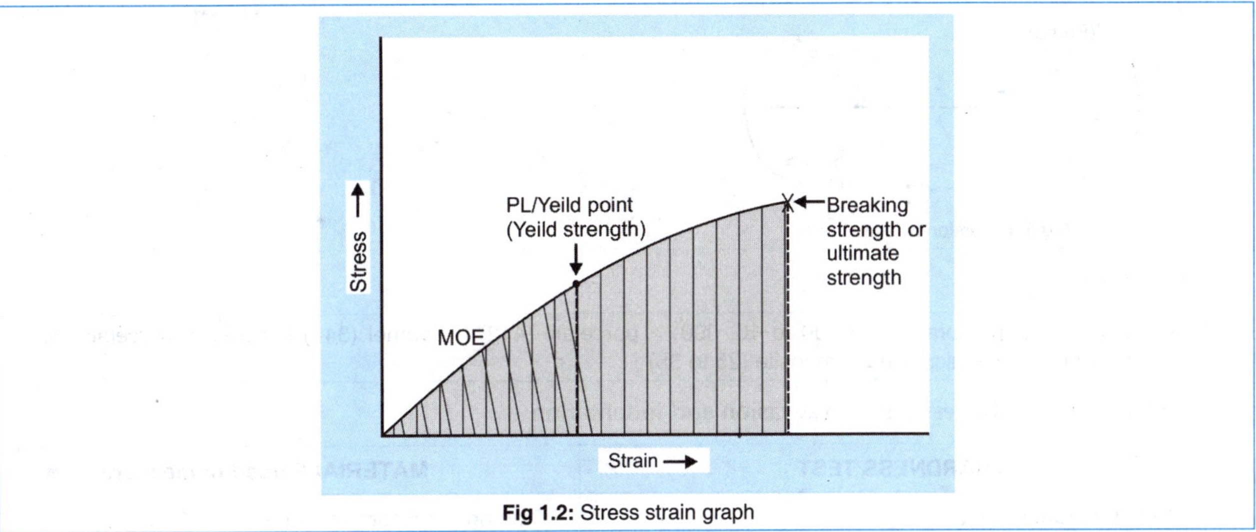

Fig 1.2: Stress strain graph

- **Moe:**

• Enamel (83,000 MPa) > Amalgam (27, 000 MPa) > Dentine (17,000 MPa)

- Cote of different material in comparison to enamel (11.4):

• Type 2 GIC (closest) to enamel	*(KCET 11)*
• 2nd closest is silicate cement [Q]	
• Note: if type 2 GIC given then it is the answer, otherwise silicate • Is closest to enamel.	
• Cote of dentine = 8.3	*(PGI 12)*
• Cote of amalgam = 25	
• Note: Cote of amalgam is nearly 2.5 times of enamel	*(PGI 12)*

- COMPRESSIVE strength of:

• Dentine (266 MPa) (KCET Q) < amalgam (310 MPa) < enamel (384 MPa)

- ULTIMATE tensile strength:

• Co Cr > Au alloys { donot confuse with Tensile strength. it is a strength

- High compressive strength + low tensile strength = Brittle (ceramic and amalgam)
- Types of Stress and Force responsible:

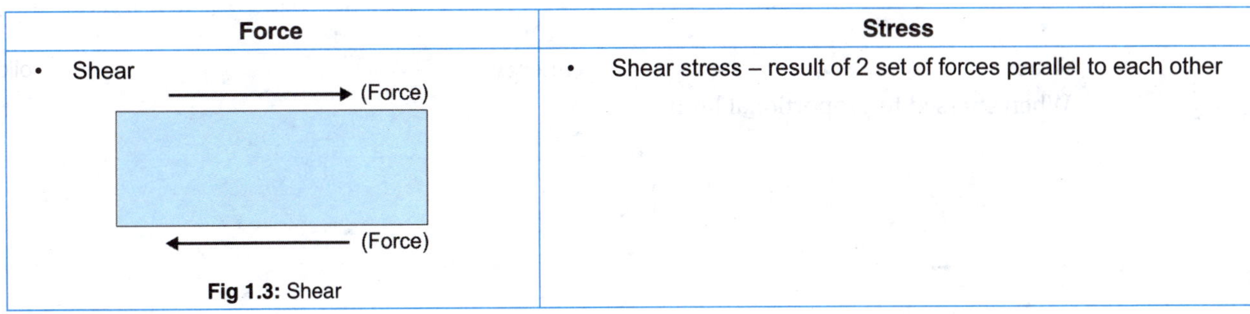

Force	Stress
• Shear (Force) (Force) **Fig 1.3:** Shear	• Shear stress – result of 2 set of forces parallel to each other

• Torsion/twisting force (Force) (Force) **Fig 1.4:** Torsion/twisting force	• Shear stress can also be produced by this force (AIPG 05)

- KHN values:

• Diamond (superabrasive) (7,000 to 10, 000) > porcelain (412) > enamel (340) (closest to porcelain PGI 05) > amalgam (90) > microfilled composite (25 to 35)

- Hardness Test: Is the resistance to abrasion and indentation

HARDNESS TEST	MATERIALS used to measure
Knoop hardness test	Diamond of Rhombic shape (TRICK: Ke Da R)
Vicker's/diamond pyramid test *(PGI 07, 11, 10)*	Diamond of square base shape (136^0)
Rockwell } Not for BRITTLE material [Q]	Diamond of conical shape
Brinells } Not for BRITTLE material [Q]	Steel ball

- **NOTE:**

• Knoop and vicker's hardness tests are the MICRO hardness tests *(AIIMS Nov. 10, AIPG 07)*
• Knoop hardness independent of Ductility of material [Q]
• Shore used for elastomers [Q]
• Barcol used for PLASTIC [Q]
• Brinell test related to proportional limit and ultimate tensile strength of dental dental GOLD alloy [Q]

- Gold is the most ductile and malleable
- Ag is the 2nd most ductile and malleable
- Enamel is stiffer and brittle than DENTINE.dentine is flexible and tougher (resistance to fracture)

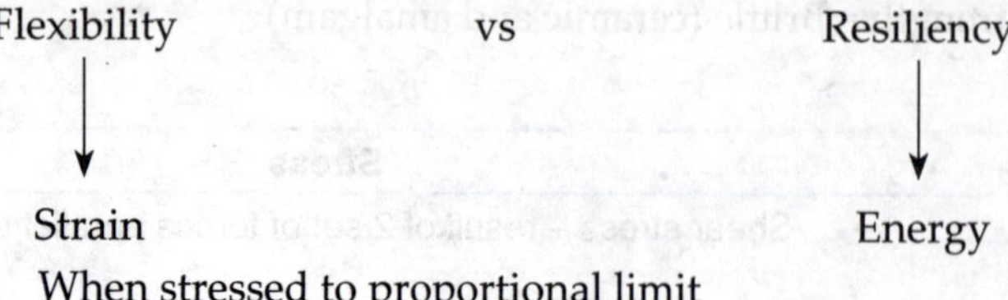

- **Brazillian Test:**

Measures the ultimate tensile strength of Brittle material

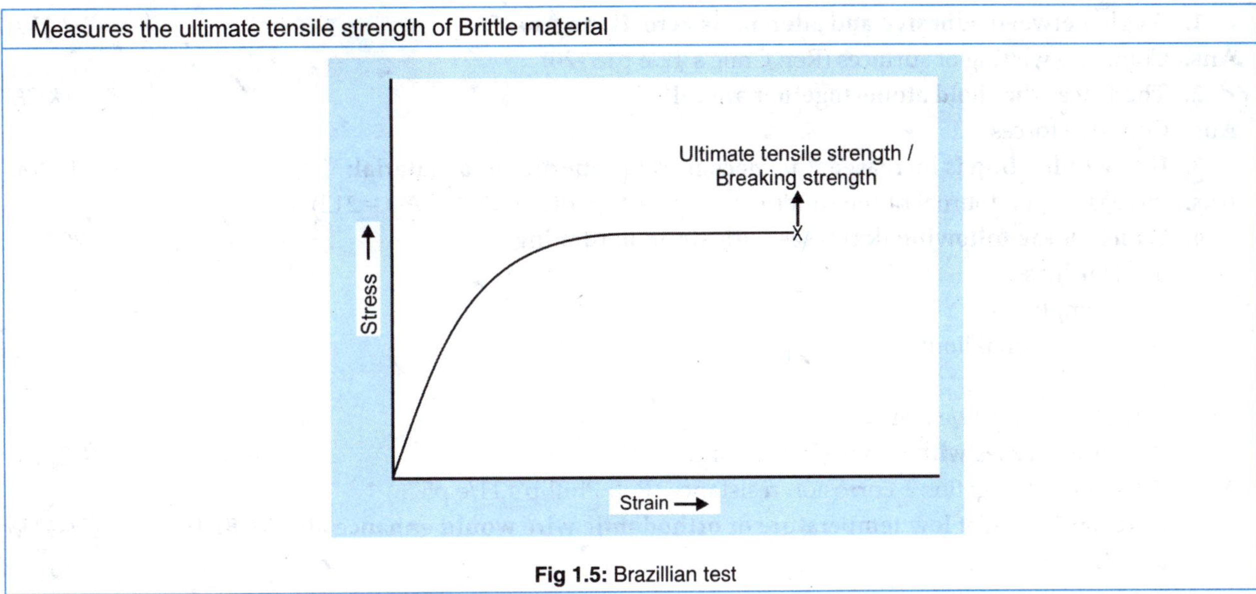

Fig 1.5: Brazillian test

- Maxwell Voigt model:

• Determine Viscoelastic behavior

- Solid solution:

• Alloy with complete solubility in BOTH solid and liquid state
• Most dental restoration are based on SOLID solution [Q]
• Simplest alloy (KCET 10)

- Eutectic alloy:

• component metal have limited solid solubility e.g Ag- Cu system [Q]
• Fusion temperature of eutectic alloy is below the melting point of either metal (KCET 11)
• Liquid → α solid solution + β solid solution

- Peritectic alloys:

• components have limited solid solubility, e.g Ag – Sn in amalgam and Ag- Pt in gold casting alloy
• Liquid + β – solid solution → α solid solution (AIIMS)

- **Concept:**

• Why there is high incidence of marginal caries around restoration? The surface energy of many restorative material is higher than tooth. so, increased tendency for surface and margins to accumulate debris.

- M.p:

• m.p of Ag – 960 ^{0}C
• m.p of Au - 1063 ^{0}C
• m.p of Ti – 1668 ^{0}C
• b.p of Au – 2200 ^{0} C

- Thermoset material – chemically set material
- Thermoplastic material – temperature affects setting

LAST 5-YEAR QUESTIONS FROM THIS TOPIC

1. **Angle between adhesive and aderend is zero. It me Ans.** *(AIPG 08)*

Ans. Complete wetting of surfaces (Ref: Craig's 12/e p18 -20)

2. **The forces that hold atoms together are called:** *(KCET 10)*

Ans. Cohesive forces

3. **If rate of loading is increased, the mechanical properties of a material:** *(AIIMS Nov. 09)*

Ans. Increases (Ref: Journal of the American Concrete Institute, 1980; 77: 1 – 212)

4. **Which of the following decreases with strain hardening?** *(PGI Dec 11)*
   a. Hardness
   b. Strength
   c. Proportional limit
   d. Ductility

Ans. d. (Ref: phillip's 11/e p74)

5. **Which decreases with surface hardening?** *(PGI Dec 11)*

Ans. Percentage elongation + corrosion resistance (Ref: Phillip's 11/e p576)

6. **Wire hardening at low temperature of orthodontic wire would enhance all EXCEPT:** *(PGI Dec 11)*
   a. Stiffness
   b. Resiliency of wire
   c. Brittleness
   d. Ductility of wire

Ans. d. (Ref: Phillip's 11/e p576)

7. **Tempering of steel:** *(PGI Dec 10)*

Ans. Increases it's toughness (Ref: Phillip's 10/e p641)

IMPRESSION MATERIAL (VERY IMPORTANT FOR AIPG)

- **Dustless alginate:** is made by coating with glycerine (if glycerine Not given in option go for Glycol/Dihydric Alcohol) *(AIIMS Nov. 09)*

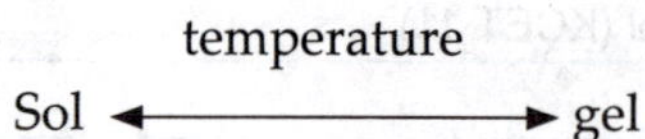

• Hysteresis is the temperature lag between gelation and liquefaction	(AIPG 07)
• Hysteresis is exhibited by AGAR [Q] not by alginate • BUT syneresis by BOTH	

- **Concept:** Controlling S.T for alginate/ZnOE

• Slight change in W/P and MIXING TIME causes marked change in physical property. So, S.T BEST controlled by adding/altering amount of " retarder" • By manufacturer. It can also be safely altered by changing TEMPERATURE of H_2O used.	
• SAME concept for gypsum products	(NEET 13)

- Agar syringe material used with → Agar tray material / → Alginate tray

- **ZnOE:**

Base paste	Reactor paste
ZnO	lanolin, resinous balsam, Eugenol/oil of cloves → ↑Ses flow (plasticizer)[Q]

- **ZnOE:**

• Is Non – H_2O based cement (KCET 12), BUT requires water for it's setting reaction:	*(AIIMS Nov. 09)*
• Produces Obtundant effect on pulp.	*(AIPG 07)*

- for Dimensional Stability:

• Of agar → stored in 2 % K_2SO_4,100 % relative humidity
• Of alginate → stored in 100 % relative humidity

- **Agar and Gypsum Hardener:** *(AIIMS Nov. 10, AIPG 07) (Important for KCET)*

BORAX was introduced into agar to improve its strength BUT it has retarding effect on setting of gypsum *(AIIMS Nov. 10)* So, an accelerator K_2SO_4 is added to agar to counter act the retarding effect of borax (AIPG 07).this 2 %K_2SO_4 is called GYPSUM HARDENER. *(AIIMS Nov. 10, AIPG 07)*

- Type 2 silicone impression material → additional silicone
- Type 1 ZnOE → HARD type 2 ZnOE → SOFT
- In NON- eugenol → HV – EBA is a substitute for eugenol (KCET)
- The MOST COMMON impression material for INDIRECT CASTING: additional polysilicone [Q]

(ALSO material of choice for OSMF patient) [Q]

- FLUORIDE release: [Q]

GIC > RMGIC > Compomer > composite

- **Stages of addition polymerization:**

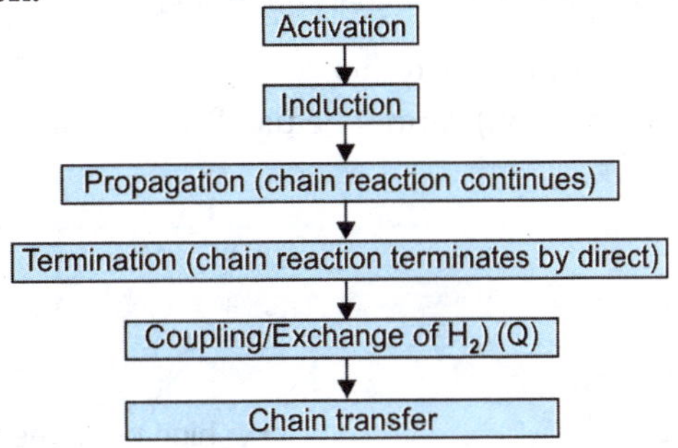

- Clinical implication of high tear strength of PolyS:

Allows their use in deep subgingival areas where removal is difficult

- Impression Compound: *(PGI 10)*

> The low thermal conductivity influences the cooling rate of this material because the outside of a mass of compound hardens fairly rapidly, whereas the inner regions remain soft. Impressions must be given adequate time to cool completely before they are removed from mouth (A favourite Q of PGI repeatedly asked)

- Polysulfide vs additional Silicone:

Polysulfide	Additional Silicone
High W.T and S.T (advantage)	Reverse of PolyS

- SNAP test:

> • Polyether shows a clearly defined W.T with a sharp transition into setting phase. This is called SNAP test

- W.T of dental materials:

Zn Polycarboxylate → 3 min
Zn PO → 5 min
Amalgam → 3-4 min

- Multiple pour/multiple casts → Addition polysilicone/polyether
- Optimal thickness of elastomeric impression material → 2- 4 mm *(KCET Q)*
- Spacer thickness – 2 mm
- Putty – Wash technique:

• To minimize the effect of polymerization shrinkage
• PUTTY Used 1st → Then wash material used
• distortion is associated with putty material

- Surfactant → is added to polyvinyl siloxane to make it hydrophilic *(AIIMS Q)*
- Multiple mix technique → heavy + light body
- Single Mix technique → medium viscocity of elastomer is used.so, single mix don't have high viscocity
- Custom Tray: used in polysulfide. {advantage – less material required. So, less polymerization shrinkage} [Q]
- Brush Heap → found in agar
- ZnOE paste → most commonly used wash/final impression for edentulous jaw. *(BHU 07)*

> Main advantage - dimensional stability. so, used for final impression

- Elastic Impression material: hydrocolloid + elastomer
- BOTH silicones (addition and condensation) cannot be used with " Latex gloves"

> Low W.T + S.T → disadvantage

- Polysulfide vs Condensation Silicone:

Polysulfide	Condensation Silicone
• Highest permanent deformation	• high permanent deformation
• High polymerization shrinkage	• Highest polymerization shrinkage

- C_2H_5OH [Q] is by product of condensation silicone is a larger molecule than H_2O [Q], a by product of PolyS (Remember)

- PolyS:

• Highest tear strength
• Trear strength: PolyS > Polyether *(PGI 11)*
• Biocompatible
• High W.T + S.T (advantage)

- Polyether:

highest cytoxicity
Stiffest (very rigid) → so, cast is difficult to remove

- Too rapid polymerization + incomplete polymerization + improper P/L
- Rough and irregular surface on impression (Very Important Q for NEET) *(AIPG 10, 07)*
- Catalyst:

PolyS – PbO_2
Condensation silicone – Sn octate
Addition silicone - chlorplatinic acid

- Addition silicone:

• Can be poured after several hours
• Pour after 20 minutes as H_2 evolves to create voids if poured before
• Called type 2 silicone impression

- FLOW of type 1 impression compound:

At 37 ^{0}C - 6 % *(AIPG 07)*
At 45 ^{0}C - > 85 %

- Of type 2 impression compound:

At 37 ^{0}C	2 %
At 45 ^{0}C	75 to 85 %

- Impression of hyperplastic tissue/flabby tissue:

Should be obtained with MUCOSTATIC technique to ensure intimate contact (AIPG 08 Q) and no pressure on tissue. So, tray with SPACER used. impression plaster used for this purpose *(AIIMS 05)*

- Additional silicone → material of choice for OSMF patient in closed mouth technique as it has excellent flow *(AIPG 08)*
- **NOTE**: (important for AIPG/AIIMS)

• Mucostatic material – ZnOE and impression plaster as they donot compress tissues during their setting reaction (impression plaster >> ZnOE)
• Also, hydrocolloid is considered mucostatic
• Mucocompressive material – ELASTOMERS, impression compound *(AIPG 07)*

- Plasticizer:

• In polyether
• Glycol ether/pthalate

- Accelerator vs retador:

Material	Accelerator	Retador
• ZnOE/ impression paste	• Zinc acetate (AIPG), $CaCl_2$, $ZnCl_2$ (AIPG 07), $MgCl_2$, $ZnSO_4$, alcohol, H_2O [Q] • PGI 11	• TRICK all oily compound • Mineral oil, waxes petroleum jelly, glycerine
• agar	• 2% K_2SO_4 (also called gypsum hardener) • Accelerate setting reaction of	• Borax ses strength and • Ces viscosity of agar
• alginate	• Ti fluoride (gypsum hardener	• Trisodium PO_4
• gypsum	• K_2SO_4, Na_2SO_4, NaCl upto 2 %, gypsum (acts as nuclei of crystalisation)	• TRICK:A B C • A – Acetate • B - Borax • C - Citrate

- **NOTE:**

* upto 2 % NaCl acts as accelerator in gypsum product BUT at higher concentration it acts as RETARDOR
* ZnOE used to make final/wash impression as it has DIMENSIONAL STABILITY [Q]

- HYDROCOLLOIDS and ELASTOMERS should be removed by sudden jerky [Q] motion as they are viscoelastic material. This is to prevent permanent deformation [Q] *[PGI]*
- AGAR: *(AIPG)*

• Has brush heap structure
• Liquefies at 70 °C to 100 °C *(AIPG 08)*
• Solidifies at 30 °C to 50 °C

- Laminate/agar – alginate method:

• Alginate → as tray material as it has poor SURFACE reproduction *(PGI 10)*
• **Note:** materials which are Hydrophillic are Not affected by saliva [Q]So, only 3 i.e agar, alginate [Q] and Polyether are Not affected by • Saliva
• Polyether has limited hydrophobicity • BUT • Alginate/agar are completely HYDROPHILIC *(KCET 2013)*

- In case of Polyether, stone cast can be easily poured but removed with difficulty. *(KCET 11)*
- In case of condensation silicone, polymerization is accompanied with repeated elimination of small molecules *(AIPG 10)*

SUB TOPIC: IMPRESSION TECHNIQUES

- Concept:

When we apply pressure while taking impression ↓ We will get denture with good peripheral seal and retention will se

- " PPS" :

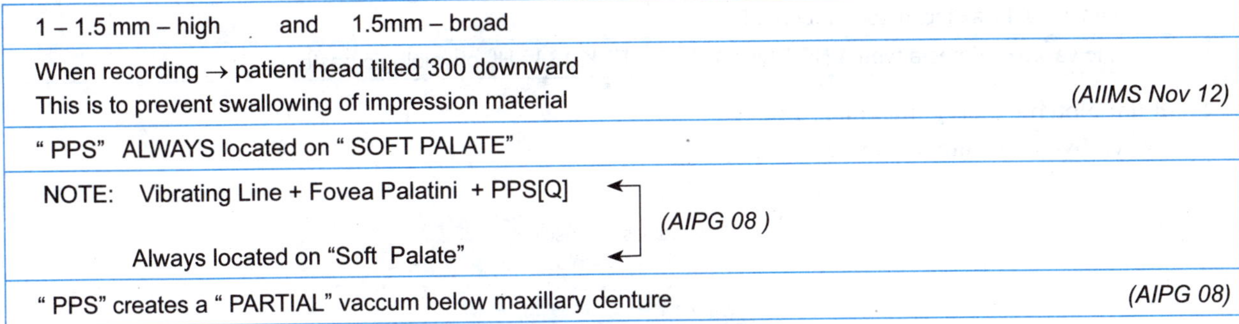

1 – 1.5 mm – high and 1.5mm – broad	
When recording → patient head tilted 300 downward This is to prevent swallowing of impression material	(AIIMS Nov 12)
" PPS" ALWAYS located on " SOFT PALATE"	
NOTE: Vibrating Line + Fovea Palatini + PPS[Q] Always located on "Soft Palate"	(AIPG 08)
" PPS" creates a " PARTIAL" vaccum below maxillary denture	(AIPG 08)

- Buccal Frenum:

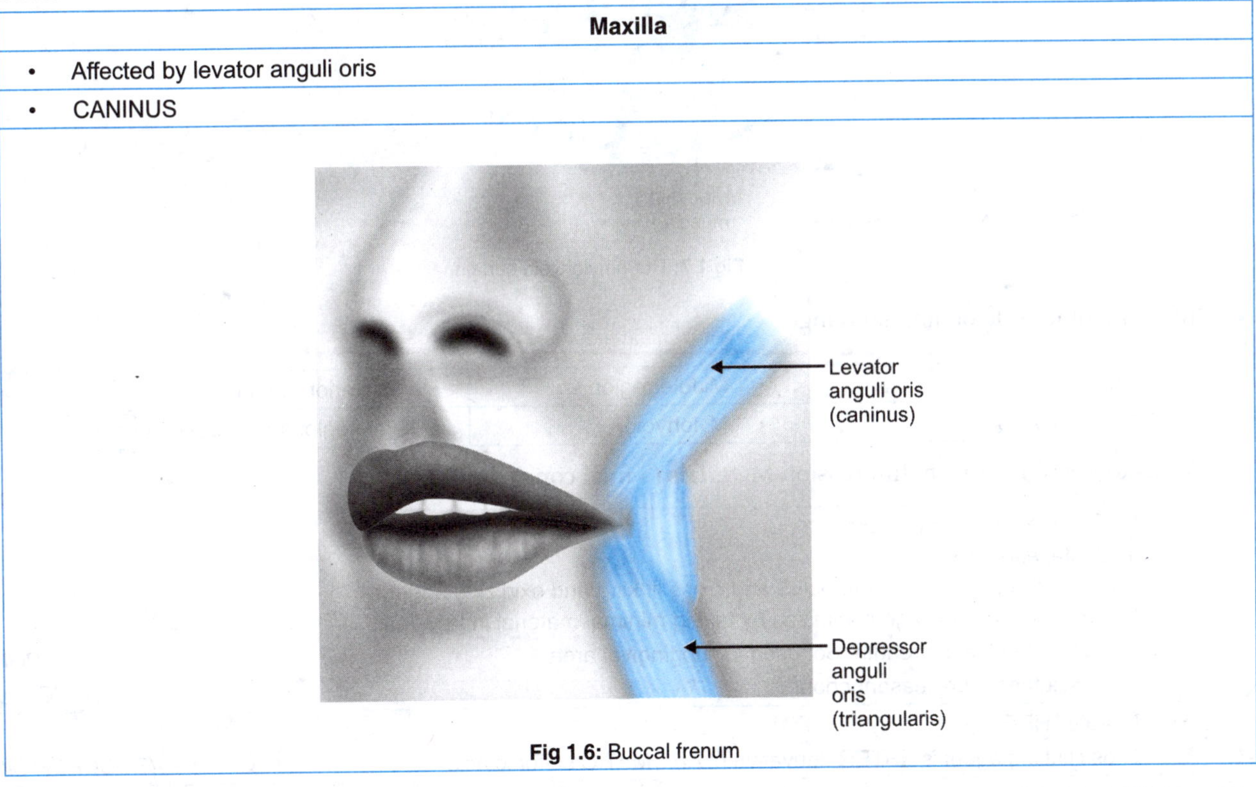

Maxilla
• Affected by levator anguli oris
• CANINUS

Fig 1.6: Buccal frenum

- **Remember:** 8 muscles form modiolus EXCEPT zygomaticus MINOR and ala Nasi *(COMEDK 07, PGI Dec 11)*
- For stability of denture tongue should rest on occlusal plane
- Massetric notch: *(AIPG 12)*

• Formed by action of Masseter on Buccinator
• (TRICK = it is " massetric notch". so, action will be of " masseter")

- Influence of CORONOID process on maxillary denture:

• CORONOID process → limits DB flange → if DB flange too thick • Denture falls during wide opening of mouth/lateral movement of mandible

- **MOUTH temperature wax:**

• Used in fluid wax technique to record PPS
• e.g Iowa wax ; Korecta type **4**(NOT type **1**) { COMEDK 13 } ; HL physiologic paste

- Hamular Notch = pterygomaxillary notch
- Retromylohyoid curtain formed by:

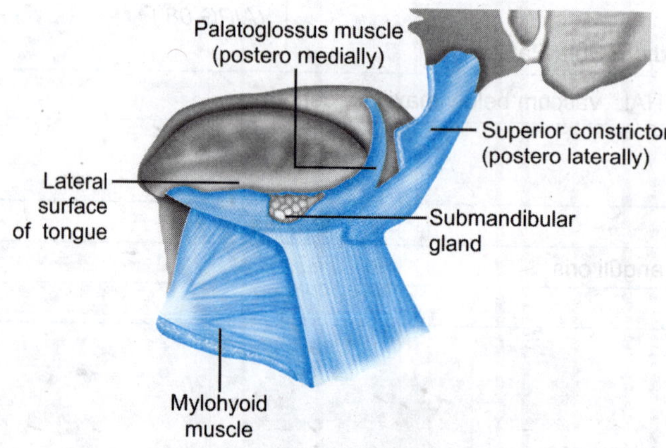

Fig 1.7: Retromylohyoid curtain

- Influence of muscle on lingual flange:

• Anterior region	• Middle region	• Posterior region
• Genioglossus	• Mylohyoid	• Palatoglossus + superior constrictor

- Points to Remember from Impression Materials (a final conclusion)

• Polysulfide/mercaptan/thiokol: 1st dental elastomer $PbO_2 \rightarrow$ gives brown color to polyS and cross linking and oxidizing agent. Polymerization shrinkage minimized by taking minimal material in tray. [Q] Shows highest tear strength. So, used in subgingival area Stains clothes + unpleasant odour	*(PGI 11)* *(AIPG 10,07)*
• POLYETHER: Cross linking agent is ESTER derivative of AROMATIC sulfonic acid	*(BOUCHER MCQ)*
• Condensation silicones polymerise by repeated elimination of small molecules	*(AIPG 10)*
• Single mix materials have lower viscosity	*(AIPG 08)*

LAST 5-YEAR QUESTIONS FROM THIS TOPIC:

1. **Working time of elastomeric impression material is defined as:** *(AIPG 10, 07)*

Ans. Time from start of mixing till just BEFORE the elastic properties have developed (Ref: Phillips 10/e p142)

2. **For ZnOE, all of the following are true EXCEPT:** *(AIPG 08)*
   a. Olive oil is used as plasticizer
   b. Addition of methylmethacrylate increases strength.
   c. Addition of o – EBA in concentration of 37 – 50 % increases strength
   d. Rosin decreases the brittleness of set cement

Ans. c (Ref: Craig's 12/e p498)

3. All of the following is used as accelerator in ZnOE except? *(PGI Dec 11)*

a. Acetic acid

b. Znic acetate dehydrate

c. Bromoglycerine

d. Calci**um chloride**

Ans. c (Ref: phillips 10/e p181)

GYPSUM PRODUCT

- ADA number = 25 *(COMED K 11)*

Property	Type 1	Type 2	Type 3	Type 4	Type 4
Other Name	Impression Plaster	1.Model plaster 2. P.O.P 3. dental plaster	1. dental stone 2. hydrocal 3. class 1 stone	Densite	Dental stone with high strength and expansion
W/P	0.5	0.5	0.28 – 0.30	0.22 – 0.24	0.18 – 0.22
S.T	4 to 5 min	All	Others have	12 to 15	min
S.E	0.15 %	0.30 %	0.20 %	0.10 %	0.30 %
Compressive Strength	800>	1300 >	3000 >	5000 >	7000
Use	Final wash	To fill flask	Construct-ion Of cast	BEST die material	Improved die material

- TRICK ⟶ to remember S.E:

• TYPE 2 = TYPE 5 = 0.30% (highest)
• Next remember Type 3 < type 1 < type 4

- Minimum requirement of SE for GP:

• ALL except type 4 and 5	• Type 4 and 5
• " 0"	• 0.10 % • Type 5 = 0.10 % *(KCET 11)*

- When G.P spatulated for longer time → set crystals breaks

↓

Leading to a weakened cast

- Factors affecting S.E of G.P: (ALL points have been asked as Q)

1. S.E is higher in α – hemihydrates in which W/P ratio is less
So, MORE powder → ↑sed expansion
S.E is higher in FINER particle size
S.E is higher with ↑sed rate of spatulation (S.T ↓ses) { OPPPOSITE to CEMENTS }

2. BOTH accelerator and retarder ses S.E so, ANTI – EXPANSION solution
K_2SO_4(accelerator)
borax(retarder), alizarin

LOWEST S.E is seen in type 4 G.P (= 0.10 %) [Q]

- H_2O of reaction for setting of G.P = 18.6 ml
- Gauzing H_2O does not react. So, S.T of G.P independent of it
- Soluble plaster:
  - Impression plaster + potato starch
  - Facilitates removal of impression from cast *(COMEDK 11)*
- Setting reaction of G.P:
  - Most accepted theory is dissolution and precipitation theory [Q].
  - According to this theory $CaSO_4$. ½ H_2O is 4 times more soluble than dihydrate. when hemihydrates is dissolved in H_2O saturated solution is formed. In this solution less soluble Dihydrate precipitates out.
- Cynoacrylate:

Low viscosity resin. Initiation of polymerization in presence of H_2O

USE:

Major: DIE hardener
Applied to wetted etched enamel, with out use of primer
↓
Moisture active resin (a favourite Q of AIIMS/AIPG)

- Fluidity measurements:
  - Type 1 and 2 (Slump Test)
  - Type 3, 4, 5 (CORE penetration test)
- **Terra Alba:** set $CaSO_4$. $2H_2O$ act as accelerator [Q]

LAST 5-YEARS QUESTIONS FROM THIS TOPIC

1. **The safest method for soaking dental cast is:** *(COMED K 11)*

Ans. Placing in a saturated solution of calcium sulfate

2. **The strength of gypsum products is generally expressed in terms of:** *(KCET 10)*

Ans. Compressive strength

AMALGAM (IMPORTANT TOPIC FOR ANY MDS EXAM)

- Composition of amalgam: (a favourite topic of PGI)

- HIGH Cu amalgam is formed by irregular + spherical particles *(KCET 10)*

	HIGH Cu	
Low Cu	**Admixed**	**Unicompositional (Best)**
Ag – 65 %	Ag – 69 %	Ag – 60 %
Sn – 29 % (PGI 11)	Sn – 17 %	Sn – 27 %
Cu - < 6 %	Cu – 13 %	Cu – 13 – 30 %
Zn - < 1 %	Zn - 1 %	Zn – 0 %

- **NOTE:** Zn containing amalgam alloys last 20 to 50 % longer than Zn free though they cause delayed expansion *(KCET 10)*
- Zn containing amalgam alloy has Zn > 0.01 %

- Hg content of " precapsulated Amalgam" – 40 to 45 % *(AIIMS Nov 11)*
- Spherical alloy = 42 – 45 % Hg [Q]
- Lathe cut = 50 % Hg [Q]

- Delayed Expansion:
  - Occurs 3-4 days after amalgam insertion and leads to pain and sensitivity (like Dry Socket → it also occurs 3-4 days after extraction)
  - Pain occurs due to pressure in pulpal direction
  - **Note:** Any pain occurring immediately is due to high points/fracture of tooth/galvanism.
  - BUT in galvanism pain is sharp and shooting *(AIPG 11, 09)*
  - REMEMBER: If pain occurs after 3 months of cast restoration is VERY characteristic of Supraocclusion

- Delayed Contraction:
  - Most modern amalgam exhibit " NET CONTRACTION". Contraction results as the particles begin to dissolve in Hg and the γ_1 phase grows.
  - γ (Ag_3Sn) + Hg → γ_1 (Ag_2Hg_3) [Q]
  - contraction continues as long as the growth of γ_1 continues i.e Hg is CONSUMED
  - high Hg → ↑ sed expansion
  - smaller particle size → ↑sed area → ↑sed consumption of Hg

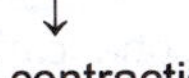

↑sed contraction

- **NOTE:** In composition of amalgam only Sn ↓ses expansion while Ag and Cu ↑Ses expansion.
- SPHERICAL amalgam requires less condensation force than lathe cut
- Phases in amalgam alloy:

γ (Ag_3Sn) → strongest phase
γ_1 (Ag_2Hg_3) → highest corrosion resistance + DOMINANT phase in well condensed low copper amalgam *(KCET 11)* γ_1 → NOBLEST phase so, highest tarnish and corrosion resistance DOMINANT phase in BOTH high Cu and low Cu amalgam Every effort should be made to keep this phase in maximum Available space in final product
γ_2 (Sn_8Hg) → very susceptible to corrosion

η (Cu6Sn5)
γ is the STRONGEST phase

- Order of Corrosion Resistance:

γ1 > γ > η > γ2
so, η is least corrosion resistant phase in high Cu amalgam as < 1% of γ2 phase in high Cu amalgam (DONOT confuse)

- Lathe cut vs Spherical alloy:

• All properties of lathe cut inferior to spherical
• Lathe cut achieves lowest compressive strength at 1 hr (AIIMS 06)

- Indisper:

10 % In admixed → ↓ses release of Hg vapour during polishing (AIPG 09)

- Compressive strength of amalgam:

After 1 week = 310 MPa
Compressive strength of amalgam at 1 hr = 80 MPa
Compressive strength of amalgam in 8 hrs = 70 % [Q]
1 hr compressive strength of spherical alloy is DOUBLE that of admixed and low Cu alloy *(PGI 12)*

- Tensile strength of amalgam:

• In 1 week = 48 to 70 MPa
• Tensile strength of admixed < low Cu

- Appearance of amalgam:

• Undermix amalgam = dull
• Adequate mix amalgam = shiny [Q]
• Over mix amalgam = soupy/sticky

- ↑Sed creep is seen with BOTH over and under trichurated amalgam
  ↓
  So, proper trichuration should be done
- Under/Over Trichuration:

In lathe cut	in spherical
Ses strength	ses strength

- BUT
  ↑ Ses CREEP in BOTH lathe cut and spherical
- **Creep and Mercuroscopic Expansion:**

" CREEP" • Is the time dependent plastic deformation which occurs when a metal is subjected to a CONSTANT LOAD near it's melting point. • Amalgam will undergo creep as it's m.p which is slightly above room temperature
CREEP → causes EXTRUSION of margin → most common cause of Marginal failure
CREEP ↓ses with increased condensation pressure

ELECTROCHEMICAL corrosion → extrusion at margins (creep)
↓
Produces further expansion ← Hg from γ_2 phase reacts with γ particles
↓
"MERCUROSCOPIC expansion"

- **NOTE:** Content of Hg is 2-3 % higher at margin
- Hg CONTENT and EFFECT:

HIGHER Hg content → Higher corrosion
HIGHER Hg content → Higher marginal breakdown

- * so, low Cu amalgam/conventional amalgam is highly susceptible to CORROSION and break down
- * elimination of γ_2 phase by η phase and LESS amount of residual Hg (42 %) made HIGH Cu alloys more resistant to tarnish and corrosion
- * content of residual Hg BEST for BEST clinical service:
  Compared to original Hg to alloy ratio, residual Hg should be usually around 50 % wt. [Q]

- Degradation of high and low copper amalgam:

most common evidence of degradation of LOW Cu amalgam
↓
MARGINAL deterioration *(AIPG 07)*

Of high Cu amalgam → BULK fracture (due to mechanical fatigue For 10 to 15 yrs)

- Marginal defect best measured by Mahler's scale
  Range of value – 1 to 11 for amalgam
- Corrosion Products:

LOW Cu	HIGH Cu
SnO + SnCl	CuO

- Penetrating type of corrosion NOT seen in high Cu AMALGAM *(AIPG 10, 09, AIIMS Nov. 09)*
- **Facts About Hg:**

- Maximum exposure of Hg (occupational) considered safe is 50 μg/m^3 of air [Q] { according to OSHA safe level for Ni is 1 mg/m^3} { PGI 11 }
- Hg absorbed from GIT, LUNGS, SKIN NOT KIDNEY [Q]
- **Absorbtion efficiency for different for Hg:**

FORM	SKIN	LUNG	GIT
• Elemental	• ---	• 80 %	• ----
• Inorganic	• ---	• 80 %	• 7 %
• organic	• ---	• ---	• 95 to 98 %

- Methyl Hg is most toxic form and absorbed 90 – 95 % from GUT [Q]
- 14 times denser than H_2O
- 65 – 85 % inhaled Hg vapour is retained in body
- Half life 55 days (NBDE Q)

• **NORMAL level in:** – Urine – 15 µg/l – Blood – 4 µg/ml
• Lower blood Hg level at which earliest non – specific symptom starts 35 ng/ ml (AIPG 07) and urine is 30 µg/ml

SUB TOPIC: CAVITY PREPARATION

- Cavity width for class 1 and 2

Material	DFG	AMALGAM	INLAY	ONLAY
Width	1/5th intercuspal (I.C) distance (most conservative)	1/4th the I.C distance	1/3rd I.C distance	>1/3rd I.C distance

- Axial wall pulpal depth (into dentine): for class 2

• Crown – 0.5 to 0.6 mm
• Root – 0.7 to 0.8 mm

- 20 retention in class 2:

• Locks – vertically oriented on AF and AL line angle (0.2 mm into DEJ)
• Groove – round, elongated structure (NBDE Q) on AF and AL line angle (0.2 mm into DEJ)
Note: grooves and coves act as 20 retention form EXCEPT class 3 and class 5 of amalgam where they act as 10 retention feature.

- 2^0 retention feature in class 3

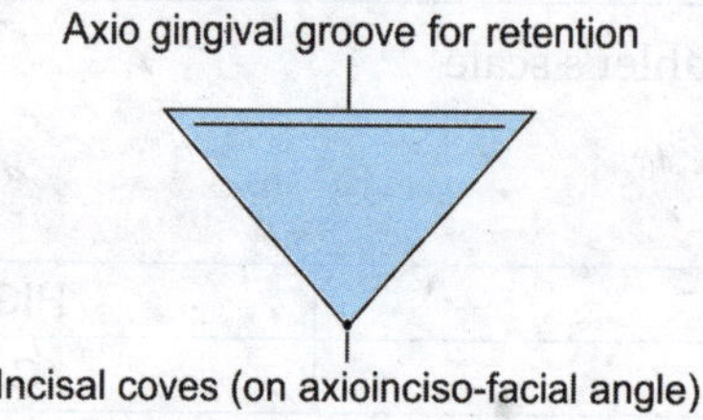

Fig 1.8: Secondary retention feature in class 3

- 2^0 retention in class 5:

• Is by placing 2^0 retention grooves on AXIAL WALL (AIIMS 11) (i.e A-G and A-I line angle)
• OR 4 coves on point angles

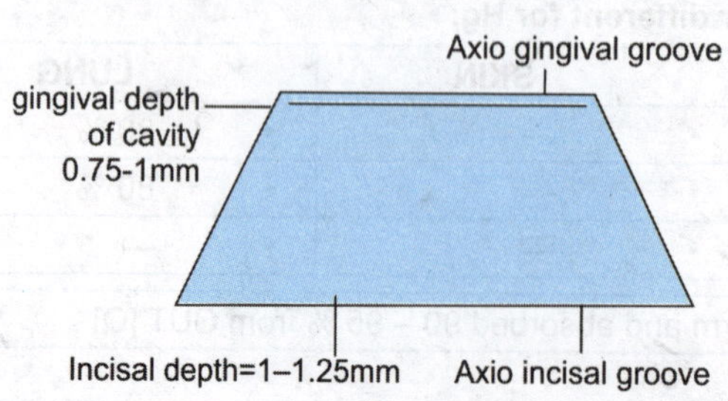

Fig 1.9: Retention in class 5

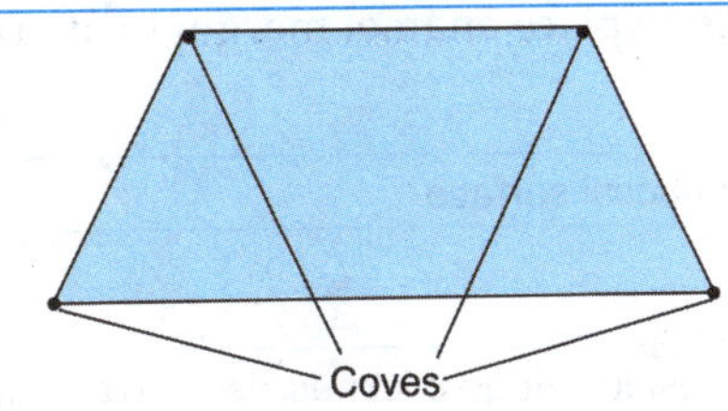

Fig 1.10: Retention in class 5

- **Internal and External line angle:**

Rounding of internal line angle → reduces stress on TOOTH
Rounding of external line angle → reduces stress on restoration (angle with apex directed outward) i.e prevents fracture of restoration i.e rounding/beveling of axiopulpal line angle prevents fracture of amalgam restoration *(AIIMS Nov 11, 06)*

- Locks and high Cu amalgam:
  Does not require locks as they exhibit less creep
- Butt joint vs Slide fit:

BUTT JOINT	SLIDE
900 butt joint for amalgam, silicate, ceramic (all 3 brittle material)	>900 cavosurface angle for CAST restoration
NOTE: 900 BUTT joint is done for silver amalgam as it has poor strength in thin sections. *(COMEDK 11)*	

- Number of line angle and point angles for class 1, class 2 and MOD:

TRICK = number of line angle increases by 3 and point angle by 2 when cavity transforms from class 1 to class 2 and class 2 to MOD

CAVITY	Class 1	Class 2	MOD
POINT ANGLE	4	6	8
LINE ANGLE	8	11	14

- Supporting cusp = centric holding/stamp cusp/functional cusp *(KCET 12)*
- cavosurface angle of amalgam cavity preparation should be at right angle *(AIPG 07)*
- BEVELS:

Produces stronger enamel margin
Provides marginal adaptation [Q]

In amalgam	In CAST restoration
Bevels are included under RESISTANCE form	NOT included in 10retention and resistance form BUT given during final cavity preparation (i.e FINISHING)

- Clearance with adjacent tooth:

• Of gingival seat	• Of facial and lingual proximal wall
• 0.5 mm	• 0.2 mm

- In class 3 preparation it is acceptable to place enamel margin in area of contact
- Reverse ' S' curve:

Has role in Esthetic → so, placed on buccal surface

- Cavity preparation in class 1:

• In amalgam/DFG when proximal residual ridge thickness is < 1.6 mm, mesial and distal wall must Diverge Occlusally
• But if this is > 1.6 mm, mesial and distal wall should converge occlusally.

- Gingival extension of restoration:

Atleast 3 mm above alveolar crest [Q]

- Concept:

Groves, locks, slots, pins → enhance retention → retention enhances Resistance form ↓ So, if 'both' options are given go for it

- Resistance form:

• It permits restoration to withstand occlusal forces.
• Includes flat pulpal floor, rounded internal line angles, inclusion of weakened tooth structure But does not include extension upto 1 mm within the dentine (AIIMS 06)

- For class 2 cavity preparation on maxillary permanent 1st molar:

• Increased chances of exposure of " MB and ML pulp horns" (NBDE Q)
• " MB" pulp horn exposed in case of 1° 1st molar *(PGI 12)*

- class 5 cavity *(Important for NEET and AIIMS):*

• Primary determinant of outline form is EXTENSION of caries *(AIPG 02)*
• External shape is related to contour of marginal gingiva
Depth of cavity → Gingivally – 0.75 to 1 mm; → Occlusally – 1- 1.25 mm/0.5 mm inside DEJ
• Direction of mesial and distal walls follow the direction of enamel rods *(AIIMS 11,08)*
• ALL walls are divergent. so, retentive grooves and coves are very important.
Note: DFG is the ideal material for class 5

- Class 3 cavity (Important for NEET and AIIMS):

• Facial, lingual and gingival walls should meet the axial walls at 90°
• Retention coves placed at axio-facio-incisal point angle.this points are placed entirely in dentine *(AIPG 07)*
• " lingual dove tail" indicated if ADDITIONAL retention needed for larger restoration, e.g CANINE

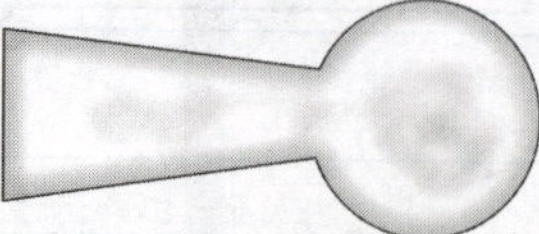

Fig 1.11: Lingual dove tail

LAST 5-YEARS QUESTION FROM THIS TOPIC

1. **Pre carve burnishing is useful for all except:** *(AIPG 12)*
   a. Removes old amalgam restoration
   b. removes excess Hg
   c. initiates carving
   d. margin of amalgam is well condensed.

Ans. a. (Ref: Sturdevant 4/e p682 – 683)

2. **When bonding of amalgam is required in orthodontic practice which of the following is selected for the purpose:** *(AIIMS Nov 12)*

Ans. 4 – META (Ref: Orthodontics – current principle and practice by grabber 4/e)

3. **Discoloured areas seen through the enamel in the teeth that have amalgam restoration are known as:** *(KCET 11)*

Ans. Amalgam blues.

4. **In case of deep carious lesion incomplete debridement is done to:** *(COMEDK 11)*

Ans. Prevent pulp exposure and allow a thin layer of a dentine to remain (Ref: Sturdevent 4/e p128)

5. **In class 2 cavity for amalgam in case of permanent teeth, axiopulpal line angle is?** *(PGI Dec 11)*

Ans. Beveled in permanent teeth (Ref: Sturdevant 5/e p746)

6. **LCOTE of amalgam as compared to tooth structure is about:** *(PGI june 10)*

Ans. 2.5 times (Ref: Phillips 11th ed pf 55, 419)

PIN RETAINED RESTORATION

- Provide MAINLY 1° retention [Q]
- SELF threaded pin:

Most retentive
Less microleakage
Causes more pulpal stress (minimal with cemented pins)
Hole diameter less than pin diameter ↓ 0.0015 to 0.004 inch → so, BEST answer is 0.002 inch *(AIPG 10)* ↓ This option is commonly given in AIPG exams
(**NOTE:** hole diameter 0.001 inch larger in cemented pin and 0.001 inch smaller in friction locked)
{1 inch = 25 mm}

- Cemented pin:

Indicated in RCT treated tooth as NO stress during pin placement *(AIPG 07, AIIMS 07)*

- Contraindication for pin retained restoration is hypoplastic tooth. [Q]
- Advantage of PIN retained restoration:

• Conservative tooth preparation
• Single visit finishing

- PIN retained restoration (Rule of Thumb)

• Pin should be 2 mm into dentine
• 2 mm within amalgam

• 1 mm from DEJ (to be safe)
• Ideal ratio = 2: 1 • Optimal = 1: 1 *(AIPG 07)*
• Two pins should not be parallel to each other [Q]
• Pin should be placed parallel to external tooth surface *(AIPG 07)*
• 0.5 mm clearance around pin should given for amalgam condensation
• 2 pins should be placed 3-5 mm apart
• 3 or more pins should be located at different vertical level
• 1 pin/missing line angle

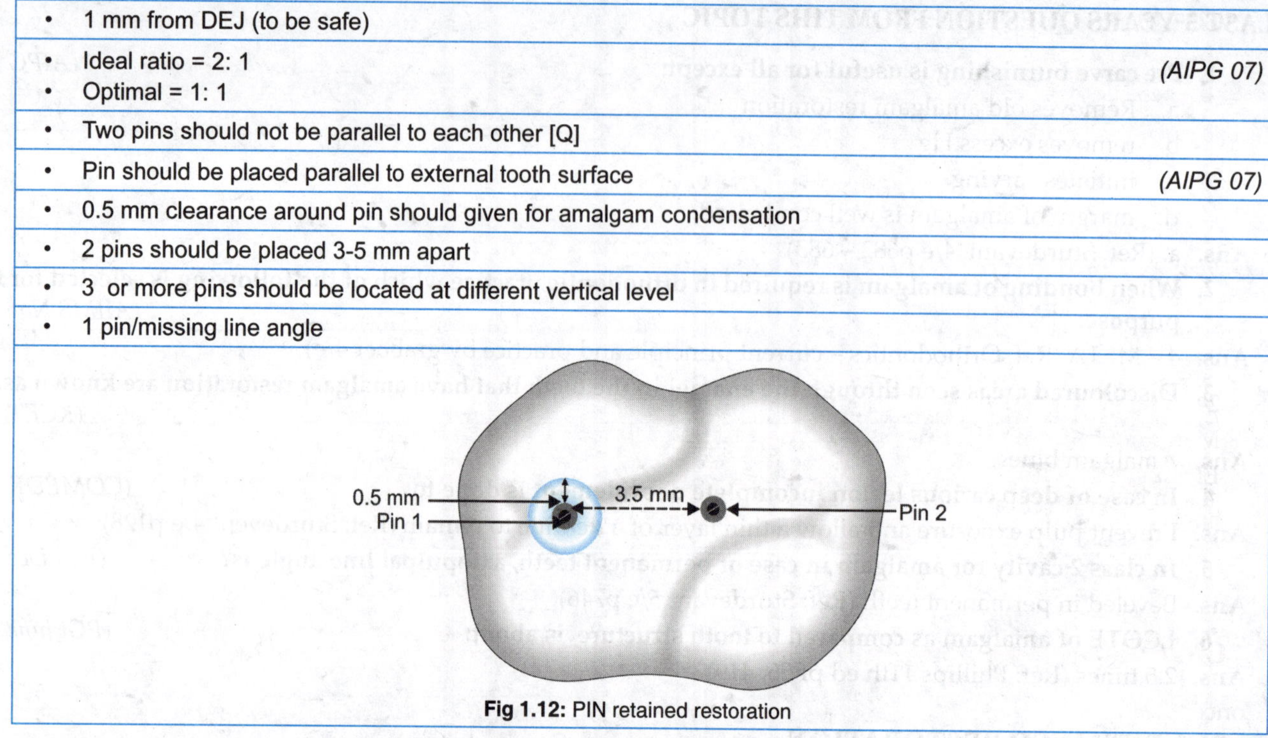

Fig 1.12: PIN retained restoration

- Pin retained restoration ↓ses strength of amalgam *(AIPG 11, 09)*

LAST 5-YEARS QUESTIONS FROM THIS TOPIC

1. **One of the following is not true regarding pin retained restoration:**
   a. Pin holes should never be prepared at different levels on the tooth
   b. A minimum of 0.5 mm clearance should be provided around the circumference of the pin for adequate condensation of the amalgam
   c. Pin hole should be located on a flat surface that is perpendicular to the proposed direction of the pin hole
   d. The pin hole should be positioned no closer than 1 mm to DEJ and no closer than 1.5 mm to the external surface

Ans. a

2. **In pin – retained amalgam restoration, failure is more likely to occur at the:** *(COMEDK 11)*

Ans. Pin dentine interface (Ref: sturdevent 4/e p783)

DFG

- It is an ideal material for class 5 cavity preparation
- Bridging:

• Voids are inherent to DFG
• Void are spaces created due to improper compaction of DFG

- Difference of cavity for DFG from that of amalgam:

• Reverse bevel + sharp line and point angle + more conservative cavity than amalgam.
• REST features are same

- **Classification of DFG:**

• Foil = fibrous gold
• Electrolytic precipitated gold = crystalline/spongy/mat gold
• Granular gold = powdered gold (KCET 11) • Powdered gold formed by atomized + chemically precipitated gold powders
• gold FOIL: is a form of DFG with highest strength and can be used in stress bearing area like External veneering • Size used commonly – 4" * 4"
• powdered/chemically precipitated/granulated (KCET Q)/ encapsulated gold: • Particle size 15 μm [Q]

- 24 karat gold = 1000 fineness
- Material providing BEST marginal seal/intergrity = DFG
- Electra alloy RV:

Gold + 0.1% Ca (COMEDK 11)
(increases strength of DFG by dispersion strengthening)

CEMENTS

Concept:

• What is the meaning of "S.T is best controlled by"? • It means controlling the setting reaction, i.e increasing the S.T, e.g for ZnOE, S.T is best controlled by adding retarders + cooling the glass slab

- Silicate cement has highest compressive strength while resin cement has highest tensile strength.
- both GIC and silicate are contraindicated in mouth breadthers
- Classification of GIC:

Type 1 – Luting cement
Type 2 – Restorative cement
Type 3 – Liner
Type 4 – Fissure sealent
Type 5 – Orthodontic cement
Type 6 – Core build up cement
Type 8, Type 9 – Posterior packable GIC for atraumatic restoration

- **Metal Reinforced Gic:**

Miracal mix/Ag cermet	Glass cermet, e.g 'ketac Ag'
• Ag – Sn alloy used	• Pure metal sintered
• NONE of the properties improved	• Fracture toughness and wear resistance improved. • Esthetic value maintained

- Type 3 GIC i.e GIC Liner:

• Maximum fluoride release after 30 days [Q] seen in type 3 GIC liner {light cured} (amongst type 1, 2, 3) *[KCET 08]*
• Initial fast release of fluoride ion from GIC, then slow release after 30 days *(AIPG 12)*

- GIC:

GIC liquid composition: • Itaconic acid, malic acid, tricarballyic acid → Plasticiser • Tartaric acid → increases W.T and decreases S.T., modifies handling properties *(AIPG 07)*
• Ionic bond present in completely set GIC *(AIPG)*
• Carboxyl group reacts with calcium in enamel and dentine *(AIPG 09, AIIMS May 11)*
• Bonding improves on clean surface provided the cleansing does NOT remove an excessive amount of Ca from tooth surface So, etching with weak acids like polyacrylic acid is recommended and stronger . Acids like phosphoric acid is contraindicated
• Treating dentine with an acidic conditioner followed by dilute solution of ferric chloride
• **Stages of GIC setting:** Decomposition → migration → gelation → hardening → maturation
• GIC should be protected against moisture and dessication – If excess moisture present – Ions like Ca^{2+}, Sr^{2+}, Al^{3+} will be lost in environment – Will Not be available for reaction – If dessicated – Ions will not have aqueous medium – Will Not migrate /react
• Bond strength = 2- 7 MPa
• Fluoride released from GIC is replaced by Hydroxyl ion *(AIIMS May 11)*

- High Viscosity GIC = RMGIC/light hardened GIC introduced in 1990 *(PGI)*
- GIC adheres to tooth surface by carboxyl group of polymer chain *(AIIMS May 10)*
- **Compomer:**
  - Properties inferior to composite BUT superior to GIC and RMGIC fluoride content:

Silicophosphate > silicate > GIC

- GIC has maximum fluoride releasing capacity BUT silicate has maximum fluoride content.So, minimum 2^0 caries associated with GIC
- bilayered/sandwich/laminated technique:

• Given by Mclean
• Increases retention form as GIC bonds both to tooth and composite

- Main disadvantage of GIC → film thickness (thick film)
- **Remember:** GIC recommended in root caries because of anticariogenic property
- After 24 hrs of setting GIC has greater tensile strength BUT less compressive strength than $ZnPO_4$
- **Concept:**

• If sufficient dentine thickness is available $ZnPO_4$ cement is ideal base
• If excavation is deep/very close to pulp then $Ca(OH)_2$ liner is indicated

- Zynomer/buffered GIC:

ZnO is added in the powder to increase pH

- Advantage of RMGIC over GIC:

• Rapid setting
• Increased esthetic { as resin increases esthetic}
• Can be finished at the time of placement (early finishing) and are • Recommended for class 5 and class 1and2 of 1⁰teeth

- Vitrabond/vitrebond:
- RMGIC base/liner *(PGI 12)*
- Resin cement = flowable resin base composite material
- NON–eugenol cement → Vanilate ester
- CERAMIC restoration/laminates are cemented using resin cement.
- e.g of chelation reaction:

ZnOE and Zn Polycarboxylate
• ZnOE cement reaction: (Autocatalytic reaction) $ZnO + H_2O \rightarrow Zn(OH)_2$ $Zn(OH)_2 + \text{eugenol} \rightarrow ZnE_2 + H_2O$ • H_2O required for reaction and also by product of reaction.

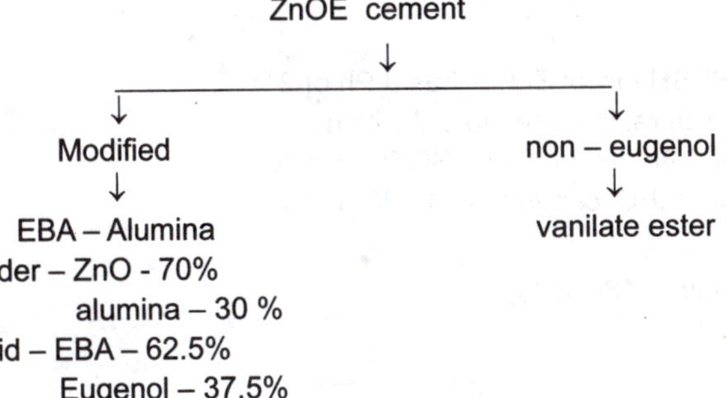

- **$ZnPO_4$ cement:**

• H_2O controls the rate of reaction
• Al is present in liquid is essential for cement forming reaction
• Liquid has H_3PO_4
• Frozen slab technique for mixing is used • It0 provides increased S.T for cementation of crown • Frozen Slab technique: • Used for mixing $ZnPO_4$ cement (COMEDK 11) used for cementation of crown. This technique will make the cement less viscous.
• Main advantage of $ZnPO_4$ → film thickness (thin film, as low as 18 μm So, is the universal luting agent)
• Range of film thickness of $ZnPO_4$ - 25 to 40 μm

- Manipulation of $ZnPO_4$ cement (used for Final cementation):

Manipulative variables	Compressive strength	Film thickness	solubility	acidity	Setting Time
↓P/L	(↓) (BHU 07)	↓	↑	↑	Slower
↑P/L	↓	↑	↓	↑	Faster
↑Mixing temperature	(↓)	↑	↑	↑	Faster
H2O contamination	↓	↑	↑	↑	faster

CONCEPT: reason is that increase mixing temperature faster the setting reaction Less amount of powder can be incorporated, So, less compressive strength.

So, with frozen slab technique: Increase S.T. So, more amount of powder can be incorporated (P/L)↑ increased compressive strength

- **Silicate cement:**

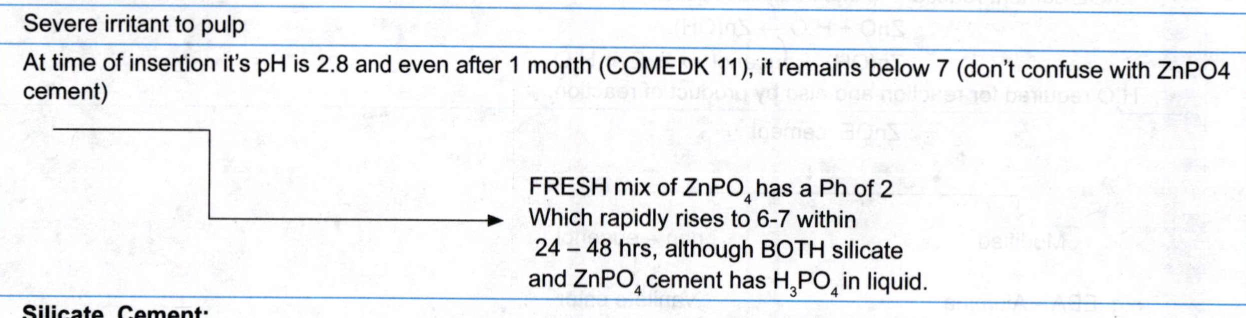

Severe irritant to pulp

At time of insertion it's pH is 2.8 and even after 1 month (COMEDK 11), it remains below 7 (don't confuse with ZnPO4 cement)

FRESH mix of $ZnPO_4$ has a Ph of 2 Which rapidly rises to 6-7 within 24 – 48 hrs, although BOTH silicate and $ZnPO_4$ cement has H_3PO_4 in liquid.

Silicate Cement:

" Strongest" of all dental cement (compressive strength = 180 MPa)

- Luting agent and their chief concern:

Luting Agent (PGI 11)	Concern
ZnOE	Less strength.so,replaced as permanent cementation agent *(PGI 10, 11)*
GIC	Solubility
$ZnPO_4$	Solubility
Composite	Film thickness

- Varnish:

• 2 – 5 μm thick
• Composition: copal rosin + 90% organic solvent, e.g $CHCl_3$[Q], C_2H_5OH
• Is semipermeable like J.E

- Concept:

Varnish and liner must for ALL cavities but base optional (only for deep cavities)

- Base:

• Maximum value for thermal protection: (0.5 – 0.75 mm)
• Base does NOT prevent microleakage and acid penetration

- Liners

THIN film liner (1- 50 μm)		THICK liners/cement liner[Q]
Solution liner	suspension liner	• 0.2 to 1 mm
Varnish	20 – 25 μm	
2-5 μm (AIIMS Nov 09)		• also called ' cement liner'
		• used for both pulpal Medication and thermal Protection

- VARNISH and ZnOE contraindicated under composite
- W.T of dental materials:

Cement	Working time
Zn Polycarboxylate	3 min
$ZnPO_4$	5 min
Amalgam	3-4 min

LAST 5-YEAR QUESTIONS FROM THIS TOPIC:

1. **A radiopaque area is observed in the dentine underlying a 3 month old class 2 amalgam restoration. Which base was used in this restoration?** *(AIIMS Nov 10, Nov 08, AIPG 08)*

Ans. $Ca(OH)_2$ (NBDE Q)

2. **To prevent damage to pulp in a deep cavity from acid etching, the cavity is lined by:** *(AIIMS Nov 10, May 09)*

Ans. RMGIC (Ref: sturdevant $4^{/e}$ p175-76)

3. **Sequence of setting of GIC is:** *(AIPG 09)*

Ans. Decomposition, migration, gelation, hardening

4. **Which of the following is true for hybrid ionomers:** *(AIPG 08)*
   a. **Release of fluoride more than compomer**
   b. **Fluoride release is comparable to conventional GIC**
   c. **More sensitive to water contamination compared to conventional GIC**
   d. **More ionic activity compared to conventional GIC**

Ans. a.

5. **A diagnosis of small occlusal cavities is most readily made by:** *(AIPG 08)*

Ans. An explorer and compressed air

6. **Which GIC developes early resistance to water intake on setting?** *(KCET 11)*

Ans. RMGIC (Ref: Phillips science of dental materials 11/e p482)

7. **For accurate interocclusal records the material of choice is:** *(COMEDK 11)*

Ans. ZnOE bite registration material

8. **Which dental cement is most kind to pulp?** *(AIIMS Nov. 09)*

Ans. Zinc polycarboxylate (Ref: Albers. Tooth colored restoratives: Principles and Techniques 9th ed pg 71 – 73)

COMPOSITE

- Composition:

Powder (initiator)	liquid – activator and inhibitor [Q]
Initiator – benzoyl peroxide (self cure) Camphroquinone (light cure, activated at 474 nm) (PGI Dec 11)	Activator – 30 amine (in self cure) Diketone (VL cure) Benzoin methyl ether (in UV – cure)
	Inhibitor - hydroquinone

- Radio opacifier added to composite → TiO2 + Zr oxide *(PGI Dec 11)*
- BIS – GMA in composite replaced methacrylate based matrix. *(KCET 10)*
- higher filler content → reduced H2O absorption
- Coupling agent → provides HydrolytiC stability (organic silanes)
- **Filler size:** (favourite Q of PGI)

• NANOfill (0.005μm – 0.01 μm) → microfill (0.01μm–0.1 μm) ↓ *(PGI 12)* • Midi fill (1μm – 10 μm) ← mini fill (0.1 μm – 1 μm) ↓ • Macro fill (10 μm – 100 μm)
• Mega fill/inserts = 0.5 to 2 mm [Q] • Inserts/mega fill are added posterior composite to improve wear resistance [Q]

- Visible light composite:

• λ range of 400 nm – 500 nm (PGI 11), i.e BLUE region predominantly at 474 nm used.
• shrinkage occurs towards light source [Q]

- Shade matching should be done within 5 sec to avoid fatigue to eye *(AIPG 12)*
- Bond:

Covalent bonds are seen in dental resins

- **Filler content:** (favourite Q of PGI)

	MICRO fill	Flowable	Packable	Conventional	Hybrid
Wt %	35 % – 60% ↓ –5%	40 % – 60% [Q] ↓ – 10%	65% – 80% [Q] ↓ –15%	75% – 80 %	75% – 85%
Volume%	30 % –45%	30% – 55 %	48% – 67 %	75% – 80%	75% – 85 %

- Microfilled composite shows more water absorption as compared to light cure composite/conventional/hybrid composite *(AIPG 07).*
- Compomer:

Polyacid modified composites *(KCET 11)* Use – for restoration in LOW stress bearing area
Recommended for patients at medium risk for dental caries
Setting reaction → 1^0 by light cure BUT acid base reaction also occurs.
NOTE: properly done composite restoration can reduce the incidence of recurrent caries.

- **Flowable composite:** Used in *(KCET 12)*

• Pit and fissure
• Class 1 restoration

- **Concept:**

Cavity preparation for composite for caries extending to root surface: When a cavity extends on to root, class 2 conventional cavity(without bevels), as bevels are only given on enamel.

- **NOTE:** Etching time for:

• Normal etching time – 15 sec
• Isolated enamel only – 30 sec
• 1^0 teeth – 120 sec (as they have aprismatic enamel)
• Etching time for fluorosed teeth extended for several minutes (60 – 90 secs according to AIIMS Nov 11)
• Sclerotic dentine etched for 30 sec = isolated enamel etching

- Curing time – 20 sec
- Enamel rod gets dissolved by acid the most in head region *(AIIMS Nov 09)*
- **NOTE:** Etching

• Increases surface area
• Increases surface free energy of enamel
• Decreases surface free energy of dentine
• Creates microporous layer (5 – 50 μ deep)
• brings about reduction in microlekage *(AIIMS 08)*

- In Acid etching GEL form is preffered over solution form for providing ease of placement over area to be etched *(AIIMS May 12, Nov. 10, 08)*
- Type of acid etching:

Type – 1 ⟶ intact periphery + removal of core

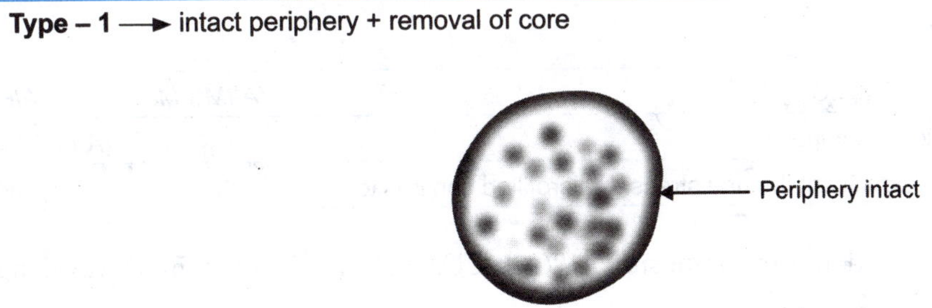

Fig 1.13: Acid etching type 1

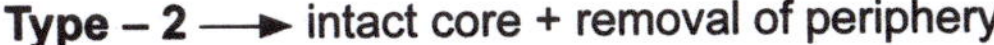

Type – 2 ⟶ intact core + removal of periphery

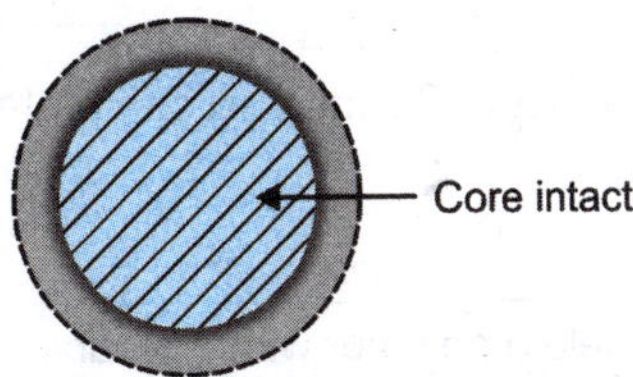

Fig 1.14: Acid etching type 2

Type – 3 ⟶ generalized roughening

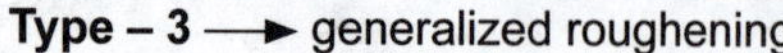

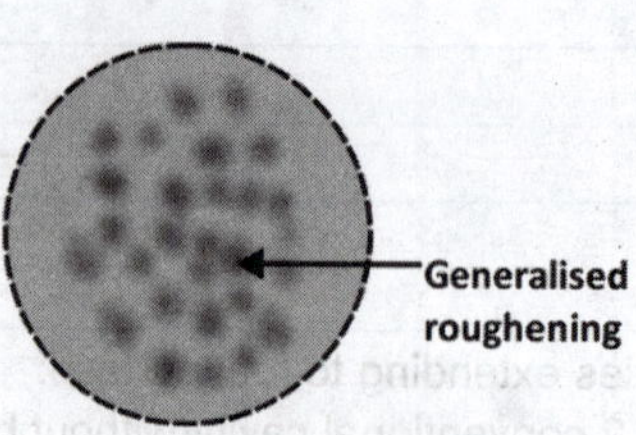

Fig 1.15: Acid etching type 3

- Etchant concentration:

> 50 % H_3PO_4 → MONO Calcium phosphate MONO hydrate	
< 30 % H_3PO_4 → Di Calcium phosphate MONO hydrate	*(AIIMS Nov 09)*

- Etchant removes/modifies smear layer primer:

• HEMA used [Q]	
• increases surface free energy of dentine+ wets the dentine surface	*(AIIMS Nov. 10, AIPG 09)*
• HYBRID layer – formed by bonding agent by co – polymerization with primer	

- Concept:

Bond strength of DBA is greater BUT clinical longevity is not as long as EBA due to H_2O content { donot confuse: in other restorations, bond strength with enamel is always greater }

- Amalgam bonding system:

4 Used	*(AIIMS Nov 12)*

- In PMMA P/L ratio:

= 3: 1 by volume	*(AIIMS May 12)*
= 2.5: 1 by wt.	*(AIIMS May 12)*

- Class 5 cavity:

• Class 5 stable erosive lesion – RMGIC	*(AIIMS May 12, 11, AIPG 09)*
• Class 5 unstable erosive lesion – composite	*(AIIMS May 11)*
• Class 5 cavity with abfraction/significant flexural stress – microfilled composite	*(AIPG 09)*

- Among lasers, only Argon laser is used to cure composite *(AIPG 10, COMEDK 11)*. it emits single wavelength [Q]
- Curing:

• Slow/soft start polymerization = QTH curing unit	*(KCET 10)*
• Rapid polymerization = PAC light cure unit	

- Depth of curing of composite by light → upto 2 mm (can correlate it with the effective depth of topical LA which is upto 2-3 mm)
- Copolymerisation:

• 2 Different monomers combine to yield a polymer with desirable property (kcet 10)
• **Remember** in addition and condensation polymerization, same monomer condenses with elimination of small molecules.

- Smear layer thickness:

Smear layer - 1-3 μm thick ↓+ 2 μm Smear plug – 2-5 μm deep

- Conservative approach for restoration:

Composite >> GIC

- Bonding Agents (favourite Q of KCET)

Total ETCH	Self ETCH Primer	All In One
3 steps(E + P + BA) 4th generation Multibottle (KCET 12)	EP + BA 6th generation	7th generation
2 step/1 bottle (E + PBA)(KCET 10) 5th generation	No rinsing for etchant. so, does'nt remove smear layer. incorporates smear plug into resin tag	
E = etchant P = primer BA = bonding agent		

- Etching:

• Head of rod → Dissolves more (more prone to acid dissolution) [Q]
• Tail and periphery → More resistant to acid dissolution

- Uses of DBA: *(PGI Dec 11)*

• Create hybrid layer for micromechanical bonding
• For desensitization of hypersensitive dentine by forming resin tags, hybrid layer and precipitation of protein/ denature protein

- Permeability of dentine depends on:

• Smear layer
• Diffusion coefficient of fluid
• Length of dentinal tubules
Not on convection of fluid *(AIIMS 07)*

- Fluoride release:

GIC > RMGIC > compomer > composite

- Curing:

• Intensity/energy required for polymerization of composite → above • 400 Mw/cm^2 [Q]
• QTH → minimum energy shouldn't be less than 300 Mw/cm^2 (300 – 1200) *(PGI 10)*

- Polymerization Shrinkage:

• volumetric shrinkage of composite + PMMA 6% • (if MMA then nearly 3 times coming to a value of 21%)
• Linear polymerization shrinkage of composite + PMMA 0.4% to 1.6%
• stress caused by polymerization shrinkage = 5 MPa *(AIPG 09, AIIMS Nov 10)*

- Polymerization stress can be minimized by:

• Soft start polymerization
• Ramped – up curing (intensity is gradually increased)
• Delayed curing (stress relaxation takes place) [Q]
• INCREMENTAL build – up

- C – Factor:

• We have to minimize C – factor to reduce polymerization shrinkage
• Class 1 = 5 class 2 = 2 class 3 = 1 class 4 = 0.5 class 5 = 0.25 [Trick = 521 number ki BUS 0.5, 0.25]
• [in KCET 2012 class 5 was asked but the answer was given as 0.5. we are sorry to say but even if it is given in sturdvent, you need to mark the same answer if Q is asked in future in KCET as they keep following their own key]

- Microleakage in composite → more as LCTE is 3 times of teeth
- Polishing:

Amalgam	Composite
SnO_2, ZnO, precipitated chalk (PGI 10), silex *(COMEDK 07)*	Al_2O_3, SiO_2

LAST 5-YEARS QUESTIONS FROM THIS TOPIC

1. While restoring a cavity, C factor is associated with: *(AIPG 12)*

Ans. Polymerization shrinkage (Ref: Sturdevant 4/e p203, 243, 479)

2. Shade matching should be done within ________ seconds to avoid fatigue of eyes to color. *(AIPG 12)*

Ans. 5 seconds (Ref: Rosensteil, land, fujimoto 06, p724)

3. While restoring a tooth with composite resin, the etched surface gets contaminated with saliva accidently. what would be done next: *(AIPG 11,09)*

Ans. Wash with water, dry area and continue restoration.

4. Class 5 cavity prepared for amalgam and composite differs in: *(AIPG 09)*

Ans. Cavosurface margin (Ref: Sturdevant 4/e p528 – 531)

5. HOW long does it take for an etched enamel to return to normal condition? *(COMEDK 11)*

Ans. 30 days (Ref: Charbeneau's principle and practice of operative dentistry 3/e p163)

6. In etching of enamel, the depth achieved is: *(AIIMS Nov 10)*

Ans. 5–50 μ (Ref: Heasmen. Restorative dentistry, pediatric dentistry and orthodontics p104)

DENTURE BASE RESIN

- COMPOSITION:

• Of heat cure is same as self cure EXCEPT presence of 3^0 amine (N,N – dihydroxy ethyl para toluidine) as an activator in self cure in liquid *(KCET 11)*
• Inhibitor prolongs self life *(PGI 09)*
• 3^0 amine = DPT (dimethyl – p – toluidine)

- **In PMMA:**

Polymer: monomer = 3: 1 (volume) 2.5: 1 (weight)

- If acrylic resin is packed in sandy state → Porosity occurs
- Properties:

All properties of heat cure are better than self cure acrylic EXCEPT greater polymerization shrinkage [Q] in heat cure acrylic. So, less stable

- Residual Monomer:

Heat cure	Self cure
0.2 to 0.5 % OR < 1 % (PGI 12)	3 to 5 %

- Concept:

In heat cure more polymerization ↓ More polymerization shrinkage ↓ Less residual monomer

- Most important disadvantage of Acrylic resin is polymerization shrinkage like composite
- Resin packed in dough state because the material will be more homogeneous and occurrence of porosity is minimized
- Curing of denture base resin:

• SLOW curing → 74°C maintained for 8 hrs
• FAST curing → 74 °C maintained for 1 ½ hrs and increased upto 100 °C • For 1 ½ hrs
• BENCH curing – 30 to 60 min

- Repair of fractured denture base:
Chemically cured resin → MORE stable → but durability decreased
- Properties of PMMA:

• Polymerization shrinkage (by volume) → 6 % • (**NOTE:** Of MMA = PMMA * 3 → 21 %)
• Polymerization shrinkage (linear) → 0.2 to 0.5 %
• Coefficient of thermal expansion → more than twice that of composite
• Compressive strength → 76 MPa
• Tensile strength → 55 MPa
• Hardness (KHN) → 15 – 18 Kg/mm^2
• Biocompatibility → good
• Thermal conductivity → poor
• Wear resistance → fair • Fatigue resistance → good
• B.P of MMA > B.P of H_2O ↓ 100.8 °C [Q]

- Disadvantage of PMMA:

Thermal properties are poor

- In resin gas inclusion porosity → seen in fluid resin porosity due to air incorporation [NOT due to heating of resin]
- Self cure are more porous than heat cure. So, to prevent porosity, self cure resins are cured under " VACUMM" pressure
- Insufficient closure of flask during packing of denture base resin results in increase in vertical dimension *(AIPG 07)*

LAST 5-YEAR QUESTIONS FROM THIS TOPIC

1. **During polymerization of acrylic resin above what temperature benzoyl peroxide form free radicals:** *(AIIMS Nov 12)*

Ans. 60°(Ref: Phillips 11/e p730)

CERAMIC

- **Composition:**

Feldspar → Basic glass former
Kaolin → Binder
Quartz → Strengthener, glass former
Metal oxide → Provide color Metallic oxide gives color to porcelain *(AIIMS 11)* The metal alloy used in PFM should NOT contain Cu/Ag as they discolor porcelain ↓ Causes greenish Discoloration *(KCET 10)*
Flux → boric oxide. Present in LOW fusing ceramic. It reduces fusion Temperature → improves fluidity, increases Cote e.g. boric oxide + (Na, K, Ca) oxide
TiO_2 + ZrO_2 → opacifier in ceramic Major advantage – Resistance to discoloration under U-V light

- PFM:

• Chemical bonding is 1° bonding
• In base metal – CrO_2 helps in bonding
• In noble metal – In and Sn oxide helps in bonding

- Porcelain teeth:

When used, sufficient interocclusal clearance should be present, i.e sufficient overjet and over bite

- Bonding of ceramic to metal occurs both by mechanical and Chemical
- Self Glazed Porcelain
- More permanent than apllied glaze
- APF gel/other topical fluorides can cause staining
- investment used for casting of ceramic → phosphate bonded
- Castable glass ceramic/machinable glass ceramic → DICOR *(KCET 10)*
- Injection moulded ceramic → IPS empress
- Glass infiltrated ceramic → inceram

- Method of decresing porosities in ceramic:

• Vacuum firing
• When porcelain is self glazed by reheating, It is the BEST method of reducing voids

- **Firing** in porcelain: (stages)

Low bisque – minimal polymerization shrinkage	
Medium bisque	
HIGH bisque – high polymerization shrinkage	*(AIPG 07)*

- High fusing = 1290 °C – 1370 °C (1300)
- (Used for denture teeth)
- Medium fusing = 1090 °C – 1260 °C (1300 – 1100)
- Low fusing = 870 °C – 1090°C (900 – 110
- Condensation shrinkage during porcelain firing is determined by particle size and shape *(AIIMS Nov. 10, AIPG 07)*
- **NOTE:**

FIRING at low temperature for a long time ↓ Decreases Porosity ↓ Gives life like appearance ↓ So, preffered
Vaccumm firing/diffusible gas like He/H_2 firing reduces porosity

- Strengthening of porcelain

• Development of residual • Compressive stress	• Distribution of crack propagation
• Aluminous porcelain • (Na K+)	• Ion exchange/chemical tempering
• Thermal tempering	• Transformation toughening, e.g. tetragonal ZrO_2 • monoclonal ZrO_2
• Thermal compatibility (increased cote of metal slightly)	

- In aluminous porcelain alumina interrupts the crack propagation by the process of dispersion strengthening
- CAD – CAM → No need for "impression" and "casting" procedure [Q]

LAST 5-YEAR QUESTIONS FROM THIS TOPIC

1. **Common between amalgam and ceramic is:** *(AIPG 12)*

Ans. High compressive strength and low tensile strength (Ref: Manapalli 2/e p372)

2. For a cast porcelain inlay, the facial wall should: *(AIPG 09)*

Ans. Diverge facially (Ref: Sturdevant 4/e p579 – 580)

3. **Ceramics fired to metals are processed by:** *(KCET 11)*

Ans. Sintering (Ref: craig's 11/e p553 -554)

METALLURGY

- Co – Cr /elgiloy:

Co – 60 %	Cr – 30 %

- In austenite (18 – 8 steel):

• 18 % Cr and 8 % Ni
• Fe is in γ form

- **Zn:** Scavenger of O_2 (Deoxidizing agent added to dental alloys) *(PGI Dec 11)*
- **Ti:** Most corrosive resistant

Others – Al, Cr	*(KCET 13)*

- Casting Difference between base metal and Au alloy:

BASE METAL	Au ALLOY
• FLUX - fluoride • (to dissolve any oxide formed e.g CrO_2) (AIPG 07)	• FLUX – borax + boric acid
• CRUCIBLE – quartz [Q]	• CRUCIBLE – carbon/clay (for high noble alloy > 40 % Au)
• SOLDER – silver	• SOLDER - Au
• PICKLING – sand blasting with Al_2O_3	• PICKLING solution – 50 % HCl (BEST), also H_2SO_4
• Casting shrinkage – 2.3 %	• Casting shrinkage – 1.5 %
• FINAL polishing - electropolishing	• FINAL polishing – rouge (Fe_2O_3)

- Sensitization and stabilization of stainless steel:

Stainless Steel ↓ 400 – 900 °C Cr Carbide ↓ Reduced Corrosion Resistance	Stainless Steel ↓ 400 – 900 °C + Ti Ti Carbide ↓ Protect Chromium Stabilization

- The only nearly pure metal used for dental casting is PURE titanium (Cp Ti) [Q] [donot confuse with DFG. It is pure Direct restorative material]
- Cp Ti is most biocompatible *(PGI 11)*
- Noble metal alloy (casting) classification:

High noble → noble metal > 60 % wt Au 40 % wt
Noble → 25 % wt of noble metal No stipulation for Au
Predominantly base metal alloy → noble metal < 25 %

- Noble metal are resistant to corrosion because they have positive EMF
- Implant material: *(KCET Q)*

• CpTi – excellent biocompatibility
• Ti alloys - Ti – 6 Al – 4 V – Because of strength issue with pure Ti, have lead manufacturer to use a Ti alloy. – Ti alloy Ti – 6 Al – 4 V has become material of choice for endosseous dental implant.

- Fluoride flux:

has KF: boric acid = 1: 1 *(PGI 09 Q)*

- **Types of flux:**

Type 1 → Prevents formation of oxide
Type 2 → Reduces already formed oxide *(PGI)*
Type 3 → Dissolves oxide e.g fluoride flux *(PGI, AIIMS)*
NOTE: Fluoride flux used during soldering of cobalt – chromium alloy/joint of 2 stainless steel wires to prevent formation of chromium oxide *(AIIMS Nov. 10)*

- **Antiflux:**

• Graphite, Pb, rouge
• Restricts flow of solder (COMEDK 11)

- Base metal vs Noble metal (e.g Au)

Base Metal	Noble Metal
• Increased hardness, strength • Increased sag resistance (resistance against thermal stress)	• Increased density, castability, • ductility

- GRAIN refiners:

• " 3 elements"
• Ir [don't confuse with In. it is NOT mentioned in PHILLIPS. In oxide helps in bonding to porcelain], Ruthenium, Rhenium
• Increases corrosion resistance and yield strength
• < 1 % for Pd alloys and much less for Au alloys

- Nickel:

Added to cast gold alloy ↓ Strengthener *(AIIMS Nov. 09)*

- Soldering vs Brazing:

Soldering	Brazing
Fusion temperature of filler material < 450 ^{0}F	Fusion temperature of filler material 450 ^{0}F

- Ideal temperature of H_2O bath for softening fluid wax 51 – 54°C
- **Heat treatment**

Softening Heat Treatment	Hardening Heat Treatment/ Age Hardening	Cold Working/Strain Hardening/Work Hardening
All Strength (Including Tensile Strength) Decreases Except Ductility (It Increases)	• All strength increases EXCEPT ductility which decreases *(PGI 11)*	• Increases strength BUT decreases ductility (PGI 11) (same improvement properties as after hardening heat treatment.
		• Grain elongation is the result of cold working
		• Corrosion resistance reduces *(PGI 10)*
	• Usually For Au Alloys	• Done for DFG, stainless steel wire

- **NOTE:** With surface hardening percentage elongation reduces
- Cold working of Dfg:

• Process of increasing strength of metal by heating below it's recrystallisation temperature OR • Process of plastically deforming a metal usually at room temperature • e.g. condensation of DFG
• REVERSED by annealing
• For DFG → cold working is characteristic BUT • For castable gold, cold working cannot be done

- Tempering of steel increases hardness *(PGI 10)*
- Wrought alloy → "cold worked" metal → hardness and tensile strength increases but ductility reduces
- Ni added to cast Au alloy → Strengthner
- Berrilium increases castability of BASE metal alloys
- Fig 16: change in properties with cold working and annealing

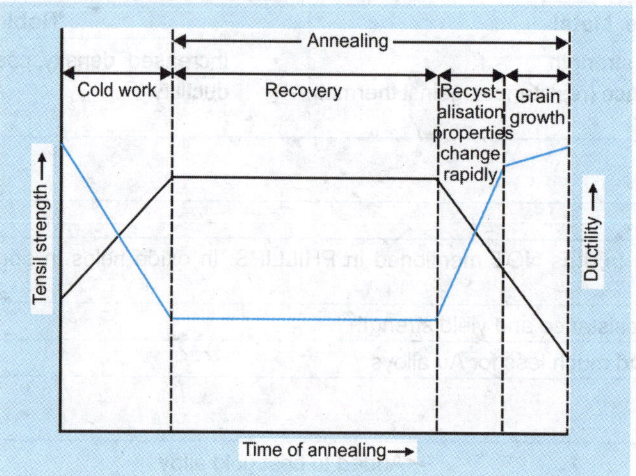

Fig 1.16: Change in properties with cold working and annealing

- Grain elongation seen in cold working:

It is the measure of ductility which increases rapidly in recrystallization phase of anneling

- Wax Pattern

• Type 1/type B	• Type 2/type C
• " DIRECT"	• " INDIRECT"

- Best technique: Direct – indirect *(PGI 12)*
- Wax Composition:

• **Paraffin:** Basic constituent – Tendency to flake (overcome by GUM DAMMAE) – Less smooth and glossy (overcome by gum dammar + carnauba/Cadelila wax)
• **Gum dammar:** Improves smoothness – Decreases flaking *(COMED K 08)*

• Carnuba/candellila wax: decreases flow • Imparts glossy surface **NOTE:** Candelilla wax may replace carnauba wax completely *(KCET 12)*
• **Ceresin:** May replace paraffin partly
• **Bee wax:** Decreases flow at mouth temperature

- Impression wax is: Bite registration/corrective wax
- Incomplete wax elimination → leaves CARBON → causes Shiny surface on cast
- Distortion is most serious problem of pattern, due to release of Internal stress
- Method to prevent Warpage in wax pattern: *(AIPG 08)*

Uniform heating of wax at 50 °C
Use of warm instrument for carving
Use of warm die
Adding wax to die in small amount
Invest the pattern immediately – Most practical method (COMEDK 11)

- Non – True wax:

Cocoa butter (to protect GIC from moisture), japan wax

- PKT -2 is wax adding instrument *(KCET)*
- Indirect spruing:

Extra Spruing → Minimizes Localized Shrinkage Porosity

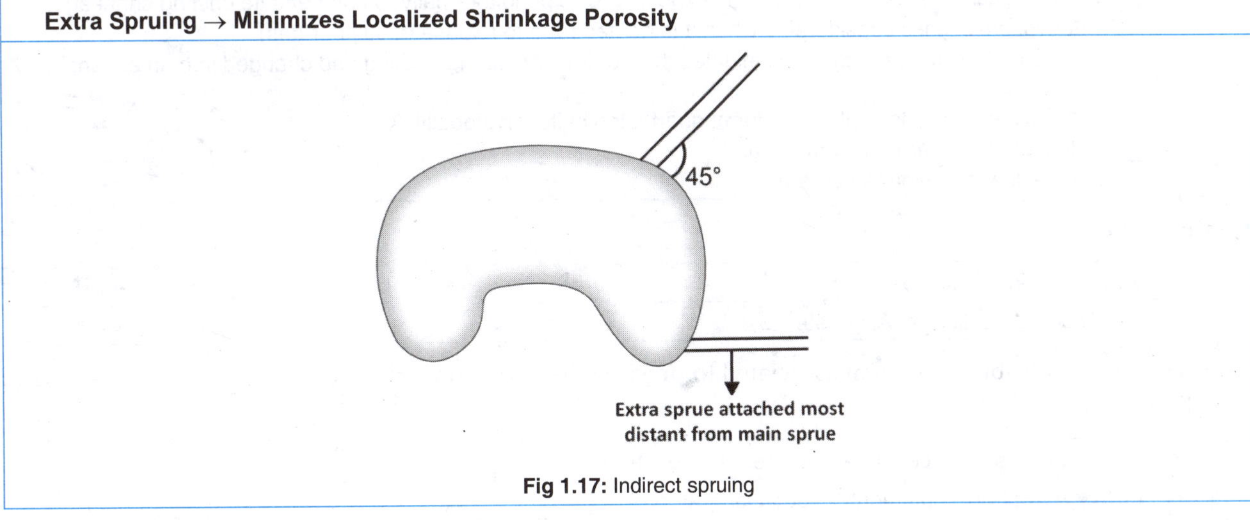

Fig 1.17: Indirect spruing

- Most common cause of incomplete casting → narrow sprue
- Turbulence of alloy in sprue → due to position of sprue
- **Ideal Sprue:** Hollow metal sprue
- sprue attachment:

• Cusp tip gives good result
• In posterior teeth ideal position is near proximal surface [Q]/just below the non functional cusp

- Investment material:

• **Gypsum bonded:** – Binder – α – hemihydrates [Q], provides strength *(AIPG 07)* – Used – casting Au alloys – Heating above 700 °C → SO_2 released *(NEET 13)* – S.E: – N.S.E – 0.5 % – H. E – 1-2 % – Thermal expamsion – 1-2 % – BEST pickling material for this investment is HCl *(COMED K 11)*
• **Phosphate bonded:** – Binder – MgO + mono ammonium phosphate – Used – high melting Co – Cr and metal ceramic – Phosphate bonded + carbon → for gold – Phosphate bonded without carbon → for base metal, Ag Pd Alloys Refractory material: quartz, cristobalite
• **Silica bonded:** – Binder – ethyl silicate/silica gel – Use – high fusing base metal partial denture alloys – GREEN shrinkage seen – Refractory material: silica – Heated upto 1200 °C
Concept: • **Refractory and investment material:** – During heating, investment material is expected to Expand thermally to compensate casting shrinkage. – But gypsum shrinks considerably when it is heated (due to release of sulphur gas) – This refractory material (Silica) eliminates this contraction during heating and changed into an expansion (AIPG 07) – " SILICA" exists in its 4 allotropic form: quartz, tridymite, crystoballite Best choice as refractory material As of low inversion temperature.

- Ring Liner:

• Permit expansion of mold
• e.g. Asbestos, cellulose, Al silicate

- Success of removable die system associated to precise relocation on working cast *(PGI 09)*
- DIE material:

• **Gypsum/die stone:** Least abrasion resistance [Q]
• **Epoxy resin:** Most commonly used in laboratory
• **Electroplated Ag:** lethal due to Ag – Poly S can be electroplated

- Porosity in cast restoration *(Very Important Topic)*

NOTE: Just remember these points, youcan easily solve any question based on this topic
• **Sub – surface porosity:** It is due to " more than rapid rate of entry" of molten alloy into the mold • [Just remember this, you can solve any question] – Cause → Large sprue diameter, high temperature (more flow)

• **Back pressure porosity:** "escape of air is prevented" due to excessive thickness of investment, too short sprue, incomplete removal of wax pattern, Inadequatecasting Pressure (AIPG 11,09). So, adjust the sprue such that there is only 6 mm (¼ inch) distance between casting ring and wax pattern
• Suck back porosity → Due to creation of " HOT SPOT" [Q] – Cause → short sprue, sprue attachment at 90°
• **Localized shrinkage porosity:** Due to long sprue
• **Microporosity:** Due to rapid solidification shrinkage. So, increases melting temperature – **NOTE:** Localized shrinkage porosity and microporosity are Not seen in denture Base Resin

- Common Cause of porosity in denture:

• High temperature (curing temperature > 100°C) → sub surface/internal porosity in " Thick Areas" of denture
• Insufficient pressure/inadequate material → voids all over the denture
• If flask is placed too soon in boiling water → porosity in thickest part of the denture
• GAS inclusion porosity → seen in " Fluid resin" due to incorporation of air. It is not due to heating of the resin

- Cavity preparation for Cast restoration:

Pulpal floor of class 2 of cast and amalgam at same level

- Bevels: Types

• Partial – involves a part of enamel
• Short – entire enamel
• Long – entire enamel + dentine partly – Most commonly used bevel
• Complete – entire enamel + dentine
• Counter/reverse bevel (given in DFG) – for cusp capping used in onlay
• Hollow ground – for base metal alloy and castable ceramic

- Most important bevel for cast inlay → Gingival bevel *(AIPG 11, 09)*
- Width of gingival bevel = 0.5 to 1 mm and merging with 2° flare
- Onlay:

• It is partly INTRACORONAL and partly EXTRACORONAL type
• At intracoronal portion → Hollow ground bevel given
• At extracoronal portion → Counter/reverse bevel given

- In inlay:

1°and 2° flare given for same function as bevel

- In onlay:

Skirts, collar (extended around entire cusp) ↓ Retention + resistance form increases

- class 2 metal restoration:

• Here A-P line angle slightly beveled
• To increase thickness of wax at this area to prevent wax pattern distortion
[**NOTE:** In amalgam this bevel prevents fracture of restoration]

- Inlay vs Amalgam

Inlay	Amalgam
• Cavosurface angle: 130^0 - 140^0	90^0 - 100^0
• Marginal metal angle: 30^0 - 40^0	80^0 - 90^0

- In inlay lap – joint present:

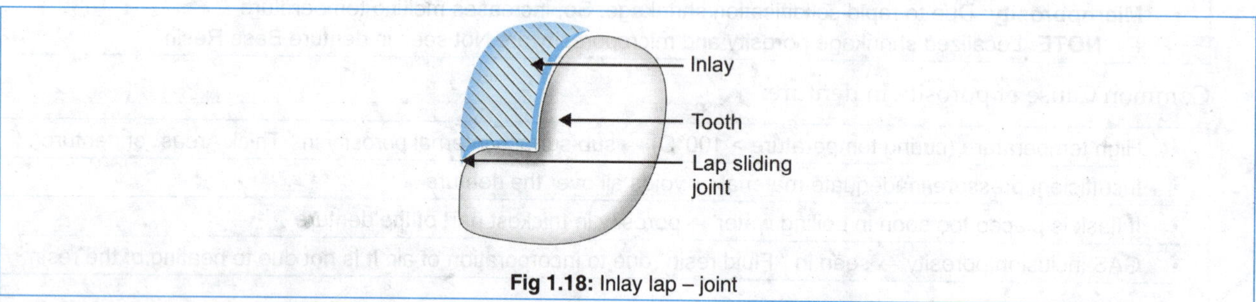

Fig 1.18: Inlay lap – joint

- Certain Clinical conditions and choice of restoration:

If no caries	→ Inlay/onlay not indicated
Short clinical crown	→ Full crown best as has better retention
RCT treated tooth	→ Ideal – crown Minimally – onlay acceptable Contraindicated – inlay

- For Inlay:

If marginal gaps/discrepancy exceeding 0.3 mm → should Not be burnished But discarded. repeat the cast

- Where to keep gingival seat?

0.5 mm below contact area for finishing

- Gingival extension of restoration:

At least 3 mm above alveolar crest

- For any Cast restoration (gold/porcelain):

All walls should diverge in inlay inorder to seat/remove wax pattern/ restoration
For porcelain/tooth coloured indirect restoration, i.e. inlay recommended gingivo – occlusal divergence > 2 – 5 ^{0} [not 2- 5^0]

LAST 5-YEARS QUESTIONS FROM THIS TOPIC

1. **Most common reason for incomplete casting when using a centrifugal casting machine is:**

Ans. Narrow sprue

2. **Which Zone of flame is used for melting alloys:** *(AIPG 10, 07)*

Ans. Reducing zone (Phillips 10/e p510, 627)

3. **Fins and spines in casting may occur because of:** *(AIPG 10)*

Ans. Rapid heating (Ref: Phillips 11/e p328)

4. **Which is not a noble metal?** *(AIPG 08)*

   a. Au

b. Ru
c. Ag
d. Osmium

Ans. c

5. One of the following is NOT true about gypsum bonded investment: *(AIPG 08)*

a. Used for gold alloys
b. 50 – 65% gypsum changes to form α – hemihydrates
c. Heating range is 500 – 700 ^{0}C
d. Heating of investment above 700 ^{0}C causes formation of SO_2 from calcium sulfate

Ans. b (Ref: Phillips 10/e p472 – 473)

6. Which is not used as antiflux: *(AIIMS Nov 12)*

a. Graphite
b. Boric acid
c. Iron oxide
d. Calcium carbonate with alcohol

Ans. b (Ref: Textbook of orthodontics – gowri Shankar 1st ed pg 761)

7. Solder and flux used for joining Elgiloy wires are: *(KCET 11)*

Ans. Silver solder and fluoride flux

8. The ideal temperature for water bath for softening fluid wax is about: *(KCET 10)*

Ans. 51 – 54 degree F

9. A casting shows round margins and smooth and shiny surface due to? *(PGI june 11)*

Ans. Inadequate wax elimination (Ref: Dental materials and their selection by William J.O'Brien 3/e p435)

CARIES

- **Difoti/Diagnodent**

Based on principle of fluorescence.
It detects the Precavitation Stage.
Detects incipient caries (proximal > occlusal) (AIIMS Nov 08,Nov 07, AIPG 11) Mainly for PROXIMAL caries.[Q]
Note: But less sensitive than Radiograph for distinguishing shallow and deep lesion.

- Pit and fissure caries vs smooth surface carie.

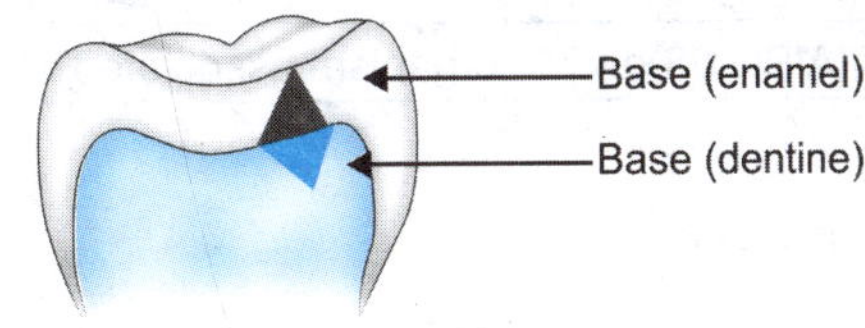

Fig 1.19: Pit fissure caries

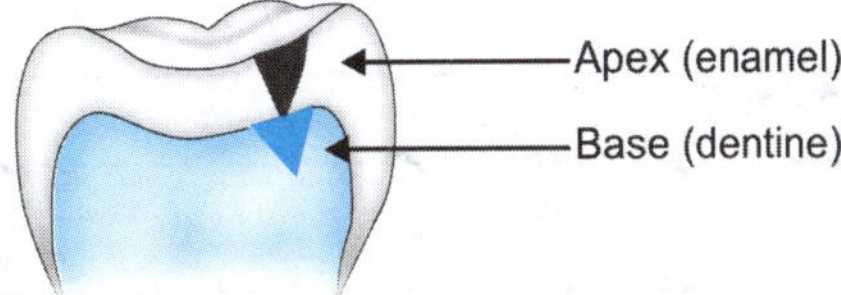

Fig 1.20: Smooth surface caries

- Forward caries:

Caries cone broad in enamel than dentine *(KCET 10, 11)*

- Affected dentine has no bacteria
- Earliest changes in incipient caries:

Loss of interprismatic/inter rod substance with increased prominence of rods

- Eburnation/sclerotic dentine:

seen in arrested caries

- The non active carious lesion is distinguished by no pain on excavation of caries *(AIIMS May 10, May 07, AIPG 07)*
- Reparative and sclerotic dentine deposition

Reparative	Sclerotic dentine
• " moderate irritant"" mild irritant, aging [Q] (attrition, erosion, caries, abrasion) • Affected odontoblasts die ↓ • This area of dentine is called " dead tract" • ↓ • Filled with air andappears Dark under microscope, i.e. In transmitted light, white in reflected ↓ • In about 15 days new odontoblasts are differentiated (AIIMS Nov 10) [Q] ↓ • Dead tracts are are sealed off at the Pulpal surface by reparative dentine formation (structurally and chemically different from 1° – 2° dentine, and being highly Atubular and impervious to most irritant)	Slowly advancing caries" ↓ Sclerotic dentine ↓ Dark in reflected light and whilte in transmitted light

- **NOTE:** In response trauma/irritant all 3 types of dentine, i.e. reparative, 2°, and sclerotic are formed
- minimum depth of demineralisation of carious lesion to be detected radiographically = 500 μm
- Minimum dentinal destruction to be evident radiographically = 40 μm
- dental caries associated with 8 serotypes of S. mutAns.

S. rattus (AIIMS/AIPG), S. cricetus, S. ferus, S. soberinus

- Streptococcus mutans and **Lactobacillus:**

Both are acidogenic andaciduric (AIPG 08)and 1° organism associated with caries

- Active caries → light brown
- Non – active caries → dark brown/black
- **Root caries:**

• Shows rapid spread
• 2° to gingival recession
• Often asymptomatic

- Arrested Caries:

Occlusal and proximal mostly

- Location of caries predominant organism: (very important in any examination)

Lactobaccilus →	Deep pit and fissure (AIIMS 05), deep dentinal caries.
S. mutans →	Pit and fissure caries (most predominant) Smooth surface caries (most predominant) Root surface caries (2nd common after Actinomyces)
Root caries →	A. Viscosus(most predominant) *(AIPG 11)* A. Naselundi(most predominant) *(AIPG 11)* S. Mutans (2nd most common)
Deep Dentinal caries →	Lactobacillus (most predominant) A. Naselundi (most predominant)

- TIME of progression from incipient to cavitated clinical caries on smooth surface = 18 month 6 month for deep pit and fissure caries:

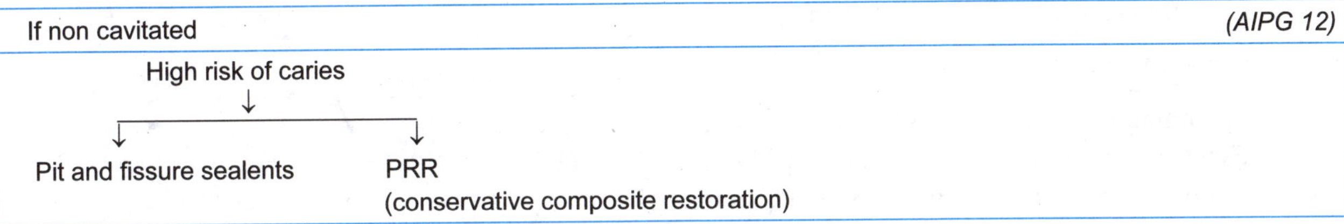

- Caries Diagnosis: Newer method of caries diagnosis

• OCT(optical coherence tomography), multiphoton imaging,infrared thermography, tetrahertz pulse imaging, TACT(tuned aperture CT), videoscope/ endoscope.
• Infrared camera–used to measure temperature drop.

- Different theories of caries:

• Chemical/acidic theory – Robertson
• Miller's chemicoparasitic theory/ Acidogenic Theory–Miller –Most Accepted. [Q]
• Proteolytic theory – Gotlieb
• Proteolysis chelation theoy – Schartz and Martin [KCET 2009]
• Auto immune theory – Burch and Jackson.
• Sulphatase theory – Pincus.

- Stephen Curve:

• recorded the ph values of plaque in situ BEFORE,DURING and AFTER the glucose rinse. *(AIPG 2008)*
• Plot between ph (on y-axis) and time (after glucose rinse) (on x- axis).
• Average ph in: – Caries free people – 7.4 – Carie prone people – 5.5
• The curve showed that plaque ph falls to low value within 2-3 minutes of a glucose rinse: – Caries free group – never below 5 – In caries prone group– 4.5-5
• Maxillary anterior Teeth exhibited greater drop in ph than mandibular anterior teeth.

- Generation of sealants:

• 1st – uv based
• 2nd- chemical cure
• 3rd- visible
• 4th- F⁻ releasing. [Q]

- Caries activity test:
- Synder's test:
  - Colorimetric test. [Q]
  - Principle – measures salivary microorganism ability to form acid in carbohydrate media.
  - Medium has indicator – Br (green ph -5.4 → yellow ph 3.8) [Q]
  - Measures

Color change	yellow	yellow	yellow
Caries activity	marked	Definite	Limited
Time	After24 hrs	48hrs	72 hrs

  - **Advantage:** Simple, low cost.
  - **Synder test** – Measure speed/rate of acid production. [PGI].
  - Method/Yard Stick of detection is by Ph change. [PGI]
- Lactobacillus count test:

No of organism/ c.c	Degree of caries activity
0-1000	Little or none
1000-5000	Slight
5000-10000	Moderate
>10000	Marked [KCET]

• The caries detection dye used to stain infected dentin contains–1% acid red solution in 0.2% proptylene glycol.
• Two tone dye stains immature plaque as red and mature plaque as Green.
• The dye used in salivary reductase test – Diazoresorcinol *(KCET 2012)* • Measures the activity of the reductase enzyme present in salivary bacteria.

- Dyes used in staining fracture line in a suspected tooth – 2% iodine [Q]
- Carisolv vs Caridex: They are alternative chemico-mechanical method for removal of caries.

Carisolv	x [PGI]
• 0.5% NaOcl,	• 1%Naocl *(AIIMS 12)*
• Leucine,lysine,glutamic acid and erythrosine dye.	• Glycine
• PH - 11	• PH -11(alkaline PH)
• Gel	• Sol
• 5-15 mints required	• 5-15 mints

- Caries Vaccine:

• IgA based. IgA is exceptionally resistant to digestion by proteolytic enzyme so highly effective in oral environment which contain microbial protease.
• Indications: patient Receiving radiation of Head andNeck, xerostomia, chronically sick children, sick patient, mentally and physically handicapped patients.

- Caries activity studies:

• **Vipeholm Study:** Gustafsson 1954 – -5 yr study of 436 adult in a mental institution of the Vipeholm Sweden. – Purpose of study: to find out does the increase in carbohydrate intake increases dental caries.effect of Sticky form of sugar on caries. Effect of non sticky form of sugar on caries. – Conclusion- physical form of sugar is more important than amount of sugar.
• **Hopewood study:** Sullivan and Harries. – Studies of dental status of children b/w 7-14 yrs at Hopewood house, – New South wales → longitudinal studies for 10 yrs. – **Conclusion:** Sparten diet (without fluoride and unfavourable oral hygiene) reduces dental caries.
• **3. Turku Sugar Study:** Scheinin and Makinen – AIM – compare cariogenicity of Sucrose, Fructose and Xylitol. – Basis of study – Xylitol not metabolized by plaque microorganism. [Q] **Conclusion:** – Fructose –less cariogenic than sucrose. – Xylitol - Non Cariogenic/Anticariogenic. Inhibits growth of st. Mutans

- Sorbitol:

• Poly alcohol sugar substitute.
• Lack enzyme to metabolize except mutans (But Even Slow)
• BEST method to reduce caries. [Q]

LAST 5-YEAR QUESTIONS FROM THIS TOPIC:

1. **Streptococci is important organism in causing dental caries as it :** *(NEET 13, AIPG 12)*

Ans. Produces extracellular polysaccharides

2. **Streptococci are acidophilic and aciduric. In this acidophilic means.** *(AIPG 12)*

Ans. Can survive in acid (Ref: Jawetz 23/e p65)

3. **Which of the following is false regarding dental caries:** *(AIPG 12)*
   a. **Infectious and transmissible**
   b. **Not caused by microbes**
   c. **Causes breakown of organic structure**
   d. **Possible without sucrose**

Ans. b. (well known fact)

4. **Bacteria are normally most populated in which area of teeth:** *(NEET 13, AIPG 12)*

Ans. Proximal

5. **Caries assessment tool CAT developed by AAPD defines high risk group as all except:** *(AIPG 12)*
   a. Visible plaque on anterior teeth
   b. Atleast 1 area of demineralization
   c. Enamel hypoplasia
   d. Children with special health care needs

Ans. b (Ref: Mcdonnald)

6. **Interproximal lesion Usually Begins:** *(AIPG 11, 09)*

Ans. Gingival to contact area (NBDE Q)

7. **Which is NOT true regarding S. mutAns.** *(AIPG 10)*
   a. Acidogenic and aciduric
   b. Requires specific conditions for growth
   c. Requires carbohydrate for metabolism
   d. Do not multiply easily

Ans. d (Ref: Clinical textbook of dental hygiene and therapy by Ireland, 2006 p77)

8. Which of the following is cariostatic? *(KCET 10)*

Ans. Molybdenum and vanadium

9. **Which of the following translucent area on hydration of tooth surface disappears?** *(PGI Dec 10)*

Ans. Incipient carious lesion (Ref: Sturdevant 4/e p408)

10. **Best method for caries reduction is:** *(AIPG 08)*

Ans. Substitute sugar by alcohol based sugar.
Ex- sorbitol.

11. **Most cariogenic sugar is:** *(AIPG 08)*

Ans. Sucrose

12. **Bacteria which adhere to tooth andcause caries is due to:**

Ans. They produce extracellular polysaccharides.

INSTRUMENTS AND MISCELLANEOUS

- Bur Description:

Bur Number	Length	Diameter
• No. 245 (inverted cone)	3 mm	0.8 mm (COMEDK 11)
• No. 330 (smaller and pear shaped bur) • Used for the most conservative amalgam preparation.	1 mm	0.8 mm

- **Antirust agent:**

• 2 %Na Nitrite [it's NITRITE not NITRATE] (AIPG 07)

- Formula for instruments:

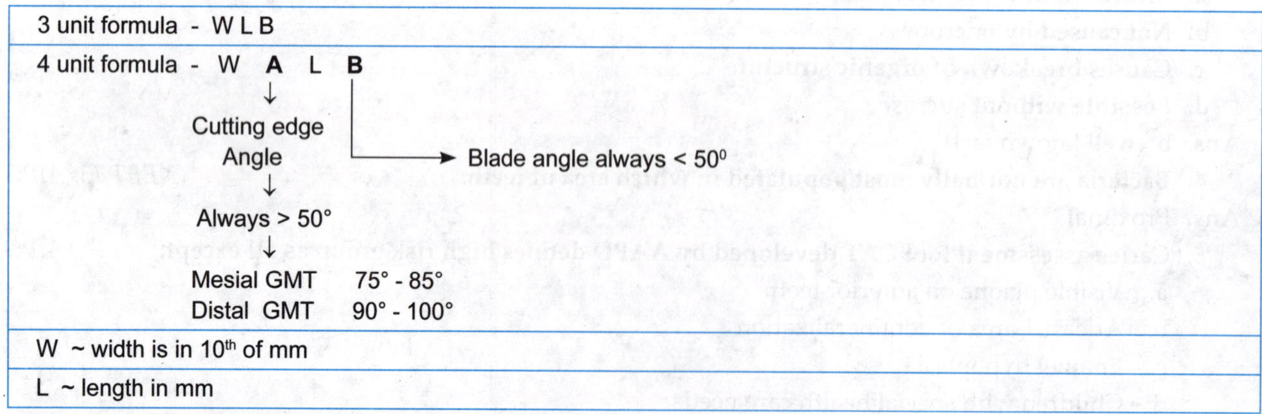

- Increased number of flutes → Decreases cutting efficiency
  ↓
  Increases smoothness/cutting efficiency

- Caries:

HARD caries	SOFT caries
Removed at high speed	Removed by bur at slow speed

- Enamel Bevel – given by GMT which is a type of Chisel [Q]
- Noise levels in excess of 75 decible → causes hearing damage *(AIIMS 06)*
- Enamel hatchet + GMT → chisel
- Angle former → excavator
- Thickness of matrix band (CLASS 2):

0.002 inch/0.001 inch ↓ Same as diameter of self threated pin

- Burs:

Carbide	Steel
• Increases cutting efficiency	• Decreased cutting efficiency
• Used at high speed	• Used at low speed
• Less heat production	• Produce more heat
	• Used for finishing

- **Thickness** of rubber dam:

Rubber Dam	Thickness	Trick to Remember
• Thin	0.006 inch (AIPG 07)	6
• Medium	0.008 inch	8
• Thick	0.010 inch	10

- Distance between 2 holes in rubber dam = 6.3 mm
- Thick rubber dam provides better retraction of gingiva → so, used in class 5 cavities
- Concept: A rubber dam does not require anything to pass
- Isolation:

• Isolate at least 3 teeth at a time for operative procedure
• For RCT isolation of the tooth being treated is enough

- Size of diamond abrasive:

" coarse" = 125 μ to 150 μ *(AIPG 07)*

- Abrasive hardness:

Diamond > boron carbide > SiC

Macro Abrasion	Air Abrasion	Micro Abrasion
12 fluted composite finishing bur	95% alumina in powder	Acid + abrasive ↓ ↓ HCl SiC
	Average particle size = 27 μ/even 20 μ given in AIPG, AIIMS may 09 [25 μ to 30μ given in Philips]	

- Air Abrasion:

• Contraindicated where risk of embolism e.g extraction socket, subgingival caries and pulmonary disease. Not deep caries

- Limit of Eccentricity:

• LIMIT of eccentricity of an aerator bur beyond which it stops working → 0.02 mm	*(AIPG 10)*
• BUT when question is asked according to ISO standard it is 0.03 mm	
• A major factor to determine eccentricity is SPIRAL angle	

- Principal of Balance (for instrument)

• The cutting edge of the blade should be nearer to the long axis of the handle for proper balance
• For optimum " ANTIROTATIONAL tendency" the blade edge must not be off the axis by more than 2 mm [Q]

- Pressure applied:

• SLOW speed rotator instrument → 2-5 pound
• HIGH speed → 1 pound with H_2O coolant as high heat is generated
• Ideal pressure → 2 – 4 pounds
• Condensation pressure for amalgam → 3 – 4 pounds

- Cavity preparation and temperature rise:
  ↓
  Not > 60 °C/130 °F
- factor influencing cutting efficiency of a bur:

Fig 1.21: Factor influencing cutting efficiency of a bur

- Rake angle:

• Negative rake angle = good for bur (long life)
• Positive rake angle = increased cutting efficiency
• [H – file has positive rake angle → so, good cutting efficiency]

- Cracked tooth syndrome:

• Diagnosed by – Best by rubber wheel test	
• Immediate Rx – splinting and relieve occlusion	*(COMEDK 13)*
• Rx of choice – Cast restoration	

- Bitewing with RVG:

Best for detecting proximal caries

- Crocus cloth = Pumice
- Heat content of propane [Q] and butane is highest

- Sterilisation:

• Gentlest method for sterilizing hand piece is EXTOX gas (ethylene oxide)
• Dry heat – Not recommended *(AIPG 10)*
• Autoclave – most rapid BUT causes dimming of fiber optic(AIIMS 06)
• Chemical vapour pressure: • Used for ceramic bearing hand piece BUT might impair others

- Important Values: *(Very Important)*

• Etching creates a depth of 5 to 50 μ
• Minimal dentinal destruction to be evident on radiograph = 40 μ
• Minimal depth of demineralization of lesion to be evident on radiograph = 500 μ
• Depth of maximum demineralization in enamel caries = 15 – 25 μ *(PGI june 11)*

- Wedge:

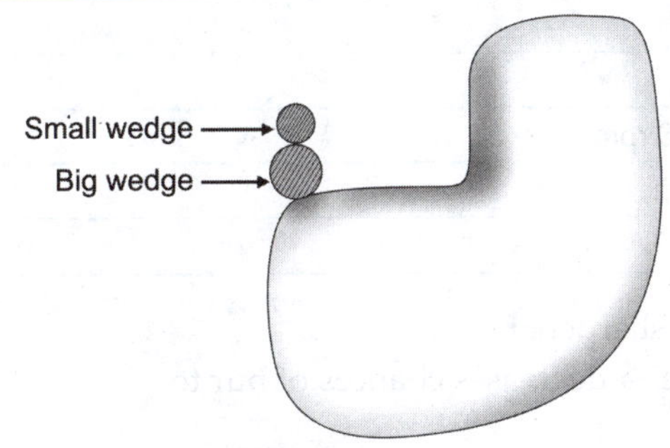

Fig 1.22: PIGGY back – used in gingival recession

Double wedge:
- Useful in facio – lingually wide proximal box *(AIPG 12)*
- One wedge facially and other lingually

Wedge wedging:
- Used in maxillary 1st premolar
- One wedge placed perpendicular to other

- Seperator:

SLOW	RAPID	
• Use of rubber/Cu Wire/orthodontic wire	• Wedge principle	• Traction principle
	• e.g. ELLIOT Separator [Q]	• e.g. ferrier double bow separator

- Chisel:

• **Straight/curved/biangle chisel:** – e.g. Wedelstat chisel [Q] with 4 unit formula
• **Enamel hatchet:** – Cutting edge parallel to long axis of handle and beveled on 1 side
• GMT

- Differentiating features of enamel hatchet from chisel: *(AIIMS 06)*

• It has a larger, Heavier blade.
• It has a cutting edge in a plane that is parallel with the axis of the handle.
• The blade does not curve (this curve is seen in GMT).

- Excavator:

• Ordinary hatchet
• Hoe
• **Angle former:** – 4 unit formula – For sharpening line angles/obtaining retention form in dentine ↓ for DFG
• Spoon excavator

- Speed:

• Low - < 8000 rpm
• Medium – 20, 000 to 45,000 rpm
• High – 45, 000 to 1 lakh rpm
• Ultra high → 1 lakh rpm

- Horning machine: Mechanical sharpener *(KCET 02)*
- In Bur → increased edge angle → decreases chances of bur to
- Fracture
- Change in bur neck diameter, shape and size of the bur and clearance angle affects efficiency of bur But not taper of bur head/height of bur head *(AIIMS 06)*
- For better efficiency and longer shelf life of a carbide bur, it should be rotated fast before entering cavity. *(AIPG 11, 09)*
- Rubber dam clamp:

1° teeth	Incisor and canine	1st Molar	2nd Molar
	' O' ivory	2, 2A ivory	26, 27 3 ivory

2° Teeth	Premolar	Partially erupted Molar	Fully erupted molar
	2, 2A ivory	154 A, 8A ivory	14, 8 ivory

- Critical/Non Critical instrument:

• **Critical**: Contact/penetrate/cut tissues e.g. endodontic file, scalpel
• **Semi Critical**: Which touch mucosa BUT donot cut/penetrate tissue e.g. air/water syringe tip, suction tip, handpiece
• Non-critical: Surface disinfection is adequate • e.g. X-ray stand, light source

- Laser:

Argon laser:	Used in composite curing Greater degree of polymerization/greater depth of Polymerization.	*(PGI Dec 11)*
Nd – YAG	1064 nm 1st laser used for dentistry Pulsed Nd – YAG ideal for soft tissue procedure and root Canal sterilization Converts dentine debris into an ionized gas leaving Debris on wall of canal (Plasma Effect) Used in Devitalisation pulpotomy + canal preparation + Laser welding	
CO_2	Used in laser welding Ideal for soft tissue and useful in cutting Fibrous tissue as in gingivectomy	
Er YAG (2.94 µ) + Er, Cr: YAG (2.79 µ)	Highest absorption of H_2O Ideal for hard tissue	
YSGG	Waterlase system	*(AIIMS May 09)*

- Polishing Agent:

Restoration	Polishing Agent
• Amalgam	• TiO, ZnO, Chalk (PGI)
• Composite	• Al_2O_3, SiC
• Noble metal alloy	• Fe_2O_3 (rouge)
• Co–Cr (base metal)	• Electropolishing
• Natural teeth	• Zr Si [Q]
• Stainless steel	• CrO → Whitening agent
• Denture/artificial teeth	• Pumice

- After amalgam polishing, the metal surface is flattened. This layer is called as Beilby's layer *(AIIMS May 11, 08)*
- Agents for treating hypersensitivity are: NaF, SnF_2, potassium nitrate *(AIIMS 08)*
- 2 % NaF is commonly used in iontophoresis *(AIIMS 06)*
- While restoring a tooth, following rules should be followed for maintaining aesthetics: *(AIIMS 06)*

• All anterior teeth should be restored in a single appointment
• Apparent size of the tooth can be increased by alteration in the height of contour of the tooth.
• Apparent length of the tooth can be increased by placement of developmental grooves on the tooth.

LAST 5-YEAR QUESTIONS FROM THIS TOPIC

1. **It is essential to lubricate dam before applying it. Which of these is not a suitable lubricant?** *(AIIMS May 11, AIPG 09)*
   a. Shaving gel
   b. Liquid soap
   c. Scrub gel
   d. Vaseline

Ans. d (Ref: Sturdevant 5/e p467)

2. **Which is the wrong way to apply dam using a wingless clamp?** *(AIIMS May 11, AIPG 09)*
   a. Put the clamp on the tooth, and then pull the dam over it.
   b. Place the dam on the tooth with fingers and then position the clamp over it.
   c. Attach the dam over the clamp and frame outside the mouth, and then put the assembly over the tooth using clamp holders over the dam.

d. Place the dam over the clamp and frame outside the oral cavity and then on tooth using a holder under the dam.

Ans. c. (Ref: Sturdevant 5/e p471)

3. **Interdental papilla are seen protruding beneath the rubber dam mostly when:** *(AIIMS Nov 11)*

Ans. Holes are placed too close (Ref: Sturdevant 5/e p469)

4. **FACIAL occlusal line in maxillary arch is formed by:** *(KCET 11)*

Ans. Non supporting cusps (Ref: Sturdvent 4/e p38)

5. **Right rear operator position refers to:** *(KCET 11)*

Ans. 11 O'clock position

6. **The disadvantage of winged rubber dam retainer is that it interferes with the placement of:** *(KCET 11)*

Ans. Matrix band

7. **Which of the following items in the dental operatory cannot be classified as a semi critical item?** *(KCET 11)*

a. Suction tip
b. Hand piece
c. Endodontic file
d. Water syringe tip

Ans. c.

8. **Function of water retraction system is:** *(KCET 10)*

Ans. Retracts water whenever spray is stopped

9. **Rubber dam is particularly adaptable to primary 2nd molar because the:** *(KCET 10)*

Ans. Cervical constriction of crown favours its retention

10. **Which of the following laser is is having a wavelength in the visible light spectrum?** *(PGI Dec 11)*

Ans. Argon (Ref: Skinner's 11/e p412)

11. **Safe level of Ni according to OSHA in clinics is?** *(PGI June 11)*

Ans. 1 mg (Ref: Sturdevant 5/e p165)

PROSTHODONTICS

- Working condyle/laterotrusive condyle
- Non-working condyle/mediotrusive condyle
- Bennet movement

Bennet movement
• concerned with Working Side
• It is 1- 1.5 mm/side

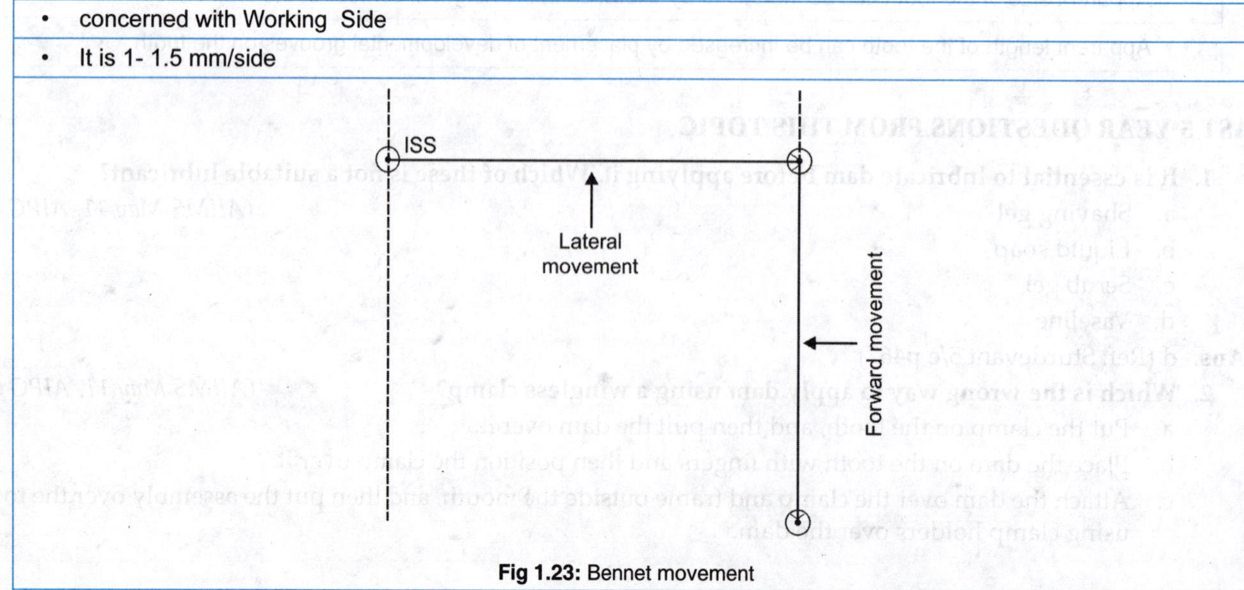

Fig 1.23: Bennet movement

- Bennet angle:

• Concerned with Non-working condyle [angle with saggital plane]
$L = \frac{H}{8} + 12$ (value around 15°)
• Bennet angle in edentulous patient is set at 30°

- Border Movements:

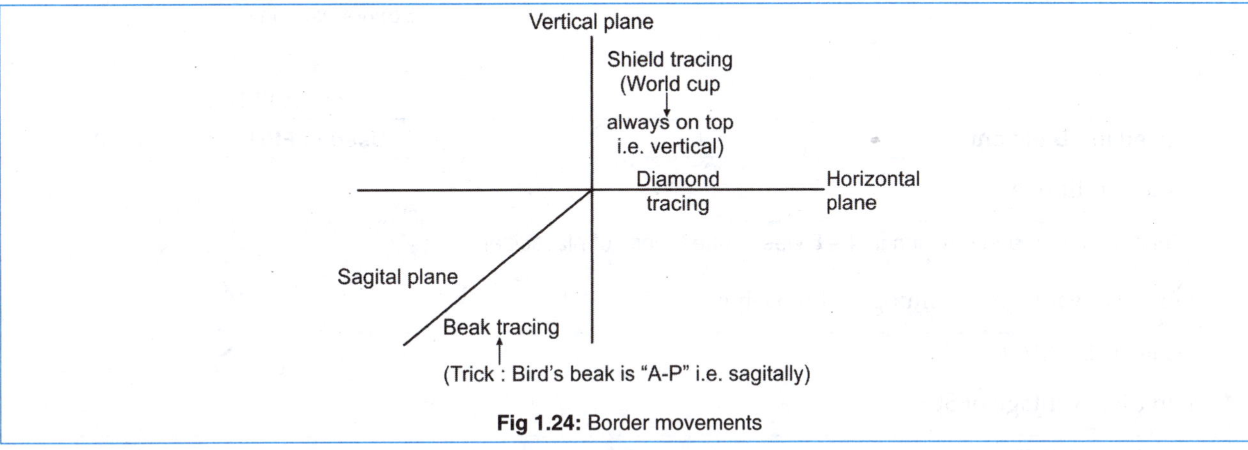

Fig 1.24: Border movements

- Vertical jaw relation:

• **Closest speaking space (silverman' s space):** – Used for measuring Vertical dimension – Physiologic method – Value 1 – 2 mm (measured in premolar area) – " ch, s, j"
• **Niswonger's method:** is physiologic method VDR = VDO + Freeway Space → 2-4 mm **NOTE:** When it is Not mentioned in question whether asking about VDR/VDO then take it as " VDO".

- Centric Relation:

• Patterson and Needle house method = functional method
• Graphic/arrow point tracing – Apex should be sharp – Pantograph → 3D → 6 styli used

- Discrepency between centric relation and centric occlusion:

0.5 to 1.5 mm → also called freedom from centric *(AIIMS 05, Nov 11)*

- Thickness of inter – occlusal record – 2 mm
- Orbitoaxial opening is determined by lateral pterygoid relining technique:

Open Mouth Method	Functional Method
• Boucher	• Winkler
• Tissue conditioner used	• ZnOE used

- **Note:** If there is CR and CO discrepancy then it needs NEW denture face bow:

Arbitary Facebow	Kinematic Facebow
Attached to maxilla	Attached to mandible ↓ UNSTABLE ↓ So, not used in CD ↓ Used in FPD
Used in CD patient	**Used in FPD**

- Tissue conditioner:

Tend to harden and roughen in 4 – 8 weeks due to loss of plasticizer

- Main disadvantage of relining and rebasing:

Change in " CR"

- Main disadvantage of SCD:

• Natural tooth wear
• Denture fracture
The main reason for sequel with SCD is difficulty in obtaining balanced occlusion

- Immediate denture:

• No anterior try in
• Frequent need of relining
Occlusal correction done after 48 hrs when swelling, inflammation subsides

- Jiffy denture is interim immediate denture hinge movement possible upto:

• 20 – 25 mm
• 12° – 15° (13°) → Rotation of condyle in TMJ

- Condylar inclination – 20 - 25°
- Average intercondylar distance in CD patient = 110 mm
- Relationship of denture base that resists the dislodgement of denture in horizontal direction is stability (AIIMS 06)
- Problems in new denture bearers:

Problem	Cause
• Soreness on slope of ridge	• Deflective occlusal contact
• Soreness on crest	• Increased vertical dimension resulting in heavy contact
• Generalized soreness of basal seat area	• Increased vertical dimension
• Increased salivation following insertion of CD	• Due to reflex parasympathetic stimulation of salivary gland

- Deflective occlusal contacts results in denture becoming loose several hours after wearing. *(AIPG 08)*

- Anterior deprogramming device:

• [Used in jaw relation and BRUXISM]
• In some patients protective reflex are well established, such patients will not allow their mandible to be manipulated and hinged easily.
• If tooth contact can be prevented, they will forget those reflexes and manipulation becomes easier.
• The teeth can be kept apart with cotton roll, leaf gauze (plastic)/a small anterior deprogramming device made of autopolymerizing acrylic resin (also known as lucia jig)

- **NOTE:** Ideal support for implant – lamellar bone in patients requiring lingual frenectomy:

Denture fabricated before surgery to act as stent and prevent relapse

- Biting Force: Measured by Gnathodynometer [Q]

In natural teeth – 20 kg (KCET 11)/ 44 pound/600 N
Maximum biting force in natural teeth - 45 kg
In CD patients - 6 – 8 kg/13 – 16 pound/110 N (KCET 10) → Maximum biting force

- Metallic Denture:

Advantage	Disadvantage
• Increased weight enhances stability of the denture	• Increased weight of a maxillary denture causes denture to fall
	• Less margin of error permissible in PPS area

- Appointment of Asthmatic patient is preffered in LATE morning/afternoon (AIIMS 06) patient type:

Phylosophical	Critical/exacting	Skeptical/hysterical	Indifferent
Best patient	Precise	Unrealistic expectation	Blaming nature
	Above intelligent	Most difficult to manage [Q]	Little concern for treatment

- Denture cleanser:

Na perborate is the main component (AIIMS May 12. direct pick from a Q bank)

- Denture adhesive:

• Synthetic salt of gontrez *(AIIMS Nov 12)*
• Good ionic adherence

- Shunting effect in CD:

If occlusal plane is lowered in posterior region → denture instability

- Die hardener:

Improves abrasion resistance of dies BUT not hardness
e.g. cynoacrylates (AIPG 10, 07 Q), acrylic resin, lacquers, polystyrenes

- Mastication vs bruxism:

Mastication	Bruxism/Parafunctional Habits
• Force generated in vertical direction	• Force generated in horizontal + vertical direction
• Intermittent and light force	• Prolonged + excessive force

- **Contraindication for relining and rebasing: [Q]**

Excessive ridge resorbtion + change in vertical dimension >> discrepancy between centric relation and centric occlusion

- Haspburg Jaw:

Class 3 → Progressive malocclusion

- Arrangement of artificial teeth depends on ridge shape and arch form *(AIPG 08)*
- Atwood classification of ridge:

Classification	Description of ridge
1	Pre – extraction
2	Post extraction
3	High well rounded *(COMEDK 11)*
4	Knife edge [Q]
5	Low well rounded
6	Depressed

- Implant: *(Very Important Topic for PGI)*

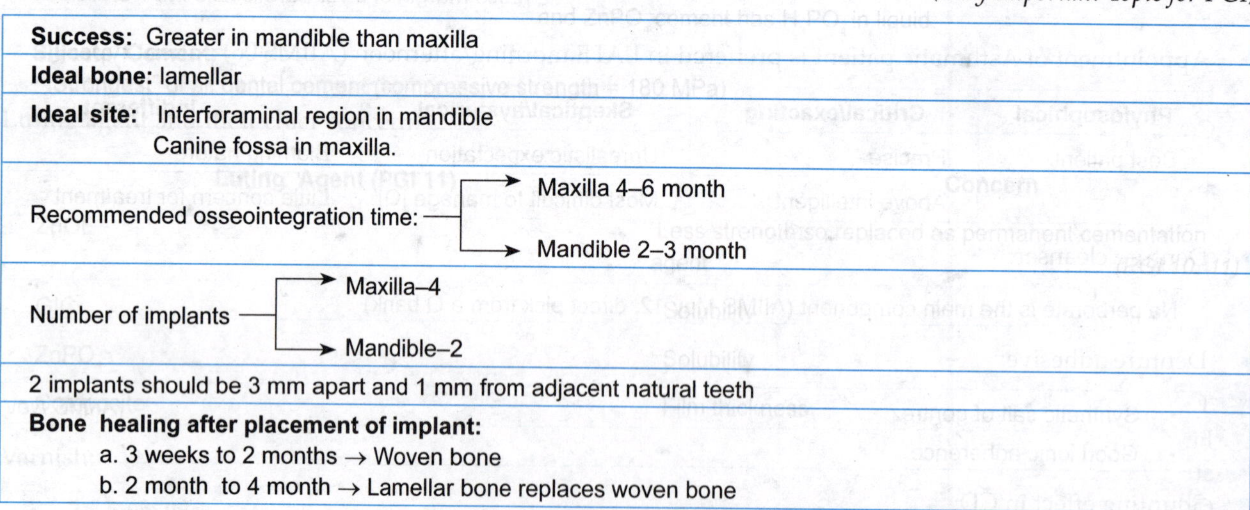

Success: Greater in mandible than maxilla

Ideal bone: lamellar

Ideal site: Interforaminal region in mandible
Canine fossa in maxilla.

Recommended osseointegration time: → Maxilla 4–6 month; → Mandible 2–3 month

Number of implants → Maxilla–4; → Mandible–2

2 implants should be 3 mm apart and 1 mm from adjacent natural teeth

Bone healing after placement of implant:
a. 3 weeks to 2 months → Woven bone
b. 2 month to 4 month → Lamellar bone replaces woven bone

- Epulis fissuratum is the tissue reaction commonly seen due to overextension of labial flanges of complete denture *(AIPG 08)*
- Rx of papillary hyperplasia:

Cryosurgery

- Rx for hyperplastic ridge:

Use of tissue conditioner for several week before making impression

- Factors affecting tooth preparation:

Factor	Higher resistance → Lower resistance
Dislodging forces	Habits → eccentric interference → anterior guidance
Taper [Q]	Minimum → 6° → Excessive
Diameter [Q]	Small (premolar) → Large (molar)
Height [Q]	Long → average → short
Type of preparation [Q] **NOTE:** U grooves are more resistant than V type	Complete coverage ↓ Partial coverage ↓ Pnlay coverage
Luting agent [Q]	Adhesive → GIC → $ZnPO_4$ ↓ PolyC ↓ ZnOE

- For abutment selection:

Shape of root + crown: Root [most important factors]

- Crown: Root

• Minimal = 1: 1
• Optimum = 2: 3 (COMED 13)
• Ideal = 1: 2

- Lateral incisor cannot be used as abutment as it has insufficient pericemental area. *(AIPG 07)*
- Concept:

"B – L width" of occlusal surface of constructed crown should be narrow to transmit forces parallel to long axis of root of abutment. so, that better tolerated by pdl.

- Taper:

• Taper of 3° - 6° is allowable (KCET 11) (3°/wall) in tooth preparation for crown
• For ceramic inlay taper > 2 - 5° (KCET 12)

- Occlusal offset → given for structural durability [Q]
- Functional cusp bevel→ provides adequate bulk to the restoration in area of heavy occlusal contact→ provides structural durability
- Good ridge support required for FPD [Q]
- If canine is missing abutments used is:

Central incisor + lateral incisor + 1st premolar [Q]

- Resistance:

Increased length/height + decreased diameter = "greater resistance" So, premolar has a greater resistance than molar

- Grove should be atleast 1 mm wide

- Cusp Reduction:

Material	Functional Cusp	Non – Functional Cusp
Cast gold	3.5 mm ↓+ 0.5 mm	1 mm ↓+ 0.5 mm
Metal ceramic + amalgam	2 mm	1.5 mm
All ceramic	2 mm	2 mm

- Angulation of functional cusp bevel:

• Full veneer crown	• 3/4th crown
• Parallel to inner Inclines of cusp of opposing teeth	• 45degree angle to long axis of tooth

- Indication of partial veneer crown:

• Tilted tooth
• Where aesthetic is desired [with normal length and shape of tooth]

- **Concept:**

If full veneer given in tilted tooth larger destruction of tooth material may take place.

- Modifications 3/4th crown: (facial surface intact)

Reverse 3/4th	Proximal/mesial half crown	7/8th crown with extension on buccal surface
Lingual surface intact	Distal surface intactsurface	Mesio buccal cusp intact
Indication – lingually Inclined tooth to prevent excess tooth reduction due to complete veneer crown	Indication – tilted abutment (mesio – distally)	Retention and Resistance is better than 3/4th as more surface is Covered

- So, in tilted tooth → go for 3 /4 th crown→ better aesthetic + conservative
- Compared to ALL ceramic, poor colour matching is main disadvantage of PFM
- Fracture of PFM→ mainly due to inadequate design fabrication of restoration (NBDE Q)
- Tooth Reduction:

PFM	ALL CERAMIC
-Labial and incisal " more" - less lingual reduction - metal thickness – 0.5 mm cervical and 0.3 mm elsewhere	" less" [1.2 to 1.4 mm]

- **Finish line:**

• **Shoulder:** – Labial surface of PFM and every where in all ceramic (AIIMS 06) – Inferior marginal adaptation compared to chamfer – Prevents fracture of restoration by providing 90° cavosurface – Margin (AIPG 11, 09)
• Shoulder with bevel: Superior marginal adaptation
BUR → Chamfer→ round end tapered/torpedo diamond BUR → Shoulder → flat end tapered, end cutting bur

- Any crown is indicated in case of gross carious destruction but contraindicated in case of uncontrolled caries
- All ceramic → incisal edge sloping towards lingual (not straight)
- This bevel (17°) necessary for stress distribution
- PFM → wing formation/vertical wall → increases retention and resistance
- Aesthetic laminates:

• Labial reduction – 0.3 to 0.7 mm
• Margin – long chamfer, subgingival
• Incisal preparation – incisal overlap
• Occlusion – canine guided
• Tooth preparation – labial to contact *(PGI 10)*
• Obtains adhesion from bonding interface from dentine adhesive, luting agent, etched enamel, and silane coupling agent *(AIIMS 08, AIPG 07)*

- Stainless steel:

• Occlusal clearance – 1 mm
• Margin – feather edge + subgingival

- For temporary restoration: among various material ZnOE is most commonly used
- Natural glaze/self glaze → more permanent than applied glaze
- For gingival retraction under chemicomechanical method:

Chemicals under astringent groups are used for cardiac patients (like hypertensive), e.g. 8% $AlCl_3$(AIIMS 06), Alum, tannic acid
Adrenaline is contraindicated But must be substituted with other agents like astringent ($AlCl_3$) [Q] [plain cord not used]
Tissue coagulant like $ZnCl_2$ should be avoided

- Types of FPD:

Fixed – fixed most commonly used
Fixed – movable/stress broken FPD → used in pier [Q]/tilted abutment ↓ (pier abutment Is lone abutment)
Cantilever: Situation → Replacement of lateral incisor with canine; → Replacement of 1st premolar with 2nd premolar and 1st molar

- RCT treated tooth with short root is contraindicated as abutment
- Resin bonded bridge:

Show micromechanical retention
Very minimal tooth preparation
Types: • Rochet bridge → 1st designed prosthesis • Maryland bridge → created by etching retainer • Virginia bridge → loss salt technique followed [don't confuse with Lost Wax technique used for fabricating cast restoration given by **Taggart**] [Q]

- Connector: Non rigid

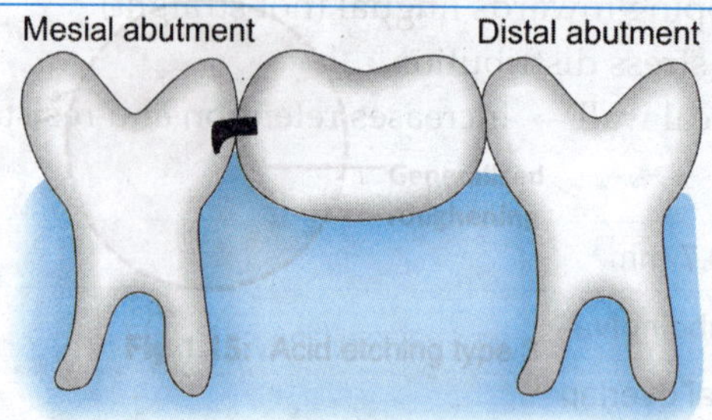

Fig 1.25: Non rigid connector

(AIIMS Nov 09)

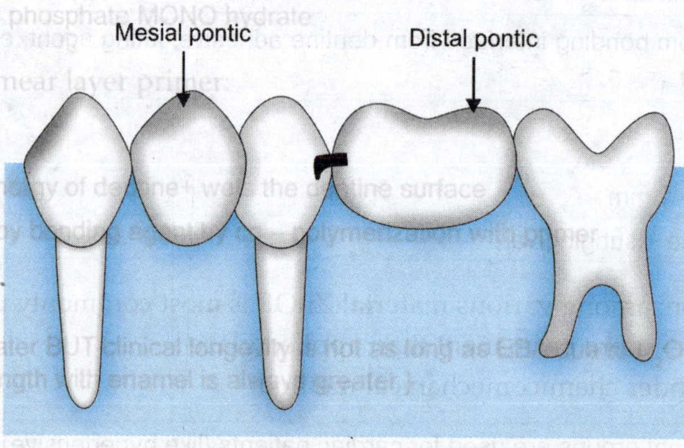

Fig 1.26: Pier abutment (AIIMS Nov O7,05, definition)

Pier abutment has a mesial and distal pontic

Conclusion: Key hole should always be prepared on mesial abutment tooth on their distal side (PGI 11)

- Pontic:

  - **Modified ridge lap used in:**
    - Anterior (AIPG 08) + premolar of both maxilla and mandible (AIIMS 06)
    - Maxillary posterior
    - So, pontic of choice in both anterior and posterior maxilla [Q]
  - **Ovate pontic:**
    - Only maxillary anteriors + premolar
    - Both modified ridge lap and ovate pontic have Good aesthetic and good hygiene
  - **Spheroidal/egg shaped/conical/heart shaped/bullet shaped pontic:**
    - Design of choice in Posterior Mandible [Q]
  - Sanitary/hygienic/ fish belly[Q] ponitic for posterior mandible
  - **Prefabricated pontic:**
    - Trueponti c and long pin pontic – for maxillary posterior
  - Saddle pontic is the Least hygienic pontic (KCET 11)
  - Faciolingual width of pontic should be smaller (2/3rd of missing tooth) while Mesio – Distal width should be same
  - Pontic in gingival area should be convex Mesio Distally and concave Bucco Lingually (for cleaning)

- Post and Core:

  - Canal should be obturated with GP not silver cone [Q]
  - Length of dowel is equal to crown length/2/3rd root length [which ever is bigger]
  - Diameter 1/3rd of diameter of root/1 mm tooth structure should suround it

• **Ferrule effect:** 1-2 mm of tooth structure should be left for this effect
• **Anti Rotational groove:** Given on thickest portion of root on Lingual side (AIIMS 06)
• Leave 4 mm of apical fill [Q]

- DIE:

• Epoxy resin (most commonly used in laboratory) and electroplated dies are dies with improved Abrasion Resistance
• **Die spacer:** 25 μ to 40 μ for luting cement

- Bucco lingual edentulous space requiring cross arch stability RPD preffered
- Too great bone resorbtion → RPD preffered as FPD requires proper ridge support
- Pulp capped tooth should not be used as Abutment
- Tooth with greatest pericemental area:
- Maxillary 1St Molar (433 mm^2) (Manipal)
- in RPD:

• Mclean functional impression which is dual impression technique is used
• ALTERED cast technique/DUAL impression procedure indicated in DISTAL extension (kennedy 1 and 2)
• Master cast made using anatomic impression (1stimpression). This anatomic master cast is altered according to functional impression /PHYSIOLOGIC impression which is made later (2nd impression)

- Principals of Design of Rpd:

• Conventional rigid design causes stress to be evenly distributed
• Stress equalization using Stress Breaker
• **Physiologic basing:** Based on functional record of soft tissue using mucocompressive technique. Thus, no difference in compressibility. So, abutment tooth is protected from extra stress
• BROAD stress distribution → Achieved by increasing the number of direct retainer, Indirect retainer, Rest, area of base

- Major Connector: (very important)

- **Mandibular**
  - Lingual bar: 1st prefferance in mandibular major connector
    - 8 mm of vertical space is required

  Modifications:
  - **Sublingual bar:** Used when height of floor of mouth does'nt allow superior margin to place 4 mm below the gingival margin. So, place inferior to lingual bar
    - Contraindicated in high frenal attachment (NEET 13) and tori
  - **Lingual plate:** Lingual bar with thin metal extension on the tooth.
    - Used when sufficient vestibular depth is Not available/High frenal attachment (NEET 13)
    - **Advantage:** Stabilizes periodontally weakened teeth and where there is need for addition of one/more anterior teeth (AIIMS 05). In case of excessive ridge resorbtion in kennedy class 1 (AIIMS 07)
    - **Cingulum bar:** Used in case of anterior crowding, diastema and when some indirect retention is required [splint the periodontally weekened teeth]
    - **Double lingual bar:** Cingulum bar attached with lingual bar
  - **Labial bar:** Used when severe lingual inclination [Q]
- **Swing lock bar:** Modification of the lingual plate which is hinged to labial bar.
- **Indication:** Missing key abutment, teeth with questionable prognosis, unfavourable teeth contour, anterior teeth with excessive labial inclination [Q]

- **Maxillary:**
  - **Antero:** Posterior strap /closed Horse Shoe: is Best design
  - Can use in almost any situation

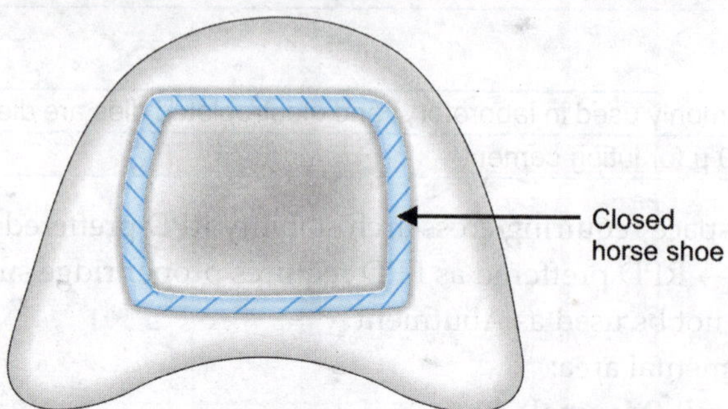

Fig 1.27: Closed horse shoe shaped major connector

  - **Horse Shoe shape/U shaped:**
    - Least rigid so, least desirable.also least desirable in case of Distsal extension RPD (KCET 11). can't use in any situation
    - Only used in case of Tori (KCET 11)

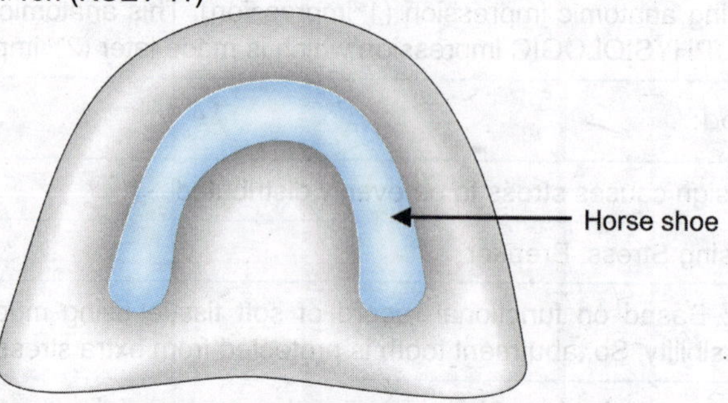

Fig 1.28: U shaped major connector

  - Single palatal strap → suitable rigidity without bulk *(KCET 11)*
  - Used in kennedy class 3
  - Single Palatal bar → most commonly used but least logical
  - Complete Palate /Palate Plate → maximum retention [Q]
  - Indicated when anterior and posterior teeth are to be replaced Bilaterally

- Repair of fractured major connector is contraindicated

- Relief under maxillary major connector is generally not required *(KCET 11)*

- Co – Cr is best suited for major connector as it has adequate strength in thin sections

- Tissue stops should be prepared on Distal extension RPD to stabilize the framework. It's an integral part of minor connector. Is of 2 mm^2 dimension

- **If major connector is flexible:** *(AIIMS O7, 05)*
  - Causes pdl breakdown
  - Residual ridge resorbtion seen because of no distribution of force

- **The purpose of " beading" in major connector:**
  - Formed by scraping the maxillary cast creating a groove not more than 0.5 mm [Q]
  - It provides intimate tissue contact of the major connector. so,prevents food entrapement

- Retention in RPD:

• **Primary retention**	• 2°/passive retention
• **Direct retainer**	• By intimate relation between minor connector and Guiding plane [Q]
	• Proximal plate [Q]

- Direct retainer *(Important topic for KCET)*
- **TYPES:**
  - Extracoronal
  - Intracoronal/internal attachment:
    - Mainly given for aesthetic reasons. abutment tooth shoud have a sound pdl + should fill all the criteria of abutment tooth + should be avoided in Distal extension cases without stress breaker (i.e can be given in distal extension cases with stress breaker)
    - Used in tooth supported prosthesis *(PGI 12)*
- **Clasp Passivity:** It should be passive until dislodging force is applied
- Circumferential clasp provides greater Stability due to "Rigid Shoulder" which is absent in bar clasp
- **Distal extension** case and choices of direct retainer:
  - As in distal extension case there are high forces on abutment. So, we have to protect it from damage. choice of direct retainer are as follows:

1. Circumferential clasp:

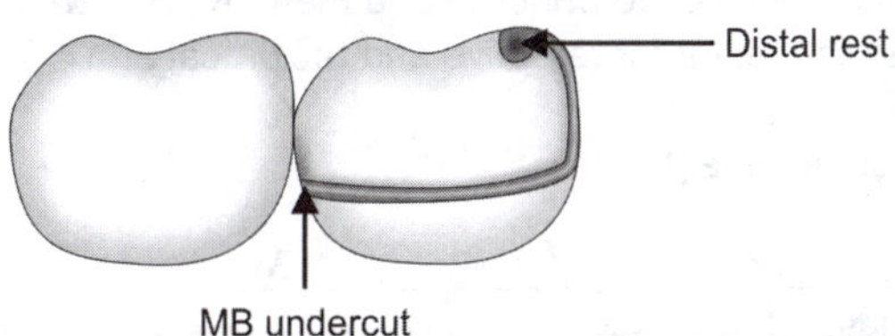

Fig 1.29: Circumferential clasp

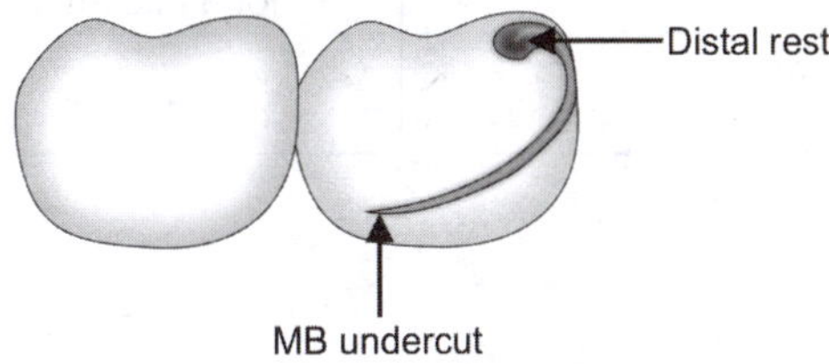

Fig 1.30: Circumferential clasp

Single circlet clasp:
- High forces on abutment as very Rigid. So, can't be used
- *Reverse circlet clasp:*
  Can be used with opposite rest, i.e. MesiaL rest involving distobuccal undercut.

2. Bar Clasp:
- Fulcrum line shifts mesially so, less force on the abutment.
- But if only mesio – buccal undercut is retentive, then use

RING clasp:

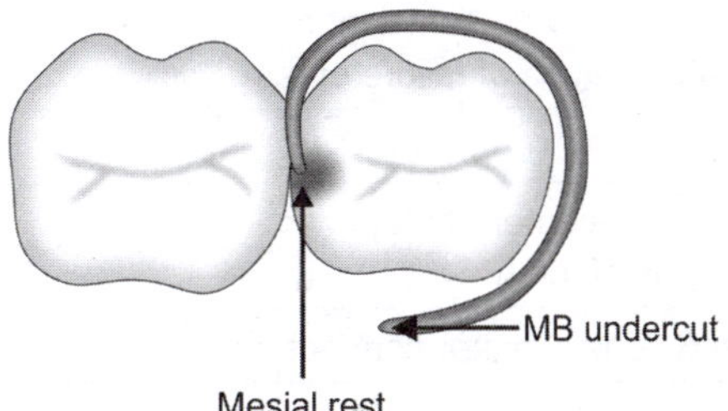

Fig 1.31: Ring clasp

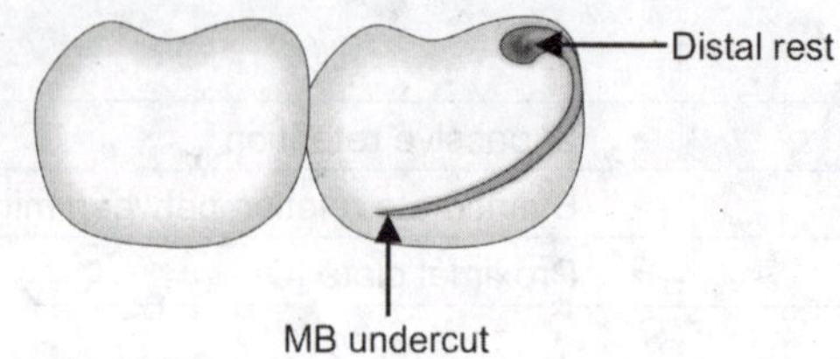

Fig 1.32: Combination clasp

Indications are:

- Tipped molar (KCET 12)
- Mandibular molar tipped mesio – lingually [Q]
- Maxillary molar tipped mesio – buccaly [Q]
- Back action clasp is a modification of ring clasp

– Hair Pin/Reverse action/Fish Hook clasp: Uses mesial rest and engages same mesio – buccal undercut

– **Combination clasp:**

Flexible retentive arm of wrought alloy. So, less force on the abutment

– **Embrassure clasp:** is always used with 2 occlusal rest

– **Multiple clasp:** indicated when denture replaces entire half of the dental arch/when EXTRA retention is needed (KCET) as in case of periodontally weakened principle abutment (KCET 08)

– HALF and HALF clasp: 2 minor connector for retentive and reciprocal arm

– Advantage is DUAL retention [Q]

– Indication is the isolated rotated abutment

- Circumferential vs bar clasp:

Aker's/Circumferential clasp (Trick: Ac)	Bar clasp/Roach
• Most logical	• Plaque accumulation and gingivitis due to increased food accumulation
• BUT decalcification of enamel and risk for caries is increased	

- Contraindication of BAR clasp:
  - Shallow vestibule
  - Large soft tissue undercut

• RPI system given by Kroll
• Minimum number of clasps required for a RPD = 2
• Round Clasp is more flexible than Half round clasp, i.e. C – clasp
• Terminal end of retentive arm is the Only flexible component of clasp
• Reciprocal arm is rigid and placed in middle 3rd of crown *(AIPG 08)*

- Rest and Rest seat:

• Marginal ridge reduced by 1.5 mm to provide sufficient bulk • Insufficient Reduction is the greatest cause of failure of rest
• Rest provides " Support"
• Floor of rest seat must incline towards center of tooth • This transmits forces along long axis of tooth
• Angle formed by occlusal rest and vertical minor connector is $< 90^0$

- Order of preference and success of rest:
- Occlusal > Lingual > Incisal

For maxillary canine (Lingual) ↓

Mandibular canine (Incisal) ↓ Unfavourable leverage forces ↓ Also some orthodontic tooth movement seen

- **Indirect Retainer:**

- Distal extension is subjected to Additional rotational forces. So, it requires additional unit (other than Direct Retainer) to resist these forces away from edentulous ridge [Not towards ridge]
- So, Indirect Retainer Is given
- [**NOTE:** in tooth supported kennedy class 3 and 4, movement of denture away from soft tissue is prevented by direct retainer]

- **Fracture of Indirect Retainer:** It is the 1st visual indicator of need for relining and rebasing

- **Forms of indirect retainer:**
  - *Positive rugae support:* It is less effective. tooth support is always better than soft tissue support
  - *Auxillary occlusal rest:* Given on mesial fossa of 1st premolar (most commonly)

Location: as far as possible from fulcrum line (AIIMS O7,05). This provides BEST leverage advantage against dislodgement.

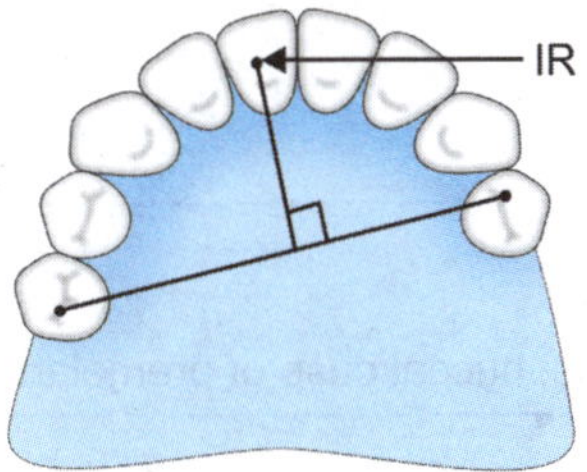

Fig 1.33: TRIPOD effect is best seen in kennedy class 2

- **E.g of indirect retainer:**
  - Proximal plate of minor connector
  - Linguo plate/cingulam bar
  - Reciprocal arm of clasp

Mechanism of action of Indirect retainer → Class 2 lever

Where as

Distal extension case is an, e.g. of class 1 lever

- **Non–anatomic teeth:**

Ideal for FLAT ridge (AIIMS 07, AIPG 07) and Parkinsonism

SOME MORE NOTABLE POINTS FROM PROSTHODONTICS

- PPS + fovea palatine + vibrating line → Movable soft palate

- Acrylic teeth vs Porcelain teeth

Acrylic Teeth	Porcelain Teeth
• Chemically bond with denture base (greatest advantage)	• Mechanically via pins/diatoric holes
• Less brittle • High resilience and toughness [Q]	• Very brittle/chipping occurs on impact [Q]
• Wear can result in decreased VDO	• Excellent abrasion resistance
• Tooth contouring/occlusal adjustment/repolishing is relatively easy	• Tooth contouring/occlusal adjustment is Difficult and may loose glaze
• Easy to grind	• Difficult to grind • Difficult to position/retain in limited interarch space

- The mesial inner inclines of lingual cusp of maxillary 1st premolar is the most common initial Supracontact at resting centric position.
- Selective grinding:

• "cusp" should be reduced only when the interference is in Both centric and eccentric position [Q]
• Prematurity in centric position only – requires reduction of opposing Fossa and Ridge [Q]

- **Curve of occlusion:**

• **Curve of Wilson:** – Medio- lateral curve – Formed due to lingual inclination of mandibular posteriors – Concave in mandible – Convex in maxilla – Is a transverse curve
• **Curve of spee:** – AP curve – Runs through cuspal tip of canine, buccal cusp of premolars and molars and passes through head of condyle
• **Curve of monsoon [Q]:** – Lateral curve – Each cusp and incisal edge forms a cicle of 8 inch diameter with center at glabella – Has concavity facing upwards
• **Curve of antimonsoon:** – Lateral curve – Teeth anterior to 2nd premolars involved – Convexity facing upwards
• **Pleasure curve:** – Monsoon + Antimonsoon curve in posterior region

- **Incisal guidance:**

Denture will be more stable as the angle approaches closer to "zero"

- For selective grinding and for clearly detecting discrepancy in occlusion
- Remount on articulator with new inter-occlusal record
- **NOTE**: It's an NBDE Q which has been asked in NEET 13. So, be thorough with all NBDE questions to crack NEET/AIIMS

- Interim immediate denture/JIFFY denture:

• Single visit extraction

- **In Overdenture:**

• Anterior abutments are preffered over posterior abutments because anterior region is more prone to resorbtion

- Concept: Implant placement

• Implant placement without surgical template, which is based on the ideal diagnostic wax-up, leads to loss of control of exact implant positioning during the surgical intervention and will lead to increased aesthetic failure. Thus, surgical template is the most important tool for accurate placement of implant (also angulation)

- Tooth most likely causing lateral balancing interferences: premolars (NBDE Q)
- CD patients have a preference for which tooth while chewing hard food – premolars
- Denture stomatitis/denture papillary hyperplasia:

• Usually associatedwith wearing denture at night
• More common in Diabetics and Women

- **Proximal groove :**

For anterior tooth	Posterior tooth
Parallel to incisal 2/3rd	• Parallel to long axis of tooth
	• MOLAR 3/4TH crown placed in buccal half with bucco lingual divergence

- **Ferrule:** Main advantage is to prevent vertical root fracture
- **New Concept:**

• The use of Single Tooth Implants in restoring missing tooth is an attractive option Both for patient and Dentist
• Today is even preffered over 3 unit bridge

- **In Co – Cr – Ni alloy/elgiloy:**

Minimum of 12 % Cr is required for passivation [don't confuse with 18/8 stainless steel]

- The average distance between upper and lower sulcus in anterior region is 36 – 39 mm (38 mm) (AIPG Q, AIIMS 05)
- Anterior lingual border forms 2° peripheral seal in mandible (NBDE Q)
- The posterior determinant of occlusion has the greatest effect on the restoration of which tooth? (NBDE Q)

Ans. Mandibular 2nd molar

- **Indication for Non-Rigid Fpd:**

• Short span FPD replacing 1 tooth
• Retainers cannot be prepared to be drawn together without excessive tooth reduction
• Tilted FPD abutment
• Pier abutment

- Occlusion:

• GROUP function/unilateral balanced occlusion: – Non balancing side contacts – Working side contacts from canine to 3rd molar – Distribution of occlusal load – E.g ceramic veneer and aesthetic laminates – Seen in middle age group (30 – 40 years)
• Canine protected occlusion/canine guided occlusion: – Also called as mutually protected/organic occlusion – Cuspid rise in protrusion – Working side contact occurs mostly in canine – Disocclusion of posterior teeth on working side – Used in porcelain veneer – Usually seen in young adults
Conclusion: Keneddy class 1 → Bilateral balanced occlusion Keneddy class 2 → Unilateral balanced occlusion and Balanced occlusion
In FPD in posterior pontic avoid Balancing side contact (AIIMS 06)

- The usual 1st STEP in occlusal adjustment is to eliminate prematurities in centric relation (NBDE Q)
- NESBIT appliance:

It is single tooth replacement/unilateral partial denture

- While recording protrusive interocclusal record:

• Lateral condylar guidance is set at 0^0
• Horizontal condylar guidance is set at 25^0
• Lower member of articulator moved forward approximately 6 mm/during protrusion of condyle minimum anterior displacement of condyle is 6 mm (PGI 12)
• **Concept:** Relief generally Not required under maxillary major connector But is necessary below mandibular major connector.

- Height of contour:

• Term height of contour was given by " Kennedy"
• 1ST device to measure height of contour was used by Fortunati

• Minimum width of palatal strap – 8 mm
• Width < 8 mm → then it is a palatal bar
• Width of lingual bar → 4 mm

- Abutment tilted > 20° ◎ Extract/Modify
- Implant:

• Minimum bone required for predictable implant success = 10 mm
• Minimum bone width = 5 mm
• Maximum bone: implant angulation for wide crest 30° • For narrow crest 20° • [Maximum tilt of abutment allowed is 24°]
• Available bone height is most important for implant success

• Survival rate of implant – 5 to 10 years
• Width of keratinized gingiva around implant is 1.5 mm *(PGI 12)*

- **Applegate's Rule for classification of edentulous span:** *(Very Important for KCET and COMEDK)*

• **Rule 1:** Classification should follow rather precede extraction
• **Rule 2:** If 3rd molar is missing and not to be replaced then it should not be considered in classification.
• **Rule 3:** If 3rd molar present and to be used as abutment then it should be considered in classification.
• **Rule 4:** If 2nd molar missing and not to be replaced then should not be considered in classification.
• **Rule 5:** The most posterior edentulous area always determines classification.
• **Rule 6:** Edentulous areas other than those which determine classification are considered as " Modification" space.
• **Rule 7:** Extent of modification is not considered. It is the number of additional edentulous areas which are taken into account. *(AIIMS Nov 07)*
• **Rule 8:** There can be no modification area in class 4 [Q]

LAST 5-YEAR QUESTIONS FROM THIS TOPIC

1. **While setting condylar guidance on a 3 pin articulator, the incisal pin is:** *(AIPG 12)*

Ans. Out of contact with the guide table (NBDE Q)

2. **The chamfer finish line is used in:** *(AIIMS May 10, May 08, AIPG 07)*

Ans. Lingual surface of PFM (Ref: Shillinburg 3/e p132)

3. **The replacement of missing part/artificial substitute is called as:** *(AIIMS May 10, May 08, May 07, AIPG 07)*

Ans. Prosthesis (Ref: Nallaswamy 1/e p810)

4. **A porcelain laminate veneer during adhesion gets bonding interface from:** *(AIIMS May 10)*

Ans. Composite resin matrix, luting agent, etched enamel and silane coupling agent

5. **A patient with complete denture complains of pain while swallowing. There is overextension of the denture in the distolingual aspect. The muscle involved is:** *(AIIMS Nov O9)*

Ans. Superior constrictor (Ref: Winkler, prosthodontics 1988 p76)

6. **A complete denture patient with poor neuromuscular control wants correction of denture. it may be achieved by which of the following?** *(AIIMS Nov O9)*

Ans. Interocclusal records are made and corrected on articulator (winkler. essentials of complete denture prosthodontics 2/e p328)

7. **After complete denture fabrication, if teeth are in end to end relation in patient, it can be corrected by:** *(AIIMS Nov O9)*

Ans. Grinding of the inclines so that the upper teeth move buccally and lower tooth move lingually.

8. **A patient has come for relining and rebasing. You do relining if:** *(AIIMS Nov O9)*

Ans. If the patient is poor and cannot afford new denture (Ref: Nallaswamy 1/e p2003, p239 -48)

9. **In an edentulous patient, the average distance between the upper and lower sulcus in the anterior region is:** *(AIPG 08)*

Ans. 38 mm

10. **To transfer the axis orbital plane we require:** *(AIPG 08)*

Ans. Either arbitrary/kinematic face bow (Ref: Bouchers 8/e p243)

11. **Retentive arm in a clasp always points towards:** *(AIIMS Nov 11)*

Ans. Occlusal (Ref: Stewart. Textbook of RPD 2/e p67 – 68)

12. **For strength and rigidity, the vertical height of a finished lingual bar should be atleast:** *(KCET 11)*

Ans. 4 mm

13. A reliable guide for positioning maxillary anterior teeth in CD patient is: *(KCET 11, NEET 13)*

Ans. Incisive papilla

14. Articulated diagnostic casts help in the following EXCEPT:

a. Diagnostic wax up to evaluate outcome
b. Detailed analysis of occlusal plane and occlusion
c. Fabrication of wax patterns for casting
d. Performing mock tooth preparation

Ans. c.

15. Height of contour term was coined by: *(KCET 11, COMEDK 11)*

Ans. Kennedy

16. The functional occlusal force applied to the periodontal tissues during one deglutition is for a duration of:

Ans. 1 sec

17. The 1st person to employ mechanical device to determine the relative parallelism of tooth surface was: *(KCET 11)*

Ans. Fortunati

18. Occlusal offset in an anterior partial veneer crown may generally be necessary to provide: *(KCET 11)*

Ans. Structural durability

19. Mode of failure during dislodgement of prosthesis cemented with zinc polycarboxylate cement is usually seen at the: *(COMEDK 11)*

Ans. Cement prosthesis interface (Ref: Phillips 11/e p112)

20. Hanau H_2 articulator has an intercondylar distance of: *(KCET 11)*

Ans. 110 mm (Ref: Wrinkle 2/e p23)

21. The technique to produce limited removal of epithelial tissue in the sulcus while a chamfer finish line is being created in tooth structure is called: *(COMEDK 11)*

Ans. Gingettage (Ref: Shillingburg 3/e p268)

22. The ultimate finish line which produces an acute margin of metal is: *(COMEDK 11)*

Ans. Knife edge (Ref: Shillingburg 3/e p132)

23. Schubiger attachment has a screw base common to the: *(COMEDK 11)*

Ans. Gerber attachment (Ref: Wrinkler 2/e p23)

24. While arranging artificial teeth, the labial surfaces of the maxillary central incisors are usually ________ in front of the posterior border of the incisive papilla: *(NEET 13, KCET 10)*

Ans. 8–10 mm

25. Torus mandibularis is common on which area: *(KCET 10)*

Ans. Lingual, premolar area

26. Functional cusp bevel has to be placed in following cusps EXCEPT: *(KCET 10)*

a. Mesiopalatal cusp
b. Distopalatal cusp
c. Distolingual cusp of mandibular molar
d. Distobuccal cusp of mandibular molar

Ans. c.

27. Wing preparation for metal ceramic restoration helps in: *(KCET 10)*

Ans. Retention and resistance.

28. During recording centric relation, compound occlusion rims with styli in maxillary arch are used in: *(KCET 10)*

Ans. Needles house technique

29. Mechanism of action of indirect retainers resembles: *(KCET 10)*

Ans. 2nd class lever.

NOTE: Distal extension RPD is an example of 1st order lever.

30. Which of the following case is contraindication for FPD? *(PGI Dec 11)*

Ans. Patients with high caries index

31. Which of the following is the most biocompatible material for dental prosthesis? *(PDI June 11)*

Ans. Commercially pure titanium (Ref: Peterson 2/e p189)

32. Margins for all ceramic are? *(PGI June 11)*

Ans. Shoulder on both buccal and lingual (Ref: Rosenstiel 3/e p175)

33. Which of the following position of mandible is in non-interfering occlusion? *(PGI June 11)*

Ans. Centric occlusion (Ref: Boucher's 12/e p277)

34. In tooth preparation procedure, the foremost principle is: *(PGI Dec 10)*

Ans. Conservation of what is remaining (Ref: Nallaswamy 1/e p567)

35. During jaw relations protrusive records are used for: *(PGI Dec 10)*

Ans. Condylar measurement of both side (Ref: Winkler 2/e p195)

36. Golden proportion rule applies: *(PGI Dec 09)*

Ans. 62 % (Ref: Sturdevant's 5/e p628)

37. The success of removable die system is based upon: *(PGI Dec 09)*

Ans. Precies relocation of the die in the working cast (Ref: Shillinburg 3/e p314)

38. Inter papillary distance is equivalent to: *(PGI June 09)*

Ans. Distance between the corners of mouth (Ref: Nallaswamy 1/e p234)

SOME MORE IMPORTANT POINTS FROM DM + OD + PROSTHODONTICS

- Addition polysilicones → type 2 silicone impression
- Silicone impression materials → have Low W.T and S.T
- In $ZnPO_4$ cement → 'Al' present in liquid which is essential for cement forming reaction
- Activator in composite:

• Diketone in VL cure composite
• Benzoin methyl ether in UV cure composite

- Glycol ether/phthalate:

Plasticizer in polyether

- Glycol dimethacrylate → cross linking agent in denture resin → provide craze resistance [Q]
- Bevel:

• LONG bevel → most commonly used
• Reverse/counter bevel → given in Onlay/DFG

- Microporosities and localized shrinkage porosities are Not seen in dentine base resin
- Tooth Reduction:

• In all ceramic → labial and incisal reduction → 1.2 – 1.4 mm
• In PFM → labial and incisal reduction → 1.5 – 2 mm

- Functional cusp bevel = 2 mm
- Wing formation in PFM → for retention and resistance (Not aesthetic)

- Resin Bonded bridge: main advantage is that it is Conservative [Q]

• Rochette → is 1st design [conical perforations seen]
• Maryland → tissue surface of retainer is etched
• Virginia → based on "Lost Salt technique" [Q]

- Pontic:

• Sanitary/hygienic/fishbelly pontic → posterior mandible [Q]
• Ovate/spheroidal/heart shaped → posterior mandible [Q]
• Prefabricated pontic (true/long pontic) → posterior maxilla

- Major connector:

Labial BAR → Used when Excessive lingual inclination [Q]
Swing lock bar: Modification of linguoplate hinged to labial bar. It is used in: 1. Excessive labial inclination 2. Missing key abutment 3. Teeth with questionable prognosis/unfavourable contour

- Tissue stops and beading:

Tissue stops	Beading
Part of minor connector [Q]	
Given in distal extension Cases	For positive intimate contact
2 mm² in dimension [Q]	0.5 mm [Q] of wax is removed

• Palatal strap width → 8 mm
• Lingual bar → 4 mm
• Tripoding is used in → class 3 keneddy *[PGI Q]*

- Indirect retainer based on → class 2 lever [Q]
- Implant: *(Very important for PGI)*

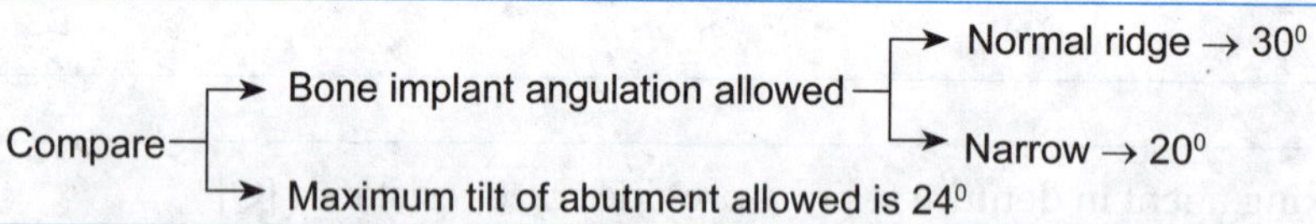

• Minimum width of keratinized gingival around an implant → 1.5 mm [Q]
• Minimum width of bone around implant periphery > 0.5 mm [Q]

- Hardness test:

• Only microhardness test is suitable for brittle material, i.e. Knoop and Vicker's method.
• Brinnel used to measure proportional limit and ultimate tensile strength of dental gold alloys.

- Mercury /(Hg):

Low blood level – 35 ng/ml → symptoms starts At which non – specific Low urine level – 30 µg/ml → symptoms starts

- Compressive strength of dentine (268) < amalgam (310) < enamel (384)

- Denture:

Deflective contact occurring on working side → Apply BULL's law[Q] ↓ Grind upper buccal (BU) and lower lingual (LL)

- During lateral excursion:

Balancing side contact occurs on BUL * LLB Buccal cusp of upper lingual — lingual cusp of lower buccal
Working side contact occurs on → LUB * BLL

- Interferences in centric relation:

Antero posteriorly (A-P ly)

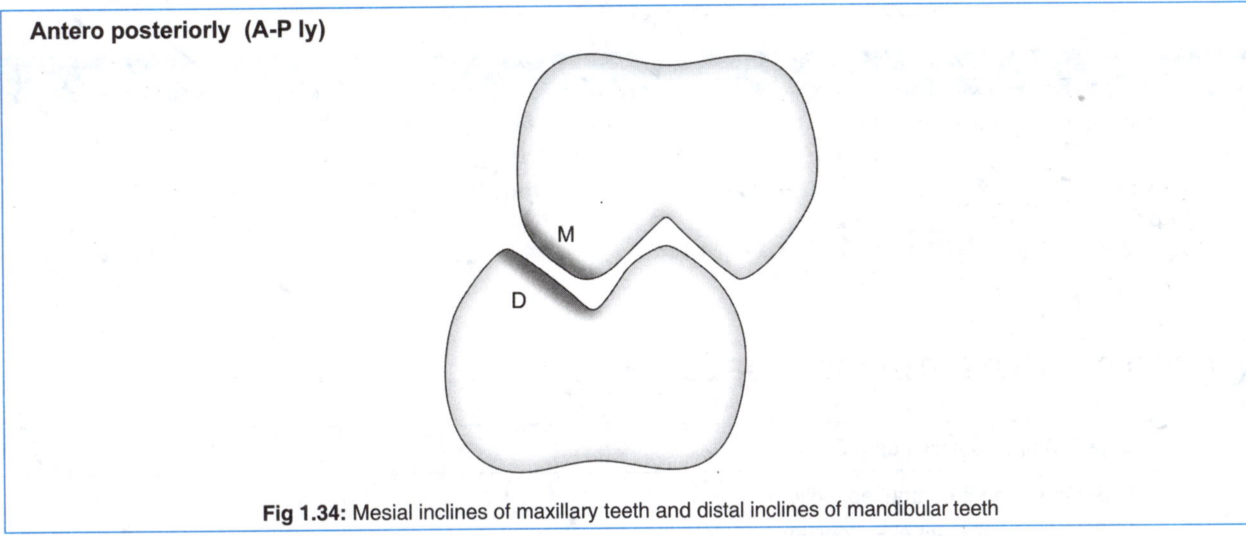

Fig 1.34: Mesial inclines of maxillary teeth and distal inclines of mandibular teeth

- Loosening of denture while smiling → inadequate relief of buccal frenum [Q]
- Gauze of wax:

Relief wax → 20 gauze
Gauze of sprue used for casting → 8 – 12

- Disadvantage of autoclave → causes fibro optic dimming
- 24 karat = 1000 fineness
- Fluoride flux → KF + boric acid (1: 1) [Q]
- Bennet movement → 1 – 1.5 mm/side
- Bennet angle → 15° [30° in edentulous patient]
- Lingual flange in mandibular denture is characteristic 'S' shaped due to action of mylohyoid muscle [Q]
- Tissue Conditioner → tends to harden in 4-8 weeks
- Fluidity measurement of gypsum product:

β – hemihydrate	α – hemihydrate
Slump test	core penetration test

- Stages in addition polymerization: (KCET Very Important)

Termination → by direct coupling/exchange of hydrogens
Chain Transfer → active stage is transferred from active radical to inactive molecule

- Indisperse → 10 % indium admix → decreases Hg vapour

CHAPTER

2 Dental Histology

Topic

- Development and Growth of Teeth
- Enamel
- Dentine
- Pulp
- Cementum
- Bone
- Oral Mucosa

DEVELOPMENT AND GROWTH OF TEETH

• Dental lamina is active upto 5 year
• CAP stage: Inner enamel epithelium (IEE) and Outer enamel epithelium (OEE) just formed. OEE Cubiodal IEE Collumnar Enamel knot and chord like temporary structures appear in this stage Enamel knot: May stimulate cusp growth by directly folding enamel organ. *(AIPG 12)*
• Bell stage: Stage of "Histo differentiation". Organising influence of IEE n dental lamina/Visce versa IEE, OEE, stratum intermedium, stellate reticulum; all 4 layers are seen Note: Stratum reticulum: Is albumin rich So, swollen up. Stratum intermedium: Absolutely required for enamel development Rich in alkaline phosphatase and mitochondria
Advanced bell Stage: Hers develops [Q] Dental hard tissues formed [Q] Future DEJ formed [Q] **Note:** Zone of reflection = cervical loop forms hers

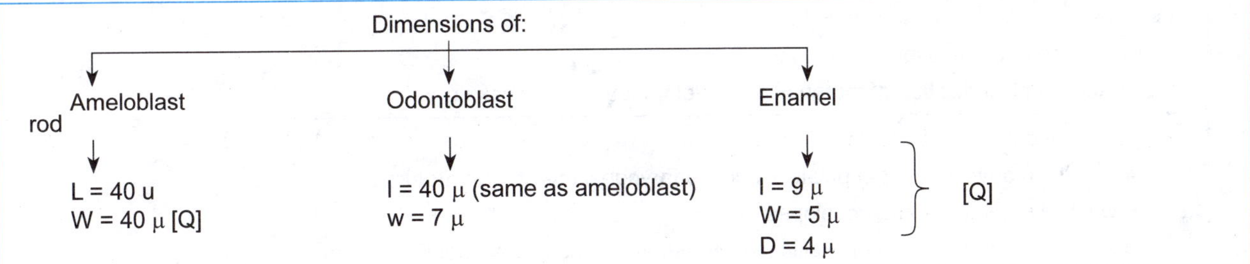

- Lip furrow band:
  Vestibular lamina forms vestibules

Membrana Pre-formitiva: Separates enamel organ from dental papilla. Seen in bell stage.

Morphologic stage of tooth development:
Is determined by epithelial part of tooth germ, i.e. Enamel organ.

Stages of tooth development Vs result of disturbance

Stage	Defect Arising
• Initiation	Defect in Number • Anodontia • Super numerary teeth • Fused/Geminated teeth
• Histo differentiation	Reaches highest in bell stage Dentinogenesis Imperfecta Atypical dentine/Osteodentine ↓ Due to vit. A Deficiency
• Morphodifferentiation	Mainly seen in advanced bell stage • Shape of teeth altered • Talon cusp • Hutchinson's incisor • Dens in dente • Macrodontia
• Apposition	[Q] Characterized by deposition of matrix and calcification Enamel hypoplasia Hypo calcification Concrescence Intrinsic staining Interglobular/soft dentine/Malacotic teeth *(AIIMS 06)*

- Calcification of enamel:
  Proceeds from cusp/incisal edges towards cervical line
  Also from DEJ towards surface
  Note: both amelogenesis and dentineogenesis starts at cuspal tip.

- Hypoplasia of systemic origin = Hypoplasia of chronologic origin

- Amelogenin and Enamelin protein: 2 major Ca^{2+} bindingprotein
  Amelogenin is low molecular weight, is secreted by ameloblast. It is predominant protein of enamel matrix.
  Note: enamel proteins do not contribute to structuring of enamel as does collagen in dentine and bone.

- Ameloblast with villous surface: associated with resorption of organic matrix

Ist evidence of 1° dentition → 2 mo i.u. 1 st evidence of 2° dentition → 4 mo i.u. 1 st macroscopic indication of morphologic development → 11 week i.u
• i.u. life and important events 4 weeks i.u development of palate + buccopharyngeal membrane ruptures 6 weeks i.u dental lamina developes 8 week i.u pulp + 1st sign of ossification + alveolar process developes 10 weeks i.u TMJ developes (1st component)
• Fusion of mandibular symphysis = 18 month postnatal

LAST 5-YEAR QUESTIONS FROM THIS TOPIC

1. **Resorption of deciduous maxillary central incisor starts at:** *(AIIMS Nov 10)*

Ans. 4 years

2. **During cap stage signalling in odontogenic epithelium is done by:** *(AIPG 12)*

Ans. Enamel knot (Ref: Orban's 12/e p26)

3. **Enzymes which play an important role in calcification are:**

Ans. Alkaline phosphatase and pyrophosphatase. *(COMEDK 10)*

4. **The cell of enamel organ that are characterized by an exceptionally high activity of enzyme alkaline phosphatase:** *(KCET 12)*

Ans. Stratum Intermedium

ENAMEL

• Specific gravity of enamel = 2.8
• Order of mineralisation Enamel > Dentine > Bone > Cementum ↓ ↓ ↓ ↓ 96% 70% 65% 45%
• No. of rods → lower incisors → 5 million → Upper 1st molar → 12 Million
• Prisms/rods: are longer and wider at cusp.
• Body of rod towards occlusal/cusp while tail is towards CERVICAL region
• Width of enamel: 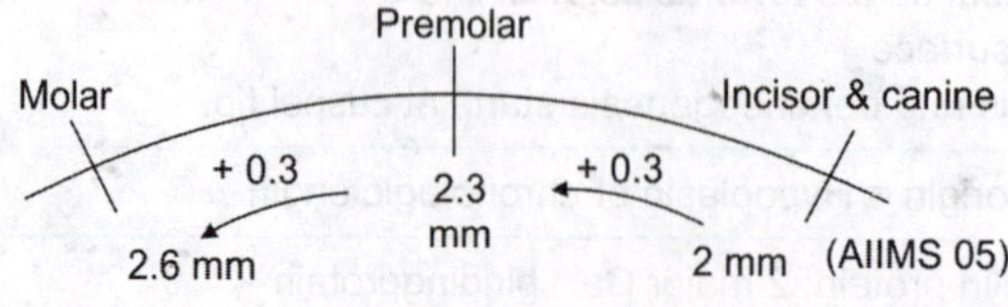 **Fig. 2.1:** Width of enamel

Life cycle of ameloblasts :

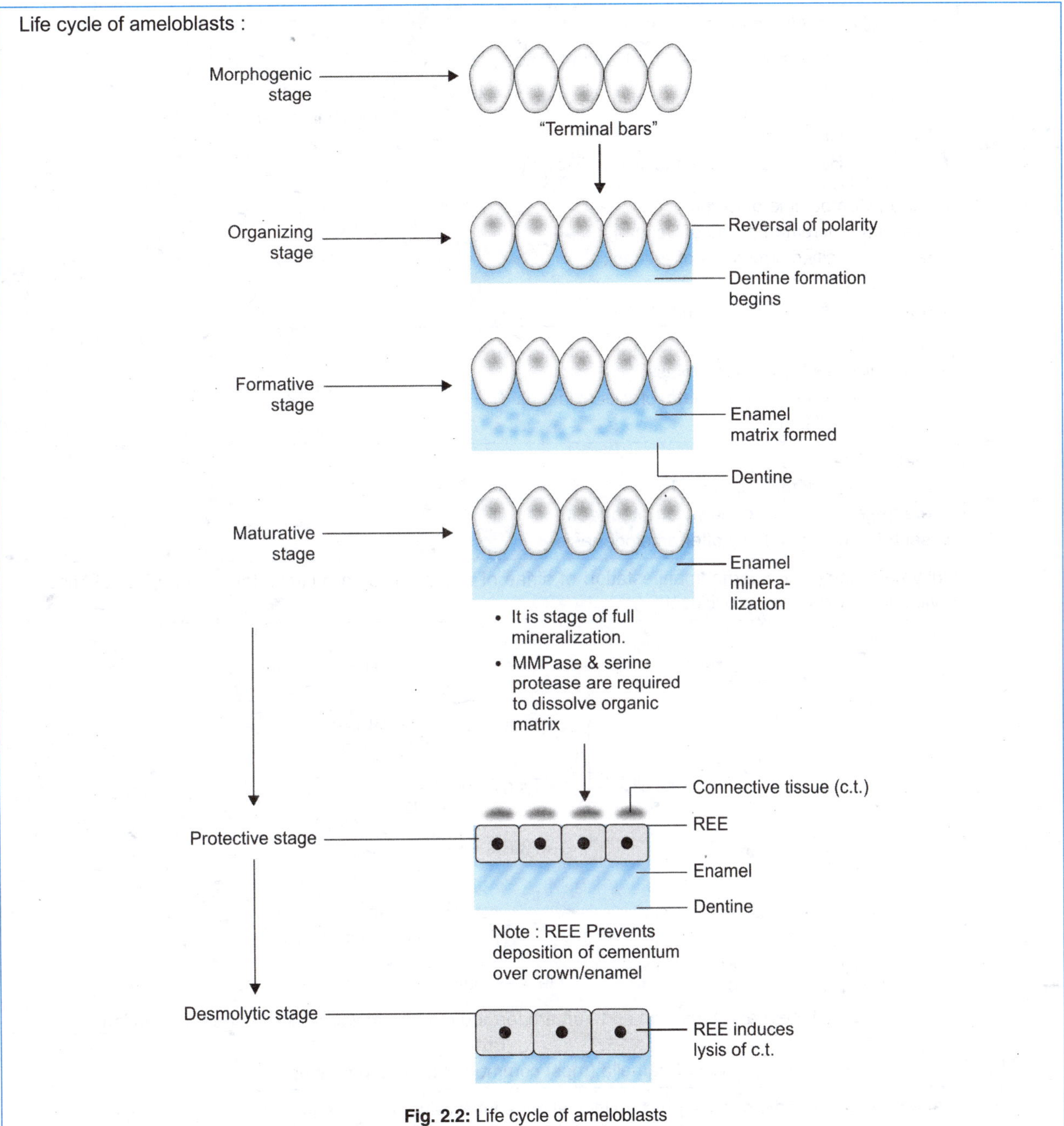

Fig. 2.2: Life cycle of ameloblasts

- Each ameloblast contributes to 4 different rods
- Rate of formation of enamel → 4 micron/day
  Diurnal rhythm corresponds to cross striation *(KCET 10)*
- Neonatal lines are "enlarged" stria of Retzius.
- Hunter schruger band: Optical phenomenon. Viewed in reflected light in longitudinal ground section. It is produced due to change in direction of rods

- Incremental lines: All are hypocalcified

  Enamel { Stria of Retzius—Major (Neonatal line); Cross striation — Minor; Horizontal incremental line of Pickerill } — Demonstrated in ground section

  Dentine { Contour line of Owen
  Cementum { Incremental line of Salter
- Other hypocalcified structures of enamel:
  Trick = "I L–T"
  Incremental lines, Lamella , enamel Tufts

- Enamel surface:
  It is structure less/Rodless/Prismless.
  Hyper mineralised e.g. Perikymata, cracks, rodends.
  Has thickness of 30 μ *(AIPG 07)*

- Enamel Cuticle:
  Called as Nasmyth membrane [Q]
  Covers the entire crown of newly erupted teeth.
  It is secreted by Ameloblast after amelogenesis

- Perikymata: they are external manifestation of striae of retzius. They are circumferential horizontal lines more in cervical region and less in occlusal

Tufts and Lamella

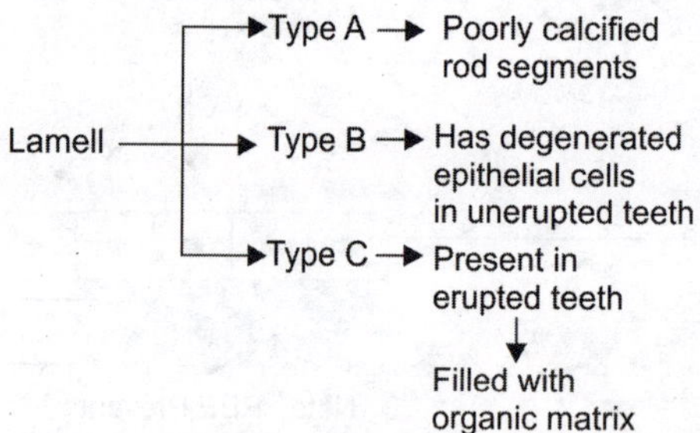

Fig. 2.3: Lamella

Note: Type A and B lamella and Tuft are formed during amelogenesis i.e. before eruption
But
Type C lamella (most commonly) formed post eruption.

- Gnarled enamel: Bundle of rods, on cusp/incisal edge inter twine more irregularly

- Enamel pearl = Enameloma:
  Excess mass of enamel derived from misplaced ameloblast. Seen commonly in Maxillary 2nd molar

- Enamel developmental defect:
  Permanent anterior most commonly affected.
  Mostly occurs in middle 1/3 rd of upper Incisors
  → Regional odontodysplasia–shows poorly calcified/ moth eaten enamel Maxilla 2.5 times more affected than mandible
  → Fluorosis: Permanent anterior teeth commonly affected
  → Odontoma :

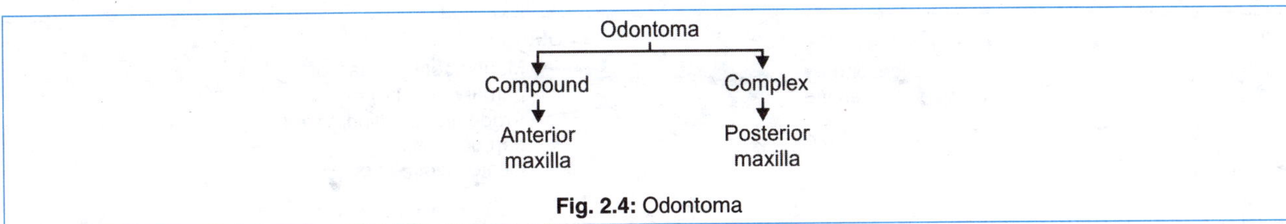

Fig. 2.4: Odontoma

LAST 5-YEAR QUESTIONS FROM THIS TOPIC

1. **The Primary tooth is whiter than the permanent tooth because:**

Ans. The difference in crystalline structure of enamel makes the refractive index different (Ref: Wheeler 12/e p50) *(AIIMS Nov 10)*

2. **Non-acidic non amelogenin enamel protein responsible for Hydroxyapetite formation is:** *(AIPG 12)*

Ans. Sheathlin (Ref: Tencates 5/e p197-200)

DENTINE

- 1st formed dental tissue. It determines shape of crown and no. And size of root.
- Classification of dentine

Classification of dentine

1°

2°/ adventitious dentine

3°

Mantle

Circumpulpal (dentine formed prior to root completion)

Intratubular/ peritubular

High mineralized

9% more mineralized than intertubular dentine

Intertubular

"Abundant"

Forms main bulk of dentine

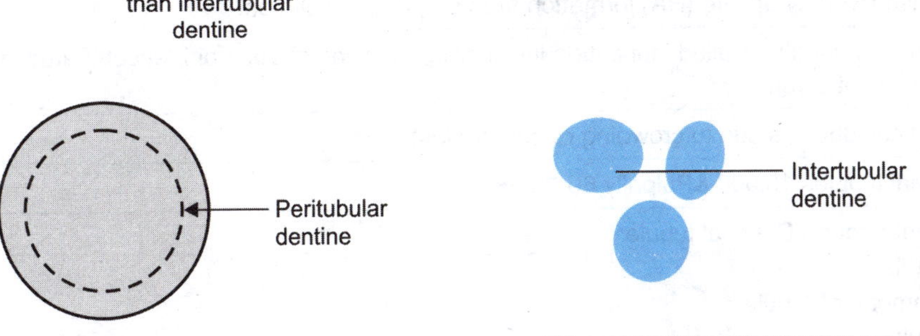

Fig. 2.5: Classification of dentine

2° dentine → Has fewer dentinal tubules than 1° dentine

Reparative → has fewer and more twisted dentinal tubules than normal dentine

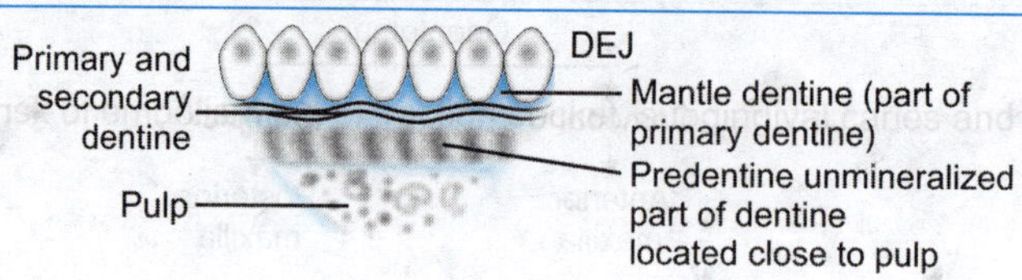

Fig. 2.6: Dentine

- **Sclerotic/transparent** dentine:
  Due to refractive index
  Most commonly seen in apical 1/3 rd of root and midway between DEJ and Pulp surface.
- Interglobular dentine:
  Hypocalcified area formed due to defective fusion of Calcospherite
  Seen in Vit. D deficiency and X-linked Hypophosphatasia
- Dead Tract: Term given by sir Wilfred fish
  Balck in Transmitted light and white in Reflected light
  Note: Opposite is seen in sclerosis
- Osteodentine/Atypical dentine:
  Has cell inclusions"
  Seen in vit A deficiency.
- Tomes granular layer/Tomes layer: granular layer on root at CDJ due to coalescing of dentinal tubules
  Note:
  Tome's process is projection of ameloblasts in enamel matrix
  Tome's Fibers is odontoblastic process
  Tomes granular layer dentinal tubules at CDJ.
- Hardness of dentine 1/4 th of enamel
- Dentine formed faster than Enamel
- Non-collagenous protein of Dentine: "Dentine Phosphoprotein" (PHOSPHORYN)
  ↓
  PP–H
  → Is phenotypic Marker of dentine
  → Absent in Pre-dentine and Mantle dentine [Q]
  → Present in Circumpulpal dentine [Q]
  "Unique"
  → This seems to be transported directly to the dentine mineralization front. Binds Ca^{2+} with strong affinity and might induce Hydroxy apatite (HA) formation from $Ca_3(PO_4)_2$ solution.
- Incremental lines of dentine: Called inbrication line/incremental line of von ebnir accentuated incremental line is called Contour line of owen
- S-shaped dentinal tubule is due to crowding of odontoblast.
- Coronal dentinal tubules 15,000 &Pulpally 60,000
- Fluid movement through Dentinal tubule:
  $F \alpha D^4/L$
  Where D = diameter of tubule
  L = length of tubule
- Odontoblastic process: Consists of few organelles and cytoskeleton network of microtubules and microfilaments
- DEJ is straight in cervical region
  S-tubules are straight in root

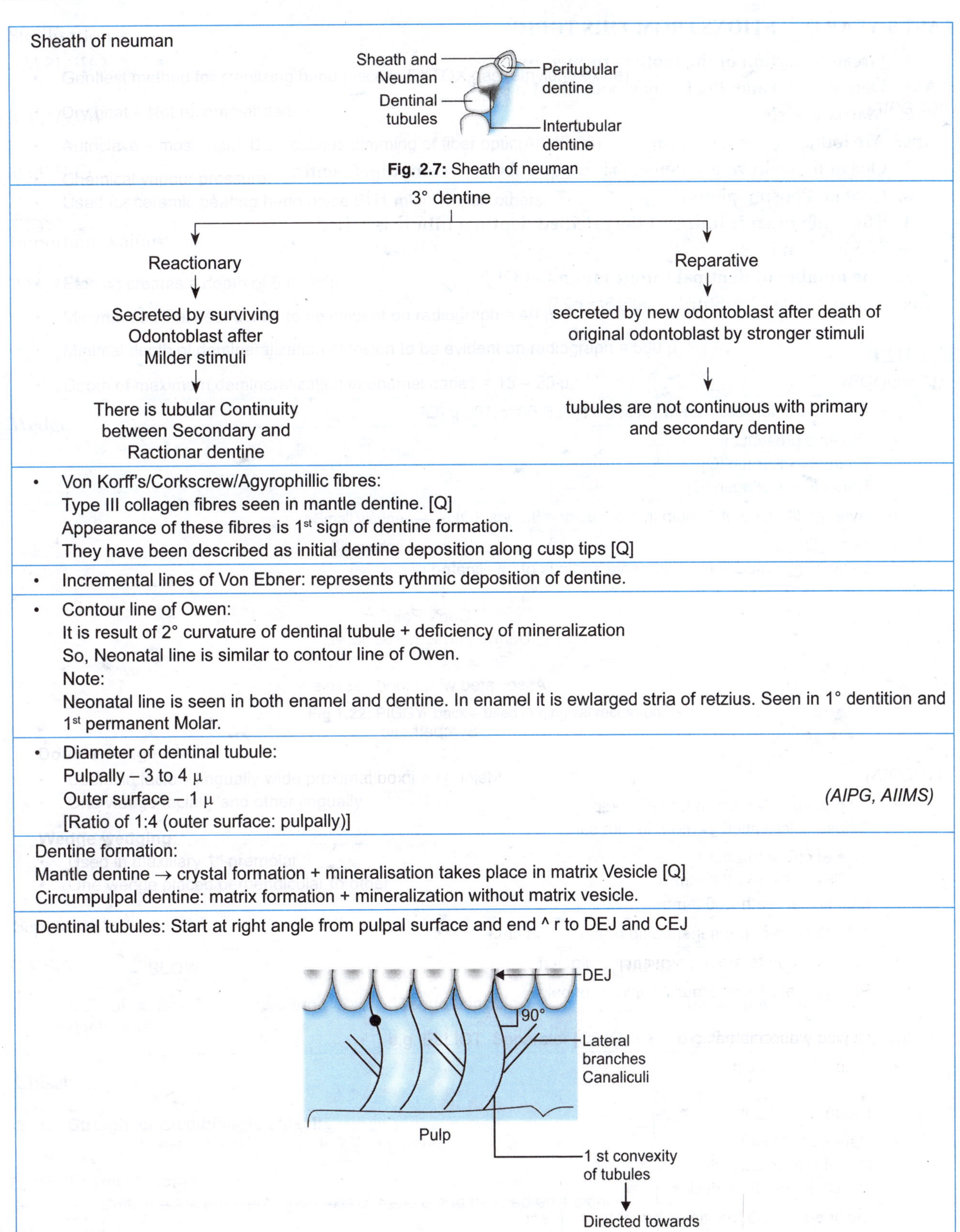

Sheath of neuman

Sheath and Neuman
Peritubular dentine
Dentinal tubules
Intertubular dentine

Fig. 2.7: Sheath of neuman

3° dentine

- Reactionary → Secreted by surviving Odontoblast after Milder stimuli → There is tubular Continuity between Secondary and Ractionar dentine
- Reparative → secreted by new odontoblast after death of original odontoblast by stronger stimuli → tubules are not continuous with primary and secondary dentine

- Von Korff's/Corkscrew/Agyrophillic fibres:
  Type III collagen fibres seen in mantle dentine. [Q]
  Appearance of these fibres is 1st sign of dentine formation.
  They have been described as initial dentine deposition along cusp tips [Q]

- Incremental lines of Von Ebner: represents rythmic deposition of dentine.

- Contour line of Owen:
  It is result of 2° curvature of dentinal tubule + deficiency of mineralization
  So, Neonatal line is similar to contour line of Owen.
  Note:
  Neonatal line is seen in both enamel and dentine. In enamel it is ewlarged stria of retzius. Seen in 1° dentition and 1st permanent Molar.

- Diameter of dentinal tubule:
  Pulpally – 3 to 4 μ
  Outer surface – 1 μ
  [Ratio of 1:4 (outer surface: pulpally)] *(AIPG, AIIMS)*

Dentine formation:
Mantle dentine → crystal formation + mineralisation takes place in matrix Vesicle [Q]
Circumpulpal dentine: matrix formation + mineralization without matrix vesicle.

Dentinal tubules: Start at right angle from pulpal surface and end ^ r to DEJ and CEJ

DEJ
90°
Lateral branches Canaliculi
Pulp
1 st convexity of tubules → Directed towards Apex

Fig. 2.8: Dentinal tubules

LAST 5-YEAR QUESTIONS FROM THIS TOPIC

1. **Greatest portion of the tooth is formed by:** *(AIIMS Nov 09)*

Ans. Dentin (Ref: Faller the Human body, 2004/e p394)

2. **Matrix vesicles:** *(COMEDK 09)*

Ans. Are found in mantle dentin

3. One of the following statements is unique about circumpulpal dentin: *(COMEDK 10)*

Ans. Contain Phosphophoryn

4. **The inner organic lining of the calcified dentinal tubule is called,** *(KCET 12)*

Ans. Lamina Limitans

5. **The number of dentinal tubules found at DEJ:** *(PHI June 09)*

Ans. 15,000-20,000 (Ref: Sturdevant's 5/e p25)

PULP

• Diameter of largest arterial vessel in PULP 50 to 100 μ [Q]
• Proteins present in: Enamel → Keratin [Q] Dentine → Collagen [Q]
• Average life time of 1° pulp in oral cavity = 8.3 yrs. [Q]
• Nerve fibres: Large myelinated fibres/free nerve endings of myelinated nerve ↓ "Carry Pain" Unmyelinated nerve fibres ↓ Associated with blood vessels ↓ Sympathetic ↓ Major type in pulp.
• Pulp stones → more in Coronal pulp. Diffuse calcification → more in root canal
• Size of apical foramen. Maxillary teeth → 0.4 mm Mandibular teeth → 0.3 mm
• Total volume of permanent pulp organ = 0.38 cm3
• Propioreceptors are not present in pulp. [Q] *(AIPG 12)*
• Pericytes are found around capillary of pulp ↓ Capillary associated fibroblasts [Q]
• 1° function of pulp ↓ Production of dentine
• Remnants of Hers: In PULP form Denticles In PDL forms Cementicles
• Molar pulp are 3 to 4 times larger than incisor Longest pulp–in canine

- Layers of pulp:

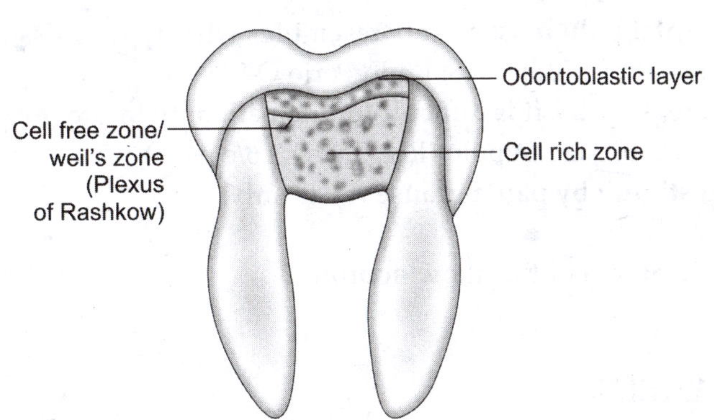

Fig. 2.9: Layers of pulp

- Most numerous cells in pulp → fibroblast
  2nd most numerous cells → Odontoblast
- Diffuse calcification of pulp is a type of Dystrophic Calcification
- True denticles – contain dentinal tubules
  False denticles – do not contain dentinal tubules
- Picket fence appearance seen in :
  Tome's process and OKC
- Phleboliths: Thrombi in angiomas may eventually calcify. Such Lesions feel hard on palpation
  Phlebectasia: Marked dilated and tortuous submucosal vein.
  Phlebectasia at the base of the tongue is called Caviar Varices
- Pain sensation in pulp is carried by:
  - Large myelinated nerve fibres
  - Free nerve endings of myelinated nerve fibres
- Defence cells of pulp:
  - Histocytes/macrophages–Irregular cells with small blunt process. In inflammation the cells have granules and vacuoles in cytoplasm, nuclei large, have prominent nucleolus demonstrated by intra vital dye like toluidine blue. Macrophages are characterised by presence of phagosomes

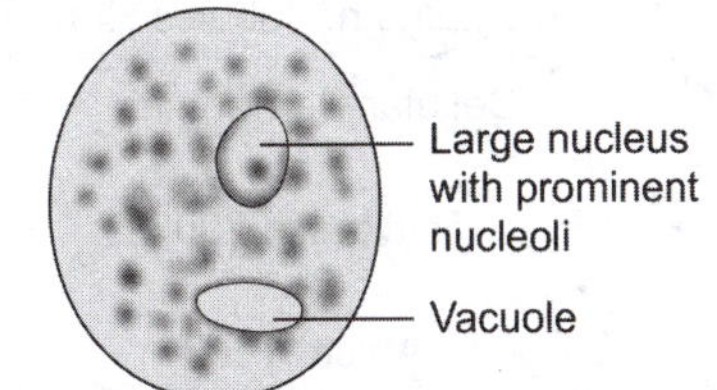

Fig. 2.10: Histocytes/macrophages

- Lymphocytes and eosinophils – can be seen in normal pulp.
- Most cells–seen in inflammation, have round nucleus, have darkly stained granules in cytoplasm.
- Plasma cells–nucleus is small and concentric in cytoplasm chromatin of nucleus is adherent to nuclear membrane giving cartwheeL appearance. Have packed RER

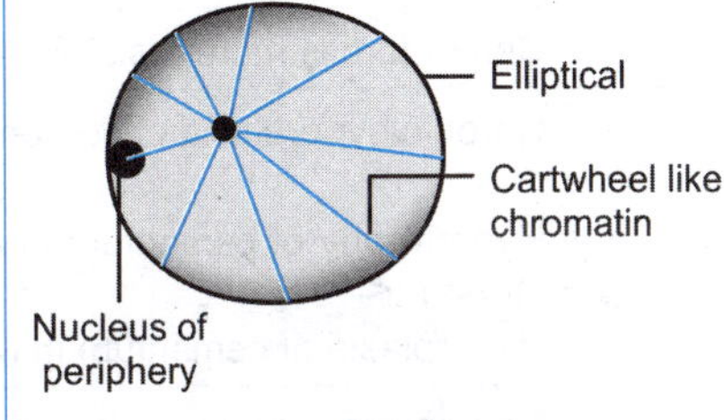

Fig. 2.11: Plasma cells

Parasympathetic fibres are not seen in pulp.

Highest pressure of Blood in Pulp

LYMPH capillaries (of PULP):
Absence of Basal Lamina adjacent to endothelium

LAST 5-YEAR QUESTIONS FROM THIS TOPIC

1. **Histologically, the dental pulp most closely resembles what type of tissue?** *(AIIMS Nov 10)*

Ans. Loose connective tissue (Ref: NBSE 1978, Endo-Perio Q-91)

2. **In a patient with acute pulpitis, it is difficult for the patient to locate the pain. This is because:** *(AIPG 12)*

Ans. Less propioreceptors are present in pulp (Ref: Shafer's 6/e p476)

3. **Pulp responds to all stimuli by pain because it has only:**

Ans. Free nerve endings

4. **The subodontoblastic plexus of Rashkow occupies?**

Ans. Cell free Zone of weil *(COMEDK 10)*

PERIODONTAL LIGAMENT

Canal of hirshfield and zuckerland: Perforation/canals present in interdental bone. These perforations are for vessels and nerves
Width of PDL – 0.15 to 0.38 mm
Intermediate plexus formed at centre of PDL is an area of rapid remodelling of fibres (An Older Concept)

LAST 5 YEAR'S QUESTIONS FROM THIS TOPIC

16. **Which is a feature of aging PDL:** *(AIIPG 12, 10)*

Ans. Increased scalloping in cementum and bone.

17. **Epithelial cell rests of Malassez are seen in:**

Ans. PDL *(COMEDK 09)*

CEMENTUM

• Hyaline/Intermediate layer: Separates dentine from cementum contains neither feature of Dentine/cementum. Contains no tubules Hers becomes trapped here.	
Cellular Cementum ↓ Thickness 200 μ ↓ Apical 1/3rd Cellular mixed fiber cementum ↓ Resorption lacuna [Q]	Acellular Cementum ↓ thickness of 20 μ ↓ Coronally 1/3rd
• Cementum is more resistant to resorption than bone as it is avascular	
• Chronic hyperplasia of cementum is associated with chronic periapical inflamation While Hypertrophy of cementum is associated with improved junctional qualities. (Condition is found in tooth with great stress) Hyperplasia of cementum in Non-functional tooth is characterized by reduction in number of sharpey's fibers.	
• Cementum contains only collagen fibre i.e. sharpey's fibre (Extrinsic Fibers) and Intrinsic Fibers both are collagen fibres. No elastic/other fibres [Q]	
• Thickness of cementum = 20 – 200 mm 20–50 μ → CEJ 50–200 μ → APEX (cellular)	

• "Cementum" Acellular cementum is the 1st formed cementum. Cellular cementum formed during tooth eruption when tooth reaches the occlusal plane. So, it is the cellular cementum contributes in Root Lengthening Acellular cementum → Contains more Extrinsic collagen fibres Cellular cementum → More Intrinsic fibres
• Cementum → Avascular, No Nerve supply (Insensitive)
• Cemental resorption: Occurs after trauma/excessive occlusal forces
• Least calcified cementum → cellular cementum Least Calcified Tissue → Cementoid (Not a type of cementum)
• Cementoid: Under normal condition, growth of cementum is a rhythmic process. As a new layer of cementoid is formed, old one calcifies. Cementoid layer lies on Cementum and lined by Cementoblast
• Cementoid and osteoid: Both are unmineralised organic matrix containing tissue
• Cementum → Cementocytic canaliculi have proper orientation towards PDL. → Deeper lying cementocytic lacuna may be empty
Bone → No such orientation and No such degeneration of osteocytes
• Intrisnsic fibres → run // lel to CDJ Extrinsic fibres → run perpendicular to CDJ

LAST 5-YEAR QUESTIONS FROM THIS TOPIC

1. **Less calcified among the type of cementum is:** *(AIIMS May 10 AIPG 10)*

Ans. Cellular cementum (Ref: Orban 11th p182-183)

2. **Which is the most common type of CEJ seen in teeth?** *(COMEDK 10)*

Ans. Cementum overlapping enamel.

3. **Cellular cementum is?** *(COMEDK 10)*

Ans. Less calcified than a cellular type.

4. **Intermediate cementum is:** *(KCET 10)*

Ans. Poorly defined zone near CDJ

BONE

• Alveolar bone proper (ABP) II Cribriform Plate as it is pierced by blood vessels and nerves
• Lamina dura: It's a radiographic manifestation of bundle bone. It is more calcified. Part of ABP → PDL fibers are inserted here
• Coupling: Inter dependency of osteoblast and osteoclast in bone Remodelling [Q]
• Collagen: → Triple – helix configuration (3 polypeptideα – chain) → Contain GYLCINE residue → Vit. C dependent enzyme required Prolylhyroxlase, LYSYL hydroxyvlase → The formation of collagen occurs "Extracellularly"
• ABP = Cribriform plate
• Reversal line is cessation of osteoclastic activity. Resting line is cessation of ostoblastic activity.

- Alveolar process:

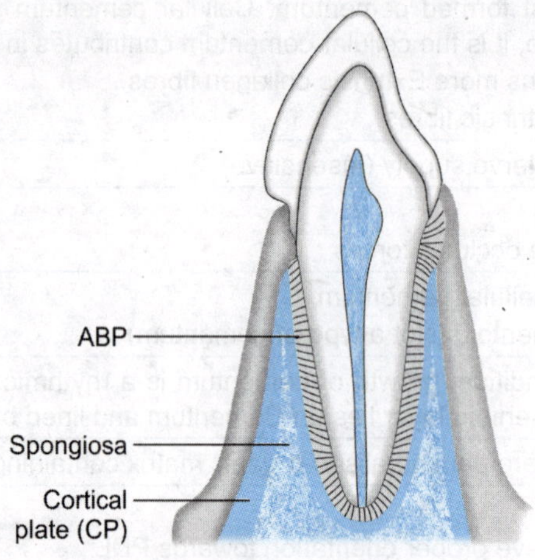

Fig. 2.12: Alveolar process

- Spongiosa: or Trabecular Bone
  → Cancellous portion
  → Less. Thicker in mandible because of thicker cortical plate
  → Yellow/fatty marrow fills space.
  → Types

  Type I (Mandible)
  ↓
  – Trabeculae regular, thicker (So, few in number)
  – Ladder like pattern
  → Type II (Maxilla)
  ↓
  Trabeculae "Irregular" Thin (So, more in number)

- Bone turnover/Remodelling:

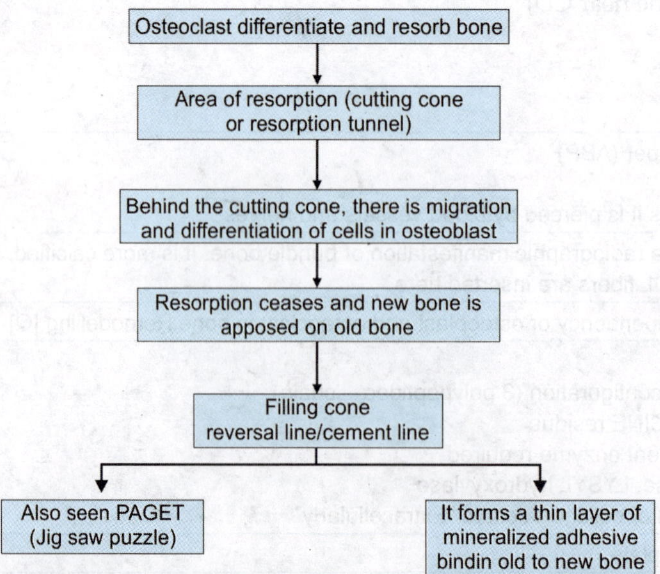

- Osteoclast:
  Peripheral to ruffle border there is a clear zone containing contractile proteins (Actin/Myosin) and is responsible for attachment of odontotoclast

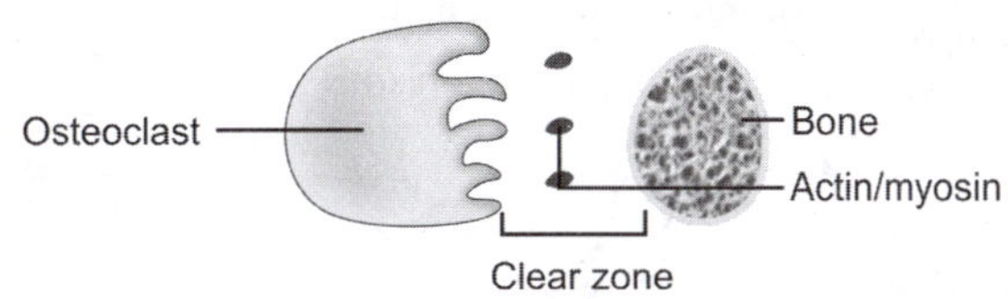

Fig. 2.13: Osteoclast

LAST 5-YEAR QUESTIONS FROM THIS TOPIC

1. **Radiographically the levels of normal interproximal alveolar crest corresponds to:** *(AIPG 11)*

Ans. CEJ of adjacent teeth

ORAL MUCOSA

- Masticatory Mucosa → "Keratinized" e.g. gingiva, hard palate, vermillion border
  Note: All others are lining mucosa i.e. Non-Keratinized.
  Specialized mucosa: Dorsum of tongue, tastebud.

- Layers

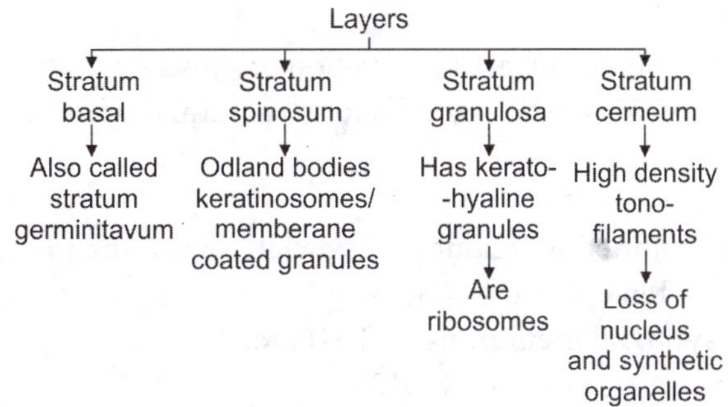

- Difference between p-Keratinised and O–Keratinised
  p-Keratinised
  - S. Corneum
  - Pyknotic nucleus i.e. incomplete removal of nucleus and synthetic organelles
  - Few synthetic organelles

  O -Keratinised
  - S. Corneum
  - Nucleus
    ↓
    Absent
  - No Synthetic organelles

Note: Non-Keratinized epithelium neither has stratum granulosum and stratum Corneum + Retain Nuclei

LAST 5-YEAR QUESTIONS FROM THIS TOPIC

1. **Level of sensitivity to pain is least in:** *(AIPG 12)*

Ans. Buccal mucosa (Ref: Oral Development and Histology by James Avery 2001, p282)

2. **Fovea palatine represent:** *(AIPG 12)*

Ans. Orifice of minor palatine salivary gland (Ref: Gray's anatomy 40/e p564)

3. Sulcular membrane acts as a semipermeable membrane through which: *(AIPG 11)*

Ans. Bacterial products pass into gingiva + fluid from gingiva seeps into sulcus

4. Attached gingiva is: *(AIPG 11)*

Ans. Resistant to masticatory force

5. Indifferent fibres are: *(AIPG 11)*

Ans. Collagen fibres

6. Buccal mucosa is: *(COMEDK 09)*

Ans. Non-Keratinized

7. Which papillae are completely Keratinized

Ans. Filliform (Ref: Ten Cate oral histology 4/e p380)

8. The glands of Von Ebner empty into a deep groove running around. *(COMEDK 09, KCET 12)*

Ans. Circumvallate papilla

9. Collagen fibrils have a transverse striation with a characteristic periodicity of: *(COMEDK 09)*

Ans. 64 nm

10. Tuft cells function as receptor cells in: *(AIPG 12)*

Ans. Excretory duct of salivary gland

11. One of the following groups of fibres in the lamina propria of the gingiva, help to bind the free gingiva to the tooth: *(COMEDK 10)*

Ans. Circular

12. The functions of myoepithilial cells may be: *(KCET 10)*

a. Initiating contraction
b. Support for the end piece during active secretion of saliva
c. Provide signals to the acinar secretory cells for structural organization
d. All of the above

Ans. d

13. Nerve endings of TMJ, confined to ligaments associated with the joint?

Ans. Golgi tendon organs (Ref: Ten Cate's 6/e p390-395)

14. The internal B cells of synovial membrane of TMJ are: *(COMEDK 11)*

Ans. Fibroblast like (Ref: Fonseca 1/e volume 04, p13)

15. Which of the following type of collagen is present in maxilla-cranial suture *(PGI June 11)*

Ans. Type I (Ref: Carranza 1s 10/e p69)

16. Epithelium of nasal, tracheal and Nasopharyngeal mucosa *(PGI June 10)*

Ans. Resemble Psuedostratified epithelium histologically (Ref: Inderbir Singh 4/e p207)

CHAPTER

3 Dental Anatomy

Topic

- Deciduous and Permanent Dentition
- TMJ
- Chewing Cycle

DECIDUOUS AND PERMANENT DENTITION

- Anterior teeth → MD width> Crown length [Q]
- Decidous canine → Mesial slope > Distal Slope

(Note: Opposite in permanent maxillary carine) + 2nd premolar)
In Ist premolar mesial slope > Distal slope)

Deciduous molar	Permanent Maxillary molar	Permanent Mandibular molar
ML cusp of lower Ist molar longest and sharpest (AIIMS may 10, may 07)	ML cusp of Ist molar longest and Sharpest	MB cusp of Ist molar longest and Sharpest

- Number of cusp:

	Deciduous (1°)	Permanent (2°)
Ist M	4	5 (4 in maxillar Ist M)
2nd M	5	4

- Number of roots: (Note: it is same in permanent teeth)

	Maxillary	Mandibular
1° Ist M	3	2
1° 2nd M	3	2

- Maxillary 20 LI has a longer root than central incisor *(COMEDK 07)*

- Roots of permanent Ist maxillary M:

Palatal	Mesio buccal	Disto buccal
• Longest	• Narrowest	• Smallest root
• greatest buccal curvature	• greatest distal curvature. So, endodontic Rx is very difficult in this root	• Most commonly resected
• Longest root to show facial and • Lingual concavity		

- Maxillary permanent Canine with its long root has maximum sensory receptor *(AIPG 04)*
- In mesial ½ of canine there is less convexity than distal ½ *(AIPG O2)*
- Lingual root of permanent maxillary molar is longest *(KCET-07)*
- Pulp canal and pulp chamber are broader in 1° teeth, apical portion of the canal is much less constricted
- Pulp horn of deciduous teeth corresponds to number of cusps:

2° Maxillary M	Major cusp → 3	4 pulp horn
2° Mandibular M	Major cusp → 4	5 pulp horn
Maxillary CI		3 pulp horn

- MB pulp horn is largest in 1° Ist M → Most commonly exposed during cavity preparation *(PGI Dec 12)*
- Ist PM (Maxillary) has sharp demarcation between pulp chamber and Root canal *(AIPG 03)*
- Maxillary Ist PM has steepest curpal inclines *(AIIMS may 07)*
- Crown completion of both upper and lower Ist molar → 2½ to 3 years
- By 2-2½ years all 1° teeth have erupted
- By 3-4 years all 1° teeth have completed root formation (i.e. root formation of 1° teeth occurs 1 to 1½ years after eruption)
- Eruption of 1° teeth

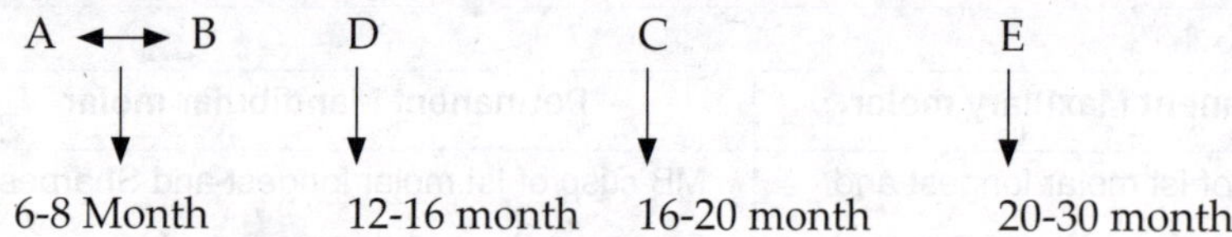

- Crown completion of permanent teeth:

Teeth	Maxilla (in yrs)	Mandible (in yrs)
CI	4–5	4–5
LI	4–5	4–5
Canine	6–7	6–7
Ist PM	5–6	5–6
2nd PM	6–7	6–7
Ist M	2½-3 *(COMEDK 07)*	2½-3
2nd M	7–8	7–8
3rd M	12–16	12–16

- Root completion of permanent anteriors:

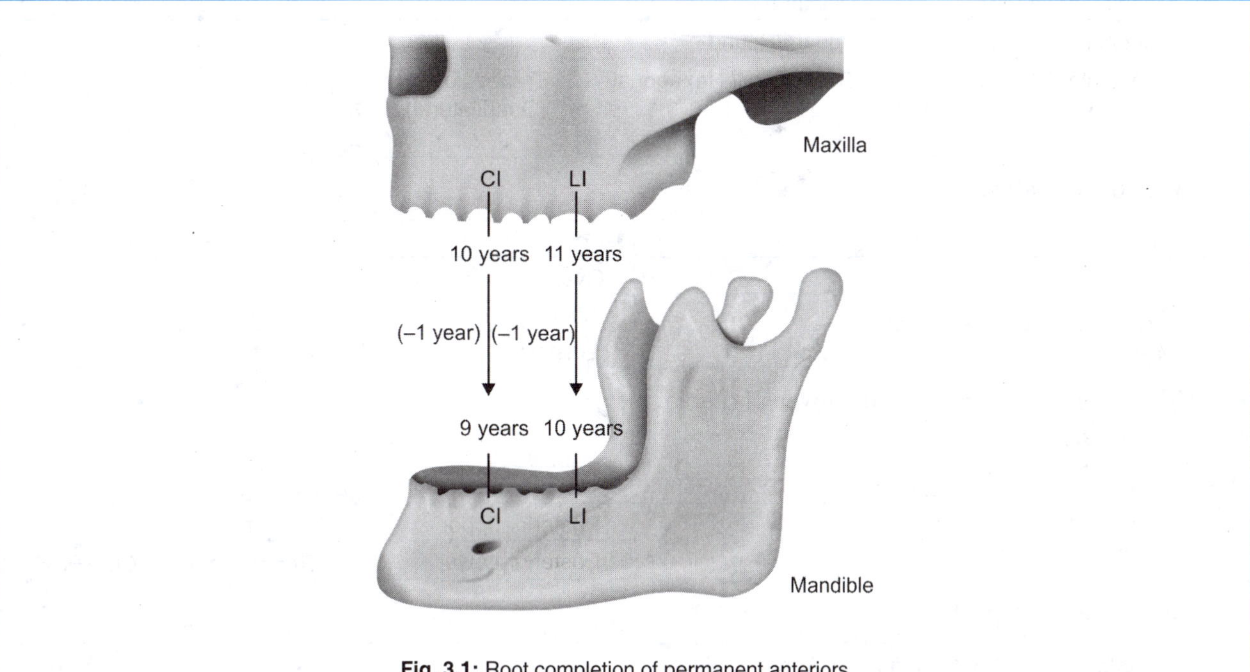

Fig. 3.1: Root completion of permanent anteriors

- Ist 2° teeth to erupt in oral cavity → Mandibular Ist M
- Ist 2° teeth to calcify = Maxillary Ist M
- 6 year M → Ist M
- 12 year M → 2nd M
- Point angle Vs line angle:

	Point angle	Line angle
Anterior teeth	4	6 *(COMEDK 09)*
Posterior teeth	4	8 *(KCET 08)*
Class II cavity	6	11

- Permanent Posterior teeth:

Mesial marginal ridge (MMR) higher than distal marginal ridge (DMR) except mandibular Ist PM [Q] (In mandibular Ist PM DMR located more occulsally) [Q]

- **Maxillary Ist PM:**

• Lingual cusp → Mesial and Distal slopes equal and meet at 90°
• Lingual cusp tip mesial [Q] to buccal cusp tip • (also for 2nd maxillary PM)

- Steepest cusp: Maxillary Ist PM (Don't confuse with ML cusp of upper M which is largest)

Tooth	Occlusal form	Access cavity	Cervical cross section
Maxillary Ist PM	Hexagonal [Q] *(KCET 08)*	Ovoid	Kidney [Q] / Eileptical
Maxillary 2nd PM	X	Ovoid	Ovoid / elliptical

Maxillary Ist M	Rhomboid	Δr	Rhomboid
Mandibular Ist PM	Diamond		
Mandibular 2nd PM	Square/Round		
Mandibular Ist M	Trapezoidal/ Hexagonal	Trepezoidal/ Rectangular (Quadilateral) (QQ) *(AIIMS 05)*	

- **Shape of Alveolus:**

Incisors	Δr
Canine	Oval
PM	Kidney [Q]
M	3 distinct

- Alveolar process is thinnest at: Lower CI (Labial plate)
- Proximal aspect:

Anterior	**Δr / Wedge**	
Posterior	Posterior upper	Trapezoidal
	Posterior Lower	Rhomboidal *(COMEDK 10, 09)*

- **Buccal / Labial aspect:**

All anterior/posterior teeth appear Trapezoidal [Q]

- **Dense in Dente:**

Most common in → maxillary Taurodontism
Most commonly → maxillary Ist M
Dens evaginatus / Leong's PM → Lower PM

- Corner teeth / Eye teeth → maxillary permanent canine
- corner stone of dentition → maxillary permanent Ist M
- Maxillary permanent Ist M:

At obtuse angle = oblique ridge cusp, i.e. (ML and DB cusps)
Oblique ridge seens from DB to ML cusp. *(KCET 05)*
At acute angle = Opposite to obtuse angle cusps
4 major cusps are separated by H-shaped grooves *(KCET 10)*

- Heart shaped occlusal form → 3rd maxillary M
- Furcation involvement maximum in mandibular permanent Ist M
- Facio lingual (FL) and MD inclination:

Posterior teeth with maximum FL and MD inclination	Maxillary 2nd M
Teeth with maximum FL inclination	Maxillary CI (28°)
Teeth with maximum MD inclination	Maxillary canine (17°)
Teeth with minimum FL inclination	Maxillary Ist PM

- Teeth with minimum MD inclination → mandibular LI
- Mandibular incisor → B/L Symmetrical with incisal edge to line bisecting tooth
- Canine → cusp tip of maxillary canine lies labial and mesial Cusp tip of mandibular canine lies LINGUALLY .

- Maxillary canine are retained for longest period *(COMEDK 06, PGI Dec 10)*
- Cervical line curvature: greatest on mesial surface of maxillary CI (3.5 mm) and is least on distal surface of posteriors
- Transverse Ridge:

(Prominent) 1° teeth → Mandibular Ist M
2° teeth → Maxillary Ist PM and Ist M → "Steepest cusp"

- Lingual fossa deepest in →Maxillary permanent LI → also associated with dense in dente
- Developmental groove in maxillary permanent lateral incisor and lower incisors creates accessibility problem and worsens prognosis after pdl Rx.
- Maxillary permanent lateral incisor → commonly has abnormal relation to adjacent teeth.

• Smallest teeth → Mandibular CI
• Smallest premolar (PM) → Lower Ist PM

• Upper Incisor → MD > BL width
• Lower incisor → BL> MD width

- Mandibular Ist PM has lingual tilt of 30°
- Maxillary Ist PM has pronounced developmental groove on MMR *(AIPG 03) (KCET 06) (COMEDK 06) (AIPG 03)*
- Mandibular Ist PM is the smallest
- Y' shaped occlusal groove is seen in mandibular 2nd premolar *(AIPG 07) (AIIMS May 07) (KCET 11)*
- Maxillary LI and 3rd M shows greatest variation in mass of crown *(AIPG 05, 07) (AIIMS May 10)*
- Maxillary permanent Ist molar:

• Cusp of carabilli seen in 60% population on mesial half of ML cusp.
• ML cusp is the most primitive cusp.

- Ideal occlusion:

• Maxillary Ist M → Buccal inclination
• Maxillary 2nd and 3rd M → Disto Buccal inclination

- Dryopithecus pattern:

ML cusp joining DB cusp along central fossa in mandibular Ist M (Oblique Ridge)

- 1° canine tip is sharper than 2° canine
- Trigone pattern of 1° cusp involves: ML, MB, DB cusps
- Primitive tooth form having single conical crown and a single root, is called Haplodont *(AIPG 07) (AIIMS May 10)*
- Human teeth are both THECODONT (inserted in socket) and Bunodont (having conical cusp) *(KCET 05)*
- Maxillary 3rd molar and mandibular CI have only 1 antagonist in opposing arch (others have 2 antagonist in centric occlusion)
- MD diameter of maxillary permanent Ist M greater Lingual due to cusp of carabilli + ML cusp (Rest posterior teeth opposite)
- Accessory Canal:

• Among anterior teeth accessory canal most common in mandibular permanent CI
• posterior accessory canal most common in mandibular 2° Ist M

- Lingual cusp of upper posterior and Buccal cusp of lower posterior are called supportive or functional/ Holding/ Stamp cusp / Centric cusp [Q]

- **Cusp – Fossa relation:**

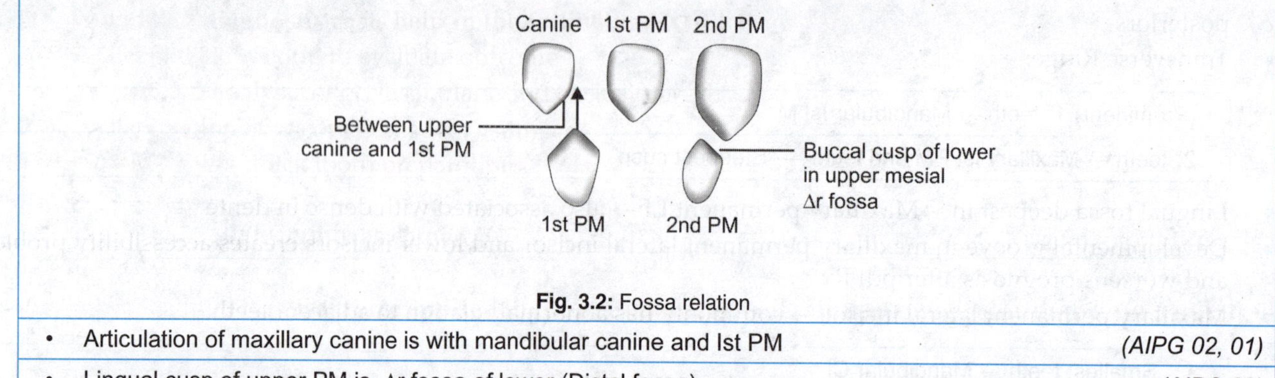

Fig. 3.2: Fossa relation

- Articulation of maxillary canine is with mandibular canine and Ist PM *(AIPG 02, 01)*
- Lingual cusp of upper PM is Δr fossa of lower (Distal fossa) *(AIPG 02)*

- Permanent Mandibular canine has Mesial surface of crown is almost parallel to long axis and root. *(AIPG 02)*
- The presence of horizontal overlap in the molars prevents (Cheek biting)
- Desmodont is another name for PDL
- Total number of occlusal contact points in dentition = 138
- Centric stops: are areas of contact that supporting cusp makes with the opposing teeth.
- Contact area of teeth (imp.):

Lower:

Mandibular CI, LI→ Both mesial(M) and Distal (D) at incisal / 1/3rd

Mandibular canine → M → Incisal third

D → Cervical to junction of incisal and middle third

Incisal 1/3rd (same)

Cervical to junction of incisal and middle 3rd.

Fig. 3.3: Contact area of mandibular teeth

Upper:

- CI→ M→ Incisal 1/3rd (PGI june 09)
  D→ junction of I 1/3 and M 1/3rd
- LI and → M → Junction of I and M 1/3 rd
- Canine D→ Middle third

Middle 3rd

Incisal 1/3rd

Lateral incisor + canine

Incisal and middle 1/3rd

Fig. 3.4: Contact area of maxillary teeth

• Mesial outline of mandibular canine when viewed labially from contact area to apex is relatively straight
• Maxillary PM → M and D (cervical to junction of occlusal and middle 1/3rd) (AIPG 01) from occlusal aspect
• anterior teeth have contact centered labio lingullary
• posterior teeth have contact areas slightly buccal to BL (Except contact between Ist and 2nd M and 2nd and 3rd M where contact is centered BL) • So, overall contact is centered BL except PM's → facially located
• **Note:** adjacent contact should be +ve opposite arch contact should be passive

- Mandibular 3rd M resembles mandibular 2M.
- **Embrasure:** (for permanent teeth)

• Smallest embrasure → between CI
• Widest incisal embrasure → LI and canine
• Largest embrasure → between canine and Ist PM (But in AIPG 02 correct option was not give. Then go for Ist and 2nd PM)
• Posterior teeth largest embrasure → Lingual (Except maxillary Ist M) → due to large ML cusp

- Curvature of cervical line in most teeth approx. 1mm less distally than mesial
- Curve of Wilson touches the buccal and the lingual cusp of mandibular teeth *(AIIMS Nov. 06)*

LAST 5-YEAR QUESTIONS FROM THE TOPIC

1. **Establishment of occlusion at Ist M during maturation of dentition occurs by:** *(AIPG 12)*

Ans. Late mesial shift (Ref: Pediatric dentistry, principles and practice by muture, and sivakumar, 2009, p108)

2. **Alignment of teeth in a curve from anterior to posterior is called is called** *(AIPG 12)*

Ans. Curve of von Spee (Ref: woefel 5/e p108)

3. **Enamel calcification is usually not completed at the time of eruption of a tooth. It gets completed after eruption when the tooth comes in contact with saliva for** *(AIPG 12)*

Ans. 2 years (Ref: Public Health dentistry by marya, 2011, p354)

4. **The eruption of teeth in active and passive phases was defined by** *(AIPG 12)*

Ans. Gottlied and orbans (1933) (Ref:Atlas of cosmetic and reconstructive periodontal surgery by cohen, 2007 p259)

5. **According to brearly and mekibbon (1973) commonly ankylosed teeth in deciduous dentition are:** *(AIPG 12)*

Ans. Mandibular Molar (Ref: McDonald and Avery Dentistry for the child and adolescent)

6. **Dentine islands are frequently found in root canals of which of the following permanent teeth:** *(AIPG 07, 10, AIIMS May 10)*

Ans. Maxillary 2nd PM and Mandibular canine

7. **True about 1° teeth:** *(AIPG 09) (AIIMS Nov. 10)*
   a. Calcification of 1° teeth is almost complete at birth
   b. Calcification of all 1° teeth and permanent incisors is complete at birth
   c. Calcification of all permanent teeth starts at birth
   d. Calcification of all permanent and primary teeth except 3rd M is completed at birth

Ans. a (Most appropriate)

8. **Pulp of mandibular 1° Ist M contains:** *(AIPG)*

Ans. 4 Pulp horns and 3 root canals (AIIMS) (Ref: Dental anthropology by Simon Hilson 1/e p60–66)

9. **Minimum number of lobes from which tooth developes is** *(AIIMS May 12) (COMEDK 07)*

Ans. 4 (Ref: Wheelers 8/e p239)
(**Note:** 1 lobe is required for development of deciduous tooth) *(PGI Dec. 10)*

10. Resorption of deciduous maxillary CI starts at: *(NEET 13, AIIMS Nov. 10)*

Ans. 4 years

11. Cusp of carabelli of the maxillary Ist M is on: *(KCET 11, COMEDK 10)*

Ans. Mesiolingual cusp (Ref: wheeler's dental anatomy physiology and occlusion 6/e p65, 21)

12. In a dried skull, holes on lingual aspects of the deciduous teeth are called: *(COMEDK-11, 09)*

Ans. Gubernacular canals (Ref: Tencate's Oral histology 7/e p270)

15. Any one of the 3 rounded protruberances seen on incisal ridges of newly erupted incisors in called. *(KCET 09)*

Ans. Mamelon

16. Enamel development defects are most common in: *(PGI Dec 11)*

Ans. Permanent anteriors (Ref: Dinical text book of dental hygiene and therapy by Robert Irrland/66)

17. Which permanent teeth is first to calcify: *(PGI Dec 10, June 10)*

Ans. Maxillary permanent Ist M (Ref: wheeler's 8/e p53)

18. Which primary teeth is most commonly ankylosed? *(PGI Dec 08)*

Ans. Mandibular 2nd M (Ref: Shafer 4/e p69)

TMJ

- Articular Disc: central portion of articular disc is avascular and devoid of nerve. So, has limited reparative capacity *(AIPG 03)*
- Functional articular surface:

• Posterior slope of eminence and anterior aspect of condyles are functional articular surface. Not the mandibular fossa.
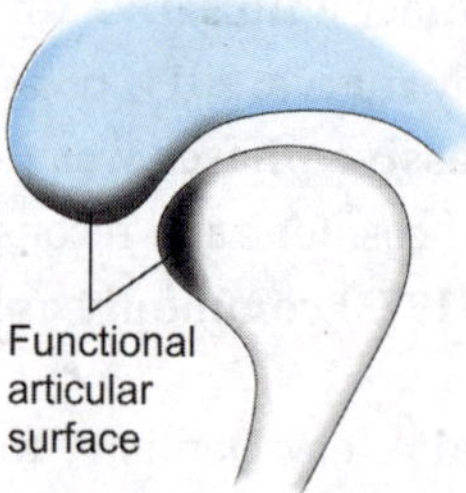 **Fig. 3.5:** Functional articular surface
• In a disease free TMJ, posterior end of the articular disc remains at 12O' clock position *(AIPG 04)*

- Upper compartments show – gliding movement
- Lower compartments show – gliding + HINGE movement

LAST 5-YEAR QUESTIONS FROM THE TOPIC

1. Nerve endings of TMJ, confined to ligaments associated with the joint? *(COMEDK 11)*

Ans.: Golgi tendon organs (Ref: Tencate's oral histology 6/e p390-95)

2. The intimal B cells of synovial membrane of TMJ are: *(COMEDK 11)*

Ans. Fibroblast (Ref: Oral and maxillofacial surgery: TMJ disorders by raymonds J. Fonseca I/e p13 vol 4)

CHEWING CYCLE

- **Dimensions:**

• Average vertical dimension = 16–20 mm
• Average lateral dimension = 3-5 mm
• Duration of cycle = 0.6 to 1 sec, depending on food, occlusion speed
• Functional occlusal force applied to PDL during 1 Deglutition is for 1 sec
• The jaw is stationary / pauses for approx. 1000 msec before the next cycle begins.
• The chewing force reaches the maximum in CO and last for 40 to 170 msec.

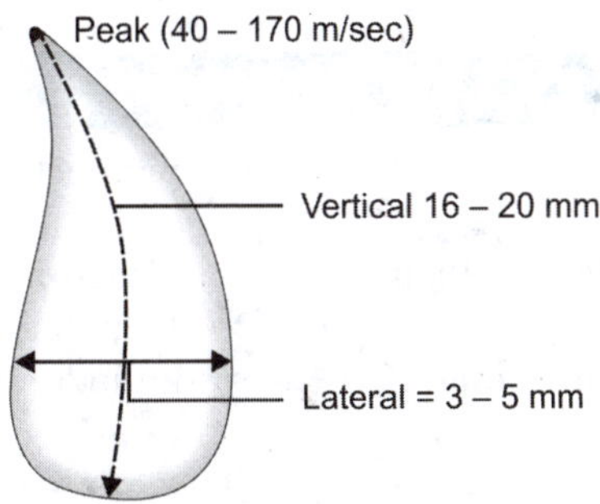

Fig. 3.6: Chewing cycle

CHAPTER

4 Endodontics

Topic

- Anatomy of Pulp
- Endodontic Microbiology
- Diseases of Pulp and Periradicular Tissues Their Diagnosis and Treatment Plan
- Endodontic Treatment of Primary and Young Permanent Teeth
- Biomechanical Preparation of Canal, Disinfection and Obturation
- Bleaching
- Traumatology
- Endodontic Surgery and Miscellaneous

ANATOMY OF PULP

- Innervation of pulp:

Nerve bundle that enters the pulp consists principally of sensory afferent nerves of trigeminal nerve and sympathetic branches of superior cervical ganglion. Each bundle consists of my and unmyelinted nerve. As nerve bundle ascends coronally, the myelinated nerve gradually lose their myelin sheath .So there is a proportional increase in unmyelinated nerves in coronal aspect of teeth. Most of the nerve bundles terminate in subodontoblastic plexus as free, unmyelinated nerve endings and small numbers of nerves pass between odontoblastic cell bodies to enter the dentinal tubules.
C fibers are 80% in pulp (0.3 to 1.2 μm in diameter) They conduct THROBBING + ACHING pain. Conduction velocity is 0. 4–2m/ sec
A Δ fibers (2–5 μ in diameter) conducts sharp PRICKING pain (COMEDK 11) with velocity of 6 to 30 m/sec

- Collagen fibers in pulp:

Pulp has type 1 and type 3 collagen **Note:** ALL oral hard and soft (gingival) tissues have type 1 (predominantly) and type 3 collagen

- Maxillary central incisor → pulp is SHOVEL shaped + has pulp horn [Q]
- Pulp chamber:

LARGEST pulp chamber → maxillary 1st molar
LARGEST pulp chamber in single rooted teeth → maxillary canine
sharp demarcation between pulp chamber and canal in posterior teeth BUT is indistinct in single rooted teeth, (e.g. maxillary 1st premolar)

- Mandibular 1st molar:

MB orifice below MB cusp
ML orifice below central groove
Distal orifice placed centrally bucco lingually

- Root bifurcation:

SUDDEN disappearance of canal RDIOLUCENCY indicates canal BIFURCATION
Among single rooted teeth, bifurcated canal are commonly seen in MANDIBULAR 1st premolar (KCET 12). Next in line are mandibular incisors and canine
NOTE: MAXILLARY central incisor and canine are least common teeth to show bifurcated root canal [Q]

- Teeth and percentage of occurrence of canal:

TEETH with accessory canals	Percentage of teeth
2 canals in mandibular premolar	10–25 %
DB_2 canal in mandibular 1st molar	30 %
2 canals in mandibular incisors	41 %
Maxillary 1st molar with MB_2 canal	84 %
Maxillary 1st premolar 3 canals *(PGI june 12)*	6 %

- %age of 2 canals in mandibular premolars: 10 to 25%

1st premolar → 23%
2nd premolar → 12%

- In maxillary 1st molar: MB_2 Canal is located lingual to MB canal
- Mandibular 1st molar:

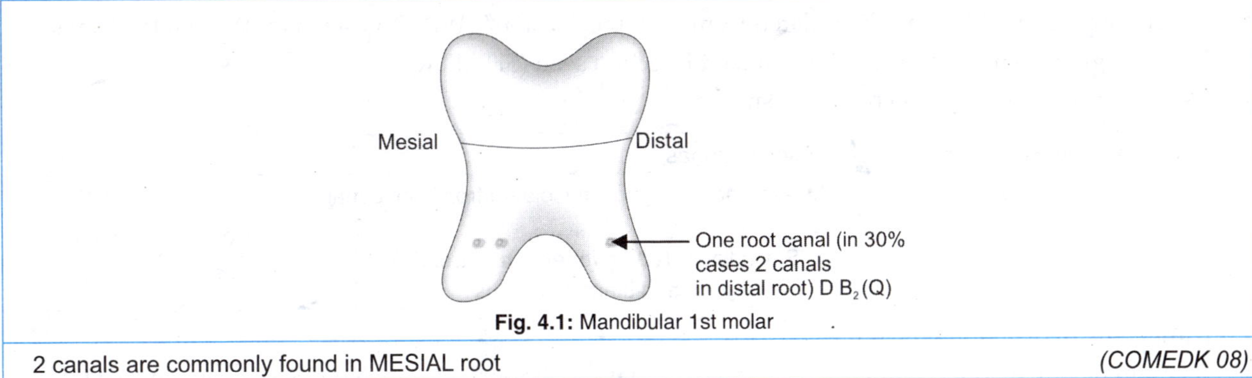

Fig. 4.1: Mandibular 1st molar

2 canals are commonly found in MESIAL root *(COMEDK 08)*

- C-shaped canal:

Mandibular 2nd molar show C–shaped canal (most common)
Also seen in mandibular 3rd molar and maxillary 3rd molar

- Major diameter = apical foramen
- Minor diameter = apical constriction

(COMEDK 09)

LAST 5-YEAR QUESTIONS FROM THIS TOPIC

1. The maxillary 1st premolar will typically demonstrate which type of pulpal configuration? *(COMEDK 10)*

Ans. a DOUBLE root with 2 root canals

ENDODONTIC MICROBIOLOGY

- Sample of root canal taken by sterile adsorbent paper points *(KCET 06)*
- FISH ZONE:

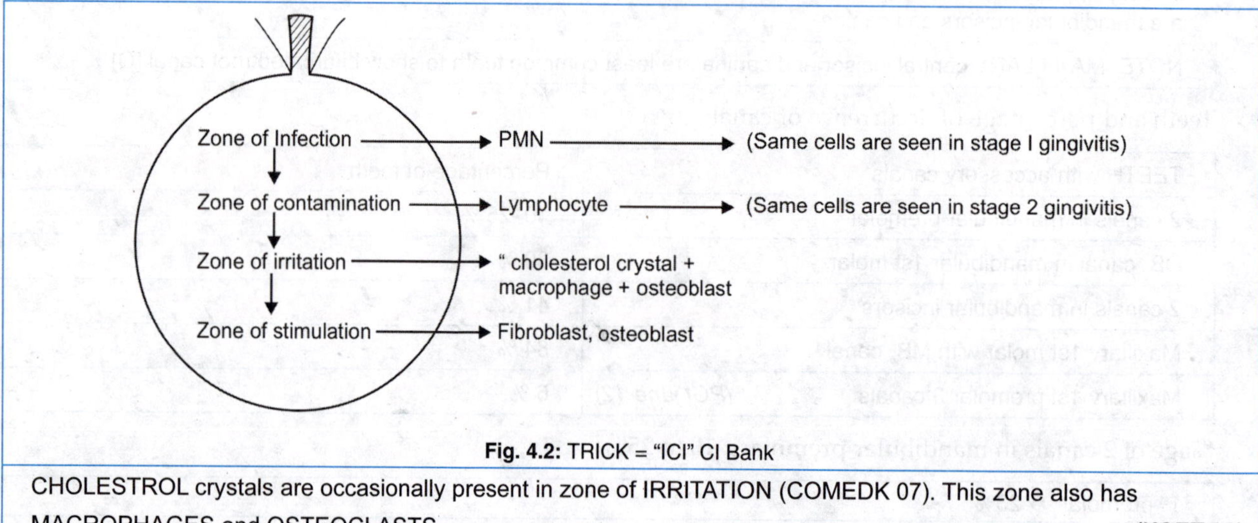

Fig. 4.2: TRICK = "ICI" CI Bank

CHOLESTROL crystals are occasionally present in zone of IRRITATION (COMEDK 07). This zone also has MACROPHAGES and OSTEOCLASTS *(KCET 06)*

- Important cytokinins in apical periodontitis:

IL–1 (mainly) [Q] + TNF–α

- "Micro organism will always be isolated from periapical lesion" (WRONG statement) → NOT always
- Peripical granuloma → NOT sterile → mixed infection seen (SHAFER)
- ROOT canal and various micro–organisms:

Organism ABSENT in root canal → Pseudomonas
Most common organism isolated from root canal ↓ S. viridians (NOT pyogens)/α - streptococci and staphylococcus

- Pathogenicity of endodontic flora:
- As gram negative flora dominates. So, endotoxin plays an important role. No role of exotoxin (AIPG)
- Biofilm:

One of the basic mechanisms of survival of bacteria in time of starvation.
E. faecalis produces intracanal microbial BIOFILM
It Can tolerate a Ph up to 11.5 *(KCET 10)*
Normally it is resistant to Ca $(OH)_2$. So, combinations are used

- The strain of yeast found in root canal: C. albicans [Q]

In RCT, Failure is caused by E. faeclis (AIIMS 08, AIPG 07)
Flare up is caused by bacteriods

- Viruses isolated from root canal:

{TRICK = these viruses are seen with lowered number of T–CELLS}
CMV, EBV, HIV

LAST 5-YEAR QUESTIONS FROM THIS TOPIC

1. **Which of the following is not a major component of endodontic pathogenic mechanism?** *(AIPG 10)*

Ans. Exotoxin (Ref: Cohen 8/e p464)

DISEASES OF PULP AND PERIRADICULAR TISSUES THEIR DIAGNOSIS AND TREATMENT PLAN

- The diagnosis of pulpal disease is obvious but is sometimes obscure
- Cold test is used to indicate vital pulp
- Heat test is not meant to test pulp vitality
- Thermal test:

Heat test → 65.5°C
Cold test → 5°C

- EPT: *(AIIMS 06)*

Can be normal in degenerative pulp
It is more sensitive for pulp tissue than gingival tissues
It brings about response by stimulating nerve endings
• **Note:** Vitality should be rechecked after 2 weeks and then 1 month
For PFM → EPT is contraindicated, instead cold test With CO2 snow/"TRIGIDENT "is test of Choice. (Temperature of dry ice/CO2 snow is–78°C) {COMEDK 08}
POSTERIORS require more current for EPT due to bulkier tooth
False negative response to EPT is seen in: • Recently traumatized tooth • Recently erupted tooth with incomplete root formation • Patient under sedative drugs

- Percussion test:

PERCUSSION test → is the test of INTEGRITY of Pdl (PGI 05)
CONCEPT: "percussion" tells about the status of the "periodontium" surrounding the tooth. NOT about whether tooth is vital/not Pulpal inflammation may/may not be present.
The diseased tooth is examined last in percussion.
POSITIVE vertical percussion ——— endodontic lesion
POSITIVE Lateral percussion ——— periodontal lesion (PGI 08)

- Cyst differentiated from granuloma by injecting Poly Acrylamide dye [Q]

- Endoray:
  - Film holder to position film for projecting X–ray in endodontic procedure.
- Snap-a-ray film holder ideally sterilized by autoclave *(KCET 12)*
- Digital imaging (commercially available):

• RVG
• Flash dent
• Sense-a–ray

- Radiographically the latent period of an acute periapical abscess is 10–15 days *(AIIMS 05)*
- Radiopaque irregularity associated with root of tooth indicates subgingival calculus *(PGI 07)*
- GCF: can be either exudates/transudate. But if both options are not given then go for " exudate"
- Transudate: Specific gravity < 1.012 *(KCET 12)*
- DNA micro processing uses DNA computer
- Acute closed pulpitis:

Is the most intense pulpal pain
It is so severe because pulp is bound by RIGID dentine *(COMEDK 05)*

- Concept: Diseases of pulp:

HYPEREMIA of pulp/focal reversible pulpitis: tooth is more sensitive to thermal and electrical test. pain is INTERMITTENT • CHRONIC pulpitis: the pulpal response to thermal and electric stimuli is " REDUCED" • ACUTE apical periodontitis: shows MARKED tenderness to percussion(PATHOGNOMIC), negative EPT (features similar to periapical abscess) • Chronic apical periodontitis (periapical granuloma): very mild tenderness to percussion. so, it's NOT the pathognomic sign	
IRREVERSIBLE PULPITIS *(PGI 05)*	REVERSIBLE PULPITIS/hyperemia/focal reversible pulpitis
Prolonged, severe pain (THROMBING) referred pain is common pain is intermittent/continuous BUT spontaneous. pain often continues when cause is removed pain may be caused by sudden temperature change especially COLD	No referred pain
Tenderness on percussion seen *(PGI June 10)*	Tenderness on percussion absent
Postural pain seen	NO postural pain
PULP TESTS: EPT–normal to elevated HEAT test–acute pain COLD test–pain relieved by cold sometimes	PULP test: EPT–normal HEAT–normal to exaggerated COLD–exaggerated
Acute pulpal degeneration = irreversible pulpitis So, most definitive sign of diagnosis patient history of unprovoked spontaneous pain *(AIIMS 05)* Treatment of choice is pulpectomy *(COMEDK 11)*	

- Internal resorption/odontoclastoma:

Result of odontoclastic activity
Result of odontoclastic activity
Usually ASYMPTOMATIC *(COMEDK 10)*
H/P: Granulation tissue with multinucleated giant cell (OSTEOCLAST) [Q] (like other inflammatory resorption) The presence of granulation tissue accounts for profuse bleeding when pulp is removed At least part of pulp must be vital for resorption to take place. Commonly coronal pulp is necrotic and apical 3rd vital.

NO chance of internal resorption after successful RCT as pulp is removed
Rx of INTERNAL resorption: PULPECTOMY should be done + Ca $(OH)_2$ dressing.
{NOTE: osteoclastoma = central giant cell granuloma}

- According to INGLE usual percentage of success in endodontic cases is 90–95%
- If RCT is performed on vital pulp, prognosis will be better than necrotic pulp
- Pulpal fibrosis: does not require any Rx till it becomes symptomatic (as fibrosis itself is a protective response)
- Rx of barodontologia
- Restore the cavity with varnish/sub base of ZnOE and base of $ZnPO_4$
- Rx for pulp polyp → extraction/endodontic therapy
- Prognosis of external root resorption vs internal root resorption:

EXTERNAL root resorption	INTERNAL root resorption
Prognosis is guarded (NOT good) and tooth becomes weak and even lost	Prognosis best before perforation

- Cracked tooth syndrome:

Mimics the STABBING pain seen in TRIGEMINAL NEURALGIA	*(COMEDK 12, 08)*
Elicited mainly when pressure is RELIEVED	*(COMEDK 05)*
URGENT treatment → selective grinding of opposing cusp (relieve occlusion)	*(COMEDK 13)*
DEFINITIVE treatment → FULL coverage crown	

- Phoenix abscess has symptoms similar to that of an acute infection. It is associated with a non vital tooth, has periapical radiolucency and is tender on percussion *(AIIMS 06)*
- Trephination: [Q]

  It is artificial sinus made in bone, a procedure to relieve pain.

  This is done by perforating cortical bone by engine driven burs/hand operated trephine to release the building pressure and exudates around root apex of a tooth.

  Time needed for osteogenesis in case of periapical lesion is 6–12 months

  Austin syndrome: pain in TMJ + headache.

LAST 5-YEAR QUESTIONS FROM THIS TOPIC

1. **A tooth tested non vital in vitality test showing periapical radiolucency shows the presence of sinus tract clinically. What should be the treatment for sinus tract?** *(AIIMS May 11)*

Ans. No treatment (Ref: Goldberg, et al. Odontogenic sinus tracts, Quintessence international, 2009, 40 p13–18)

2. **A radicular cyst is always associated with:** *(AIIMS Nov 10, May 09)*

Ans. Non vital tooth/teeth (Ref: Q 76 NDBE dec 1977 endodontology and periodontology)

3. **What is the term for radio opaque area found at the root apex of a young permanent tooth involved with a chronic pulpitis?** *(AIIMS Nov 10, AIPG 11)*

Ans. Apical condensing osteitis (Ref: Q- 89 NDBE 1978 endodontology and periodontology)

4. **A patient has an infectious process associated with the maxillary right lateral incisor. The tooth is deeply carious and non-restorable. His temperature is 102 °F. The patient has not been able to chew for the past 24 hours from the right side of the face. The treatment of choice would be:** *(AIIMS Nov 11, 08)*

Ans. Incision and drainage

5. **Pulp vitality tests usually used to check?** *(PGI Dec 10, June 08)*

Ans. Afferent nerve fibers (Ref: Walton and torabinejad p57)

{Trick: Vitality has "A" so, it's Afferent nerve}

6. ALL of the following tests are used to determine the status of the pulp except: *(KCET 11)*

a. Heat test
b. Cold test
c. Electric test
d. Anesthetic test

Ans. d (Ref: Grossman's endodontic practice 12/e p70)

7. Application of COLD/the electric pulp tester can be used: *(KCET 10)*

Ans. To test tooth under treatment for pulpal anesthesia

8. A pulp vitality test which uses the principle of measuring the velocity of RBC in capillaries: *(KCET 12)*

Ans. Laser Doppler flowmetry

9. Pulp oximetry is used to measure: *(PGI June 12)*

Ans. Oxygen saturation

10. HOT tooth refers to: *(PGI June 12)*

Ans. Tooth which cannot be anaesthetized

ENDODONTIC TREATMENT OF PRIMARY AND YOUNG PERMANENT TEETH

- Direct pulp capping and Ca $(OH)_2$ pulpotomy are contra indicated in primary tooth
- Ledermix:

Has Demeclocycline (AIIMS may 09) + Prednisolone + Triamcelanone in Ca $(OH)_2$ (TRICK: DPT-C)
It's a DIRECT pulp capping agent with corticosteroids and antibiotics. It reduces pulpal inflammation

- Pulpotomy is contraindicated in case of: *(AIIMS 05)*

Mobility
Pain on percussion
Periodontitis involving pulp

- Pulpotomy:

In SWEET technique of devitalisation pulpotomy FORMOCRESOL saturated cotton pellet is placed over the amputated pulp stumps for 5 minutes *(COMEDK 05)*
BUCKLEY's solution used in devitalisation pulpotomy is composed of cresol, formaldehyde, water and glycerin *(AIIMS 06)*
FERRIC sulfate pulpotomy: Ferric sulfate = MONSEL's solution Done for 10–15 sec [Q] It is a type of preservative pulpotomy Also used as haemostatic agent [Q] CVEK's PULPOTOMY/PARTIL pulpotomy: Done in young permanent tooth (for completion of root development)

- Apexification:

Ca $(OH)_2$ → fill the entire canal (time taken for apexification is 6 to 24 months)
MTA → Composition: tricalcium silicate, dicalcium silicate, Tricalcium aluminate, CaSO4 dihydrate Bismuth oxide used in pulpotomy, DPC, APPEXIFICATION immature teeth (PGI 06, KCET 08 Q), in case OF PERFORATION of tooth it's a root end filling material (KCET 08) NOT root canal filling material (PGI 09) Fill in apical 3 to 4 mm (single step procedure) Obturate with thermoplastic GP technique Powder: liquid ratio = 3 : 1 (AIPG 11) (same ratio for PMMA volume wise) Ph of set MTA is 12.5 (AIPG 10)

Mechanism of action of MTA:
1. Induces expression of OCN (osteocalcin gene)
2. Induces cementoblast to form hard tissue

LAST 5-YEAR QUESTIONS FROM THIS TOPIC

1. **The type of laser used in pulpotomy procedure is:** *(COMEDK 10)*

Ans. Nd: Yag laser (according to the official key given)

2. **High rate of failure after direct pulp capping in primary teeth is due to:** *(KCET 12)*

Ans. High cellular content of pulp

BIOMECHANICAL PREPARATION OF CANAL, DISINFECTION AND OBTURATION (VERY IMPORTANT TOPIC FOR ANY EXAM)

- GLASS bead sterilizer:

Used at 425 °F for 15 sec (Range is 425 °F–475 °F) *(KCET 08)*
ABSORBENT paper point is sterilized by glass bead sterilizer
HOT salt sterilizer used at 425 °F for 10 sec
Hottest part is present on periphery while lowest temperature is at center
To sterilize immerse at least 14 inch below salt
Main disadvantage of glass bead sterilizer is that ONLY small instruments can be sterilized

- Access cavity:

Maxillary molar triangular shaped access cavity
Mandibular molar with 3 root canal trapezoidal access cavity
Mandibular molar with 4 root canal rectangular access cavity *(AIIMS May 11, 08)*

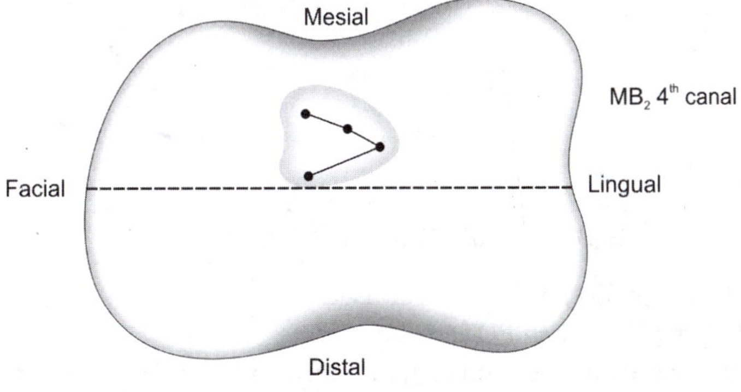

Fig. 4.3: Access cavity

CONCEPT: Access opening in both upper and lower molar are always on mesial half of occlusal surface.
Perforation with bur is common in mandibular central incisor > mandibular premolar
In creating access opening through a PFM crown diamond is used for ceramic while carbide is used for metal *(AIPG 07)*

- Exploration of canal orifice of Mandibular 1st molar:

MB orifice present under MB cusp and is explored from MB cusp side (SAME side)
ML orifice is present below the central groove and is explored from DB direction (OPPOSITE side)
The DISTAL orifice is explored from MESIAL side (OPPOSITE side)

- Standardization of instrument:

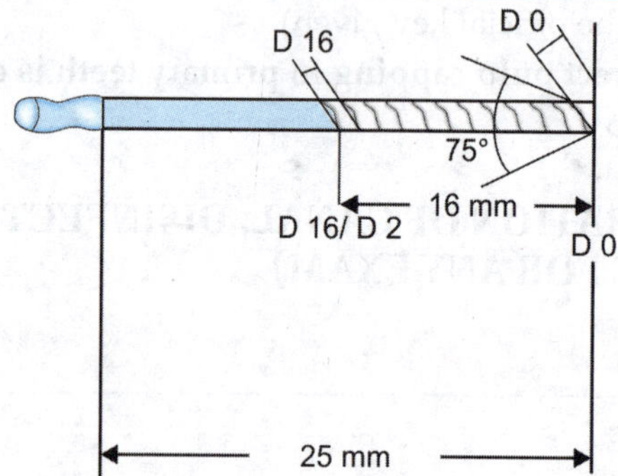

Fig. 4.4: Standardization of instrument

According to ISO standardization files and reamers should have a taper of 0.02 mm/mm	*(KCET 08, 05)*
Instrument numbered from 1 to 100 1. Each number denotes tip diameter in hundredths of mm 2. $D_0 = D_1$ = diameter at tip 3. $D_{16} = D_2$ = diameter at 16 mm from the tip of the instrument (KCET 12, 11)	
Tip angle of an endodontic instrument should be 75 50	*(KCET 06, COMEDK 12)*
Handle of instrument has color coding: Pink → 6 Grey → 8 Purple → 10 White → W → 15 Yellow → Y → 20 Red → R → 25 Blue → B → 30 Green → G → 35 Black → B → 40 Repeat again from W, Y ,R, B, G, B 45, 50 ,55, 60 (PGI 06), 65, 70	*(PGI 06)*

- To locate canal orifice DG–16 endodontic explorer used
  In calcified canal SHARP explorer with EDTA used
- Endodontic instruments should be used with ¼ th to ½ turn and withdrawn with a pull stroke to prevent fracture (1/3rd turn was the answer in NEET 13.
  It was a direct from a Q bank)
- Case:
  When a calcified canal cannot be located/instrumented then the dentist must proceed with the understanding that an unexplored/unfilled canal is worse than a perforation *(KCET 06)*

- Reamers and files:

CONCEPT: With respect to difference between REAMER and FILES Most of the companies make reamers and files with same blank. They are mainly different with respect to number of flutes. *(AIIMS 06)*
NOTE: blank determines cutting efficiency and fracture resistance
No. of flutes: 1. In files–1 1/2 to 2 1/2 flutes/mm 2. In reamers - 1/2 to 1 1/2 flutes/mm
Cutting actions of: 1. Reamers–they are twisted 1/4 to 1/2 turn 2. Files–they are withdrawn without any turning
The IDEAL instrument that is used to widen the canal is FILE (as less likely to break than reamer)
Instrument for cutting dentine EFFICIENTLY REAMER
More chances of "debris" to be pushed is "FILES" [Q]
RASP = RAT tail file
REAMERS used in PUSHING–rotating motion FILES used with RASPING/PULLING motion
K–file: called work horse of endodontic

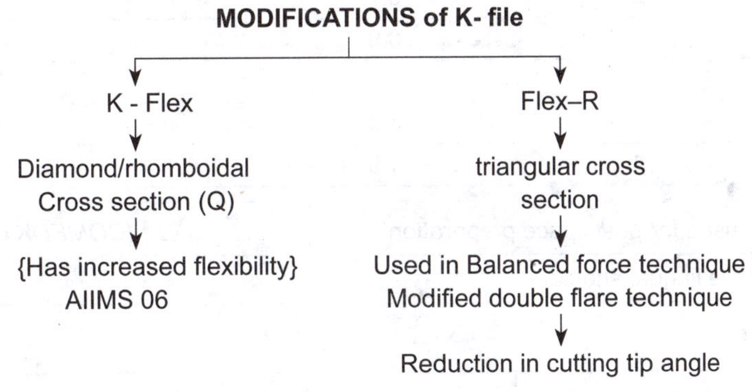

- H-file:

H-File has SPIRAL flutes, positive rake angle with 60° - 65°. So, they are aggressive cutters, but there are greater chances of fracture. (AIIMS Nov 11, KCET 08) so, can't be used in curved canal.
H–File has "TEAR DROP" single helix, Christmas tree appearance.
Clinician should use H- file only in 1 direction i.e. PULLING and never in TORQUING motion. *(AIIMS 05)*
It is used to FLARE the canal *(PGI 05, COMEDK 05, KCET 09)*
Modifications of H–file: *(COMEDK 12)* Safety H–file–has non cutting side Hyflex–S shaped design Unifiles–double helix design S–File–double helix design

- Group 2 non–rotatory endodontic instruments used with HAND piece:

ENGINE DRIVEN	ULTRASONIC and SONIC
Giromatic Uses K Files/reamers in root canal with 90º reciprocating arch with a speed of 3000 cycles/min	Produces movement of K file between 0.001 to 0.004 inch at a frequency of 25 to 30 KHz No. 15, 20 K file used *(PGI 12)*
Can be used for canal opening but shouldn't be used for canal preparation.	Along with cutting it improves mechanical, thermal, bactericidal and cleansing ability of irrigant solution (by cavitation and acoustic streaming) [Q]

- Group 3 rotatory endodontic instrument used with hand piece:

SLOW speed rotator hand piece instrument:
E.g. GG drill/peso reamer → set of 6
GG drill → 0.5 to 1.5 (tip diameter)
Pesoreamer → 0.7 to 1.7 (tip diameter)
BOTH GG drill and peaso reamer are made of carbon steel, so aggressive cutter BUT inflexible. So, used in SLOW SPEED.

NUMBER of instrument	GG DRILL (KCET 07) (tip diameter)	PEASO REAMER (tip diameter)
1	0.5 —(+0.2)→ ↓ + 0.2	0.7
2	0.7	0.9
3	0.9	1.1
4	1.1	1.3
5	1.3	1.5
6	1.5	1.7

PEASO REAMER is used for post space preparation *(COMEDK 06, KCET 11, 12, AIPG 12 ,07)*

GG drill used to remove lingual shoulder

- Ni–Ti instrument:

Are flexible because of their super elasticity *(COMEDK 09)*
Can be used in PURE ROTATION motion in curved canal
Disadvantage: no VISUAL indication of fracture
Tapered instrument → they have same diameter at tip. Instrument are developed with a taper of 2%, 4%, 6 %
2% taper = diameter increases by 0.02 mm/mm So, 4% taper = diameter increasing by 0.04 mm/mm
Advantage: preparing canals of wider diameter without enlarging the canal at working length.
LAND area of certain files: this feature is incorporated to reduce canal transportation and support cutting edge.

- NiTi Vs stainless steel:

Q–Advantage of NiTi over stainless steel in endodontic: it's SUPERELASTICITY *(PGI June 12)* Rotatory stainless endodontic instrument fracture when cyclic loading leads to metal fatigue.
NiTi instrument can withstand several hundred flexural cycles before fracture in endodontic setting but at higher number of cyclic loading

- Canal exploration:

Canal exploration: 8, 10 K file used
In calcified canal–6 K file, C+ file, profinder

- Electronic apex locator:

Electronic apex locator is used in endodontics to determine the working length *(COMEDK 10)*
High accuracy, powerful and useful adjunct to radiograph but NOT an alternative.
Classification: (remember the one asked in exams) Multiple frequency apex locator (3rd generation) e.g. root ZX (AIIMS 04), TriAuto ZX, Propex 2

- Wein modifiction of working length determination by radiograph:

1. Reduce length by 1 mm if NO root + bone resorption
2. Reduce length by 1.5 mm if bone resorption
3. Reduce length by 2 mm if both root and bone resorption

- Balanced force technique:

Uses Flex–R file (with triangular blank)
Technique: 1st engage the canal by clockwise 90° direction with LIGHT apical pressure. Then instrument is rotated COUNTER clockwise 180° - 270° with SUFFICIENT apical pressure.

- Crown-down technique/step back = telescoping technique: *(COMEDK 09)*

Coronal 2/3rd preparation with 15, 20, 25 H file GG drill to flare Apical segment preparation with 10, 15 no. file coronal segment Advantages: ZIPPING is less, working length less likely to change, better penetration of irrigant.

- Zipping:

Transportation of apical portion of canal
Lesser seen with crown down technique

- Double flare technique (by both crown down and step back):

K file used
Meant for straight canal

- Modified double flare technique:

Meant for curved canal [Q]
Flex–R file used

- Mesio buccal root in maxillary molar is most difficult to prepare as has greatest distal curvature and narrowest of all
- In BMP final "2–3 mm" apical part of cavity preparation is most crucial. This is a region where leakage of sealing agent occurs and this is the region where accessory canals are most commonly present *(PGI Q)*

- Concept: Root canal preparation:

RETENTION form: provided by 2–3 mm of parallel walls at the apical 3rd of preparation to provide tug back of the master cone
RESISTNCE form: provided by parallel walls of apical seat to preserve the integrity of natural apical constriction and prevent overfilling/over extrusion. Resistance to overfilling is the primary objective of resistance form i.e. it prevents extrusion of master cone. *(AIIMS 06)*
"APICAL COLLAR" = RETENTIVE form (usually nearly 2 mm of parallel walls at apical region) KEY word is TUG back
Blood seen at end of paper point indicates INCOMPLETE removal of pulp *(PGI 05)*

- Activity of all disinfectant is reduced by organic debris/Blood.
- Gold standard of irrigant solution:

H_2O_2 + NaOCl (best for removal of smear layer) *(KCET 06)*
NaOCl should be used last to avoid surgical emphysema caused by H_2O_2
NaOCl can dissolve pulpal tissue *(COMEDK 10)*

- Sodium hypochlorite accident:

EMERGENCY during treatment
Cytotoxic and caustic effect seen on periradicular tissues
So, a lower concentration of 0.5 to 2.5 % preferred with light pressure *(COMEDK 11)*

- Ultrasonic instrument:

Ultrasonic instruments use → NaOCl as irrigant *(COMEDK 07)*
FILE size used with ultrasonic handpiece for irrigating root canal: 15 and 20 *(PGI june 11)*

- Sonic instruments use → H_2O as irrigant
- H_2O_2 as irrigant has limited antibacterial activity
- EDTA irrigant solution:

Removal of smear layer is done by 17 % EDTA irrigant solution *(AIPG 07, KCET 07)*
Also dissolves pulp stone
It has a Ph of 7.3 [Q]

- CHX digluconate as "irrigant":

Highly active against E. faecalis. Also active against C.albicans
Sustained activity due to it's property of "SUBSTANTIVITY"
BUT does not remove smear layer

- RC prep = EDTA + urea peroxide (used in calcified canal) *(KCET 07, COMEDK 06, COMEDK 09)*
- EDTA C = C stands for cetavlon
- MTAD:

Recently used irrigant *(PGI 08)*
Mixture of Tetracycline isomer like DOXYCYCLINE (AIIMS may 09), ACID (citric acid) and detergent
Advantage: removes smear layer effectively + highly effective against E. faecalis

- Gauze of needle used for irrigating canal: 27 (according to Ingle and Cohen) *(PGI June 11)*
- Intracanal Medicament:

The 2 intracnal medicament recommended is endodontic practice are Ca (OH)2, CHX

- 0. 1 % benzoate and citric acid can kill E. fecalis Also 2 % CHX used as intracanal medicament is effective against E. faecalis
- **NOTE:** E. faecalis is normally resistant to most of the intracanal
- Medicament; it can tolerate a pH up to 11.5
- Root canal sealer:

Root canal SEALER move coronally after proper BMP. It should be NON–TOXIC and NON–IRRITANT (IDEAL requirement)
CONCEPT: Root canal sealer ALL of the materials used to seal root canal i.e GP, sealers, cements irritate periradicular tissue (Q if allowed to escape from canal)

- **Sealers:**

ZnOE based: Grossman sealer, tubliseal, wasch sealer, roth sealer [Q], EWT (extended working time) (TRICK: all sealers starting with name belong to this category)
Ca $(OH)_2$ based: - sealapex, apexit, CRCS
GIC based: ketac endo
RESIN based: AH–26 [Q], AH plus, diaket, endorez [Q], real seal (contains UDMA resin { AIIMS may 09 })
ENDOREZ: hydrophilic, good adptation to canal wall in presence of moisture so, reduces micro leakage
AH–26: very toxic when prepared. But after 24 hrs of placement has lowest toxicity among endodontic sealer. Reason for toxicity is release of small amount of FORMALDEHYDE.
AH plus: modified form of AH–26 .formaldehyde NOT added

- Lentulospirals are used for application of root canal sealer *(KCET 05)*
- Ca $(OH)_2$:

Was introduced in endodontics by HERMANN
Is used as intracanal medicament between appointments because of ANTIMICROBIAL property [Q]

- Medicated sealer:

The basic ingredient is ZnO but usually they contain other contraindicated ingredients like para–formaldehyde which is highly irritating to periapical tissues.
So, use of medicated sealer is controversial and NOT clinically recommended

- Ultracal:
- Commercially available, non settable Ca $(OH)_2$ based intracanal medicament.
- Three mix MP triple antibiotic paste:

Consists of Metronidazole + Minocycline + Ciprofloxacin	*(AIPG 12) { TRICK MMC }*
It is very effective in eliminating intra canal microbes	
Most important disadvantage is that minocycline causes discoloration of tooth	*(AIPG 12)*

- Cementum is An ideal apical seal after obturation *(AIPG 10, 07)*
- Best material for obturating root canal:
- GP with sealer

- While best technique is warm vertical condensation technique

Bowman introduced GP
Bowen introduced Bis GMA

- GP:

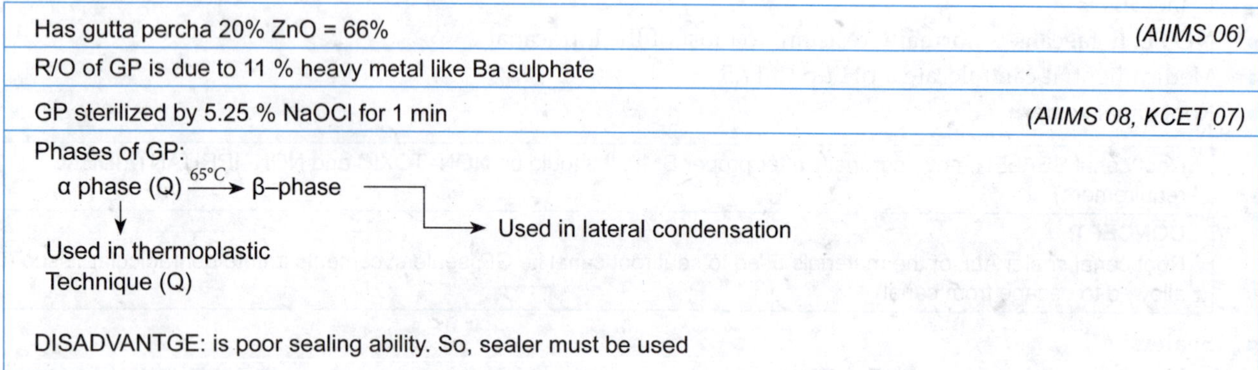

Has gutta percha 20% ZnO = 66%	(AIIMS 06)
R/O of GP is due to 11 % heavy metal like Ba sulphate	
GP sterilized by 5.25 % NaOCl for 1 min	(AIIMS 08, KCET 07)
Phases of GP: α phase (Q) —65°C→ β–phase → Used in lateral condensation; α phase ↓ Used in thermoplastic Technique (Q) DISADVANTGE: is poor sealing ability. So, sealer must be used	

- Protaper system:

S2 = 0 .20 mm

	DIAMETER	TAPER
F1	0.20 mm	0.07 mm
F2	0.25 mm	0.08 mm
F3	0.30 mm	0.09 mm

S2 = F_1 *(AIPG 10)*

- Lateral condensation technique:

Most commonly used but NOT best technique to obtain 3D seal (for this best technique is VERTICL compaction)

- Vertical condensation/Schilder's technique:

Causes vertical root fracture

- McSpadden compactor:

Flutes of McSpadden compactor are similar to flutes of H file in reverse	(COMEDK 05)
It is an OBTURATING instrument in VERTICAL compaction	(COMEDK 10)

- JS quickfill:

Mc Spadden compactor with GP Coated	(COMEDK 08)

- Endotec:

MARTIN developed it	
Combines best of lateral and vertical compaction technique	(COMEDK 08).
Device contains battery powered, heat controlled spreader .	

- High heat obturation technique:

Is OBTURA 2
Temperature reduces from 200 °C to 70 °C [Q]

- Thermo plasticized GP injection technique:

e.g. OBTURA 3 (cooling to temperature of 71 °C) (same for OBTURA 2) *(COMEDK 08)*
disadvantage: voids can be seen if vertical compaction not combined
Indication: Obturation for • Internal resorption • Perforation • Complex root anatomy (most important) • Open apex (obturation done with apical barrier)

- Thermafil is a SOLID core carrier (thermolpasticised GP technique) used for OBTURATION of root canal *(COMEDK 08)*
- Sectional method of obturation used for POST and CORE [Q]
- Chemically plasticized GP technique:

Chemical used is chloroform, xylol, eucalyptol
Disadvantage: shrinkage Poor apical and lateral seal So, not recommended

- Primary GP cone must fill the apical 3rd tightly *(COMEDK 05)*
- Ag points discovered for fine torturous canal (KCET 12, 11). no longer used due to corrosion [Q]
- Wrigly appearance of master cone is due to SHORT cone (AIPG 07) in the canal
- Concept: healing is better in under filled than overfilled canal
- RCT failure most common reason is inadequate obturation of main canal *(AIIMS 08)*
- Temporary filling materials:

Minimum depth = 3 mm *{ AIIMS nov 10, AIPG 09 }*
Optimal depth = 4 mm
ZnOE: most commonly used but prone to LEAKAGE
Cavit: ZnO + $CaSO_4$ + $ZnSO_4$ (hydrophilic nature, so, superior seal)
IRM: resin based ZnOE cement (also called KALZINOL) [Q]
TERM: UDMA containing resin

- Endodontic retreatment case:

Has poorer prognosis than original treatment *(PGI 06)*
Removal of GP in RE-treatment cases: • Files–for poorly condensed GP (hand instrument used) *(PGI 06)* • Rotatory instrument for removal of GP–in straight canal and when GP is well condensed (PGI) .new PROTAPER universal system was introduced consisting of D1 (to remove filling from coronal 3rd), D2 (to remove filling from middle 3rd), D3 (to remove filling from apical 3rd) • Solvents–chloroform most commonly used and most efficient. • Other solvents are–eucalyptol, xylitol
SILVER CONE removed with steiglitz pliers *(KCET 07)*

- Retrieval of broken instruments from root canal:

• Masseran kit *(KCET 05)*
• Brassler endo exter kit
• SIR (separated instrument retrieval)

LAST 5-YEAR QUESTIONS FROM THIS TOPIC

1. **A protaper F_2 series GP when cut 1 mm in apical position of canal, the diameter of the tip of GP point is:** *(AIIMS Nov 10, AIPG 09)*

Ans. 0.33 mm (Ref: cohen 8/e p256)

2. **When estimating working length using parallel technique radiograph, how much enlargement of image is allowed?** *(AIIMS Nov 10)*

Ans. 1 mm

3. **The most important criteria in using irrigating solution is** *(AIIMS May 10, Nov 11, KCET 07)*

Ans. Volume of irrigant (Ref: textbook of endodontics by grossman 12/e p264, 266, 270)

4. **After endodontic treatment, the apical foramen is closed due to deposition of:** *(AIIMS May 10)*

Ans. Cementum (Ref: INGLE 5/e p653)

5. **Alternate contact points along the shaft are seen in:** *(AIPG 10)*

Ans. Real world endo (Ref: endodontic topics 2005, 10, p176–178)
{NOTE: alternate cutting edge is present in RACE }

6. **The most important criteria while using irrigating solution is:** *(AIIMS nov 11, AIPG 10, 07)*

Ans. Volume of irrigant

7. **Primary/master cone of GP point used for obturation of root canals is defined as:** *(AIPG 12)*

Ans. Cone with snug fit (Ref: Endodontology by Bergenholtz p291)

8. **Which instruments can be used for flaring canals during endodontic retreatment?** *(PGI June 11)*

Ans. K–file (Ref: textbook of endodontics by Nisha garg 1/e p113 and INGLE 5/e p475)

9. **What is the taper of 20 number GT file?** *(PGI June 11)*

Ans. 0.06, 0.08, 0.10, .012 (Ref: textbook of endodontics by nisha garg 1/e p120)

10. **What is the recommended speed for rotatory NiTi instruments?** *(PGI June 11)*

Ans. 150–300 rpm (Ref: textbook of endodontics by nisha garg 1/e p120)

11. **A child comes with an avulsed tooth kept in dry enviorment for 1 hour. It is kept in sodium hypochloride solution for 10–15 minutes. What should be done next?** *(PGI June 11)*

Ans. Placed in 2% NaF for 20 minutes/in 2 % SnF_2 for 5 minutes

12. **Fall in alkalinity of $Ca(OH)_2$ when used as a root canal dressing starts at:** *(PGI June 10)*

Ans. 1 week (Ref: sturdvant's 4/e p128 -129)

13. **During cleaning and shaping in endodontic procedure, files are kept in which cleansing agent?** *(AIIMS May 12)*

Ans. Sodium hypochlorite (Ref: textbook of endodontics by Grossman 11/e p188–189)

14. **In Ingle's method of endodontic working length determination, safety allowance is for: (COMEDK 10)**

Ans. Possible image distortion/magnification (Ref: Ingle endodontics 5/e p514)

15. **Reference points in endodontics in posterior teeth are:** *(COMEDK 10)*

Ans. Cusp tip (Ref: Ingle endodontics 5/e p392)

BLEACHING

- Calcific Metmorphosis:

One of the cause of tooth discoloration
Characterized by rapid deposition of hard tissue in root canal following trauma
Tooth appears more " OPAQUE" due to tertiary dentine deposition

- Mcc–Inns solution:

Used for removal of " ENDEMIC–fluorosis"
Mc inn's technique: 5 parts 30% H_2O_2 + 5 parts 36 % HCl + 1 part diethylether This is micro abrasion technique
KROLL → "MICROABRASION technique → "18 % HCl *(PGI dec 10, COMEDK 08)*
Indication of microabrasion: Fluorosis stains/any stains–limited to depth not more than 0.2 to 0.3 mm

- Techniques to remove Intrinsic discoloration:

1. AI or DI is impossible to eliminate
2. For fluorosis microabrassion is done
3. For tetracycline stain NIGHTGAURD bleaching + In–office vital bleaching done

- Non Vital bleaching (Trick: Without Ticket)

A. Walking bleach = Na perborate + Superoxol (method of choice as requires less time as well as no special equipment required) NUTTING: gave combination of walking bleach i.e 30% H2O2 + Na perborate Combination of sodium perborate + water in walking bleach was given by Spasser WALKING bleach = home bleach
B Thermo catalytic method = 35 % H2O2 + heat Thermo catalytic technique given by STEWART
Indication for non vital bleaching: 1. Mild flourosis and tetracycline stain 2. In severe discoloration before giving veneer crown
Contraindication of non vital bleaching 1. Superficial stain 2. Carious tooth/resin restoration 3. Hypersensitive tooth 4. Children with large pulp 5. Exposed root surface 6. Pregnant/Lactating women
Some POINTS about WALKING BLEACH: *(AIIMS 06)* NON–vital IN–office bleaching procedures for endodontically treated teeth *(COMEDK 10)* Appointment is completed in 1 or 3 appointments Water/saline with sodium perborate powder is used to make paste It uses a mixture of sodium perborate and hydrogen peroxide The use of eugenol as temporary seal after the process is avoided
STEPS in intracoronal/NON–vital bleaching: Canal obturated with GP ↓ GP terminated 1 mm below CEJ In case of gingival recession GP is sealed 1mm below level of recession *(AIIMS may 12, nov 10, AIPG 09)* ↓ Seal orifice of canal with 1 mm intracoronal PROTECTIVE barrier over GP to prevent percolation of bleaching agent to apical area [Q]. Commonly used material is GIC, RMGIC, CAVIT, MT (superior)
NOTE: WALKING BLEACH: use of eugenol as temporary seal is avoided as composite is used as permanent restoration.

AFTER intra coronal bleaching: (NON–vital bleaching) 1. If the question is asked about doing esthetic restoration immediately, then " apply CATALSE" to the teeth immediately after bleaching (AIIMS nov 11) to eliminate the H2O2 residue and prevent it's radicular penetration. SIMPLY speaking catalase removes residual O2 . ALSO Na Ascorbate (derived from Vit. C) is powerful antioxidant useful for eliminating residual O2 following intracoronal bleaching 2. If Q is asked about best treatment planning after bleaching NOT mentioning about immediate requirement of esthetic restoration then mark the answer as "WAIT for 1 week " [Q]
Side effects related to NON VITAL bleaching: 1. External cervical resorption–if proper protective barrier is not given then it leads to diffusion of bleaching agent through dentinal tubule into periodontium. *(KCET 12, 11)* 2. Acute apical periodontitis–if canal is not properly obturated

- Vital bleaching:

Power bleach = 35 % H_2O_2 + HEAT (similar to thermo catalytic method. only difference is that power bleaching is done on VITAL teeth)
Night guard = 10 % carbamide peroxide (AIPG 12, KCET 07 ,KCET 06) (7 % urea + 3 % H2O2) [Q]. Also called as MATRIX bleaching
HAYWOOD and HAYMAN gave nightguard bleaching
Indication for vital bleaching: 1. Discoloration of pulp 2. Dentine discoloration *(COMEDK 13)*
Contraindication for vital bleaching: 1. Superficial enamel discoloration 2. Defective enamel formation 3. Severe dentine loss 4. Presence of cries 5. Discolored composite

LAST 5-YEAR QUESTIONS FROM THIS TOPIC

1. **After intracoronal bleaching if patient desires an immediate esthetic composite restoration, then before doing acid etching** *(AIIMS Nov 11)*

Ans. Rinse with catalase immediately (Ref: bleaching techniques in restorative dentistry by greenwall Lindap 162)

2. **Macroabrasion is:`** *(COMEDK 10)*

Ans. The removal of localized superficial white spots and other surface stains/defects (Ref: textbook of operative dentistry by Chandra 1/e p371)

TRAUMATOLOGY

- In 1° teeth fracture commonly occurs at 1–2 ½ years (when child starts walking)
- In 2° teeth fracture commonly occurs at 8–11 years
- Maxillary CENTRAL incisors are most prone to injury
- Number of radiographs recommended by IDT (international association of dental traumatology):

• 90° horizontal angle with central beam through tooth
• Occlusal view
• Lateral view from mesial/distal aspect of tooth

- Ellis fracture:

ELLIS and DEWEY class	EXTENT of fracture
Class 1	Enamel
Class 2	Enamel + dentine
Class 3	Enamel + dentine + pulp
Class 4	Non-vital tooth
Class 5	Avulsion
Class 6	Root fracture with/without Crown fracture
Class 7	Displacement of tooth without Fracture of crown/root
Class 8	Fracture of crown en mass
Class 9 *(KCET 12)*	DECIDUOUS tooth fracture

- Stunned pulp = Traumatized pulp which is not capable of positive response to tooth vitality tests for 6–8 weeks after injury *(AIPG 12)*
- If severe blow to a tooth occurs, then pupal death will occur regardless of treatment as all forces are transferred to pulp only.
- "Contusion" is due to blunt trauma of soft tissue:
- Concussion, subluxation and luxation:

Concussion	Subluxation	Luxation
No mobility/ displacement Only increased Sensitivity To percussion *(KCET 10)* ↓ Pulp vitality should Be checked after 10–12 days *(AIPG 07)*	No displacement but increased mobility *(KCET 11)*	BOTH mobility and displacement

- "Intrusive luxation":

1. Developing immature teeth with open apex → NO TREATMENT required → spontaneously re erupts
2. Permanent teeth with closed apex → orthodontic extrusion initiated as soon as possible, delaying no more than 2 to 3 weeks post trauma. as it cannot re erupt spontaneously

- Exrticultion = avulsion
- Media for transport of avulsed tooth:

IDEAL media to transport avulsed tooth is → in SOCKET
NATURAL media → MILK (low fat) (COMEDK 08) is the best media for storage of avulsed tooth
NOTE: HBSS (COMEDK 12) = milk > H_2O (for storage of avulsed tooth)
LEAST desirable medium for storing tooth is WATER *(AIIMS nov 11)*
CONCEPT: extra oral time is the most important factor for prognosis of avulsed tooth. if the time is < 20 min then prognosis is good

- Rx of avulsed tooth before reimplantation:

The most important factor for the treatment of avulsed teeth is extra oral time and not the presence/absence of debris

EXTRA ORAL TIME

- < 60 minutes
  - Closed apex → Rinse debris With water/ Saline. Replant gently
  - Open apex → Tooth soaked in doxycycline/minocycline For 5 minutes, debris rinsed off. tooth replanted
- > 60 minutes
  - Closed apex → PDL removed by placing in acid for 5 minute EMDOGAIN/ fluoride Applied on root Surface. Replanted
  - Open apex → Replanted in same manner as closed apex Only RCT By Apical approach

NOTE: in case of extraoral time > 60 minutes
2.4% NaF applied for 20 minutes
OR
2% SnF_2 applied for 5 minutes *(PGI 11 June)*

Prior to reimplantation, tooth is soaked in 3% citric acid to remove Pdl (AIPG 12) if extraoral time > 60 minutes .

- 5 Minutes in " Endodontics" (In avulsed tooth with extra oral Time > 60 Minutes):

CITRIC acid applied for 5 minutes
DOXYCYCLINE applied for 5 minutes
2 % SnF2 applied for 5 minutes

- Trumatology periods:

1. Avulsion → splint for 7–10 days/1-2 weeks
2. Root fracture → splint for 4–6 weeks (cervical 1/3rd root fracture splint for 4 months) *(AIIMS 09)*
3. Subluxation → splint for 2–3 weeks
4. Luxation → splint for 2–6 weeks
5. Fractured root gives negative EPT for 6–8 weeks
6. Pulp vitality in case of trauma should be rechecked after 2 weeks and again after 1 month
7. Following trauma blood flow returns to normal in may be as long as 9 months *(COMEDK 11)*

- Root resorption:

Inflammatory Resorption	Replacement Resorption
Failure of re–implantation (main reason Q	Tooth becomes " ANKYLOSED " [Q]
	Success of re–implantation [Q]

- Dental injury and observation period prior to orthodontic tooth movement:

Type of dental injury	Observation period prior to orthodontic tooth movement
1. Crown and crown/root fracture without/with pulpal involvement 2. Concussion/subluxation/extrusion/lateral luxation (minor injury)	3 Months *(AIPG 12)*

1. Root fracture (AIPG 12) 2. Severe lateral luxation 3. Intrusion 4. Avulsion and replantation	1 year if no ankylosis occurs
Immature traumatized teeth	Await for radiographic sign of continued root development. observe for 6 months, 1 year and 2 year
Auto transplanted teeth	3–9 months, i.e. after pdl healing

LAST 5-YEAR QUESTIONS FROM THIS TOPIC

1. In the root fracture of the apical 1/3rd of the permanent anterior teeth, the teeth usually: *(AIIMS Nov 10, 08)*

Ans. Remain in function and are vital (Ref: Q-75 NDBE 1978 endodontology and periodontics) in an avulsed tooth, maximum revascularization will occur with the treatment of? *(AIIMS May 10)*

OR

2. In avulsion the following increases success rate: *(AIPG 10, 07)*

Ans. Doxycyline (Ref: Cohen 8/e p637)

3. The radiograph of a traumatized tooth is necessary to: *(AIIMS Nov 09)*

a. Assess the stage of root development
b. Determine the presence/absence of root fracture
c. Have a base from which comparrision can be made with future radiographs
d. All of the above

Ans. d (Ref: grossman. textbook of endodontics 12/e p362)

4. Which of the following causes most damage to the protective layer of the tooth? *(AIIMS May 09)*

Ans. Intrusion

5. An 8 year old child reports with avulsion of central incisors due to trauma 20 minutes back. on inspection the teeth are contaminated with debris. What should be done? *(AIPG 11, AIIMS Nov 11)*

Ans. Clean the root surface with saline and reimplant

6. The greatest frequency of pulpal necrosis is encountered in the following type of luxation injury of permanent anterior teeth: *(KCET 12)*

Ans. Intrusion

7. Enamel infarction can be detected by: *(KCET 12)*

Ans. Fiber optic light source

8. Which test is NOT done immediately after trauma? *(PGI Dec 12)*

Ans. Vitality test

9. 1 hr back a child comes with ELLIS class 3 # with small pulpal exposure .trearment of choice is: *(PGI Dec 12)*

Ans. DPC

ENDODONTIC SURGERY AND MISCELLANEOUS

- Endodontic surgery:
  Because of inaccessibility endodontic surgery should be avoided on lingual surface of molars
- Antibiotic of choice in endodontic surgery:

Penicillin is drug of choice in endodontic surgery
If allergic to penicillin give AZITHROMYCIN

- Flaps:

Commonest cause of tearing of flap during surgery is mishandling of tissues during retraction *(AIPG 07, KCET 06)*
To prevent dehydration of periosteal surface of flap, it should be irrigated frequently with saline (0.9 % NaCl) not with water as it is hypotonic
PARTIAL thickness flap more prone for dehydration. so, require more irrigation
SEMILUNAR flap: Advantage: minimal bone damage High healing potential Disadvantage: heals with scar formation

- TEV–DEK suture:

"Polyester suture with Teflon coating ". Coating provides minimum friction, allowing suture to pass easily through the most friable tissue.
Originally developed for heart transplantation.
Non stick surface, hence less bacterial adhesion and faster healing. also there is reduced dead space in the braided form.
Removal–minimum after 48 hrs and maximum 96 hrs i.e 48–96 hrs *(AIPG 11 ,09)*

- Prolene:

Low coefficient of friction (least adherent to tissue) *(AIPG 12)*
Tissue reactivity is extremely low (less thrombogenic, used in vascular and plastic surgery

- Plastic suture: very good tensile strength
- One visit RCT:

Indications: In patient with heart valve as they require repeated regimen of prophylactic antibiotic .
• **CONTRINDICTION of ONE visit RCT:** – Painful, necrotic tooth with no sinus tract [Q] – Teeth with severe anatomic anomalies (PGI 08) – Asymptomatic non vital molars with periapical radiolucency and no sinus tract . – Patient who have apical periodontitis and severe pain on percussion – Most–retreatment

- Post and core → 4 mm of GP left
- Apicoectomy → 3 mm apical area cut *(COMEDK 05)*
- Endodontic implants:

Is metalic extension of root with the objective of increasing root to crown ratio.
Thus indicated in case of periodontally weakened tooth, tooth with short root/resorption of root apex. *(COMEDK 07)*

- Laser:

3. Characteristics are – Monochromatism – Collimation – Coherence
LASER used in WATERLASE system (hydrokinetic technology)  YSGG laser

- CPR instruments: They are non surgical endodontic ULTRASONIC instruments. types:

CPR 1: (medium to high intensity) used to remove retained post and core and crown and bridge.
CPR 2: (medium to high intensity) used to remove bulk of restoration and dentine islands (AIPG 10), PULP stones [Q]
CPR 3–8: low intensity. used for removal of broken instruments from canal

- Chraley Hose: *(KCET 09)*

MYOSPASM of muscle due to overstretching, which is already strained due to sustained mouth opening during RCT.

LAST 5-YEAR QUESTIONS FROM THIS TOPIC

1. **For making antirotational groove, the minimum offset of the edge from the bur axis should not be greater than:** *(AIIMS Nov 09)*

Ans. 2 mm (Ref: rosensteil 3/e p283, 323, 329, 331, 335)

2. **Root end filling material of choice is:** *(AIPG 10, 07)*

Ans. MTA (Ref: cohen 9/e p756–760)

3. **Cardiac pain may be transmitted to the jaw due to overlapping of:** *(KCET 11, 12)*

Ans. 5th cranial nerve, 3rd cranial nerve and 1st thoracic nerve (according to the key given in exam)

4. **In molecular biological methods in endodontic the process of annealing the complementary bases of two single stranded DNA is known as:** *(KCET 09)*

Ans. DNA–DNA hybridization

CHAPTER 5

Pedodontics

Topic

- Caries and Restorative Dentistry
- Child Psychology
- Miscellaneous

CARIES AND RESTORATIVE DENTISTRY

- CAT in pedodontics stands for caries risk assessment tool

Nursing caries	Rampant caries
• ECC (term given by Davies)	• 10/more lesions/year (Rapid appearance of New lesion) *(KCET 10)*
• It is a specific form of rampant caries	• Early pulpal involvement of teeth which are immune to decay (lower incisors are involved)
• Occurs in 71 months of age/younger	
• A specific pattern of involvement is seen the maxillary is followed by molars are involved. Significantly mandibular is are not involved.	• Proximal surface of lower anterior teeth and development of cervical type of caries is very characteristic *(PGI 05)*

Note: Abnormal feeding habits (Major reason)

- Dental caries in child and Adolescent:

S. mutan s → major and most virulent of caries producing organism transmitted from mother to infant.

- **MDSMD (Maternally derived streptococcus mutans disease):**

Has been recently used to describe childhood caries
Kissing–main method of transmission

- **Maximum ↑se in number of micro-organism in mouth is seen at:**

Eruption of deciduous teeth as it provides virgin environment for microorganism.

- Window of Infectivity:

1st – 19-13 Month with eruption of 1° teeth
2nd – 6-12 year c eruption of 2° teeth

- Surface of molar susceptible to dental caries:

Occlusal–all expect 1st 1° molar (Distal surface is involved)
Note: on proximal surface below contact point is involved.

- Chronic peraipical infection in 1° Molar is Ist manifested as furcation involvement
- Most common cause for gingival fistula is chronic apical lesion

Note: Fistula → is a chronic condition
Sinus → is an acute condition

- Laser Doppler flowmetry:

"Promising pulp vitality tests for young children"
Vital teeth show regular signal

- Laser used for Devitalization Pulpotomy "Nd-YAGG"

• Class II on 1° Molar should be more wide B–L [Q] to place gingival margin in self cleansable area (This is because 1° teeth have broad point contact)
• Due to "Cervical constriction" gingival wall should not be too gingival (in 1° teeth)
• enamel rods are directed occulsally in 1° molar → so, no need of beveling gingival seat
• In 1° Molar MB pulp horn is too high → avoid going too deep
• Pulpal infection → 1° teeth → earliest change → furcation involvement → 2° teeth → earliest change → widening of pdl

- Rubber dam thickness:

Children → 5" x5"
Adult → 6" x 6"

- Direct pulp capping vs Pulpotomy:

Direct pulp capping	**Pulpotomy**
• Exposure of pulp during cavity preparation traumatic exposure in a clear field i.e. Non-infected case	• Carious pulpal exposure, i.e. infected case.

- In DCM:

$Ca(OH)_2$ should be in direct contact
So, $Ca(OH)_2$ – followed by varnish over entire cavity – followed by base

- Concept:

• "Sealants" can be applied in all individuals in both fluoridated and Non-fluoridated areas. Expanding the use of pit and fissure sealents significantly ces the incidence of caries compared to fluoride and other preventive measure.
• Pulp mummification: – "Devitalization Pulpotomy" contains p-formaldehyde → Causes devitalization → Fixes the entire coronal and radicular pulp tissue.

- Root canal filling material for 1° teeth:

• KRI paste → Iodoform (80%) + Camphor + p-chlorophenol + methol + ZNO
Advantage → Resorbs along with root + less irritating

- Margin of stainless steel → 0.5 to 1 mm subgingival
- Stainless steel crown: discovered by Brearly
- **Composition of stainless steel crown:**

• Austentic type → Rocky mountain and Unitek Fe – 70%, Ni – 10%
• Ni based crown → "3M crown" Fe – 10% [Q] Ni = 70%

- Carisoly and caridex:

both contain NaOCl at pH 11
Carisolv has 0.5% NaOCl

- Esthetic crown:

• Poly carbonate crown: can be easily adjusted
• Strip crown: most commonly used crowns in pediatric practice (KCET 10)
• Pedo jacket
• Fuks crown
• New millennium crown – very expensive + brittle
• Nusmile crown: durability + full coverage
• Cheng crowns: pure resin facing less time consuming + single visit required

- Sugar substitute:

Caloric → Xylitol/sorbitol
Non-caloric → Saccharin/Aspartame → (AIPG 04)

- Gingivitis in children is peak between 6-7 years (at puberty)

• Rx for rampant caries: child should completely restrict sugar intake for 21 days
• Rx for caries susceptible individual: Reduced sugar intake to meal times → "Not in between"

- M-B pulp horn of 1° First molar → Largest in both maxillary and mandibular teeth → Commonly exposed during cavity preparation

LAST 5-YEAR QUESTIONS FROM THIS TOPIC

1. **In a 6 year old child, caries status can be judged by:** *(AIIMS Nov. 10)*

Ans. Past caries experience (Ref: Bowen and tabak, cariology for the nineties)

2. **In stainless steel crown on deciduous molar with overhanging margins, gingival pain and inflammation occurs due to:** *(AIPG 12)*

Ans. Plaque retention (Ref: Pedodontics by Arthi Rao, 2008, p225)

3. **Radiographically, chronic pulpal infection of 1° molars is noted as** *(AIIMS May 12, AIPG 11, 09)*

Ans. Changes in furcation area (Ref: Shobha tendon I/e p333)

4. **Most common caries seen in 1° Ist M.**

Ans. Proximal surface below the contact (Ref: Pediatric dentistry by Koch and poulsen 2/e) *(AIPG 11)*

5. **"High viscosity saliva may lead to increased caries in children" this statement is:**

Ans. Really true *(AIPG 11)*

6. Most common cause of gingivitis in children below 5 yrs of age:

Ans. Local irritants *(AIPG 10)*

7. The "Window of infectivity" period in which there is growth of microorganisms in mouth of a newborn? *(PGI June 11, COMEDK 11)*

Ans. 19-33 months (Ry: Shobha Tandon 2/e p196)

8. On examining of a 9 year old child, caries prevalence will mostly be found in *(PG Dec 10)*

Ans. Occlusal surface of Ist M (Ref: Shobha Tandon 1/e p94)

9. Obturation of deciduous tooth can be done with:

Ans. Iodoform paste

10. Prophylactic odontomy was proposed by: *(KCET 09, 12)*

Ans. Hyatt

11. The valuable test for evaluating caries activity in very young children is: *(KCET 10)*

Ans. Swab test

12. Which pulp horn is most likely to be exposed during cavity preparation on 1° molars? *(KCET 10, PGI 2012)*

Ans. MB of Ist M

13. Occult disease refers to disease that *(COMEDK 11)*

Ans. Presents no clinical sign/symptom (Ref: White and pharoh 5/e p267)

14. A 4 year old presents with labio lingual caries affecting only maxillary incisors and involving molars Case report: *(COMEDK 12)*

a. The diagnosis would be:

Ans. Type II ECC

b. The most probable cause of such condition is:

Ans. Consumption of cariogenic food

c. The number of S. mutans colony forming units (CFU) per unit of saliva will be:

Ans. > 10,00,000

CHILD PSYCHOLOGY

- Fear of Separation from parents → 2–3 (Preschool going children)
- Fear:

• Innate → without stimuli/previous experience
• Subjective → most difficult to overcome [Q] transmitted from friends, family members.
• Objective → Fear due to one's own experience

- Cases:

• A child patient demonstrates resistance in dental office → Anxiety [Q]
• A 4 year old child who is aggressive in his behavior in dental stress condition → Fear Reaction (NBDE Q)
• A 6 year old demonstrating fear in dentistry → Subjective fear [Q]
• Basic fear of 2 year old during Ist dental visit to dentist is → fear of separation from parents [Q]

- Fear Management:

• Best method of communicating with a fearful deaf child → Euphemisms/word substitutes/reframing [Q]
• Best way to help a frightened child to overcome his fear → Identification of his fear [Q]
• Effective way of fear management: – Reconditioning – Explanation – Reassurances

- Classification of child psychology theories:

Psychodynamic theory	Behavioral theory
• Psychosexual/psychoanalytic theory → Sigmund Freud	• Hierarchy of needs → Masler
• Psychosocial theory → Eric Erickson	• Social learning theory → Bandura
• Cognitive theory → Jean piaget	• Classical conditioning → Pavlov
	• Operant conditioning → skinner

- Barbiturates may cause paradoxical hyper excitability rather than sedation in some children.
- Frankel's behavior rating scale:

• Definitely negative (–) refuses Rx cries forcefully
• Negative (–) Reluctant to accept Rx [Q]
• Positive (+) Accepts treatment but may become unco-operative
• Definitely positive (++) Good rapport with dentist

TSD (tell show do) → Addleson
Modeling → Bandura
Desensitization → Joseph Wolpe
Home → Jordan
Dental home concept → Arthur Nowak

- Maternal behavior vs child's behavior

Maternal behavior	Child's behavior
• Over protective	• Sky, submissive
• Over indulgent	• Aggressive, demanding shows temper tantrum
• Authorative	• Evasive and dawdling
• Rejecting	• Aggressive, disobedient
• Under affectionate	• Well behavior • cries easily

• Newborn/neonate → birth to 28 days
• Infancy → till 1 year
• Toddler → 1-3 year
• Preschool going → 3-6 years [Q]

- **Behavior shaping:**

Desensitisation/TSD	Modelling	Contigency management
Indicated in: • child > 3 years [Q] • fearful child [Q] • Ist visit [Q]	use live models filmed models posters audio visual aids	Re – inforcement

- **Phobia:** Fear of a single object:

• Acrophobia → height
• Xenophobia → stranger (PGI 12)
• Claustrophobia → closed space, e.g.: dental clinic [Q]
• Agoraphobia → open space
• Anthrophobia → people

- Wrights classification of child behavior:

• Hysterical/uncontrolled → show temper tantrums → e.g. pre-school going children on their Ist dental visit
• Defiant/Obstinate → spoilt/stubborn → siren like cry
• Timid/shy
• Stoic → physically abused child → accept any Rx without facial expression
• Whining type: → complaining type
• Tense co-operative → Borderline between negative and positive.

- Home + physical restraints = aversive conditioning
- Jean Piagets's cognitive theory stages:

• Sensorimotor → 0 to 2 years
• Pre-operational → 2 to 6 years [Q] → symbolizes
• Concrete operational → 7 to 11 years [Q]
• Formal operational → 11 to 15 years – Invisible audience – Personal fable

- Dosage of midazolam in children:

ORAL	IM
0.25 to 1 mg/kg	0.1 to 0.15 mg/kg

- **IQ level classification:**

IQ range	Grade
> 140	very superior
129–139	Superior
110–119	High average
90–109	Average
80–89	Low average
70–79 (Comedk 08)	Borderline impaired
52–68	Mild retarded

36–51	Moderate retarded → can be trained to perform self help skills
20–35	Severe retarded
<19	Profound retarded → require custodial care

- Terrible "TWO" = Pre-cooperative stage [Q] → Separation fear
- Cornerstone of behavior management: TSD
- Euphemism:

• Raincoat → Rubber dam [Q]
• Pudding → alginate
• Whistle → High speed aerator (AIPG COMEDK 09)
• Motorcycle → low speed
• Tooth paint → sealant
• Vacuum cleaner → suction
• Cavity fighter → topical fluoride
• Statues → study models

- Freduian stages:

Oral → 1–2 yrs
Anal → 2–3 yrs
Phallic (Oedepus and electra complex) → 3-5 yrs [Q]
Latency → Personality and skill development (PGI 12) + mixed dentition phase genital

- > 3 yrs Child → TSD HOME

LAST 5-YEAR QUESTIONS FROM THIS TOPIC

1. **In a 6 year old child, fear of dentistry is due to:** *(AIIMS May 10)*

Ans. Subjective fear

2. **Retraining approach in a pediatric patient, all are true, Except:** *(AIPG 12)*
   a. Avoidance
   b. De-emphasis and substitution
   c. Distraction
   d. Discrimination

Ans. d

3. **A papoose board is used for immobilization of:** *(KCET 09)*

Ans. Whole body

4. **Behavior modification includes all of the following except:** *(KCET 09)*
   a. TSD
   b. Desensitization
   c. Modeling
   d. Home

Ans. d

5. **Mentally retarded child will have an intelligence quotient (IQ) in the range:** *(KCET 09)*

Ans. 69 and below

6. **According to American association of mental Deficiency classification scheme, IQ range of 36-51 is:**

Ans. Moderate (Ref: Shobha Tandon 1/e p538) *(PG June 09)*

7. **Which of the following extremes of parental behavior were manifested either in extreme Dominance/ Indulgence?** *(COMEDK 09)*

Ans. Overprotection (Ref: Shoba Tandon pedodontics 1/e p14)

8. **Fear of strangers and fear of separation from parents for the children will be diminished by** *(COMEDK 10)*

Ans. 3rd birthday (Ref: Pinkham JR pediatric dentistry: Infancy through adolescence 3/e)

9. **A "Parent" asks the dentist, 'Is the treatment necessary?' after initial examination and explanation about treatment required. The behavior of parent is termed as?** *(COMEDK11)*

Ans. Hostile (Ref: McDonal 5/e p46)

MISCELLANEOUS

- Route of sedation:

Most common route of sedation – inhalation in adult and children
Oral route is most easy and used for premedication in behavior management
Subdermal – route is not used for premedication in children
2nd common route in → Adult → i.v.
→ children → submucosal

- Entonox:

50% N_2O + 50% O_2
On conscious sedation generally used concentration is 65% N_2O + 35% O_2

- Dietary instructions in case of conscious sedation:

(1) Clear liquid→ stopped up to hrs [Q] before the procedure.
(2) No milk/solid → Reasons: "Vomiting" during/immediately after a sedative procedures

- Child tooth brush compared to adult:

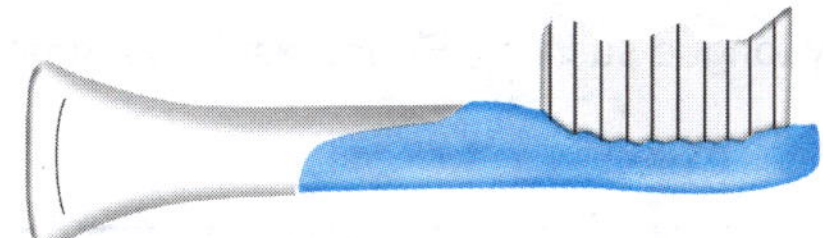

Fig. 5.1: Smaller head size of brush

Bristles are soft bristles as in Adult.
Rounded bristle end is preferred.

- Flossing is considered in fully erupted permanent dentition
- But Tooth brushing should be initiated with the eruption of 1st tooth
- Brushing technique best for young children/mixed dentition period/ young Adult is FONES
- Leukemia is seen in Down (High Risk), Kleinefilter but not in "Turners"

- Natal Teeth:

seen in Ellis-van-Creveld/ chondroectodermal dysplasia, Sotos syndrome, cleft plate, Pierre Robin, Pachonychia congenital
Not seen in VAN der woud syndrome *(AIIMS 11)*
Natal teeth, if possible retain it because of importance of growth and uncomplicated eruption of adjacent teeth.
90% of precociously erupted teeth are deciduous (1° teeth) out of which 85% are mandibular incisors

- **Rate of Eruption:**

During rapid emergence (time of gingival emergence) → 1-10 μ /day
to reach occlusal place → 75 μ/day

- F– absorption takes place mainly in GIT (Stomach) *(NEET 13)*

F absorption α 1/(pH of stomach) (greater in acidic pH)
"F in bones" → greater concentration in cancellous bone
F in any form is C/I in chronic renal failure

- Porter's appliance: [Q]

"Soldered W-lingual arch"
it's a reminder appliance used in children with thumb sucking habit.

- Gene:

HOX → patterning of limbs e.x- polysyndactyly
SSH → organogenesis
MSX→ Homebox gene plays an important role in tooth development. Lack of MSX results in arrest of tooth development in Bud state.

- Bilabials:

are sound made with compression of lips
e.g. → b/p/m are 1st to be mastered by child
Fluid sounds that are produced by tongue such as /R/ are last to be mastered.

- Speech development:

Speech delay till → 24 month
Speech retarded till → 36 month

- By what age child can sit without support → 6 month [Q]
- Approximate age be which child begins to walk without support → 12 month – 15 months
- Reflex:

Monro/Startle reflex disappears by 3-4 months [Q]
Rooting reflex disappears by 7-8 months

- Number of fontaneles present at birth: '6'

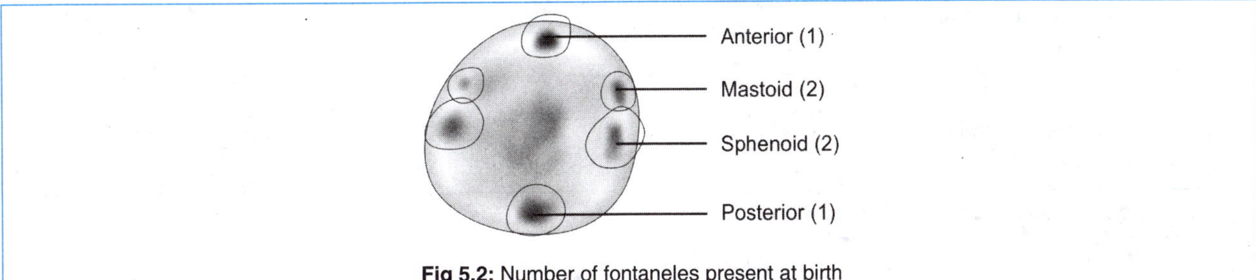

Fig 5.2: Number of fontaneles present at birth

- Interdental spacing in deciduous dentition:

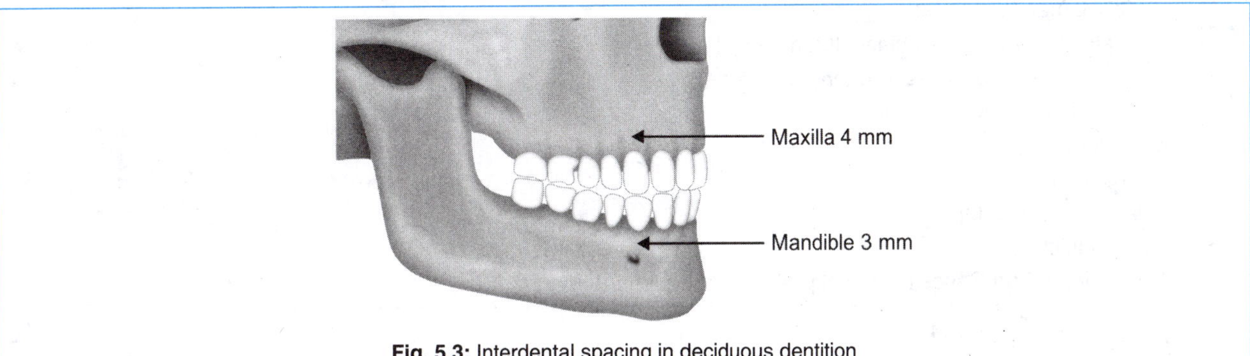

Fig. 5.3: Interdental spacing in deciduous dentition

- Growth spurt:

Time of greatest influence of environment or heredity on organ.

- Autism/Kanner's/Asperger's syndrome:

Serious physical disorder of early childhood, lack of mental and emotional development.
Lack of attachment and response to parents and other human beings.
Lack of speech and language development, temper tantrums
Motor development is defective while sensory is intact.
They have parrot like repetitive speech.

- In cleft palate patient, before grafting expand the arch.
- Cerebral palsy:

Non progressive disorder features → persistence of certain Neonatal reflex, pdl problems, caries, malocclusion, bruxism, trauma.
Types: • **Spasticity:** most common sudden violent involuntary contraction of muscles with marked hyper tonicity. • **Athetosis:** slow worm like purposeless involuntary muscle contraction [Q] Basal Ganglia involved. • Ataxia • Rigidity
Spastic cerebral palsy patient presents with spastic tongue thrust, constricted mandible and maxillary arches → class II div 2 malocclusion (75% cases) → usually with a U/L – crossbite Excessive drooling of saliva and difficulty in swallowing.

- Down's syndrome:

1° defect → extra chromosome present given by Jane, Trupin, Gautier
→ Head: Brachycephalic [Q] Large anterior fontanelle [Q] Open sutures
→ Eyes: Upward (Mongoloid) slant [Q]
→ Muscles: Hypotonic + hyper mobility [Q]
→ IQ: 25-50
→ ORAL manifestations: Hypoplasia of maxilla → class III tendency [Q] Macroglossia Scrotal/ fissured tongue Anterior + posterior cross bite Microdontia, conical teeth delayed eruption [Q] periodontitis **Note:** Other than Caries all dental problems are present [Q]

- Dentitia tarda → related eruption of 1° teeth
- Dentitia precox → precocious dentition
- **Rigafede disease:**

Ulceration of ventral surface of tongue due to natal/neonatal teeth.

Erythroblastosis foetalis: Blue green color 1° teeth only affected staining due to haemolysis of RBC → Bilirubin + biliverdin formed ↓ deposited in dentine of teeth ↓ Rh hump seen
(2) **Tetracycline stain:** Yellow/Yellow brown/segmentation of dentine. Teeth fluoresce Yellow under UV light [Q]
(3) Cystic fibrosis: due to tetracycline used in Rx of this disease
(4) Porphyria: purplish brown teeth red urine hypersensitivity to light

- **"Intrusive injury"**

After intrusive injury tooth re-erupts in 6 months (FULLY ERUPT) and they often re-erupt within 3-4 weeks after injury.

- Acid etch composite is the emergency Rx of choice in case of traumatic injury of tooth.
- Oblique ridge: Extend between DB to ML cusp (of maxillary Ist Molar)

- Features of 1° Dentition:

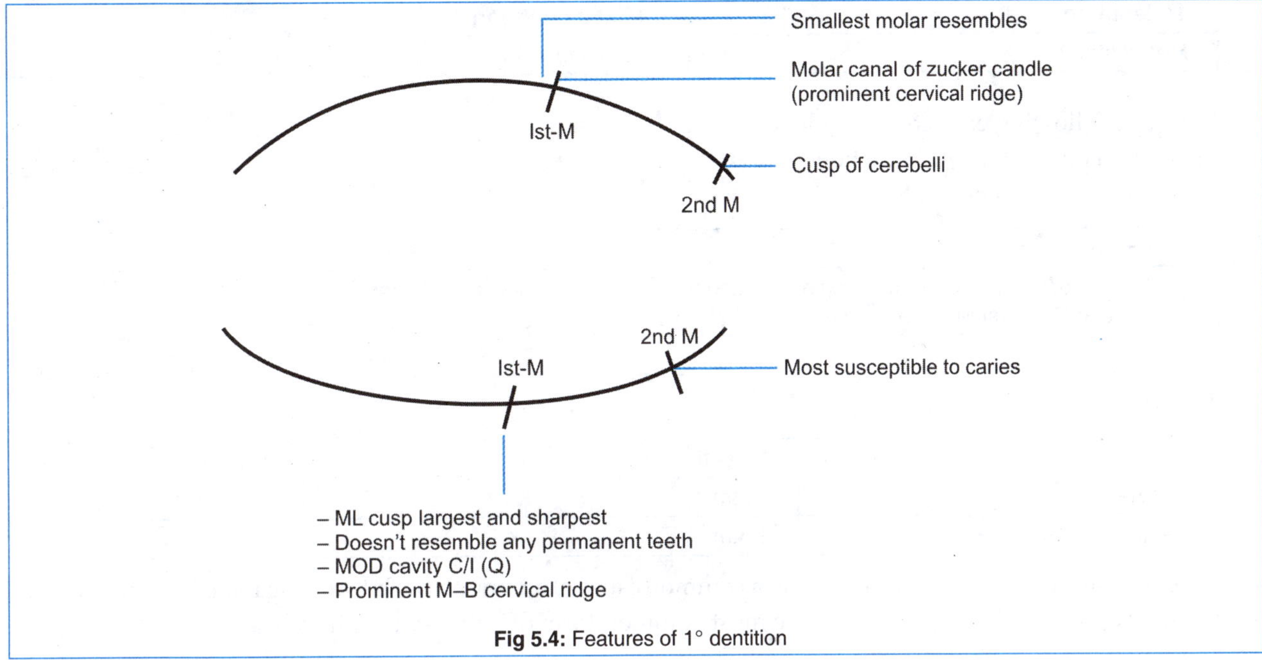

Fig 5.4: Features of 1° dentition

- Successional teeth → 2° teeth having 1° predecessor
- Accessional teeth → 2° teeth having NO 1° predecessor
- Teeth usually erupt when ½ to ¾th of root completed (Boucher MCQ) teeth usually erupt when ¾th of root completed (Profit)

  It takes 2 to 3 years for root to be completed after eruption of tooth (Profit)
- Minimum number of lobes for 2° teeth – 4
- Minimum number of lobes for development of 1° incisors → 1
- 2° cementum is characteristically Absent in 1° teeth (Present only in 2° teeth)
- Alveolar atrophy is rare in 1° teeth but present in 2° teeth.
- Metabolic disorder causing mental retardation:

PKU	Galactosemia
	→ Disorder of galactose metabolism
	→ Leads to galacitol accumulation in lens
	→ Results in cataract

- Fusion of mandibular symphysis: at 18 month
- Ist book on child dentistry → Hurlock [Q] father of pedodontics → Robert Bunan
- Father of pedodontics in INDIA → Dr B.R. Vaclier
- Thixotropic property → present in APF gel

- Normally:

1° dentition	Mixed dentition
Mesial step found	Flush terminal found

- Bone loss following extraction is more during Ist 6 months
- Black stain on tooth is due to actionomyces
- Number of developmental lobes:

Permanent teeth	1° teeth
All 2° teeth develop from 4 lobes except 3 cusped mandibular PM & Ist M (it developes from 5 lobes)	1° incisors = 1 lobe
	1° 2nd M = 5 lobes

- **Thickness of:**

	1° teeth	2° teeth
Enamel	1 mm	2-3 mm
Dentine	1 mm	2 mm

- Over retained anterior 1° teeth are the most common cause of anterior cross bite during mixed dentition period [Q]
- Petitmal epilepsy/absence seizure is the most common form of epilepsy in children.

LAST 5-YEAR QUESTIONS FROM THIS TOPIC

1. **All of the following syndromes are associated with natal teeth, except:** *(AIIMS May 11)*
   a. CL
   b. Van der woude syndrome
   c. Ellis-van creveld syndrome
   d. Sotos syndrome

Ans. b (Ref: Walker pediatric gastro intestinal disease pathophysiology, diagnosis vol 1.)

2. **A mother is worried about green stains on recently erupted upper anterior teeth of her child, which do not get removed after tooth brushing, these stains are due to:**

Ans. Chromogenic bacteria *(AIIMS Nov. 10, AIPE 11)*

3. **Which of the following is true about calcification of teeth?** *(AIIMS Nov. 10)*

Ans. Calcification of 1° teeth is almost complete at the time of birth (Ref: wheeler's DA 8/e p51)

4. **The seizures with no aura, no tonic/clonic phase that occurs a symptomatic in children with several times in a day is:** *(AIIMS May 10)*

Ans. Petit mal epilepsy/Absence seizure (Ref: Harrison 15/e p235)

5. **The most common cause of # of the root tip of 1° molar during extraction is:** *(AIIMS Nov. 09)*

Ans. Root resorption between the apex (Ref: Damle pediatric dentistry 3/e p178-80)

6. **Fluoride absorption in child takes place mainly in:** *(AIIMS Nov. 09)*

Ans. Intestine (Ref: Damle pediatric dentistry 3/e p259-60)

7. **Which one of the following is a space maintainer?**

Ans. Willet's appliance (Ref: Tandon textbook of pedodonties 2/e p459) *(AIIMS May 09)*

8. **All of the following are contraindications of serial extraction, except** *(AIIMS May 09)*
   a. Open bite
   b. Flaring of anteriors
   c. Severe space deficiency greater than 10 mm

d. Nasal stenosis

Ans. c. (Ref: Tandon Text book of orthodontics 2/e p475)

9. Children with thumb sucking habit have:

Ans. A long face, convex profile. (Ref: Tandon textbook of pedodontics 2/e p500)

(AIIMS May 09, NEET -13)

10. All of the following are considered normal variations of TMJ function in a child Except: *(AIPG 12)*

a. Occlusal wear
b. TMJ pain with no clinical signs and symptoms
c. joint sounds
d. Limitation/deviation of mouth opening

Ans. b

11. A 3 year and 7 month old child with history of traumatic intrusion of 51-IOPA reveals fore shortening. The Rx is: *(AIPG 12)*

Ans. Wait and watch

12. True about knee to knee position when applied to child management: *(AIPG 12)*

a. It is a practical method for babies upto 18 month
b. Operator secures child's hands while mother steadies the child's head.
c. Accompanied with gloved finger and plastic sleeved pen light/torch.
d. Can be used at home for brushing teeth of infant

Ans. b (Ref: Pediatric dentistry by mutur p171)

13. An 8 year old child with large front teeth having jagged margins seeks consultation. What is the treatment plan:

Ans. Assure and send him back *(AIPG 11, 09)*

14. A young child of 7 years age is seen with indurate ulcers, lyphadenopathy and fever the likely treatment is: *(AIPG 11, 09)*

Ans. Symptomatic treatment

15. A 6 year old patient reports with greenish blue swelling distal to deciduous 2nd molar. Treatment would be:

Ans. No treatment, only observation

16. An 8 year old HIV positive child reports with periapical abscess of deciduous mandibular Ist molar which needs to be extracted, what procedure should the dentist follow:

Ans. Send patient for CD4 measurement and take physician consent before treatment *(AIPG 10)*

17. In a child, failure of IAN block is caused by: *(AIPG 09)*

Ans. Angle (Position) of needle (Ref: Mcdonald 8/e p273)

18. Total period of adolescence in boys is:

Ans. 5 years (Ref: Essential pediatrics by OP Ghai 6/e p66) *(PG Dec 11)*

19. H_2O is not used as a storage medium for avulsed tooth because: *(PG June 11)*

Ans. It is hypotonic and causes rapid cell lysis (Ref: Shobha tendon 2/e p596)

20. Objective sign of IAN is checked in:

Ans. Same side U/L from midline till molar *(PG June 11, Dec. 12)*

21. Which type of injury is last common in children?

Ans. Complicated crown fracture (Ref: Mc Donald pedodontics 8/e p479-480, 485-486)

22. The distal shoe appliance is used: *(KCET 09)*

Ans. When 2nd primary molar is lost and Ist permanent molar has not erupted.

23. The reasons for maxillary permanent canine impaction could be all except: *(KCET 09)*

a. Long development period
b. Dubious course in eruption

c. Occupies several developmental positions in succession
d. A symmetrical development

Ans. d

24. Eruption of Ist permanent molar causes: *(KCET 09)*

Ans. Early mesial shift

25. According to Ellis and Davey classification a fracture of 51 involving dentine and associated loss of vitality is classified as:

Ans. Type 9 *(KCET 09, 12)*

26. Recently added in the centre of pediatric treatment triangle is: *(KCET 09)*

Ans. Society (Ref: Medonalld 7/e p34)

27. The best alternative storage medium for avulsed teeth in case culture media are not available is: *(KCET 09)*

Ans. Milk (Ref: Medonald 7/e p488)

28. Percentage of APF used is: *(KCET - 09)*

Ans. 1.23%

29. Which of the following is an indication for serial extraction? *(COMEDK 09)*

Ans: Class I with severe mandibular anterior crowding.

30. Pacifier Sucking is an, e.g. of: *(COMEDK 09)*

Ans. Non-nutritive sucking (Ref: Shobha tendon 1/e p429)

31. For a 3 year old child, a removable space maintainer is fabricated, what is the biggest disadvantage of this appliance? *(COMEDK 09)*

Ans. Child may not tolerate wearing.

32. "Guidance of Eruption" is another term for:

Ans. Serial extraction (Ref: Pinkham pedodontics 2/e p340) *(COMEDK 09)*

33. Mayne space maintainer represents which of the following type of space maintainers? *(COMEDK 09)*

Ans. Non-functional

34. Which of the following is true about thermal and electric pulp tests after trauma? *(COMEDK 09)*

Ans. It may take up to 9 months for normal blood flow to return *(Ref: Cohen 9/e p612)*

35. Which medium of storage for avulsed tooth is best for prolonged extra oral periods? *(COMEDK 10)*

Ans. HBSS

36. The fears that are produced by direct physical stimulation of the sense organs are: *(COMEDK 10)*

Ans. Objective fear

37. The principle that 'The stimulus must be altered to elicit a change in the response' is applied in: *(COMEDK 10)*

Ans. Retraining (Ref: Medonald 8/e p47)

38. A severely incapacitating disturbance of mental and emotional development that causes problem in learning, communication and relating to others is: *(COMEDK 10)*

Ans. Autism (Ref: McDonald 8/e p543)

39. If the use of a technique on a child is objectionable enough that the child will cooperate in order to avoid it, that technique will come under *(COMEDK 10)*

Ans. Aversive domain (Ref: McDonald p46)

40. Class II preparation for amalgam restoration in 1° teeth requires: *(KCET 10)*

a. Arch length deficiency in comparison to total tooth material
b. Patient with straight profile
c. Absence of sufficient growth to overcome the jaw base-tooth size discrepancy.
d. Class II and III malocclusion with skeletal abnormality

Ans. d

41. During what stage of development is peer group identity strongest? *(KCET 10)*

Ans. Teenager

42. Stainless steel crown are contraindicated in: *(KCET 10)*

Ans. Medically compromised patient (VSD, ASD)

43. Caries excavation using carisolv: *(KCET 10)*

Ans. Clinical separation of sound and carious dentin

44. How is a 2 year old positioned for an emergency examination of fractured incisor? *(KCET 10)*

Ans. On the parent's lap

45. According to Ellis and Davey classification of 51 involving dentin and associated loss of vitality is classified as: *(KCET 12)*

Ans. Class 9

46. All of the following represent a potential obstacles for daily oral hygiene for a child with special needs except: *(KCET 12)*

a. Perioral sensitivity
b. Limited manual dexterity
c. High gag reflex
d. Low pain threshold

Ans. d

CHAPTER

6 Periodontics

Topic

- Periodontal Histology
- GCF
- Plaque and Calculus
- Periodontal Diseases
- Periodontal Microbiology
- Treatment of Periodontal Disease
- Miscellaneous

PERIODONTAL HISTOLOGY

- Biological width:

J.E. + Connective tissue (C.T.) = 2 mm (vertical dimension)
↓ ↓
1 mm 1 mm

- Distance between gingival margin of restoration and alveolar crest = 3 mm
- Distance between CEJ and alveolar crest = 1.5 mm
- "Width of gingiva" required for restoration of a tooth with crown = 5 mm: *(PGI 07)*

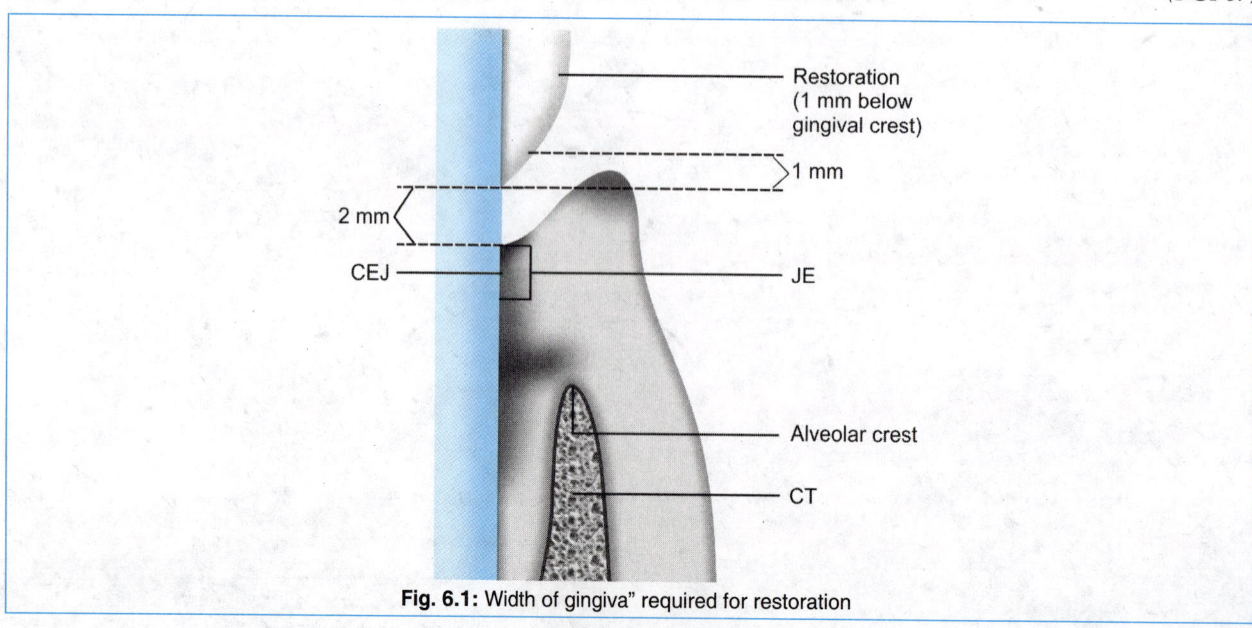

Fig. 6.1: Width of gingiva" required for restoration

So, total width of gingival required for restoration = 1 mm + 2 mm + J.E. + C.t. = 5 mm

- J.E. length: 0.25 to 1.35 mm
- J.E. is completely restored around implant and even after surgery it is derived from oral epithelium (mainly) + R.E.E
- Gingiva attached to tooth by Dento Gingival unit
- Dentogingival unit formed by: J.E. + gingival fibers
- J.E Attached to tooth By Hemidesmosomes/Internal basal + lamina
- Not desmosomes ◎ Keratinocytes are joined by them (Do not confuse)
- Non keratinocytes:

Melanocyte	Langerhan's cells	Merkel cells
Basal + spinous [Q] Layer	Present in suprabasal Layer (High level cells)	Present in deep layer
Are Dendritic cells [Q]	Absent in J.E. of normal gingival	

- Non keratinized mucosa: J.E. + sulcular epithelium + Col.
- GINGIVAL SULCUS:

Histological depth → 1.8 mm
Probing depth → 2–3 mm

- Stippling:

Appears in children after 5 years.
Absent in infancy and old age.
It is reversible
Indicates surface keratinisation

- Alveolar bone is predominantly a "COMPACT" bone [Q]
- Width of attached gingival:

Maxilla		Mandible	
Greatest	Least	Greatest	Least
Incisor Region	Premolar Region	Incisor Region	Premolar Region
3.5 to 4.5 mm	1.9 mm	3.3 to 3.9 mm	1.8 mm

- Pdl fibers (Types):

Type I collagen	Elastin + fibers (↓ses with age)
Principal fibers [Q]	Oxytalan + fibers (– regulate blood flow)
	Eulanin [Q] *(AIIMS 07)*

- Type of collagen:

Type	Area where found
Type one collagen	Bone, Gingivone, pdl
Type two collagen	Car two lage (cartilage)
Type III collagen	Reticular fibers (KCET-08, 09) Granulation tissue
Type IV collagen	Basement membrane Note: Affected in ALPORT syndrome
Type VII	Anchoring fibrils

Note: Oral hard and soft tissues are predominantly composed of type I (Mainly) [Q] and Type III collagen

- Collagen has glycine, proline, hydroxyproline [Q] (Non-essential amino acids)
- Principal fibers of pdl.:

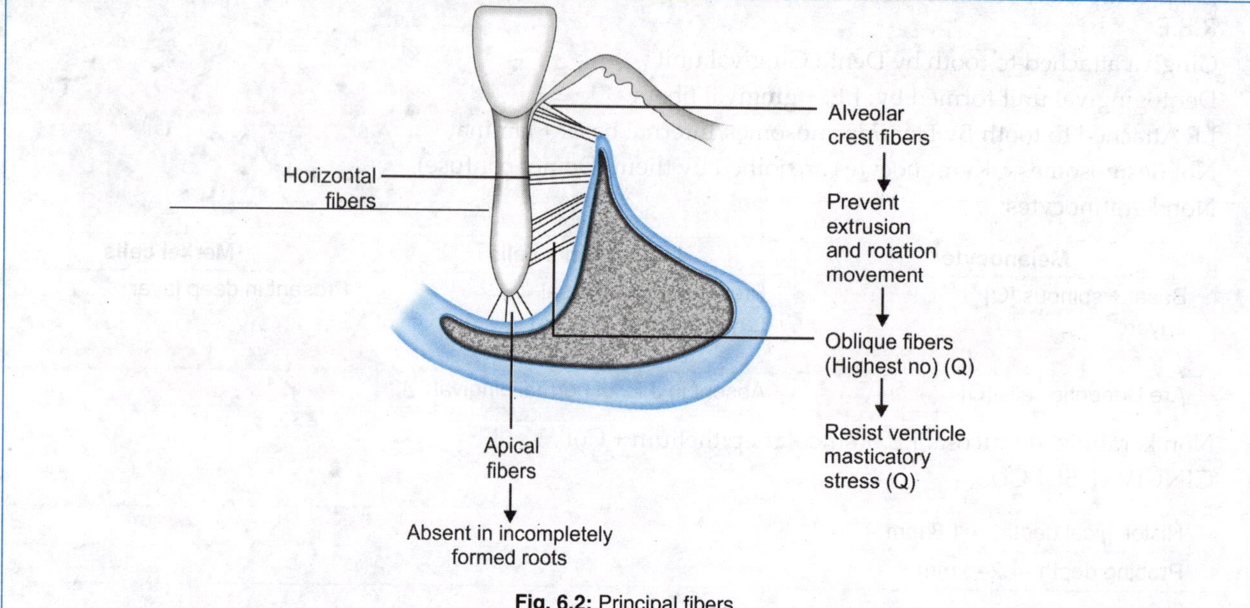

Fig. 6.2: Principal fibers

- Other principal fibers are:
  - Transseptal fibers: Seen between adjoining teeth
  - Interradicularfiber: Present in furcation area of multirooted teeth.

Note: Transseptal fibers are considered as both gingival andpdl fibers [Q]. They are constant finding [Q] They are even reconstructed even after damage to alveolar bone. They are seen after removal of granulation tissue [Q]

- Vessels in pdl are closer to Bone than to cementum.
- O_2 consmuption of normal gingival = 1.6 + 37%
- Keratin:

• Stratification specific keratin in gingival epithelium = K_5, K_{14}
• Keratin characteristic of highly proliferative epithelium = K_6, K_{16}
• Keratin present in para keratinized epithelium only = K_{19}
– Palate is most keratinized

LAST 5-YEAR QUESTIONS FROM THIS TOPIC

1. **Sulcular epithelium is?** *(PGI Dec. 11, June 10)*

Ans. Non keratinized but becomes keratinized on removal of inflammation (Ref: Carranza 10/e p52, 53)

2. **Attached gingival is considered as:** *(PGI Dec. 09, June 09)*

Ans. From the base of sulcus to mucogingival junction. (Ref: Orban's 10/e p283)

3. **The fibers of pdl which maintain neighboring teeth in contact:** *(COMEDK 12)*

Ans. Transeptal fibers

4. **Clinical gingival sulcus is measured from marginal gingival to:** *(AIIMS Nov 10)*

Ans. Apical end of the penetrated probe (Ref: Carranza 10/e p551, 552)

5. **the interdental col is more prone to periodontal disease because it:** *(AIIMS May 12)*

Ans. Is covered with non keratinized epithelium (Ref: Carranza 10/e p47)

6. **J.E. is derived from:** *(COMEDK 12)*

Ans. Reduced enamel epithelium

7. **Thickness of basal lamina is:** *(COMEDK 11)*

Ans. 300 to 400A (Ref: Carranza's clinical periodontology 10/e p52)

8. **Haversain System (Osteons) are found primarily in the:** *(COMEDK 11)*

Ans. Alveolar bone proper

9. **Basement membrane is:** *(KCET 10)*

Ans. Consists of lamina densa and lamina lucida

10. **Life preserver shaped enlargement of the gingival margin in known as:** *(KCET 09)*

Ans. McCall festoons

11. **These substances play a major role in regulating cell and cell matrix interaction in:** *(KCET 09)*

Ans. Proteoglycans

12. **Elastin fiber system present in the lamina propria consists of all the these except:** *(KCET 09)*
    a. Oxytalan
    b. Elastin
    c. Elaunin
    d. Collagen

Ans. d

13. **The following parts of gingival are keratinized except:** *(KCET 09)*
    a. Marginal gingival
    b. Attached gingival
    c. Interdental papilla in the anterior teeth
    d. Interdental Col

Ans. d

14. **Reticular fibers found in pdl consist of:** *(KCET 09)*

Ans. Type III

15. **Which of the following cell types contains a vasoactive amine that is released in inflammatory process?** *(KCET 09)*

Ans. Mast cells

GCF

- Can be either transduate/exudates
- Ig G > Ig A
- Both in CSF and GCF →↑ sed Glucose [Q]
  ↓
  Has 3-4 times ↑ sed Glucose [Q]
- T: B cell = 1:3 (reverse of peripheral blood)
- Peritron → method of measuring GCF
- It has high concentration of tetracvcline + metronidazole → 7 times of serum concentration
- Orogranulocytes → PMN reaching oral cavity through gingival sulcus

- **Leukotoxin:** Exotoxin produced by A.a

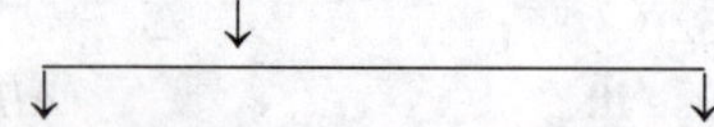

Inhibition of PMN function ↓ Killing T and B cells

A.a. produces PMN chemotaxin inhibiting factor

- IL-1 and TNF → Bone resorbing factor and key cytokines in pathogenesis of periodontitis
- GCF ↑ sed in normal mastication and NOT in TFO [Q] Smoking causes transient by marked increase in GCF
- MMPase is not an inflammatory mediator but INF is *(AIPG 12)*

PLAQUE AND CALCULUS

- Supragingival calculus vs Subgingival calculus:

Supragingival calculus	Subgingival calculus
• HA same	• HA same
• More $Ca_3(PO_4)_2$ and Brusite	• More Mg white locate
• Hard clay like	• Hard flint like

- Note:

Only pellicle do not have microorganism

- Calculocementum:

Calculus embedded deeply into cementum

- Pigmented non-cariogenic plaque causes massentric lines
- Generalized calculus formation in children with Cystic fibrosis is higher otherwise calculus formation is less common in children
- Normal distance between apical end of JE and bone is constant

Distance between apical extent of calculus and alveolar bone (crest) in pdl pocket is most constant (1.97 mm) [Q]

- Calculus → the major concern for clinician. It is not due to the mechanical irritation but due to the presence of bacteria in calculus
- In 0.5 hr – 2 hrs → Pellicle formation [Q]
- 2 hr – 4 hr → Irreversible colonization (QQ)
- Afte 1 day → 1 day is required for all the organization and maturation to reach completion after 1 day term biofilm is used → Term for mature plaque
- Amount of H2O in plaque 80%

LAST 5-YEAR QUESTIONS FROM THIS TOPIC

1. **Specific plaque hypothesis was put forward by:** *(PGI Dec. 10, June 09)*

Ans. Loesche (Ref: Carranza 9/e p105.

2. **In the etiology of which disease does microbial plaque plays the most obscure role?** *(AIIMS May 11, 12)*

Ans. Desquamative gingivitis

3. **Plaque forms after brushing:** *(AIIMS May 12, Nov 10)*

Ans. ½ to 1 hr

4. **After enamel has been exposed to bacteria, irreversible bacterial colonization takes place in:** *(AIIMS Nov 10, AIPG 09)*

Ans. 2-4 hrs (Ref: Carranza 9/e p98-100)

5. **According to Glickman, maximum plaque accumulation is seen in:** *(AIIMS May 12, Nov 10)*

Ans. 30 days (Ref: Carranza 10/e p145-146)

6. **Content of supragingival calculus is:** *(AIIMS Nov 11)*

Ans. Hydroxyapatite andbrushite (Direct pick from a question bank)

7. **Specific plaque hypothesis states that:** *(AIPG 12)*

Ans. Only specific microbes cause caries (Ref: Microbiology for dentistry by lakshmansamarnayake 3/e p 269)

8. **Acidity of plaque in proximal area remains below normal for:** *(AIPG 12)*

Ans. 120 min (Ref: Mc Donald)

9. **Difference in the color between supragingival and subgingival calculus is related to:** *(AIPG 11)*

Ans. Hemolysis of erythrocytes

10. **Supragingival plaque undergoes which of the following changes with time:** *(AIPG 11)*

Ans. Plaque micro flora becomes more gram –ve

11. **Which of the following is a characteristic of supragingival and not of sub gingival plaque in humans:** *(AIPG 11)*

Ans. Bacterial composition is altered by dietary sugar consumption

12. **Brushite crystals forms of calculus is more common in**

Ans. Mandibular anterior (Ref: Carranza's textbook of periodontology 10/e p173. *(COMEDK 11)*

13. **Adhesion of plaque to tooth is mainly due to** *(AIPG 10, 12, NEET 13)*

Ans. Dextran

PERIODONTAL DISEASES

- Pre-pubertal periodontitis:

Occurs below 11 years.
Systemic diseaes associated → Assocaited with Neutrophil function ↓ Papillonlefever syndrome Down syndrome Chediak highaski Neutropenia Hypophosphatasia (ALP → No cementogenesis + ↓ sed Bone mineralisaton) Leukemia

- Periodontal lesions seen in HIV patients:

Linear gingival erythema/HIV gingivitis → Diffuse/marginal (more common)
ANUG + NUP

- Commonest plunger cusp → DL cusp of upper 2nd M [Q]
- Vit. B2 deficiency:

(Riboflavin deficiency) Patient presents with Chelosis + glossitis + Angular stomatitis + Delayed healing after pdl surgery + magenta colored tongue.
(Trick: MR) M → Magenta tongue R → Seen in Riboflavin

- McCalls festoons and Stillman's cleft:

Most commonly seen in canine and PM
Are a peculiar inflammatory change of marginal gingival
Traumatic occlusion as an etiological factor Never established

- LJP – 10-20 yrs (young adolescent)
- Stages of gingivitis:

Initial gingivitis/Subclinical stage I → GCF only, PMN [Q]
Early/stage II → T-lymphocyte
Established/stage III → Plasma cells characteristic [Q]
Advanced/stage IV

- Tuberous sclerosis: Triad of epilepsy + mental deficiency + cutaneous angiofibroma
- Gingival enlargement:

"Diffuse" → Leukemia, plasma cell, fibrotic, idiopathic
"Marginal + interdental" → Rest (Pregnancy + puberty [Q], drug induced, gingival abscess [Q]

- Pregnancy Gingivitis: "Factor" responsible for pregnancy gingivitis ◎ Plaque [Q]
- Changes in gingival during pregnancy are attributed to changes in hormonal level
- Phenytoin: Stimulates fibroblast + ses their degradation of collagen (fibrotic enlargement)
- Pregnancy gingivitis seen in 50-100% [Q]
- Extraction done in ANUG after 4 weeks
- Pus is a common feature of pdl disease but is only a 2° sign
- Conditional gingival enlargement:

(Trick = PAN hai) P → Pyogenic gramutoma Puberty/pregnancy (Hormonal) A → Allergic (due to peppermint (–) Chewing gum N → Nutritional (vit C. deficiency)

- Circular fibers andDentogingival fibers: predominantly affected in stage II/Early gingivitis. Also it is Ist fiber to be involved in periodontitis

OLD name	New name
Gingivosis	Desquamative gingivitis
Periodontosis	LJP

- AHGS + ANUG: Corticosteroids are contra indicated as these conditions are already immuno suppressed
- Listgarten [Q] described 4 zones in ANUG:

Bacterial Zone → Neutrophil rich zone → Necrosis zone → Spirochaetal zone (Intermediate spirochetes are seen in maximum number)

- AHGS: seen on masticatory mucosa high temperature (102°F) + vesicle eruption are present
- Note: Apthous ulcer is seen only on lining mucosa
- Pseudomembrane:

Un detachable in syphilis
Difficult to remove in diphtheria

- ANUG is common in adolescent

- Leukemic gingivitis resemble ANUG
- Toxin type and bacteria:

Trick = ENG (read like CNG) EN → Endotoxin GN → Gram negative
Endotoxin is associated with gram negative bacteria.

- Probable etiology of gingivosis is deficiency of estrogen and testosterone.
- Note: In menopause there is low level of Estrogen, testosterone, progesterone. These result in thinning of oral mucosa, burning mouth, gingival recession, xerostomia, altered taste sensation, bone resorption. Desquamative gingivitis is also seen.
- Other conditions in which desquamative gingivitis is seen: most commonly lichen planus, cicatricialpemphigoid/ benign mucous membrane pemphigoid.
- Periodontal abscess: Formed in pdl along lateral aspect of root/soft tissue lateral wall of pocket.
- Pdl pocket wall is densely infiltrated by Plasma cells (80%)
- Probing pressure: 25 g/0.75 N
- TFO:

Traumatic occlusion causing "Tissue injury" is "TFO/Occlusal trauma" So, it refers to tissue injury due to excessive occlusal fore not due to deflective occlusion [Q] It doesn't cause pocket/Gingivitis because of rich blood supply to marginal gingival is sufficient to maintain it. So, TFO cause → Angular bone defect without pocket formation.
Note: All game is within periodontium (No effect on gingiva)
TFO → Excessive occlusal force → Area of compression with in periodontium → Bone resorption (Tissue Injury) → Angular bone defect → Then Repair (Stage II) → Then adaptive remodeling (Stage III) → Widening of pdl → Tooth mobility [Q]
"Furcation" are most susceptible to TFO
Coronoplasty/Occlusal adjustment: used mainly in TFO with goal of achieving a stable, non-traumatic occlusal → "Therapeutic occlusion"
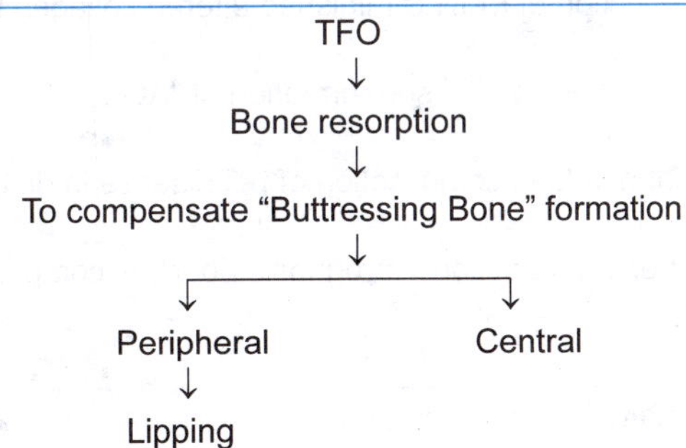

- Wall defects:

In order of involvement of walls: Facial > Lingual > Distal → Most commonly in 3 wall defect (AIIMS *Nov* 11) (2ndand 3rd molar)
Dehiscence → Facial surface most commonly involved.
One wall defect = Hemiseptum
Three wall defect = Intrabony defect
Craters are the most common type of lesion in periodontitis (2/3 rd of all mandibular defects)

- Excessive force:

Either within physiologic limit OR Beyond physiological limit "Bone resorption" (Bone is very sensitive to pressure) → leads to widening of pdl space

- Down's syndrome:

• Both chemotaxisand Phagocytosis of neutrophil is affected → so, pdl degeneration, recession, ANUG , NUP seen
• Caries incidence is low

- Bone loss pattern in LJP:

• Arch shaped mirror image destruction
Vertical bone loss in LJP and TFO (Only)
Note: Horizontal bone loss is commonly seen in LJP

- PMNs → 1° defense against periodontal pathogen
- Ist sign of:

TFO → Tooth mobility
LJP → Pathogenic migration

- Papillonlefever syndrome:

• Defect in chromosome 11
• Destructive periodontitis: Loss by both 1° and 2° teeth by 15 years
• Palmar plantar hyperkeratosis
• Calcification of duramater

- Diabetes:

Pathogenesis of pdldiseases: Bacteria responsible – A.aandCapnocytophaga
↓
Function of PMN Diminished altered collagen metabolism
↓
↑sed formation of "AGE's"
↓
Plays central role in complication of pdl disease in diabetes Young patient
↓
Rapid bone destruction + prognosis poor (as compared to old patient)

- Pocket depth:

It is base of pocket to gingival margin
Or
Coronal end of J.E. to gingival margin

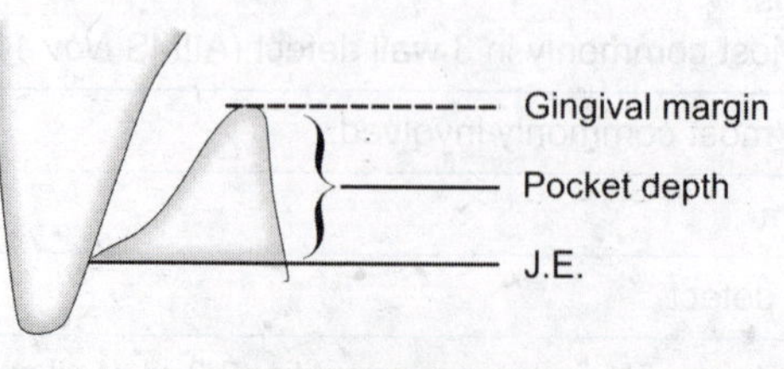

Fig. 6.3: Pocket

- Periodontometer/Periotest measures tooth mobility
- Periotron → measures GCF
- Bone morphology:

• Cannot be revealed by radiograph
• Transgingival probing [Q] + surgical exposure [Q] are definitive for diagnosis

- Note: tooth brush abrasion more common on maxillary left teeth
- Furcation:

Grade II Furcation involvement is CUL-DE-SAC
Most commonly involved tooth → Mandibular molars
Least commonly involved tooth → Maxillary Ist molar (as furcation at lowest level)
Poorest prognosis → Maxillary Ist premolar

- Most common age of gingivitis in children → 6–7 years
- Note: for caries it is 11 to 13 years (Chocolate)
- Pregnant patients:

More Pdl problems as sed prevotella intermedia but same degree of dental caries

- Periodontitis:

Characterized by sed number of plasma cells (80%) (and B-lymphocytes)
and se in number of T-lymphocytes.
Neutrophils migrate the most in gingival sulcus.
In pocket wall characteristically plasma cells present

- Lateral pdl cyst:

develops from 1/more cell rests of dental lamina [Q]
Trick for development of other cysts: (Cysts derived from dental lamina/cell rests of serre) LOG to Google L → Lateral pdl cyst O → OKC G → Gingival cyst of newborn G → Gingival cyst of adult G → Glandular odontogenic cyst [Q]

- Gingival ablation: Gingival recession due to "soft tissue" friction

LAST 5-YEAR QUESTIONS FROM THIS TOPIC

1. Which one of the following condition indicates a periodontal rather than an endodontic lesion? *(PGI Dec. 11)*

Ans. Pain to lateral percussion with wide sulcular pocket (Ref: Cohen 8/e p656-657)

2. Giant cell lesions of the periodontium are best considered as? *(PGI Dec. 11)*

Ans. Non-neoplastic reactive lesions

3. Mc call's festoon is due to? *(PGI Dec. 11, 10)*

Ans. Inflammatory changes(Ref: Carranza 10/e p370)

4. IL-1 and TNF- during inflammation are secreted by: *(PGI Dec. 11, AIIMS Nov 10)*

Ans. Activated Macrophages (Ref: Carranza 10/e p239)

5. **Aggressive periodontitis is characterized by the following major features except:** *(KCET 12)*
   a. Non contributory medical history
   b. Rapid contributory medical history
   c. Pathologic migration
   d. Familial aggregation of cases

Ans. c

Note: Pathologic migration is not a major feature

6. **Type of cells which predominate in the stage III lesion of gingivitis are?** *(PGI June 11, June 10, 09, AIPG 11)*

Ans. Plasma cells (Ref: Carranza 10/e p355, 359)

7. **Pregnancy gingivitis is at peak in which month of pregnancy?** *(PGI June 11)*

Ans. 8 months (Ref: Carranza 10/e p288, 639.

8. **Most common factor for gingivitis?** *(PGI June 11)*

Ans. Plaque (Ref: Carranza 10/e p175)

9. **Smoking increases the risk of pdl disease by?** *(PGI June 11)*

Ans. 6-10 times (ref.; Carranza 10/e p252)

10. **Which of the following represents a periodontal lesion predominantly?** *(PGI June 11)*

Ans. Pain on palpation of attached gingival of a tooth associated with exudates and deep sulcular pocket (Nishagarg 2/e p312)

11. **Association between coronary artery disease and periodontal disease has been found to be?** *(PGI June 11)*

Ans. Positively related (Ref: Carranza 10/e p316)

12. **Presence of signs of periodontitis without inflammation is termed as:** *(PGI June 09)*

Ans. Periodontosis (Ref: Carranza 10/e p507)

13. **Which of the following condition if not treated, can lead to in different course?** *(PGI Dec. 10)*

Ans. ANUG (Ref: Carranza 10/e p391-392)

14. **If a periodontal disease is continuously present and is not resolving with regular treatment, it is known as?** *(PGI June 11)*

Ans. Refractory periodontitis (Ref: Carranza 10/e p104, 409-410.

15. **Who was the Ist person to experimentally demonstrate gingivitis?** *(PGI June 11)*

Ans. Henry Loe (ref.Carranza 10/e p156)

16. **Which of following can lead to gnawing radiating pain?** *(PGI Dec. 09)*

Ans. ANUG (Ref: Carranza 10/e p392)

17. **Most common implant related disease which is mild, reversible, suprabomyand present in the soft tissue is:** *(PGI Dec. 09)*

Ans. Peri-implant mucosites (Ref: Bhalaji p317)

18. **Disuse atrophy of periodontium occurs in all except:** *(PGI Dec. 09)*

Ans. Herpangina (Ref: Shafer's 5/e p427, 474 and 1112)

19. **TFO is least likely to affect in which of the following?** *(AIIMS May 11)*

Ans. Epithelial attachment (Ref: Carranza 10/e p473, 474, 847, 853)

20. **CASE REPORT:** *(COMEDK 12)*

An18 years old male reported with chief compliant of sensitivity and deep, dull, radiating pain during chewing, intra oral examination showed sparse plaque and calculus deposits, distolabial migration of the maxillary incisors with diastema formation, mobility of maxillary and mandibular incisors and Ist molars. Prescribed radiographs showed an arc shaped loss of alveolar bone extending from the distal surface of the 2nd molar. There was vertical bone loss in the maxillary incisor region.

a. The most likely diagnosis

Ans. LAP

b. The bacterial etiology of this disease is

Ans. A. a

c. The antigens consistently associated with this disease are

Ans. HLAAG and B15

d. The host modulation therapy that may be used as adjunctive therapy for this disease is

Ans. Sub antimicrobial dose clindamycin

21. The histopathological picture of chronic gingivitis is: *(AIIMS May 11)*

Ans. Infiltration of neutrophils, lymphocytes and plasma cells (Ref: Carranza 10/e p368)

22. A grayish white membrane is present on necrotic area in ANUG, this membrane is: *(AIIMS Nov 11)*

Ans. Pseudo membrane (ref.; Carranza 10/e p391)

23. Initial clinical symptoms of juvenile periodontitis? *(AIIMS Nov 11)*

Ans. Mobility of molar and incisor teeth (Ref: Carranza 10/e p507)

24. Bluish black discoloration of gingival that has been previously inflamed is due to: *(AIIMS Nov 11)*

Ans. Bismuth (Ref: Shafer's 6/e p554)

25. The severe alveolar bone loss seen in patients with juvenile periodontitis is associated with: *(AIIMS May 12, AIPG-11)*

Ans. Impaired neutrophil chemotoxis (Ref: Carranza 10/e p510, 511, 243, 244)

26. In the soft tissue wall of a pdl pocket what changes are expected: *(AIPG 11)*

Ans. Both proliferative and degenerative changes

27. In gingivitis, the role of immunoglobulin is consistent, with increased number of: *(AIPG 11, 10)*

Ans. Plasma cells

28. Gingival clefts may be formed by: *(AIPG 11)*

Ans. Faulty tooth brushing

29. Most common clinical sign of occlusal trauma is the presence of: *(AIPG 11)*

Ans. Tooth mobility

30. A probable etiology of gingivosis is: *(AIPG 11)*

Ans. Deficiency of estrogen and testosterone

31. Delayed hypersensitivity/cell mediated immune reactions occur in patient with periodontal diseases because they often have: *(AIPG 11)*

Ans. T-lymphocytes sensitized to plaque bacterial antigens

32. Which of the following is most useful in differentiating an acute periodontal abscess from periapical abscess: *(AIPG 11, 09)*

Ans. Result of periodontal probing

33. Teeth that are least affected by periodontal disease: *(AIPG 11)*

Ans. Lower premolars and upper canines

34. On the radiograph, the mesial side of mandibular Ist molar reveled bone loss of 2-3 mm. On probing, 6 mm pocked was revealed. The discrepancy could be due to: *(AIPG 11)*

Ans. Superimposition of bone remaining on facial and lingual surfaces.

35. Which of following cell migrate into the sulcus, in largest quantity, as a result of plaque accumulation: *(AIPG 11, 10)*

Ans. Neutrophils

36. CASE report

A 30 year old male reported with chief complaint of constant radiating, gnawing pain that is intensified by eating spicy foods and chewing. He also reported a "Metallic" foul taste and an excessive amount of "pasty" saliva a general examination revealed fever and increased pulse rate. Intraoral examination showed punched out, crater like depression at the crest of the interdental gingival papillae, covered by a gray pseudomembranous slough in the upper anterior teeth (COMED K-11)

a.

Ans. NUG

b. The microbial etiology is

Ans. Fusospirochaetes

c. The infection is reported to have an increased incidence in

Ans. HIV

d. Surgical procedure for severe tissue destruction in such infection is

Ans. Reshaping the gingival

37. The most reliable indicator of gingival inflammation is: *(COMEDK 11)*

Ans. Bleeding on probing

38. According to horning and Cohen staging of oral necrotizing diseases stage on represents: *(KCET 10)*

Ans. NUG

39. Which of the following stages of gingivitis characterizes periodontal breakdown? *(KCET 10)*

Ans. Advanced lesion

40. In chronic marginal gingivitis, radiographic feature is: *(AIPG 09)*

Ans. No change (Ref. Carranaza 10/e p362, 406)

PERIODONTAL MICROBIOLOGY

- Corn Cob structure:

Supragingival plaque [Q] typically demonstrates highly specific cell to cell interaction,
characterized by inner core by gram -ve bacteria and outer surface of coccal bacteria Gr+ve

- Co-aggregation:

Occurs between different species and Genera .
Occurs between gram - ve bacteria
Test tube arrays.

- Supragingivalplaque:

1° Colonizer	2° Colonizer
Facultative anaerobes	Are anaerobes
(S. Sanguis, Viscosus)	

- Subgingival plaque → Motile bacteria (Spirochaetes + vibrio)
- A.a:

Is facultative anaerobic gram - ve rod.
Note: Majority of oral microbes are facultative anaerobes including A.a + Early plaque colonizers.

- Collagenase produced by A.a, Pg [Q] (Mostly)
- S. sanguis:

Found in sites where no attachment loss is present (Inactive site)
Prevents colonization of A.a by producing H2O2 which is lethal to A.a

- Organism directly invading Host tissue: Pg [Q], A.a, Treponemadenticola, F. Nucleatum

- Organism initiating "Puberty" gingivitis

  +

  associated with diabetes melitus

  +

  Associated with LAP

- Capnocytophaga (Don't confuse with prevotellaintermedia which is increased in pregnancy)
- Osteoclast secrete

  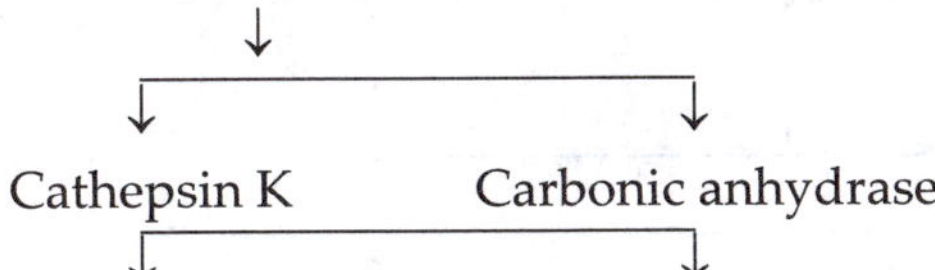

  Cathepsin K → Dissolves organic matrix

  Carbonic anhydrase → Dissolves inorganic matrix

- Bacterial adhesion on tooth is prevented by myeloperoxidase
- Radius of action of Toxin = 1.5 – 2.5 mm
- Orange complex:

Trick = INR valve
I → P. Intermediate N → F. Nucleatum R → Rectus

- Green Complex:

Trick: ACE inhibitor
A → A.a C → Capnocytophaga E → E. Corrodens

- Red Complex:

Trick: GDF fund
G → P. Gingivalis D → T. Denticola F → B. Forsythus

- Organisms predominating Late plaque → Gram-ve anaerobic rods + filaments → Pg, P.i, Fusobacterium, Capnocytophaga
- Bacteria associated with Health: (Present but does not cause disease)

S. Sangius [Q] S. Mitis A. Viscosus Capnocytophaga [Q] Niesseria [Q] Veillonella [Q]

- Bacteria Associated with periodontal disease:

Pg, Pi, A.a, Fusobacterium + 2E	
E → Eikenella [Q]	E → Eubacterium [Q]

- Organism Not present in plaque: S. Pyogens> S. Salivarius
- Organism associated with ANUG: Spirochaetes (Intermediate sized. + Fusiform bacilli
- Organism not following Koch postulates: *(KCET 13)*

M. Leprae
Gonococci
T. Pallidum (Not cultured in artificial media)

- S. Salivarius:

• Forms longest chain
• 1st organism to invade cavity
• Most common organism in saliva
• Not/ Not in high number in plaque

- Organism absent in gingival sulcus:Diptheroids
- Organism responsible for root surface caries:

A. Visocus
S. Sangius is 2nd common organism

- Facultative anaerobicmicro organism associated with LJP: A.a
- 1 gm of plaque contain " 2x10" bacteria
- Organism causing pregnancy gingivitis:

Pi + bacteriodmelanogenicus

- Note: Bacteria maximum after meal not in morning

LAST 5-YEAR QUESTIONS FROM THIS TOPIC

1. **Which of the following micro organism increase in pregnancy gingivitis?** *(PGI Dec 11, 10, June 10)*

Ans. Prevotella intermedia (Ref: Carranza 10/e p380)

2. **Which of the following is not a part of koch's postulates?**

Ans. Bacteria may/may not cause disease in experimental animals (Ref: Anathanarayan 8/e p5. *(AIIMS Nov 10)*

3. **A attachment on tooth surface can be prevented by?** *(PGI Dec. 11, June 10, Dec. 09)*

Ans. Myeloperoxidase (Ref: carranza 10/e p349)

4. **Which microorganism has 90% presence in LAP?** *(PGI June 11)*

Ans. A. a (Ref: Carranza 10/e p509)

5. **Which of the following is not a bactericidal?** *(PGI Dec. 10)*

Ans. Bicarbonate andPhosphate (Ref: Carranza's 10/e p349)

6. **Which of the following organisms is not implicated in the etiology of periodontal disease?** *(AIIMS May 11, 11, AIPG 09)*

Ans. Neisseria (Ref: Carranza 10/e p143, 156, 157)

7. **Bacteria which are not found in normal healthy periodontium are:** *(AIIMS May 11)*

Ans. Eubacterium (Ref: Carranza 10/e p143, 156-60)

8. **The bacterial flora associated with juvenile periodontitis is mainly:** *(AIIMS May 11, AIP -1, 09)*

Ans. Gram–ve anaerobic rods (Ref: Carranza 10/e p509-510)

9. **To identify the key microorganism in periodontal disease, koch's criteria have been modified by:** *(AIIMS Nov 10)*

Ans. Socransky (Ref: Carranza 10/e p155)

10. **Which of the following is not present in periodontitis?** *(AIIMS May 09, AIPG 11)*

Ans. Actinomyces (Ref: Carranza 10/e p143, 156-160)

11. **H/P Examination of the tissues in desquamative gingivitis would reveal?** *(AIIMS May 12, AIPG 11)*

Ans. Loss of basement membrane (Ref: NBDE, Endo periodec. 1977 Q-41)

12. **A bacterial enzyme capable of altering ground substance of the pdl is:** *(AIIMS May 12, AIPG 11)*

Ans. Hyaluronidase (Ref: Carranza 10/e p52, 53, 59)

13. **Pregnancy gingivitis is caused by:** *(AIIMS May 12)*

Ans. Bacteriodes melaninogenicus (Ref: Carranza 10/e p380)

14. **The attachment of the actinomyces species to the tooth surface is facilitated by:** *(COMEDK 12)*

Ans. Fimbriae

15. **Bacterial communication with each other in a biofilm is known as:** *(KCET 10)*

Ans. Quorum sensing

16. **Microorganism invades host tissue cells directly is:** *(COMEDK 09)*

Ans. P.g. (Ref: Carranza periodontology 10/e p157)

17. **Bacterial species which is protective/beneficial to the host is:**

Ans. S. sanguis

18. **Predominant microorganism isolated from localized aggressive periodontitis lesions is:** *(COMEDK 09)*

Ans. a

TREATMENT OF PERIODONTAL DISEASE

- The horizontal scrub method removes more plaque than other techniques
- Regenerative osseous surgery = New attachment
- Reattachment = Repair by Long J.E.
- Host modulatory Therapy (HMT):

Aims to reduce tissue destruction and even regenerative
• Doxycycline hyclate suppresses collagenase activity. • **NSAIDS:** Flurbiprofen inhibits PGE2 mediated alveolar bone resorption

- Anti tartar agents:

Trick = TPZ
T → Triclosan P → Pyrophosphate Z → Zn salt

- Phenytoin:

Stimulates fibroblast
ses the degradation of collagen (fibrotic enlargement)

- Coronoplasty/occlusal adjustment:

Used mainly in TFO with goal of achieving a stable, non traumatic occlusion → Therapeutic occlusion

- Rx for LJP:

Tetracyclin → "Ist choice" Augmentin → 2nd choice

- Local drug delivery (LDD):

Artisite – Tetracycline [Q] Arttidox – 10% Doxycycline [Q] Periochip – CHX [Q] Periocline – 2% minocycline Arestin (KCET 10)

- CHX:

Inhibits gram +ve ;gram –ve bacteria and yeasts (i.e. all micro flora. [Q]

- Gingivectomy contraindicated in → Pocket beyond mucogingival junction + Intrabony pocket
- Embrassure types andCleaning:

Type I → Normal → Floss
Type II → Mild to moderate → Proxa/Interdental brush ↓ Recession of papilla + concavities
Type III → Complete loss of papilla→ Uni tufted brush

- Perioaid:

It is a Δr shaped wedge attached to a handle. Keeps furcation areas plaque free. Floss is inefficient in furcation and Concave areas

- CHX:

• Used as a mouth wash – 0.2%
• Minimum amount of CHX required in mouth wash to prevent plaque formation – 0.12%

- Water irrigating device:

Dilutes bacterial products/Alters the plaque [Q] H2O + CHX can be used ↓ Significant reduction in gingivitis

- Gingival massage ses:

Keratinization, epithelisation, blood circulation in lamina propria.

- Epithelisation: (Completed in)

After gingivectomy by 1 month (or even after pdl surgery)
after curettage by 1 week (2–7 days)

- Electro surgery:

Used in → gingivectomy, pdl abscess, relocation of frenal attachment
Contra indicated → in procedures that involve closeness to bone i.e. flap andmucogingival surgery

- Ideal thickness of true gingival graft 1 to 1.5 mm
- Reverse bevel incision:

Is also called internal bevel incision.
Internal/reverse bevel incision → Removes pocket lining NOTE: External bevel incision ↓ Used in gingivectomy → Removes pocket wall

Location of internal level incision: In apically displaced and modified Widman flap, internal bevel incision is as close to tooth and close to marginal gingival
Note: Modified widman is a type of undisplaced flap.
In other undisplaced flap, incision is away from tooth and marginal gingival So, unaesthetic but removes entire pocket wall.

- Both apically positioned flap and Modified widman flap preserves pocket wall (Removes pocket lining)
- After reflection of full thickness flap, post surgical alveolar bone loss is greatest on thin facial margin.
- Partial/split thickness flap: Indicated in case of fenestration and Dehiscence (as full thickness flap is not preferred)
- Edian Majehar'stechnique: ses depth of vestibule
- Like gingivectomy entire pocket wall is removal in undisplaced flap. So, undisplaced flap is also called "Internal bevel gingivectomy"
- Periodontal surgery ↑ Pocket elimination is "Definitive"
- Autogenouscancellous bone has maximum osteogenic potential. Most of grafts have osteoconductive potential only.
- Free gingival graft is placed on periosteum (COMEDK 13). It may also be placed on bone.
- Best position of apically displaced flap is 2 mm apical to alveolar crest.
- Root resection: DB root of maxillary 1st molar is most favorable.
  Note: DL cusp of maxillary 2nd molar is the plunger cusp.
- HemisectionandBicuspidation: Mandibular molars are most suitable.
- Rx of furcation:

Furcation	Description	Treatment plan
Grade I	• Incipient lesion • No X-ray finding • Suprabony pocket • Edematous Gingiva	• Scaling + root planning • Odontoplasty • Gingivectomy for Fibrous pockets
Grade II	• Cul-de-sac • Moderate cases: Partial penetration • X-ray finding may/may not be present	Scaling + root Planning Odontoplasty GTR with bone graft. • Advanced cases: Root resection/hemi section
Grade III	• Inter radicular Bone loss • Through and through Passage of probe. • Furcation is covered by gingiva	• Scaling +root planning • Tunneling • Root resection/Hemi section
Grade IV	Grade III + Furcation not Covered with gingiva –Moderate case	Same as grade III + occlusal adjustment Advanced cases: Extraction

- Graft Types:

Graft type	Example
• Autogenous/ Autograft	Graft taken from same person e.g. → osseous coagulum, bone blend Costochondral graft etc.
• Allograft/Homograft	Graft taken from different individual of same species e.g. →Un decalcified /decalcified freeze dried bone grafts.
• Xenograft/ Heterograft	Graft from other species e.g → anorganic bone (OX-bone) kiel bone, calf bone
• Isograft	Graft from twins
• Alloplastic graft/Synthetic graft	e.g. → perioglass/bioactive glass [Q] HTR polymer

- Nature of graft material:

• **Osteogenic:** Has viable bone cells ideal bone graft e.g. autogenous cancellous bone graft.
• **Osteoinductive:** Activity induces bone formation by converting neighboring cells to osteoblast. E.g. decalcified freeze dried bone *(KCET 10)*
• **Osteoconductive:** A physical effect by forming conductive channel that favors outside cell to enter → to form bone. E.g. HA, tricalcium phosphate (TRICK = all calcium compounds)

- Root biomodification:

e.g. of New attachment material used are • Citric acid (PH = 1) • Tetracycline • Fibronectin

- For pdl related osseous defects:

Reattachment (simple repair → by long J.E.) [Q] Not an ideal procedure
Note: New attachment gives ideal result

- Ramping: done for 1 wall defect.
- steps in osseous respective surgery:

Vertical grooving
↓
Radicular blending (Osteoplastic)
↓
Flattening of interproximal bone
↓
Granulizing marginal bone (Ostectomy)

- Infrabony pocket therapy is performed 1st in pdl surgery → sub gingival curettage
- membrane used in GTR:

Biodegradable: polylactic acid (Biobrane) [Q]
Non – biodegradable: PTFE (Goretex)

- Regenerative osseous surgery:

It's a new attachment procedure [Q]

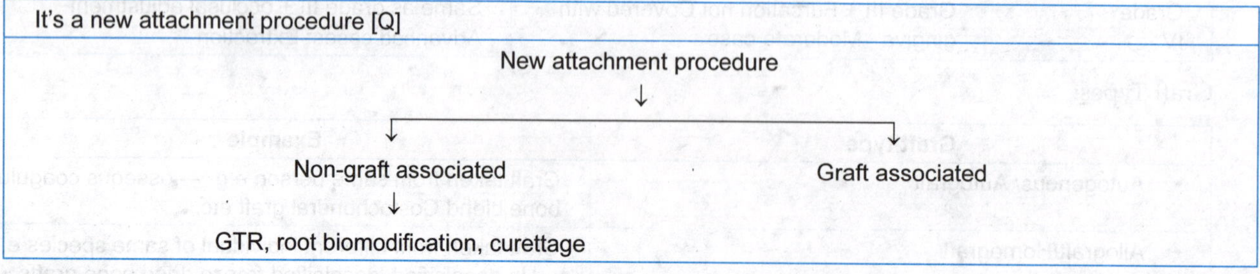

- Bone blending:

It is a technique employed for transplanting "Cortical bone" [Q] *(AIPG 10)*
Bone blend is an autogenous graft.
It is used to overcome disadvantage of osseous coagulum (bone dust from cortical bone + blood)

- Best bone:

For implant → lamellar bone
Formed after osseous fill procedure → Bundle bone
1st bone formed in response to orthodontic loading → Woven bone [Q]

- Occlusal guards:

Does not prevent bruxism.
They interfere with the effect of bruxism by dissipating musculoskeletal forces

- Periodontal dressing/pack:

• Controls infections (Bacteriostatic andfungicidal action) **Note:** It does not accelerate healing
• Hemostasis
• Controls pain by preventing food contact
Types → Eugenol based → Allergic Non Eugenol based (e.g. coepack)
Tannic acid present → causes liver damage [Q] so, should be eliminated from pdl pack composition.

- NSAIDS inhibits bone resorption in pdl disease
- Gingivectomy:

Indication:Suprabony pocket which is firm and fibrous gingival enlargement (Fibrous)

- Various antibiotic used for pdl therapy:

Amoxicillin, Augmentin, Tetracycline, Minocycline, Doxycyline, Ciprofloxacin, Clindamycin, Azithromycine, Metronidazole
Note: Erythromycin is not used (KCET 12)
1° aim of scaling and root plaining is restoring gingival health. Root plaining removes necrotic cementum [Q] and Residual cementum [Q]

LAST 5-YEAR QUESTIONS FROM THIS TOPIC

1. **The critical structure for bone regeneration is?** *(PGI Dec. 11)*

Ans. Periosteum (Ref: Biology of the periodontium by meleherandbowen pg. 508)

2. **In periodontal flap, most important factor to be considered is:** *(PGI Dec. 10)*

Ans. Amount of attached gingival (Ref: Glickman's 8/e p568)

3. **The free gingival graft is placed on:** *(PGI Dec. 09)*

Ans. On the periostium (Ref: Carranza 10/e p1008)

4. **The best way to prevent the exposure of dehiscence during surgical procedure is by elevating:** *(PGI Dec. 09)*

Ans. Partial thickness flap (Ref: Carranza 10/e p926, 1014, 1016)

5. **The type of incision in periodontal surgery depends on:** *(PGI Dec. 09)*

Ans. Width of attached gingival (Ref: Carranza 9/e p722-730)

6. **Fibrotomy to prevent rotational relapse was advocated Ist by:** *(COMEDK 12)*

Ans. Edward

7. **The soft tissue tooth interface formed after flap surgery in place of a previously denuded root surface is called:** *(AIIMS Nov 10)*

Ans. Long JE (Ref: Carranza 10/e p632-634, 968)

8. The following conditions do not create gingival defects necessitating gingivoplasty except: *(AIIMS Nov 10)*

a. ANUG
b. Desquamative gingivitis
c. Acute herpetic gingivitis
d. erosive lichen planus

Ans. a. ANUG (Ref: Carranza 10/e p914)

9. Juvenile periodontitis is associated with: *(AIIMS Nov 10)*

Ans. defect in neutrophil chemotactic activity (Ref: Carranza 10/e p507-509)

10. An 8 mm pocket depth with J.E. coronal to CEJ is: *(AIIMS Nov 10)*

Ans. Pseudopocket (Ref: Carranza 10/e p434-435)

11. Gingival manifestation and cutaneous manifestation as in leukaemic cutis has which cell predominant in acute leukaemia? *(AIIMS Nov 09)*

Ans. Monocytic (Ref: Carranza 10/e p292-294)

12. Hypercementosis of the whole dentition is seen in: *(AIIMS Nov 09)*

Ans. Paget's disease (Ref: Carranza 10/e p77)

13. Which of the following is observed in bone loss involving periodontitis? *(AIIMS May 09)*

a. Osteoblasts on tension side, osteoclasts on pressure side
b. Osteoblasts on pressure side, osteoclasts on tension side
c. Atrophy
d. None of these

Ans. d. None of these (Ref: Carranza 10/e p181, 456-462)

14. Which of the following not a feature of LJP? *(AIIMS May 09)*

a. More in females
b. B/L Symmetrical bone loss
c. Inflammatory process consistent with bone loss
d. Bone loss more rapid compared to normal

Ans. c. Inflammatory process consistent with bone loss (Ref: Carranza 10/e p229, 507-509)

15. Which of the following is least commonly affected by periodontitis? *(AIIMS May 09, AIPG 11)*

Ans. Upper canine and lower 2nd PM (Ref. Carranza 10/e p148, 170, 506-509)

16. Bone fill procedures are most successful in treating: *(AIIMS May 09)*

Ans. Narrow 3 wall defects (Ref: Carranza 10/e p460-464)

17. Resorption of thick margins resulting in plateau formation is called as: *(AIIMS Nov 11)*

Ans. Ledge (Ref: Carranza 10/e p462)

18. 3 wall defect most commonly seen in: *(AIIMS Nov 11)*

Ans. Inter proximial wall (Ref: Carranza 10/e p830)

19. In a patient with trench mouth interproximal architecture has been lost and having a history of smoking, the antibiotic/ combination required to treat this is: *(AIIMS Nov 11)*

Ans. Penicilline + Metronidazole (Ref: Carranaza 10/e p 391, 707)

20. The reverse bevel incision is made to: *(AIIMS May 12, AIPG 10)*

Ans. Remove the infected tissue in the sulcus (Ref: Carranza 10/e p928, 929)

21. Apical migration of the epithelial attachment with corresponding recession of the marginal gingival results in: *(AIIMS May 12, AIPG 11)*

Ans. A shallow sulcus (Ref: Carranza 10/e p434-436)

22. Tobacco chewing is thought to be a contributing/predisposing factor in which condition? *(AIIMS May 12, AIPG 11)*

Ans. ANUG (Ref: Carranza 10/e p396)

23. Type of bone present in the inter-radicular area is: *(AIIMS May 12)*

Ans. Cancellous (Ref: Carranza 10/e p80)

24. In response to TFO, alveolar bone has: *(AIIMS May 12)*

Ans. Osteoblast in area of tension and osteoclast in area of pressure (Ref: Carranza 10/e p469)

25. Periodontal surgery is best performed: *(AIIMS May 12)*

Ans. 4 weeks after completion of the hygienic phase (Ref: Carranza 8/e p567)

26. A drug that exerts anti collagenase activity: *(KCET 11)*

Ans. Tetracycline

27. Shelf like thickening of the alveolar margin due to peripheral butteressing is called as: *(KCET 10)*

Ans. Lipping

28. Following a flap procedure, pressure is applied to the tissue for 1 min. in order to: *(AIPG 10)*

Ans. Adapt tissue against bone

29. Indication for mucogingival surgery include the following except: *(AIPG 10)*

a. High frenum attachment
b. Shallow vestibule
c. Infrabony pockets
d. Insufficient attached gingival

Ans. c. Infrabony pockets (Ref: Carranza 9/e p851)

30. Embedding of new periodontal ligament fibers into new cementum and the attachment of new gingival epithelium to a tooth surface previously denuded by disease is called:

Ans. New attachment

31. Fibronection is used in periodontal therapy as: *(COMEDK 09)*

Ans. Biomodification of root surface

32. Interdependency of osteoblasts and osteoclasts in bone remodeling is called as: *(COMEDK 09)*

Ans. Coupling (Ref: Carranza 10/e p81)

33. Tissue destruction in periodontitis is due to: *(COMEDK 09)*

Ans. Tissue associated plaque

34. The extent of bony defects can be best estimated by: *(COMEDK 09)*

Ans. Transgingival probing

35. The most reliable indicator of gingival inflammation is: *(COMEDK 09)*

Ans. Bleeding on probing

36. Advantages of modified Widman flap are all except: *(AIPG 10)*

a. Adaptation of healthy tissue to tooth surface
b. Post operative interproximal architecture is normal
c. Conservation of bone and optimal coverage of root surface by the soft tissue
d. The procedure is feasible when grafting of bone is contemplated

Ans. b. Post operative interproximal architecture is normal (Ref: Ramjford Ash p300-302)

37. All those factors affect the height and thickness of facial and lingual bony plates except: *(KCET 09)*

a. Alignment of teeth
b. Angulation of root to the bone
c. occlusal forces
d. Mesiodistal angulation of crest of interdental septum

Ans. d. Mesiodistal angulation of crest of interdental septum

38. Which CCB can cause growth of gingival tissues? *(KCET 09)*

Ans. Nifedipine

39. Frequent periodontal abscess appears to be an important periodontal feature in: *(KCET 09)*

Ans. Diabetes mellitus

40. The predominant immune cell in the initial lesion of gingivitis is: *(KCET 09)*

Ans. PMN

41. Differential diagnosis of hypercementosis includes all of these except: *(KCET 09)*

a. Cemental dysplasia b. Cemental aplasia
c. Condesnsing osteitis d. Periapical osteopetrosis

Ans. b. Cemental aplasia

42. If an osseous fill procedure is successful, the type of bone formed in the defect is: *(AIPG 09)*

Ans. Bundle bone

43. Coronoplasty should be carried out in patients with: *(KCET 09, NEET 13)*

Ans. Sign of TFO

44. Grafts taken from an individual of the same species who is not genetically related to the recipient is:

Ans. Allograft *(KCET 09)*

MISCELLANEOUS

- Gracy curret types:

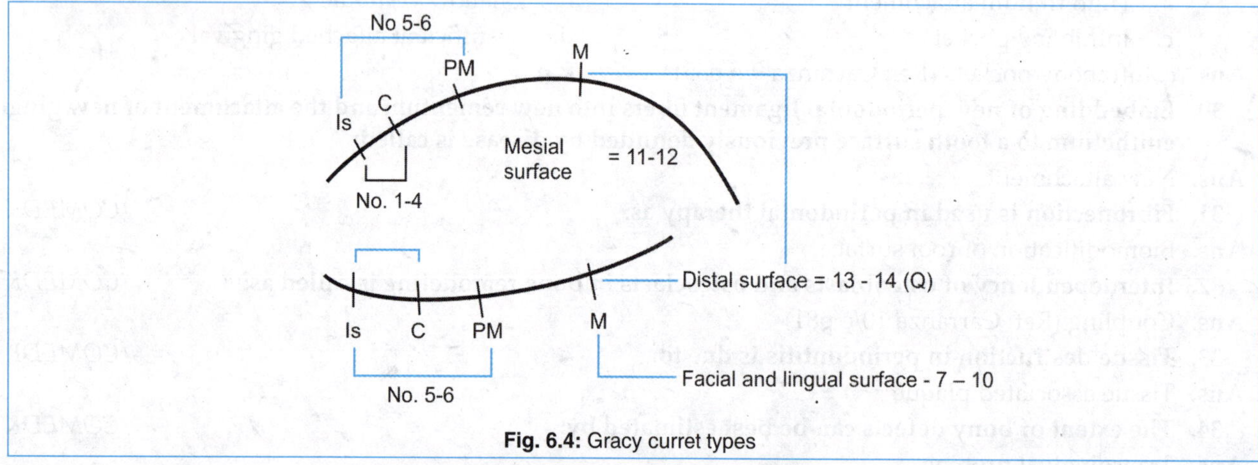

Fig. 6.4: Gracy curret types

- Difference between gracy curette and Universal curette:

Gracy curette	Universal curette
One cutting edge used	Both cutting edges are used
Blade is curved in 2 planes	Blade is curved in 1 plane
Offset -60°	Offset – 90°

- Finger rests:

→ Conventional finger rest → immediately adjacent to working area
→ Finger on finger → used for lingual surface of maxillary posterior
→ Palm up extra oral fulcrum – Maxillary right posterior (KCET-12)
→ Palm down → Maxillary left posteriors

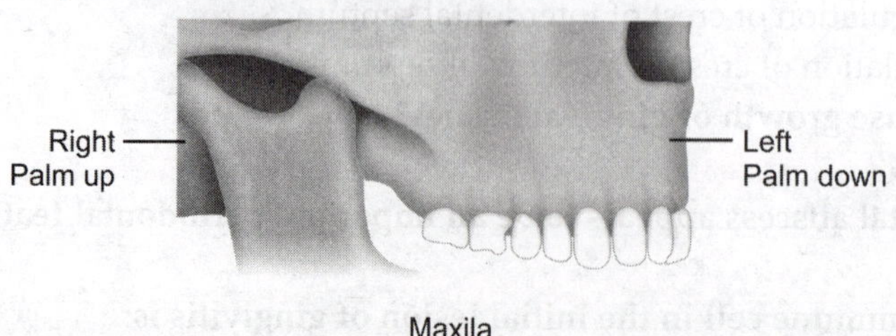

Fig. 6.5: Finger rests

- Gold standard for testing Halitosis:

"Organoleptic" rating by a judge

- BANA test:

Chair side diagnostic test for pdl risk
done in 5 mins.
Subgingival plaque of patient. ↓ Over BANA (Substrate) ↓ BANA hydrolyzed by Trypsin like enzyme ↓ Positive in (Treponema denticolla, P.g, B. forsythus) + capnocytophaga ↓ (Red complex)+ capnocytophaga ↓ blue color

- Dental endoscope: Fibro optic endoscope [Q] used subgingivally in diagnosis and Rx of pdl disease
- Evalusite:

important immunodiagnostic method.
Used for A.a, P.g, P.i.
Is a modification of ELISA [Q] → So, ELISA can be used in diagnosis of A.a

- Implant (very important for PGi)

• Interimplant distance = 3 mm from outer surface of implant
• From adjacent natural tooth = 1–1.5 mm
• From lingual plate, maxillary sinus, nasal cavity [Q] = 1 mm
• From inferior alveolar canal = 2 mm (from superior bony aspect)
• From mental nerve = 5 mm from anterior part
• From incisive canal = avoid midline of maxilla

- Occlusal adjustment:

• Grooving – Restoring depth of developmental groove
• Spheroiding – Reducing supra contact
• Pointing – restoring cusp point contours

- Nylon bristles are superior to natural bristles
- Brush type and bristle diameter:

Soft → 0.2 mm → 0.007 inch
Medium → 0.3 mm → 0.012 inch
Hard → 0.4 mm → 0.014 inch

- Composition of dentifrices:

Component	Example
Abrasive	Silica, Calcium carbonate, Al. oxide [Q] Ca3 (PO4)2
Humectant	Sorbital
Surfactant/ detergent	Sodium lauryl sulphate
Binding agent/Thickening agent	Alignate, Carrageenates, Cellulose [Q]
Anti tartar agent	TPZ
Fluoride (1100 ppm)	Sodium mono fluoro phosphate
Sweetening agent	
flavoring agent	
desensitizing agent	

- Brushing technique and conditions:

• Gingival recession → Modified Stillman
• Healing wounds after surgery → Charters
• Routine technique with /without pdl disease → Bass/Sulcular method
• Most recommended in patient with pdl disease → Sulcular *(AIIMS 12)*
• Recommended in children → Fones
• Most common brushing technique → Scrub technique
• Least effective method → Roll
ROLL method → Roll + modified Stillman method
Vibratory → Bass, charter, Stillman
Circular → Fones
Vertical → Leonard *(KCET 11)*
Horizontal → Scrub

- ADA specification for brush of brushing surface: *(KCET 13)*

Length → 1–1.25 inch
Width → 5/16 –3/8 inch
Rows → 2–4 rows
Tufts → 5–12 tufts/row

- Tooth powder:

has 95% abrasive NOTE: tooth paste has 20–40% abrasive (20–30% water present)
Dentine abraded 25 times Cementum abraded 35 times } More than enamel

- CADIA:

Measures alveolar bone density changing overtime, so, causes pdl disease Progression [Q]

- Probes:

→ Foster miller: Pressure sensitive probe also measures CEJ [Q]
→ Florida probe: Computerized/Automated probe (Also pressure sensitive)

- Wax coating on dental floss ◎ Spermacit wax
- Mercurochrome/erythrocin/two tone ◎ is Disclosing agent
- Probing pressure: 25 g/0.75 N (Q)
- Oral pigmentation:

Hg/Bismuth/Arsenic → Black line of marginal gingival
Pb → "Bluish" red/deep blue line on marginal gingival
Ag → Violet marginal line + diffuse bluish gray.

LAST 5-YEAR QUESTIONS FROM THIS TOPIC

1. **Piezoelectric hand piece works at frequency of:**

Ans. 20,000 – 45,000 Hz.

2. **The chemical that mainly contributes to halitosis is:** *(KCET 12)*

Ans. Hydrogen sulfide

3. **Concentration of CHX used in mouthwash is?** *(PGI Dec. 11, June 10)*

Ans. 0.2% (Ref: Carranza 10/e p338)

4. **The lacto peroxidase thiocynate system present in saliva is against:** *(KCET 12)*

Ans. Streptococcus

5. **Gingival bleeding index is used to asses:** *(PGI Dec. 10)*

Ans. Measures periodontal health (Ref: soben peter 2/e p156)

6. **In periodontal patients, the most frequently recommended tooth brushing technique is:** *(AIIMS May 11, 12)*

Ans. Sulcular technique (Ref: Carranza 10/e p733)

7. **Which of the following is not used as an abrasive in dentrifices?** *(AIIMS May 11, 12)*

Ans. Amylose (Ref: Glickman, periodontology 7/e p688)

8. **The antibiotic of choice in treating LAP involving primary dentition is:** *(KCET 12)*

Ans. Metronidazole

9. **Which dentrifices should be used for periodontal patients?** *(AIIMS May 11)*

Ans. Tooth pastes with minimum abrasive content (Ref: Carranza 10/e p732)

10. **A periodontometer is a device used to measure:** *(AIIMS May 12, May-09, AIPG 11, 09)*

Ans. Tooth mobility (Ref: Carranza 10/e p1080, 1101)

11. **Piezoelectric motion, which is not seen:** *(AIIMS Nov 11)*

Ans. Figure of 8 motion (Ref: Carranza 10/e p830)

12. **Tooth brush abrasions are more common on the:** *(AIIMS May 12)*

Ans. Maxillary teeth, on the left half of the arch (Ref: Carranza 10/e p184)

13. **Dental floss should ideally be used in:** *(AIIMS May 12, AIPG 09)*

Ans. Type I embrasure (Ref: Carranza 10/e p737)

14. **Which index would your use to access the severity of periodontitis in epidemiological studies of a large population:** *(AIIMS May 12)*

Ans. Periodontal index

15. **The CPITN is recorded for:** *(AIIMS May 12)*

Ans. Sextants

16. According ADA, the acceptable dimensions of toothbrush are: *(AIIMS May 12)*

Ans. 1–1¼ Inch Long, 5/16–3/8 inch wide, 2-4 rows, 5-12 tufts per row (Ref: Carranza 8/e p494)

17. The main disadvantage of Florida probe system is: *(COMEDK 12)*

Ans. Lack of tactile sensitivity

18. Ideal angle the sharpening stone must form with the face of the blade is: *(KCET 10)*

Ans. 100–110 degrees

19. Furcation involvement is best diagnosed by: *(COMEDK 09)*

Ans. Naeber's probe

20. DNA probes: *(COMEDK 09)*

Ans. Determine the presence of specific organism

21. Removal of broken curette tip from a deep periodontal pocket is facilitated by: *(COMEDK 09)*

Ans. Schwartz periotriever.

CHAPTER

7 Orthodontics

Topic

- Growth and Development
- Tooth Eruption, Occlusion and Malocclusion
- Habits
- Cleft Lip and Palate
- Diagnosis
- Cephalometry
- Model Analysis
- Skeletal Maturity Indicator
- Phonetics
- Biology and Mechanics of Tooth Movement
- Preventive and Interceptive Orthodontics
- Treatment Options
- Miscellaneous

GROWTH AND DEVELOPMENT

- Method of studying growth:

• Implant –Bjork's (KCET 06) longitudinal study	*(AIPG 2004)*
• Vital stain (Alizarin, trypon blue, Pb acetate, tetracycline) ↓ Stains Ca ↓ • Shows dynamic changes	*(AIIMS 08) [Q]*
• Radiograph–shows static changes	
• Radioisotopes–Tc–33, Ca -45, K–32 ↓ • Used in autoradiography [Q]	

- Theories of growth vs scientist:

• Sutural theory = Sicher	
• Cartilaginous theory = Scott	
• Nasal septum theory of craniofacial growth = Latham	*(COMEDK 09)*
• Functional cranial concept = Van der Klauss	*(COMEDK 05)*
• Functional matrix theory = Melvin moss	*(COMEDK 05, 04)*
• Multifactorial theory = Van Limborgh	
• Servo system theory of growth/Cybernatics = Petrovic/Chartier	
• Genetic theory = Brodie	
• Neurotropism = Behrents	

- Functional matrix hypothesis:

Hypothesis states that origin, form, position, growth and maintenance of skeletal tissues are secondary to related non-skeletal tissues *(KCET 07)*
Based on functional cranial component theory given by vander klauss *(KCET 08, COMEDK 05)*
It includes connected cellular network (CCN), mechanotransduction Epigenetic epithesis not septopremaxillary ligament development Which is a component of Scott's hypothesis *(AIPG 2004)*

FUNCTIONAL CRANIAL COMPONENT

- Functional matrix
  - Periosteal matrix e.g muscles, blood vessels, nerves,gland etc.
    → Act directly and actively upon microskeletal units [Q]
    → Pneumatic brings active and
    → Compensatory transformation
  - Capsular matrix e.g- neurocranial capsule, oro facial capsule (PGI Q)
    → Acts indirectly and passively on macroskeletal units
    → brings about
    → Passive translation
- Skeletal units
  - Macroskeletal units e.g maxilla mandible
  - Microskeletal units e.g alveolus angle,condyle gonial,mental coronoid *(KCET 06)*
    maxilla: orbital palatal

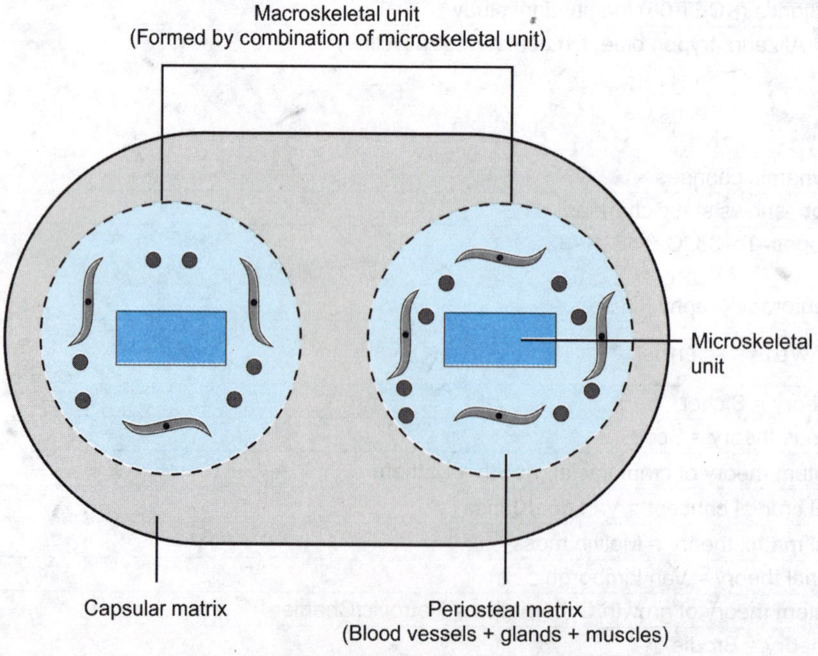

Macroskeletal unit
(Formed by combination of microskeletal unit)

Microskeletal unit

Capsular matrix

Periosteal matrix
(Blood vessels + glands + muscles)

Fig. 7.1: Functional matrix theory

- Bone remodelling theory of craniofacial growth:

Given by brash *(AIIMS 2012)*
Based on John Hunter's vital staining method
Theory states that bones grow only by interstitial growth
Other components of this theory are: • Jaws grow by deposition of bone at posterior surface called as hunterion growth • Cranial vault grows by apposition on ectocranium while resorption on endocranium

- Van–Limborgh's multifactorial theory:

• Growth under control of genetic and environmental factors
• Intrinsic genetic factor: Factor within skeleton
• Epigenetic factors: factors outside skull BUT manifests indirect influence on associated structures (PGI Dec 12), e.g. eyes, brain etc.(local epigenetic) and hormones (General epigenetic)

- Scammon's growth curve:

Neural tissue: major tissue system of body earliest to complete growth and development *(KCET 08)*
S-shaped curve/general body curve: • Birth to 2-3 years rapid growth • 3–10 years slow growth *(COMEDK 09 Q)* • > 10 years rapid growth
Mandible follows the general body curve .so, growth of body Influences growth of mandible *(AIIMS 05)*
Lymphoid tissues: e.g. thymus • Attains 200% adult size in late childhood • Involutes by 18 years to attain adult size. Show - ve growth *(AIPG 2004)*
Genital tissues: Shows no growth till puberty

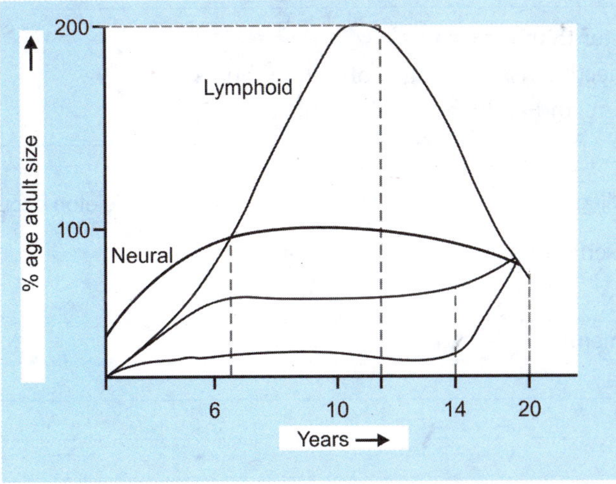

Fig. 7.2: Scammon's growth curve

- Benninghoff lines:

• Indicates natural lines of functional stress in skull
• Trajectories of maxilla: (KCET 07) Frontonasal/canine buttress Malar zygomatic buttress Pterygoid buttress
• Trajectories of mandible: Condyle to condyle through symphysis

- Wolff's law of transformation of bone:

Origially known as trajectory theory of BONE formation
Given by Meyer and cullman [Q]
The architecture of bone is such that it can resist forces brought to bear upon it with the use of as little tissue as possible. So bony trabeculae align up in response to mechanical stresses. *(AIPG 2005, COMEDK 06)*

- Cartilage:

Mandible → Primary cartilage: meckle's cartilage Mandible → Secondary cartilage: Condyle, Coronoid, Symphysis *(KCET 08)*
Maxilla → primary cartilage → nasal septum, ethmoid
Other primary cartilages: Synchondroses and epiphyseal cartilage of long bone.

- Pacemaker of growth:

Maxilla–nasal septum
Mandible–condyle

- Growth site of maxilla:

Sutures, maxillary tuberosity, nasal septum

- Growth of mandible faster than maxilla
- Intramembranous: connective tissue being replaced by bone
- 1st bone to show both i.m. and endochondral ossification:

Occipital at 8 weeks i.u
So, 1st evidence of cartilage getting converted to bone in craniofacial skeleton occurs at 8 weeks i.u. [Q]

- Ossification centers present at birth *(PGI Dec 08)*
- Only 6 centers present:

• Proximal end of humerus
• Proximal end of tibia
• Distal end of femur
• Calceneous
• Tallus
• Cuboid

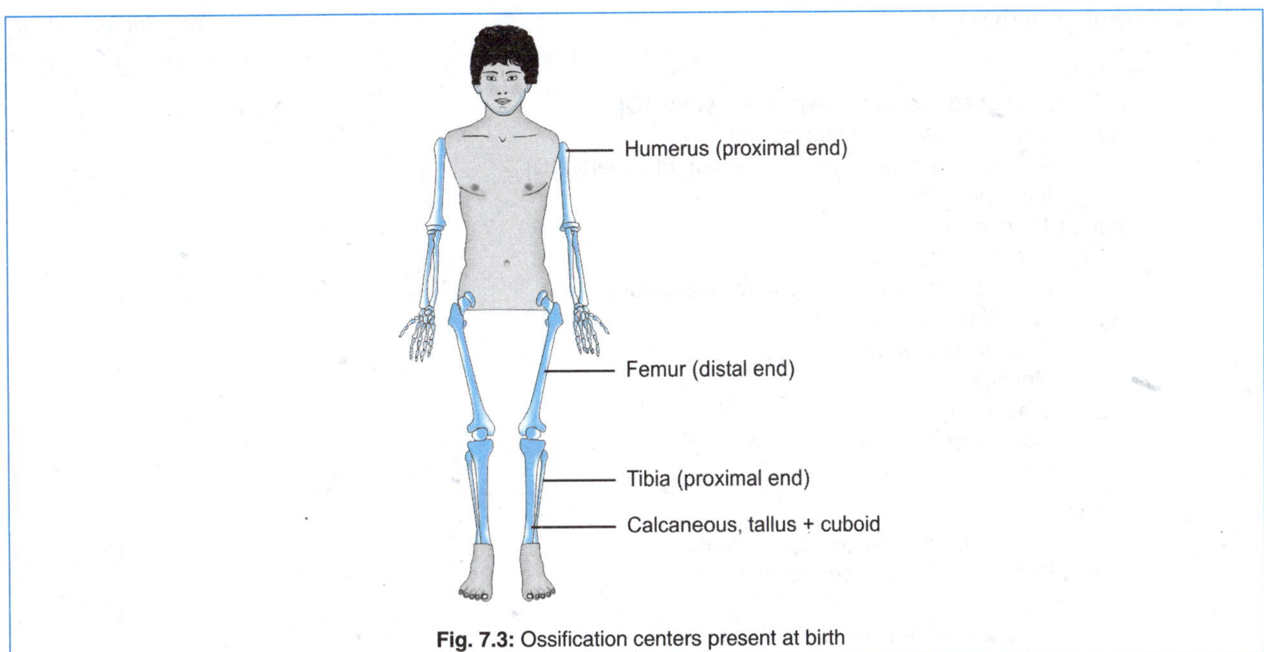

Fig. 7.3: Ossification centers present at birth

- Both i.m and endochondral growth seen in:
- Trick = SOT

Sphenoid Occipital Temporal
Concept: facial bones develop i.m (Intramembranous), e.g. Maxilla *(AIPG 2004)* Except inferior nasal concha and ethmoid which are entirely cartilaginous The structures away from face develop from endochondral ossification

- Intersphenoid 1st to ossify (at birth) *(COMEDK 08)*
- Mandible is the 1st bone to ossify *(PGI Dec 08)* {Clavicle >> mandible}
- Mandibular lingula is the site at which ossification stops in mandible *(KCET 06)*
- Fusion of mandibular symphysis at 18 month
- Spheno occipital last to ossify (17–20 years) { principal growth cartilage of cranium in childhood . causes upward and forward growth *(COMEDK 06)*}
- Ossification center:

A single ossification center for each half of mandible arises in area of future mental foramen lateral to meckel's cartilage in 6 weeks i.u life
For maxilla 3 ossification centers present = 2 in premaxilla and 1 for maxilla proper in infraorbital foramen.

- Growth spurt:

Time of greatest influence of environment/heredity on an organ
• Just before birth/Prenatal period–corresponds to most rapid growth in humans *(COMEDK 06)* • 1 years after birth • Mixed dentition phase (F = 7- 9 yr M = 8- 11 yr) • Adolescent growth phase (F = 11–13 yr M = 14–16 yr)
Absence of "sesmoid bone"–indicates delay in reaching puberty. [Q]

- Adolescent growth stages: *(Very Important for PGI)*

• For girls Total duration of adolescent growth = 3 ½ years [Q] Stage 1: Beginning of adolescent growth Appearance of breast buds (1st sign of puberty) [Q] Initial pubic hair Stage 2: 12 months later Peak velocity in height Noticeable breast development, axillary/pubic hair Stage 3: 12–18 months later Growth spurt ending Menses Broadening of hips Adult fat distribution Breast completed
• For boys Total duration of adolescent growth = 5 years *(PGI June 10)* Stage 1: Beginning of adolescent growth Fat spurt *(PGI June 10)* Weight gain, feminine fat distribution Stage 2: 12 months later Height spurt beginning Redistribution/reduction in fat Pubic hair Growth of penis Stage 3: 12–18 months later Peak velocity in height Facial hair/axillary hair growth Muscle growth Stage 4: 15–24 months later Growth spurt ending Facial hair on chin and lip appears Adult distribution of pubic and axillary hair Adult body form

- Period of ovum/germinal period : < 2 weeks (PGI Q)
- Period of embryo : 2 weeks–8 weeks *(PGI June 12, Dec 08)*
- Period of fetus : > = 9 weeks to birth
- **Note:** Gestational period is after fertilization
  ↓
  So, not fertilization period [Q]
- Gonial angle: follow BDC for KCET and COMEDK with following values

• Prenatal = 135 -150 degree according to BDC
• Soon after birth = 130–140 degree
• Adult = 110–120 degree
3-5 degree greater in female
Note: But for AIPG at birth angle is 175 degree a/c to certain Q Bank from which they directly pick. So, for neet and AIIMS go for this answer *(AIPG 2007)*

- No. of bones in skull:

• At birth = 45	*(COMEDK 06)*
• Adult = 22	

- Cranium has 3 parts:

• Neurocranium/brain case e.g Brain, eye, middle ear
• Viscerocranium/facial skeleton e.g (Trick: Vipul Can Not Make My Pet Zebra Laugh) Vomer, Inferior nasal Concha, Nasal bone, Maxilla, Mandible, Palatine, Zygomatic, Lacrimal
• Endocranium/brain supporting bone e.g sphenoid

- Body ratio:

At 2 months i.u head: body ratio is 1: 2 i.e head: lower body ratio is 1:1	*(PGI June 08)*
growth of cranial, facial and oral structures begins around 21 days i.u. (period of embryo)	*(PGI Dec 06)*

- Type of facial growth:

• Type A: middle face growth = lower face growth	*(PGI June 11, Dec 10)*
• Type B: middle face growth > lower face growth	
• Type C: middle face growth < lower face growth	

- Order of growth:

• Face: Growth is completed 1st in width and last in length (Trick: TSV: Transverse > Saggital > Vertical)	*(KCET 06)* *(PGI Dec 12)*
• Cranium: Vertical > Transverse > Saggital (Trick: VTS) {So, be careful while solving such question}	
Growth of cranium continues upto 15–18 years	
Growth of brain completed by 6- 7 years	*(AIIMS Q)*
75 % growth of brain is completed by 2 years	*(NEET 2013 Q)*

- With advancing age human profile decreases in convexity (AIPG 2006), i.e., concavity increases.
- Percentage of growth of cranial base, maxilla, mandible completed at different ages:

	1-5 years	5-10 years	10-20 years
Cranium	85 %	11 %	4 %
Maxilla	45 %	20 %	35 % (AIPG 04)
Mandible	40 %	25 %	35 %

- More than 90% brain/brain vault growth is completed by 5 years *(COMEDK 06)*
- Maximum growth of brain takes place in infancy *(PGI Dec 08)*
- Volume of cranial growth at 7-8 years is 4/5 *(PGI June 05)*
- Vertical growth of maxilla/V–shaped palatal vault formation is due to growth of alveolus
- Cranial growth is completed by 17-18 years
- In a new born child we generally see mandibular retrusion

- Meckle's cartilage:

Mandible developes lateral to it
Meckle's cartilage forms malleus, incus, sphenomandibular ligament
Disappears without contributing to the formation of mandible.

- Condyle:

Only bone showing both appositional and interstitial growth.
Bone: grows by apposition
Cartilage: grows by interstitial growth

- Drift → deposition + resorption → results in drift towards deposition Side
- Displacement → Primary: due to own growth; → Secondary: Due to growth of adjacent
- Structures
- "V" shaped pattern of groth- Ramus [Q], coronoid, condyleandpalate

Growth of maxilla	Growth of mandible
Downward and forward *(PGI June 08)*	Downward and forward

- Growth of maxillary alveolar process Vs mandibular alveolar process

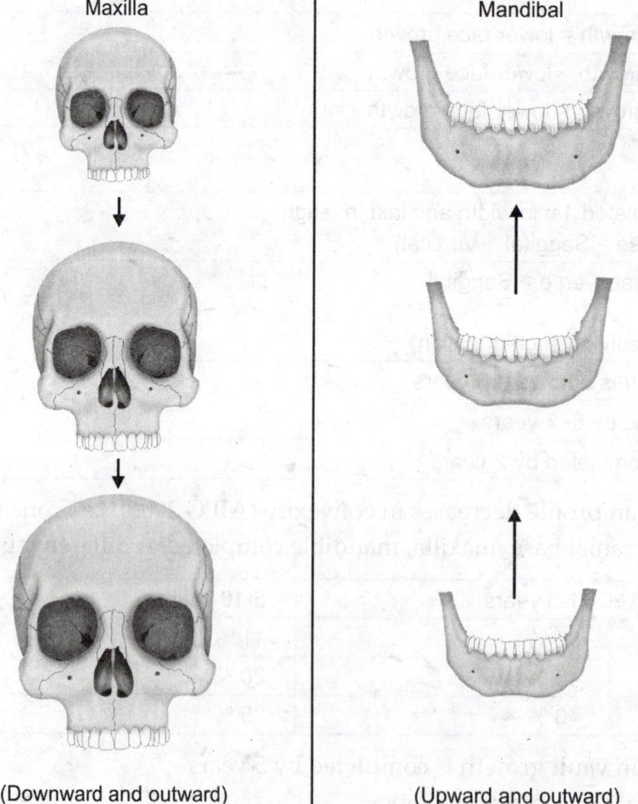

Fig. 7.4: Growth of maxillary alveolar process vs mandibular alveolar process

- If teeth do not develop, development of alveolar process will be affected *(AIPG 03)*
- After 6 years of age, lengthening of mandible occurs mainly by resorption at the anterior border of the ramus and deposition at the posterior border

- Gum pad:

Divided into 10 segments by Transverse groove *(AIPG 07, AIIMS 06)*

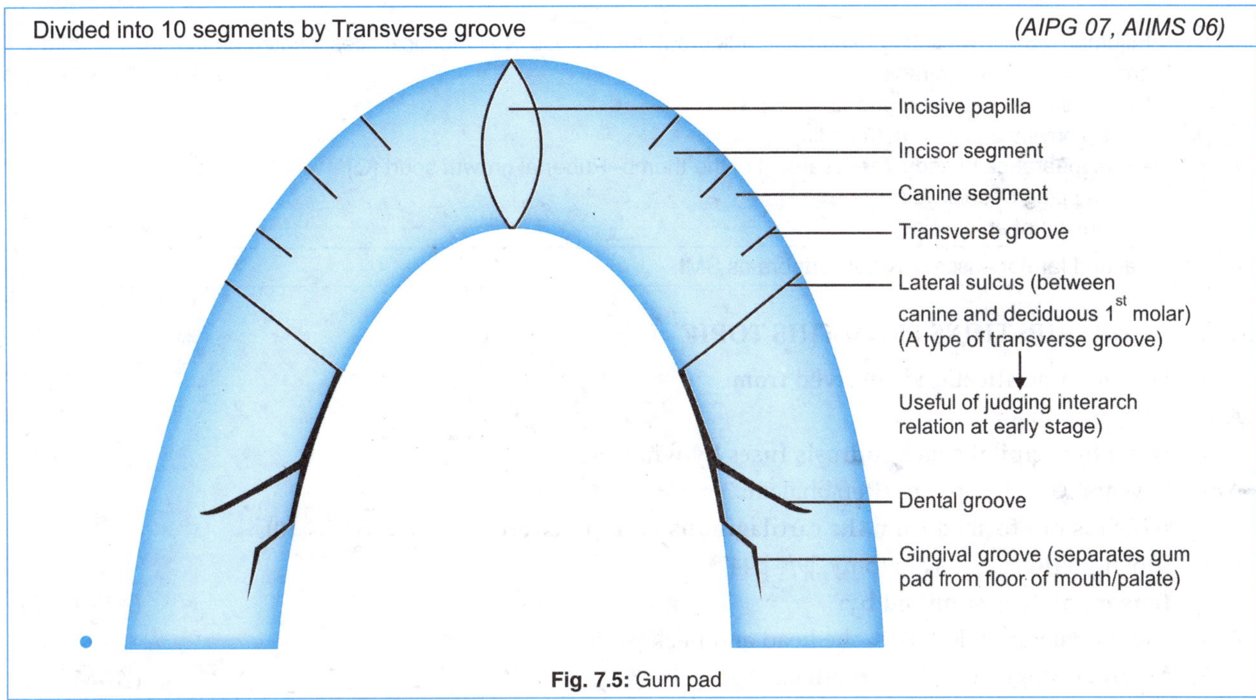

Fig. 7.5: Gum pad

- Tongue muscles oppose bucinator mechanism *(KCET 07)*
- Cartilage, nerves, muscles and cartilage derivatives: [Q]
- Trick: remember the nerves of the arch-the muscles these nerves supply will be the muscle derived from the same arch. [Very Imp.]

Cartilage	Nerve of Arch	Muscle of Arch	Cartilage Derivative
1st arch/ mandibular arch (COMEDK 08)	Mandibular	• Muscles of mastication (nerve supply of maseter/lateral pterygoid *(PGI Dec 06, June 05)* • Tensor tympani • Tensor palate (Nerve supply AIPG 2002) • Mylohyoid • Anterior belly of digastric	• Sphenomandibular ligament • Malleus • incus
2nd arch/hyoid arch	Facial	• Muscles of face (Nerve supply of bucci-nator *(PGI Dec 05)* • Platysma • Stapedius (Nerve supply AIPG 2001) • Stylohyoid • Auricular • Occipito frontalis • Posterior belly of digastric	• Stapes • Stylohyoid Process • Stylohyoid Ligament *(COMEDK 06)* • Lesser Cornua • Superior part of body of Hyoid *(COMEDK 07)*
3rd arch	Glossopharyngeal	Stylopharyngeus	• Greater cornua of Hyoid • Inferior part of body of Hyoid *(COMEDK 07)*
4th arch	Superior laryngeal	• Muscle of Pharynx • Soft palate • Cricothyroid	Cartilage of larynx
6th arch	Recurrent laryngeal	• Muscles of larynx • Except • Cricothyroid	Same as 4th arch

- SMI(skeletal maturation indicator):

• Fishman's SMI–evaluating hand wrist radiograph makes use of anatomical sites located on the–thumb, third finger, fifth finger and radius. *(NEET 2013, KCET 2005)* Uses 4 stages of bone maturation: [Q] – Epiphysis equal in width to diaphysis. – Appearance of adductor sesamoid of the thumb- Pubertal growth spurt [Q] – Capping of epiphysis – Fusion of epiphysis
Hassal and farman–uses cervical vertebra as SMI.

LAST 5-YEAR QUESTIONS FROM THIS TOPIC

1. **Muscle of mastication is derived from:** *(NEET 13)*

Ans. 1st branchial arch

2. **Spheno- occipital synchondrosis fuses by what age:** *(AIPG 12)*

Ans. 16 years {Closest option} (Ref: bhalajhi 3/e p31)

3. **Which is not formed from the cartilaginous part of viscerocranium: (AIPG 10)**

Ans. Sphenoid (Ref: gray's anatomy 39/e p447)

4. **Tensor palate is supplied by:** *(AIIMS Nov 12)*

Ans. Trigeminal nerve (Ref: BDC 4/e head and neck p155)

5. **At which stage of Nolla, s tooth start erupting?** *(AIIMS Nov 12)*

Ans. Stage 6 (Ref: Moyer's handbook of orthodontic's 4/e p111)

6. **Remodeling theory of craniofacial growth was given by:** *(AIIMS Nov 12, PGI Dec. 12)*

Ans. Brash (Ref: Textbook of craniofacial growth by Sridhar Premkumar 1/e p64)

7. **Derivative of 2nd branchial arch is:** *(AIIMS May 12)*

Ans. Muscles of facial expression (Ref: inderbir singh 7/e p115)

8. **Ossification of ulnar–sesamoid begins:** *(AIIMS May 12)*

Ans. Onset of puberty (Ref: bhalajhi 3/e p167)

9. **Neural tissue completes maturing at:** *(AIIMS May 2012)*

Ans. 6-7 years (Ref: bhalajhi 3/e p10)

10. **Which of the following is not a derivative of Meckle's cartilage?** *(KCET 13)*

Ans. Stapes

11. **What is the number of bones a neonatal skeleton has?** *(KCET 13)*

Ans. 270

12. **Premature stenosis b/w the pre and post sphenoidal parts would lead to:** *(KCET 13)*

Ans. Depression of the nasal bridge

13. **Scott's hypothesis emphasized on:** *(KCET 13)*

Ans. Nasal septum (Ref: Bhalajhi 3/e)

14. **The optimal time for a molar tooth to erupt is:** *(KCET 13)*

Ans. 2/3 rd of root is completed

15. **Sensitive period for tetracycline induced discoloration in the permanent maxillary and mandibular incisors and canines is:** *(KCET 12)*

Ans. 3 months postpartum to 7th year of life

16. **The first sign of tooth development in human being is around:** *(KCET 12, PGI Dec 06)*

Ans. 6th week i.u

17. Who proposed the trajectory theory of bone formation? *(KCET 11)*

Ans. An anatomist Meyer and a mathematician Cullman (Ref: textbook of bones and cartilage: developmental and evolutionary skeletal biology by Brian Keith Hall 1/e p410)

18. The groove separating gum pad from the palate is called: *(KCET 11)*

Ans. Gingival groove (Ref: Textbook of pedodontics by Shobha Tandon 2/e p57)

19. The Meckle's cartilage is derived from: *(KCET 10)*

Ans. 1st branchial arch

20. Into how many segments the infant gumpad is divided? *(KCET 10)*

Ans. 5 in each quadrant (Ref: Textbook of pedodontics by Shobha Tandon 2/e p57)

21. Grooves which are present in gumpad s between the canine and the 1st molars: *(KCET 09)*

Ans. Lateral groove (Ref: Textbook of pedodontics by Shobha Tandon 2/e p57)

22. In the 3 planes of space, in both maxilla and mandible, growth is 1st completed in *(KCET 09)*

Ans. Width

23. Which of the following is not a derivative of 2nd pharyngeal arch: *(COMEDK 13)*

Ans. Anterior belly of diagastric {It is supplied by nerve to mylohyoid which is a branch of inferior alveolar branch of mandibular nerve .so, derivative of 1st pharyngeal arch

24. Beginning of adolescent growth in boys is with: *(COMEDK 13)*

Ans. Feminine fat distribution

25. The medial confluence of stress lines on the medial surface of the ramus that represents the racial growth of surface of the mandible is known as: *(COMEDK 13)*

Ans. Eva point (A/C the answer key given)

26. Growth is generally completed: *(COMEDK 10)*

Ans. First in head and last in height of face (Ref: Profit 4/e p113)

27. The first evidence of cartilage getting converted to bone in craniofacial skeleton occurs during: *(COMEDK 10)*

Ans. 8th prenatal week (Ref: Bhalajhi 4/e p25)

28. Tooth eruption generally occurs when root development is completed by: *(COMEDK 10)*

Ans. 75 % completed (Ref: Pedodontics by shobha tendon 2/e p95)

29. Scammon's corve for which of the following tissue systems show an ' S ' shaped curve *(COMEDK 12, 09)*

Ans. Muscle and bone tissues (Ref: Bhalajhi 3/e p10)

30. Period of embroyo is: *(PGI June12)*

Ans. 2-8 weeks

31. Growth stops in following order *(PGI Dec 12, PGI Dec 06)*

Ans. Transverse, saggital, vertical

32. What are epigenetic factors in Van limborgh's multifactorial theory? *(PGI Dec 12)*

Ans. Genetic factors present outside the jaw

33. Time period of growth-spurts in girls occurs during: (PGI Dec 11, June 07)

Ans. 3, 7-9, 11-13 years of age (Ref: Bhalajhi 3/e p9)

34. In which of the following aspects growth is completed soon after birth and shows no further growth with age and remains in size throughout? *(PGI June 11)*

Ans. Width of oropharynx (Ref: Hoyte DA.The cranial base in normaland abnormal skull growth. Neurosurg Clin N Am 1991 ; 515-537)

35. Duration of adolescent stage in boys: *(PGI June 10)*

Ans. 5 years (Profit 4/e p109)

36. Fat spurt in adolescent stage in boys indicate *(PGI June 11)*

Ans. Beginning of adolescent stage (Ref: Profit 4/e p109)

37. Cartilages differ from bone in that: *(PGI Dec 09, Dec 07)*

Ans. Interstitial growth pattern (Ref: Profit 4/e p40)

38. The growth activity at which of these synchondrosis completed 1st *(PGI June 09)*

Ans. Intersphenoidal (Ref: Bhalajhi 3/e p30- 31)

39. Development of mandible is by: *(PGI June 09)*

Ans. 1st brnchial arch (Ref: Inderbir singh 8/e p108-109)

40. Growth of alveolar process of maxilla is in: *(PGI June, Dec 09)*

Ans. Downward and outward

41. Growth of alveolar process of mandible is in: *(PGI June 09)*

Ans. Upward and inward (Ref: Profit 4/e p46)

TOOTH ERUPTION, OCCLUSION AND MALOCCLUSION

- Mandibular permanent incisor tooth buds lie ' inferior and lingual' to deciduous incisors *(AIPG 02)*
- Nolla's stage of tooth development:

Nolla's stage
• Absence of crypt
• Initial calcification
• 1/3 rd of crown completed
• Crown 2/3rd completed
• Crown almost completed
• Crown completed [Q] ↓ Tooth starts erupting (PGI 2007, AIIMS Nov 12)
• 1/3rd of root completed
• 2/3rd of root completed ↓
• Most of the teeth pierce alveolar mucosa at this stage [Q]
• Root almost completed
• Apical end of root completed

- Permanent tooth begin to erupt when root is ½ to ¾ th (Boucher MCQ) formed OR ¾ th formed (Proffit)
- Time period required for erupting premolar tooth to move through 1 mm is 4-5 months. *(KCET 06)*
- Chronology (very imp.)

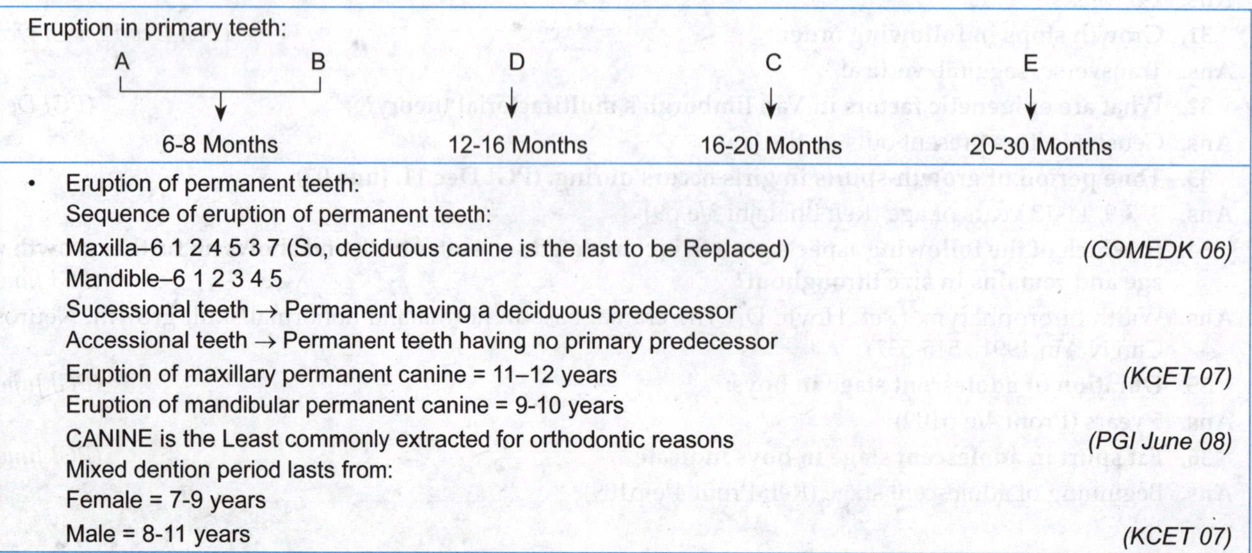

Eruption in primary teeth:

A, B → 6-8 Months; D → 12-16 Months; C → 16-20 Months; E → 20-30 Months

- Eruption of permanent teeth:

Sequence of eruption of permanent teeth:

Maxilla–6 1 2 4 5 3 7 (So, deciduous canine is the last to be Replaced) *(COMEDK 06)*

Mandible–6 1 2 3 4 5

Sucessional teeth → Permanent having a deciduous predecessor

Accessional teeth → Permanent teeth having no primary predecessor

Eruption of maxillary permanent canine = 11–12 years *(KCET 07)*

Eruption of mandibular permanent canine = 9-10 years

CANINE is the Least commonly extracted for orthodontic reasons *(PGI June 08)*

Mixed dention period lasts from:

Female = 7-9 years

Male = 8-11 years *(KCET 07)*

Supervision of child's developing occlusion is most critical at mixed dentition period = 7-10 years *(AIPG 06)*
Note: A 9 year old child has 12 primary and 12 permanent teeth [Q]
1st permanent teeth to erupt in oral cavity mandibular 1st molar *(AIPG 02)*
1st permanent teeth to calcify maxillary 1st molar
6 years molar 1ST molar
12 years molar 2nd molar
A variation of 0-6 months in eruption of molars is considered normal *(PGI Dec 09, June 08)*

- 1st evidence of calcification:
  - Permanent teeth -

Maxilla		Mandible
Central incisor = 3-4 months		Central incisors = 3-4 months
Lateral incisors = 10 months	(PGI june 12)	Lateral incisors = 3-4 months
Canine = 4-5 months		Canine = 4-5 months
1st molar = at birth	(PGI dec 12)	1st molar
1st premolar = 1 ½ years		1st premolar same as maxilla
2nd premolar = 2- 2 ½ years		2nd premolar
2nd molar = 2 ½ - 3 years		2nd molar

3rd molar → 8-10 years [Q]
Concept: Crown completion/calcification completion is 2-3 years before eruption
Root completion is 2-3 years after eruption

Crown completed $\xrightarrow{\text{2-3 years}}$ eruption $\xrightarrow{\text{2-3 years}}$ root completion
According to schour and massler the crown completion of both permanent maxillary and mandibular 1st molar is 2-3 years *(COMEDK 07)*

Rule of 4 for permanent teeth (Not 3rd molar)
At age of 4 years → all crowns have initiated
At age of 4* 2 = 8 → years all crowns are completed

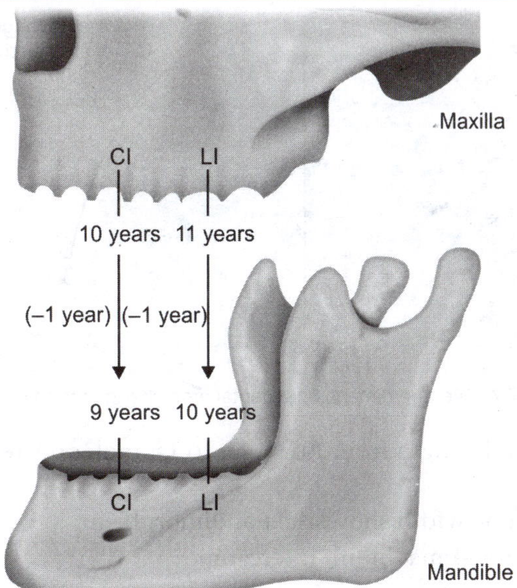

Fig. 7.6: Root completion of anteriors

Deciduous teeth calcification:
Deciduous teeth calcification: 1st macroscopic evidence of morphologic development of primary incisors occurs at 11 week in utero *(COMEDK 06)* 1st evidence of calcification at 3- 4 month i.u (AIPG 06)/14 to 17 weeks i.u (COMEDK 07) and Is almost completed at birth [Q] Completion of calcification 4-10 month after birth [Q] Cental and lateral incisor = 4 month [Q] Canine = 9 month [Q]
Rule of 6: 6 week i.u → beginning of dental development 6 month old → emergence of the 1st primary teeth
By 2 - 2 ½ years all primary teeth have erupted
By 3-4 years all primary teeth have completed root formation, (i.e. root formation of primary teeth occurs 1–1 ½ years after eruption
Following eruption, the root of the maxillary central incisors completes development by 10 years *(COMEDK 08)*

- Rate of eruption:

Time of GINGIVAL emergence 1 -10 μ/day
To reach occlusal plane 75 μ/day

- Average dimensional dental arch changes from 6 to 18 years:

Upper Arch	Lower Arch
Arch length decreases by 1 mm (PGI June 12, Dec 08)	Arch length decreases by 0-1 mm *(PGI June 12)*
Arch circumference increases by 1mm [Q]	ARCH circumference decreases by 4 mm *(PGI 12)*
Inter canine arch width increases by 5 mm (Maximum overcome by incisal liability)	Inter canine arch width increases by 3 mm
Inter molar arch width increases by 4mm	Inter molar arch width increases by 2mm

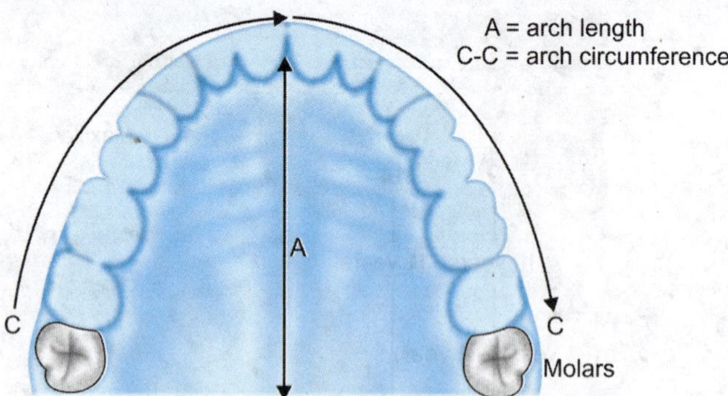

Fig. 7.7: Average dimensional dental arch changes from 6 to 18 years

- After mixed dentition stage arch length from 1st molar to 1st molar decreases due to mesial drift of permanent molars
- Increase in maxillary intercanine width shows sexual dimorphism
- M = 18 years F = 12 years → maximum intercanine
- Dimension is completed. *(COMEDK)*
- Increase in mandibular inter canine width does not show sexual dimorphism. normally completed around 9-10 years

- Safety valve:

Maxillary intercanine dimension serve as safety valve during pubertal growth spurt

- A force of 10-15 gm/cm2 is generated by lip musculature on the upper incisors *(PGI June 11)*
- Tetracycline staining: (Very Imp.) (KCET)

Sensitive/critical period for both deciduous and permanent teeth is from 1st evidence of calcification to crown completion.
Oxytetracycline and doxycycline causes less discoloration.
Minocycline causes discoloration of even fully erupted teeth as it has affinity for collagenous tissue like dentine, pulp, dermis and sclera where it gets oxidized and produces discoloration
ASCORBIC ACID–an antioxidant can block formation of discoloration.
After discontinuation of drug discoloration of teeth persist while that of skin fades easily.

- Incisal liability:

Maxilla = 7 mm *(COMEDK 05,06)*
Mandible = 5 mm

- Primate space/simian space/anthropoid space: *(AIPG 01, COMEDK 05, 07)*

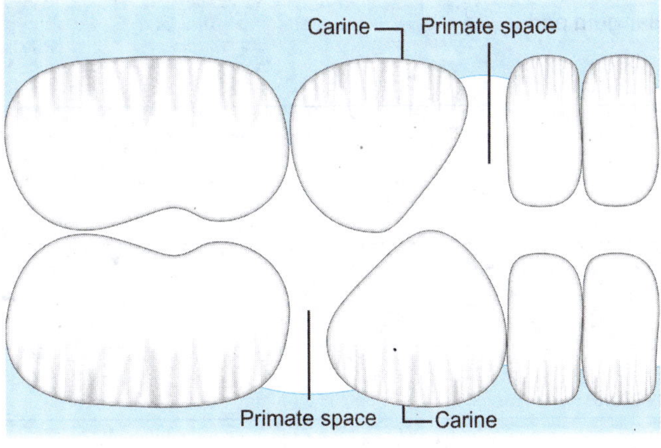

Fig. 7.8: Primate space

- Leeway space: *(KCET 08)*

Difference between sum of MD width of primary canine and molars and sum of MD width of permanent canine and premolars *(AIPG 12)*
Maximum contribution is by primary 2nd molar (PGI dec 10, june 08)
Maxilla = 1.8 mm *(AIPG 05, COMEDK 07)*
Mandible = 3.4 mm *(KCET 06, COMEDK 07)*

- Interdental spacing in deciduous dention:

Maxilla = 4 mm
Mandible = 3 mm
Absence of physiologic space indicates possibility of crowding after eruption of larger permanent teeth.

- Baume's classification: Classification of eruption of primary molars .Based on relation of distal surface of upper and lower 2nd primary molar

Primary Molar Eruption in	Permanent Molar Erupts in	Permanent Molar Later Changes to by Late Shift
Flush terminal plane	End to end (AIPG 06)	Class 1 by late mesial shift
Mesial step	Class 1	Class 3 by late mesial shift
Distal step *(KCET 06)*	Class 2	End on by late mesial shift

- Mesial step → class 3 tendency
- Mesial shift:

Early mesial shift utilizes primate space (Don't confuse with physiologic space)
Late mesial shift utilizes leeway space *(COMEDK 05)*
Lower molar should move 3-5 mm to achieve class 1 relation from end on *(KCET 06)*
Normally (do not confuse) Primary dentition mesial step is found *(KCET 07)* Mixed dentition flush terminal is found

- Self correcting anomaly:

• Pre–dental period: Retrognathic mandibular gum pad Anterior open bite Infantile swallow
• Primary dentition: *(KCET 08)* Anterior deep bite Flush terminal plane Spacing
• Mixed dentition: Ugly duckling stage End on molar relation
• Permanent dentition: – Increase overjet overbite

- Ugly duckling:

Concides with 2nd transitional phase
Term given by "Broadbent"
Seen between 8-9 years, is due to distoangular axial inclination of maxillary Incisors. *(COMEDK 07)*
Results in midline diastema
Not seen in mandible b'coz lower anteriors erupt almost simultaneously (AIPG 02)
Corrected by eruption of canine *(COMEDK 07)*

- Andrew's 6 keys of normal occlusion(AIPG 05): (Repeatedly asked in PGI)

• Molar inter-arch relationship
• M-D crown angulation
• Labio–lingual crown inclination: Maxillary incisor crown inclination + ve Mandibular incisor crown inclination – ve Maxillary and mandibular posteriors – ve
• Absence of rotation

• Tight contacts (PGI Dec 11)
• Curve of spee: according to andrew's curve of spee should be flat

- Bolton ratio is 7th key of normal occlusion *(AIPG 04)*
- 1st molar is used to identify the type of occlusion universally *(AIPG 06)*
- Homogenous population has LOWER incidence of malocclusion than heterogenous population *(AIPG 06)*
- Percentage of population affected by malocclusion:

Ideal occlusion–2-3 %
Class 1: 60-70 % [Q]
Class 2: 30 % [Q]
Class 3: 5 %
Open bite: 5 %

- APDI score:

Antero- posterior dysplasia indicator
Obtained by tabulating the facial angle ,the A-B plane angle and plus/minus the palatal plane angle
MEAN value is 81.75 3.5 *(PGI June 12)*
Highest for class 3 and least for class 2

- Malocclusion and its etiology: (Very imp.)

Malocclusion	Cause
Most common local cause of malocclusion	Premature exfoliation of primary teeth
Main cause of lower incisor crowding (Imbrication) [Q]	Arch length and tooth size discrepancy (Main cause of ectopic eruption) *(AIPG 01)* Arch length dicrepency is most commonly due to premature exfoliation of primary teeth
Development of mandibular crowding in late adolescent phase	Pressure from erupting 3rd molar
Class 2 malocclusion/	Growth discrepancy
Class 3 malocclusion	Hereditary
Most common cause of non skeletal anterior cross bite	Retained primary incisors *(AIIMS 08)*

- Prolonged retention of primary teeth might result in altered path of eruption of suceedeneous teeth *(AIPG 02)*
- Retained mandibular deciduous central incisors will result in lingual eruption of mandibular permanent incisors
- Prolonged retention of deciduous teeth is the most common cause of an anterior cross bite in mixed dentition *(AIPG 07)*
- Main causes of Class 2 malocclusion is growth discrepancy between maxilla and mandible
- Milwauke braces:

Used for scoliosis
Cause retarded mandibular growth
Results in class 2 malocclusion

- Lower tongue position:

Seen in Class 2 div 1 (Lip trap) and Class 3
Result in narrow upper arch

- Class 2 div 2 is characterized by retroclined central and proclined lateral incisor *(AIPG 05)*

- Class 3 skeletal growth pattern is characterized by: *(AIPG 04)*

Acute cranial base angle
Anteriorly positioned articular
Middle cranial fossa align posteriorly and superiorly
Dentoalveolar compensation of class 3 malocclusion is proclination of maxillary anteriors and retroclination of mandibular anteriors.

- Pseudo class 3 vs True class 3:

Pseudo class 3/habitual/functional Class 3	True class 3/anatomic Class 3
Deviated path of closure (forward) to centric occlusion Cause is functional shift (AIIMS nov 06, AIPG 01)	Normal path of closure to centric occlusion, i.e. No deviation
Normal gonial angle	Increased gonial angle (Antigonial notch is increased in ankylosis)

- Certain terms for various malocclusion:

Apertognathia = open bite
Closed bite = deep bite [Q]
Sunday bite/seen in class 2 div 1. Achieved by Dual bite = Bringing mandible forward (PGI Centric slide June 09, June 08)
Scissor bite/maxillary posteriors entirely buccal Buccal = To mandibular posteriors i.e non Mandibular segment constrained occlusion Within maxillary segment [Q]
Imbrication = lower anterior crowding *(KCET 06)*
Transposition = altered sequence of position
Perversion = impacted tooth
Labio version = labial to normal position
Liguo version = lingual to normal position
Infraversion = inferior to line of occlusion
Supraversion = supraeuption
Torsiversion rotation around it's axis *(KCET 08 = 05)*
Cross bite abnormal buccolingual relationship = Of teeth *(COMEDK 08), Malocclusion* Common in Australian Aborigines *(PGI June 08)*

- Malocclusion most common among Indian population is crowded teeth *(AIPG 06)*
- Posterior dental cross bite: more common due to displacement of maxillary than mandibular teeth
- Incomplete overbite is overjet with NO overbite
- Deep bite: *(AIIMS Nov 06)*

• Shows horizontal growth tendency
• Shows decreased anterior growth
• Shows decreased interocclusal space
Deep bite is most damaging feature of Class 2
Reduced deep bite is most damaging feature of Class 3
Vertical jaw dysplasia like deep bite, open bite is more genetically determined than other jaw dysplasias *(AIPG 2007,PGI Dec 12)*

- Crowding:

Reason for crowding: (AIIMS nov 05) • Soft food and diet → no proximal attrition • Epigenetic factor • Inbreeding
Classification: • Mild → < 2 mm → proximal stripping • Moderate 2-4 mm (AIIMS 05) → extraction of 2nd premolar • Severe crowding → 5-9 mm (KCET 06) → Extraction of 1st premolar • Extremely severe crowding → > 10 mm → serial extraction if No skeletal discrepancy [Q]

- Transposition of teeth:

Canine and premolar transposition most common *(KCET 07, AIPG 05)*
Canine to lateral incisor 2nd most common
More common on left side, unilateral (like Cleft Lip and palate)
Maxilla, more common in female
Never seen in deciduous dentition

- When all the teeth are in scissor bite, the condition is called bodie syndrome
- Dewey's modification (Very imp. For PGI)
- Modification of class 1

Type 1	Anterior crowding
Type 2	Protrusive maxillary anteriors (PGI Dec 08)
Type 3	Anterior cross bite
Type 4	Posterior cross bite
Type 5	Permanent molar has drifted mesially due to early extraction of 2nd deciduous molar/premolars

- Modification of class 3

Type 1	When maxillary and mandibular arch are separately viewed they are normally aligned, but when occluded edge to edge incisor alignment. Indicates forward moved mandible
Type 2	Mandibular incisors are crowded and lingually related to maxillary incisors
Type 3	Maxillary incisors are crowded and in cross bite

- New born infants are obligate nasal breathers
- Simon's classification of malocclusion: Various planes used and related malocclusions

• FH plane: Classification of malocclusion in vertical direction If jaw comes near plane → attraction If jaw moves away from plane → abstraction

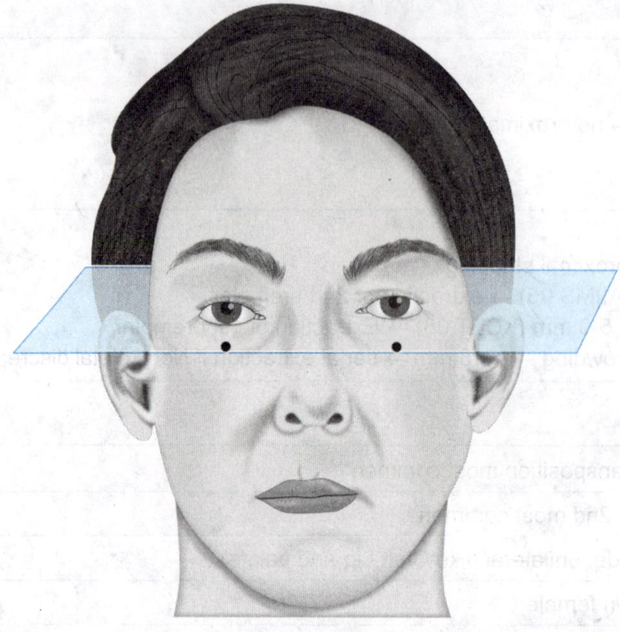

Fig. 7.9: FH plane

- Orbital plane:
  Passes through distal 3rd of canine *(AIIMS Nov 06)*
  Perpendicular to FH plane
  Classification of malocclusion in A-P direction/saggital direction
  Jaw comes near the orbital plane → retraction
  Jaw moves away from orbital plane → protraction

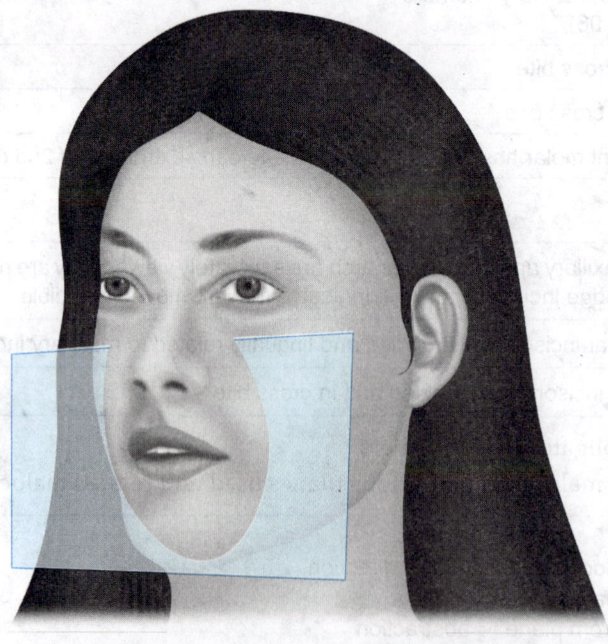

Fig. 7.10: Orbital plane

- Sagittal plane:
  A-P plane
  Classify malocclusion in transverse direction
  Jaw comes near the plane contraction
  Jaw moves away from the plane distraction

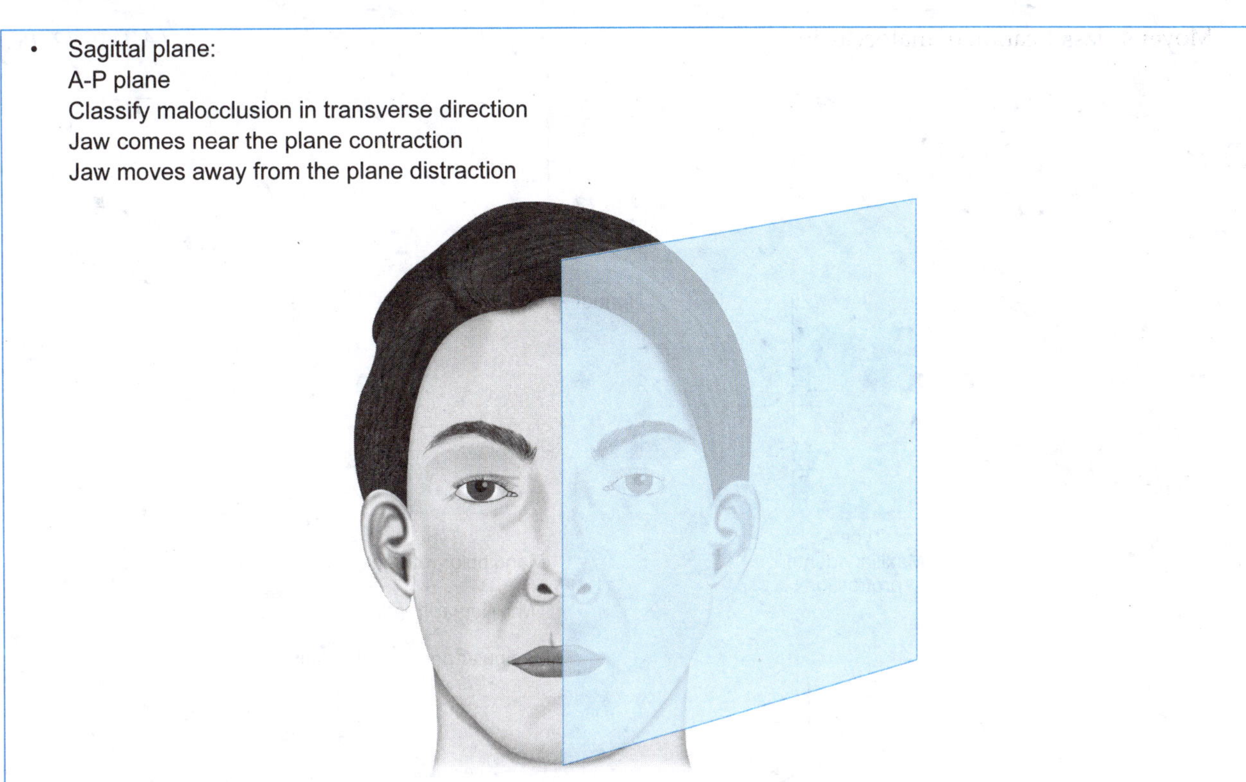

Fig. 7.11: Sagittal plane

- Ackerman–profit classification:

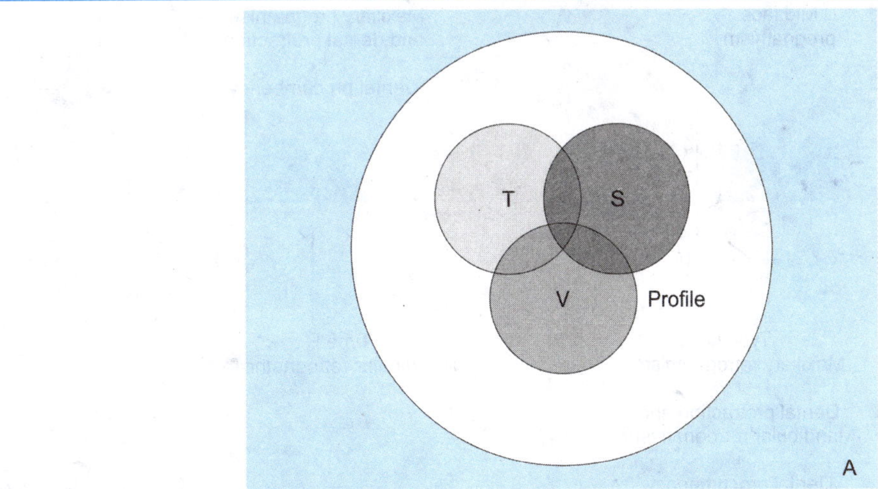

Fig. 7.12: Ackerman–profit classification

T = transverse
S = sagittal
V = vertical
A = intra–arch alignment

Malocclusion representing transverse deficiency is referred to as cross bite	*(AIPG 06)*
Outermost envelope denotes alignment	*(PGI Dec 08)*

- Moyer's classification of malocclusion: *(AIIMS 12, PGI 12)*

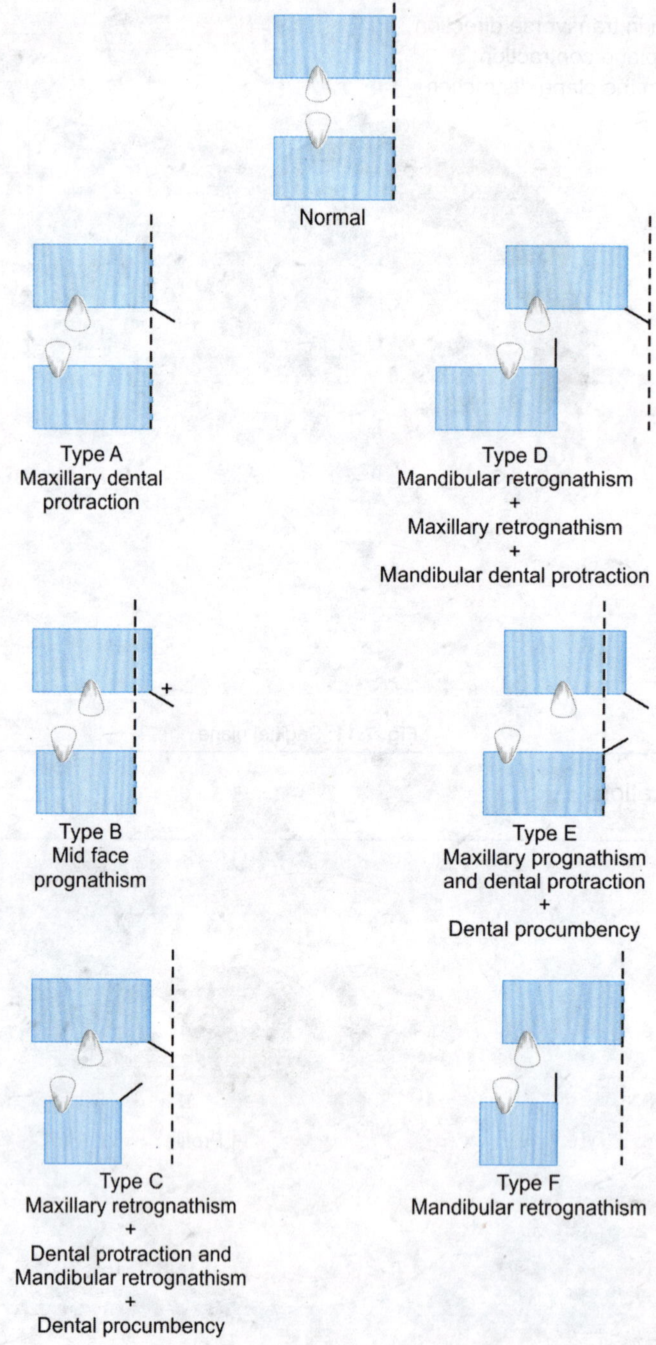

Fig. 7.13: Moyer's classification of malocclusion

- Mandibular 2nd premolar:

Tooth showing greatest variation in eruption timing
Shows greatest variation in occlusal form next to maxillary 3rd molar
3 cusp type premolar is more common
Tooth in the mandibular arch that is most likely to be displaced due to arch Size discrepancy

- Amount of space loss after premature extraction of primary teeth:

Maximum loss of space occurs by premature exfoliation of primary teeth Before the eruption of permanent teeth More in maxillary arch than mandibular arch. Maximum loss of space occurs with in 6 month of extraction of teeth *(PGI 06)* Rate of space loss after premature extraction of deciduous teeth: In maxilla: 1.5 mm/yr [Q] In mandible: 1 mm/yr [Q] *(PGI 06)*
{Note: Rate of physiological migration of teeth leading to shortening of arch Length → 0.5–0.75 μ/day due to inter proximal wear} *(PGI 06)*

Effect of Early Loss of Primary Teeth

- As primary teeth provides eruption force to the successor permanent teeth BUT it is not the only force for eruption. So, eruption will Occur but "delayed eruption"
- Most common cause of malocclusion. Crowding in permanent teeth.

- Most common cause of missing central incisors ——— supernumerary tooth [Q]
- Most common cause of missing lateral incisors ——— congenital absence of tooth [Q]
- Jaw abnormality and associated disease:

Jaw Abnormality	Disease
Underdeveloped maxilla (class 3 malocclusion)	• Down syndrome • Craniofacial dysostosis • Cleidocranial dysplasia • Achondroplasia
Under developed mandible (Class 2 malocclusion)	• Pierre robin syndrome • Treacher Collins syndrome
Under developed both maxilla and mandible	Hypopitutarism
Enlarged maxilla	Monostotic fibrous dysplasia/Leontiasis ossea
Enlarged mandible	Acromegaly
Enlarged both maxilla and mandible	Pagets disease (Maxilla >>> mandible
Asymmetric deformation of mandible	Caffey's disease (PGI)
Prominence of premaxilla	Thalassemia
Under developed premaxilla	Congenital syphilis

LAST 5-YEAR QUESTION FROM THIS TOPIC

1. **Establishment of occlusion at the first molars during maturation of dentition occurs by:** *(AIPG 12)*

Ans. Late mesial shift (Ref: Pediatric dentistry: Principles and practice by Muthu, Muthu and Sivakumar, 2009 p108)

2. **If the deciduous molars erupt in a flush terminal plane, then the most likely molar relation in permanent dentition would be:** *(AIPG 12)*

Ans. Class 1 (Ref: Bhalajhi 4/e p47, 48)

3. **Leeway space is due to:** *(AIPG 12)*

Ans. Space difference between deciduous canine and molar and their succedaneous permanent teeth (Ref: Bishara p57)

4. Which of the following event has little/no significance: *(AIPG 12)*

a. Mandibular incisors erupting before mandibular molar

b. Mandibular canine erupting before mandibular premolar

c. Mandibular 2nd premolar erupting before mandibular 2nd molar

d. Maxillary premolar and canine erupting before maxillary 2nd molar

Ans. a. (Ref: Oral development and histology by avery, steele, avery, 2002 132)

5. The eruption of teeth in active and passive phases was defined by: *(AIPG 12)*

Ans. Gottleib and orban (1933) (Ref: Atlas of cosmetic and reconstructive periodontal surgery by Cohen, 2007 p259)

6. In edge to centroid relation *(AIPG 10,07, AIIMS May 10, May 08, May 07)*

Ans. Edge is in front of centroid (Ref: Mitchell and Littlewood 1/e p168)

7. True about primary teeth is: *(AIPG 09)*

Ans. Calcification of all primary teeth is almost completed at birth (Ref: Wheelers)

8. With a flush terminal plane, permanent first molars will erupt in: *(AIPG 08)*

Ans. Erupt immediately into an end on relation (Ref: Bhalajhi 3/e p43)

9. At which stage of Nolla's tooth start erupting? *(AIIMS Nov 12)*

Ans. Stage 6 (Ref: Moyer's handbook of orthodontic's 4/e p111)

10. The optimal time for a molar tooth to erupt is: *(KCET 13, AIPG 04)*

Ans. 2/3 rd of root is completed

11. Sensitive period for tetracycline induced discoloration in the permanent maxillary and mandibular incisors and canines is: *(KCET 12)*

Ans. 3 months postpartum to 7th year of life

12. The first sign of tooth development in human being is around: *(KCET 12, PGI Dec 06)*

Ans. 6th week i.u.

13. Tooth eruption generally occurs when root development is completed by: *(COMEDK 10)*

Ans. 75 % completed (Ref: Pedodontics by shobha tendon 2/e p95)

14. Establishment of occlusion at the 1st molars during maturation of dentition occurs by: *(AIPG 12)*

Ans. Late mesial shift (Ref: Pediatric dentistry: Principles and practice by muthu and shivakumar, 2009 p108)

15. If the deciduous molars erupt in a flush terminal plane, then the most likely molar relation in permanent dentition would be: *(AIPG 12)*

Ans. Class 1 (Ref: bhalajhi 4/e p47-48)

16. Which of the following event has little/no significance: *(AIPG 12)*

Ans. Mandibular incisor erupting before the mandibular molar (Ref: oral development and histology by Avery, Steele, Avery, 2002 p132)

17. Moyer's classification type D of class 2 malocclusion there is: *(AIIMS Nov 12, PGI Nov 12)*

Ans. Retrognathic maxilla and mandible (Ref: American journal of orthodontics)

18. Lingually locked left maxillary CI in 9 years old child with good harmony of bone, the reason is: *(AIIMS Nov 12)*

Ans. Retained deciduous primary left CI

19. Malocclusion can be progressive in: *(AIIMS May 12)*

Ans. Class 3 (seminars in orthodontics–early timely treatment of class 3 malocclusion by Petr Ngan p140–141)

20. Most common cause of anterior cross bite in mixed dentition is: *(AIIMS May 10, May 07)*

Ans. Prolonged retention of deciduous (Ref: bhalajhi 4/e p105)

21. A midline diastema b/w erupting permanent maxillary incisors may indicate which of the following?

Ans. A normal stage of development before eruption of canines *(KCET 13)*

It may be related to a mesiodens/tooth size discrepancy

It may be related to high frenal attachment

22. Early mesial shift makes use of: *(KCET 11)*
Ans. Primate space not physiologic spaces (Bhalajhi 3/e p43)
23. Identify the term which indicates teeth/other maxillary structures too low down in the face *(KCET 10)*
Ans. Abstraction
24. Which is not a common finding of the deciduous dentition *(KCET 10)*
Ans. Tight contacts, absence of spacing
25. Eruption of 1st permanent molar causes: *(KCET 09)*
Ans. Early mesial shift
26. The most accepted cause for late incisor crowding: *(KCET 09)*
Ans. Late mandibular growth (Ref: Orthodontics by profit 4/e p108)
27. Which terminal plane is favorable for E/E to have class 1 molar relation *(KCET 09)*
Ans. Flush terminal plane
28. "Safety valve "Mechanism is: *(KCET 09)*
Ans. Increase in maxillary intercanine width at 12 years (Ref: manual of orthodontics kumar 1/e p123)
29. Which one of the following has maximum familial tendency *(KCET 09)*
Ans. Deep bite
30. Pigmentation of the permanent teeth may develop if tetrcyclines are given between the ages of: *(COMEDK 13)*

a. 5–7 years
b. 0.2–5 years
c. 6–10 years
d. 10–12 years

Ans. b.
31. Vertical malocclusion include: *(COMEDK 13)*
Ans. Gingivally supported DEEP bite
32. What is the amount of time required by erupting premolar to move through 1 mm of bone as measured on a bite wing radiograph? (COMEDK 12, PGI June 11 {Question was mentioned as through what amount of bone does a tooth normally erupt in 4-5 months?})
Ans. 4-5 Months
33. Clockwise rotation refers to mandibular rotation: *(COMEDK 11)*
Ans. Downward and posteriorly (Ref: Tectbook of orthodontics by gowri Shankar 1/e p71)
34. When vertical cephalometric analysis reveals increase in skeletal components of anterior face height, it is termed:
Ans. Apertognathia (Ref: textbook of orthodontics by gowri Shankar 1/e p616)
35. Tendency of drifting of posterior teeth into extraction space is more in? *(COMEDK 11)*
Ans. Maxilla (Ref: Texbook of orthodontics by gowri Shankar 1/e p515)
36. At what age maxillary intercanine dimension is essentially completed in boys and girls during growth? *(COMEDK 10)*
Ans. 18 years in boys and 12 years in girls (Ref: Orthodontics by gowri Shankar 1/e p64)
37. Displacement occurs in which direction in Angle classification? *(PGI June 12)*
Ans. Saggital
38. Colomn angle is seen in which malocclusion? *(PGI Dec 12, AIIMS May 13)*
Ans. Class 2 div 2
39. Malocclusion classified on the basis of etiology by: *(PGI Dec 12)*
Ans. Bennet (Ref: Ballajhi 3/e p78)
40. What is intramatrix rotation: *(PGI Dec 11, Dec 10)*
Ans. Movement of core of mandible in relation to mandibular plane (Ref: profit 3/e p102)

41. Molar–Incisor hypoplasia in 10 teeth at occlusal plane is due to developmental defect occurring during: *(PGI June 10)*

Ans. Birth–12 months (Ref: Shafer's 4/e p54)

42. In orthodontic analysis roll describes discrepancy of: *(PGI June 10)*

Ans. Transverse cant of occlusion (Ref: Profit 4/e p186)

HABITS

- Classification of habits:

Author	Classification
Earnest klein *(PGI Dec 12)*	• Intentional/meaningful habits (psychological basis) • Unintentional/empty habits
William james	• Useful habits • Harmful habits
Finn and sim	• Compulsive habits • Non compulsive habits OR • Primary habits • Secondary habits
Kingsley	• Functional • Muscular • Postural • combined
Morris and bohnna	• Pressure habits • Non pressure habits
Graber (classified on basis of etiology)	• Tongue thrusting • Thumb sucking

- Normal time period of various features:

Features	Normal time Period (Age)
Infantile swallow	1 ½ – 2 years
Breast feeding	1 ½ years
Thumb sucking	3 ½ – 4 years
Tongue thrusting	3 – 11 years

- Tongue thrusting:

Normal up to '3-11 years'

Abnormal perioral muscle activity is one of the patient factor for tongue thrusting

Types of tongue thrust:

Simple Tongue Thrust	Complex Tongue Thrust
Teeth together swallow [Q]/teeth contact swallow	Teeth apart swallow [Q]
Contraction of mandibular elevators	Absence of mandibular elevator contraction (e.g temporalis)
Associated with thumb sucking	Associated with stuffy nose, tonsillitis,

Note: Facial muscle contraction seen in both simple and complex tongue thrusting

Diagnosis: Tongue posture is examined: during rest, dorsum of tongue touches palate, while the tip rests against cingulum/fossa of lower incisors ↓ (So, posterior cross bite seen)
Rx: • Myofunctional therapy (Habit breaker) + muscles excercicse Developes a new swallowing pattern • Appliance therapy

- Rooting reflex was given by benjamin
- Freudian theory and different phases seen:

Oral → 1-2 years
Anal → 2-3 years
Phallic → 3-6 years (Oedipus and Electra complex seen)
Latent → 7-11 years [Q] (Development of mixed dentition and Character formation) *(PGI Dec 12)*

- Oral drive theory:

Given by sears and wise
States that prolonged suckling leads to thumb sucking

- Rooting reflex disappears around 7-8 months
- Infantile swallowing:

Seen prior to eruption of BUCCAL teeth (NORMAL till 1 ½ - 2 years)
Retained infantile swallowing is rarest finding and shows poorest prognosis
Retained infantile swallow: Patient thrusts tongue between front teeth and laterally on BOTH sides violently. Such patients will have poor, expressionless face and difficulty in Mastication

- Thumb sucking:

Prolonged suckling → Leads to thumb sucking
Thumb sucking leads to anterior open bite and maxillary constriction (KCET 07), Proclination of upper centrals *(COMEDK 05)*
Palatal crib is a habit breaking appliance used in case of thumb sucking *(AIPG 02)* Palatal crib should be worn for at least 6 month

- Causes of bruxism:

Psychological stress and occlusal discrepancy between C.O and C.R [Q]
Occlusal night gaurds are used to redistribute the forces on teeth due to habit of bruxism *(AIPG 02)*

- Mouth breadthing:

Leads to adenoid face (KCET 07)/long face syndrome
Classification by Finn: *(KCET 08)* Anatomic–due to incompetent lip Habitual–continued mouth breathing even after nasal obstruction is removed Obstructive–due to adenoids/tonsils/deviated nasal septum

It can be diagnosed using cephalometry, rhinomanometry, mouth mirror test, Massler's butterfly test/cotton test *(AIIMS Nov 06)*
Oral screen is used for treatment of mouth breadthing . It allows child to breadth through nose *(AIPG 05)*

LAST 5-YEAR QUESTIONS FROM THIS TOPIC

1. **Facial profile of a patient with chronic mouth breadthing is:** *(AIIMS Nov 09)*

Ans. Long and convex (Ref: Hason and Mason. Orofacial Myology 2/e p393)

2. **Children with thumb sucking habit have which of the following?** *(AIIMS May 09)*

Ans. Long face convex profile (Ref: Singh 2/e p590)

3. **Which of the following are not associated with complex tongue thrusting activity?** *(KCET 10)*
   a. Naso-repiratory distress
   b. Contraction of the temporalis
   c. Contraction of mentalis and lower lip during swallow
   d. Absence of contact of teeth during swallow

Ans. d

4. **Mouth breathing with enlarged tonsils and adenoids may be best described as:** *(KCET 09)*

Ans. Obstructive

5. **Bruxism is _________ during sleep:** *(COMEDK 13)*

Ans. Grinding of teeth

6. **Case study: 5 Year old residential school child walks into your clinic with the habit of thumb sucking in association with bruxism:** *(COMEDK 12)*

   Q.1. What would be probable cause?
   Ans. Psychological
   Q.2. Usually sucking digit will be having:
   Ans. Fibrous roughened callus
   Q.3. Chemical approach for reminder therapy is:
   Ans. Femite
   Q.4: Following effects are seen on maxilla except:
   a. Increase SN to ANS-PNS angle
   b. Increased proclination
   c. Increased, axillary arch length
   d. Increased SNA
   Ans. a

7. **Case study: A 6 years old female child reported with a chief complaint of proclined upper anteriors. Parents give a history of prolonged bottle feeding and a persistent thumb sucking habit. Clinical examination reveals anterior open bite with proclined upper anterior and retroclined lower anterior teeth and associated tongue thrusting.** *(COMEDK 11)*

   Q.1. Usually,digit sucking habits are outgrown by:
   Ans. 3-4 years (Ref: Balajhi 3/e p97-102)
   Q.2. In thumb sucking protraction of the maxillary teeth is seen when:
   Ans. When pollex is held upward against the palate
   Q.3. The tongue thrust seen in this case is:
   Ans. Simple tongue thrust
   Q.4: The foremost line of treatment in this patient is:
   Ans. Psychiatric consultation prior to any therapy

CLEFT LIP AND PALATE (IMPORTANT TOPIC FOR PGI)

- Highest incidence of Cleft Lip and palate:

Mongoloids [Q] > Afghan

- Cleft Lip and palate management:

At birth → give feeding plate
3-6 week → presurgical/infant orthopedics (To bring protruded Pre-Maxillary segment back into arch to obtain good Surgical repair of LIP) [Q] *(COMEDK 08)*
3-6 month → Alignment of deciduous teeth, Cleft Lip repair *(AIPG 03, COMEK 06)* Cleft Lip repair follows MILLARD rule of 10: Repair carried out at 10 weeks Weight should be 10 pound Hemoglobin should be 10 gm/dl of blood
6-18 month → cleft palate repair Done primarily to correct speech *(PGI 06, 08)* Surgery of hard palate may inhibit growth causing facial Profile to become more concave [Q] because of Maxillary retrusion only (don't confuse that There can be mandibular protrusion as mandible grows Normally while maxillary growth is retarded) *(AIPG 01)* This leads to class 3 malocclusion [Q]
2-8 years → restorative care
8-15 years → bone grafting(prefer to expand the arch before grafting) (should be done before canine eruption AIIMS 11), orthodontic treatment

- Armany proposed partial maxillary defects:

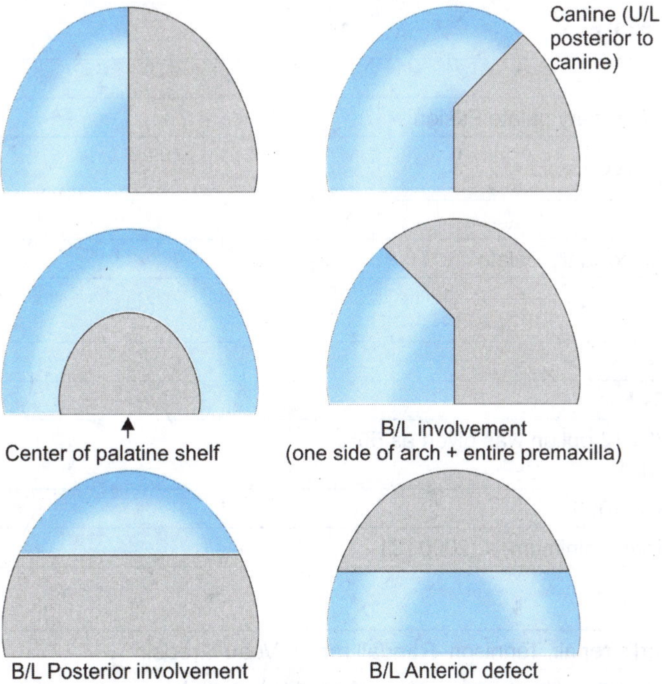

Fig. 7.14: Armany classification of partial maxillary defects

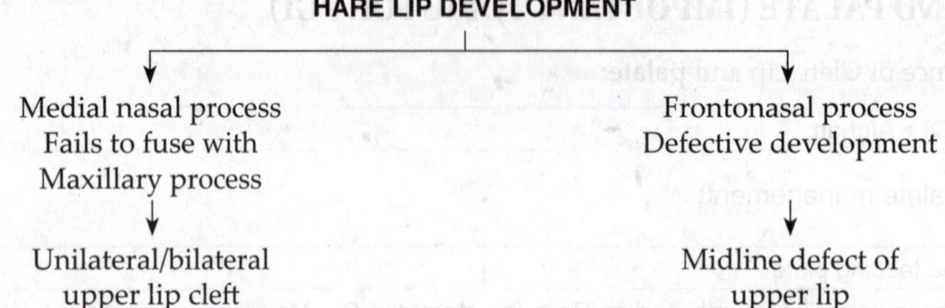

- Long face + Convex profile:

Seen in thumb sucking (AIPG 02)
and
Mouth breadthing

- Cleft palate patient concave profile
- Cleft lip and palate

Leads to maxillary retrusion
↓
Concave profile + bilateral posterior cross bite

- Cleft lip and palate maximum in mongoloids:

Cleft Lip → common in males (PGI 07) (Trick–remember the " vardhan' of 'DON' starring amithabh bacchan. He, seems to have Been operated for cleft lip)
Cleft palate → common in females
Unilateral clefts → seen in 80 % cases
Among unilateral cleft, left side cleft is more common as seen in 70% cases *(PGI 08)*
Combination of Cleft Lip and palate are more common than isolated .seen in 50 % cases *(PGI June 12)*

- Cleft Lip formation between:

4-8 weeks i.u
Coincides with the time of primary palate Fusion

- Cleft palate formation between:

8-12 weeks i.u.
Coincides with fusion of secondary Palate

- Occurrence rate of:

Cleft Lip alone → 15%
Cleft palate alone → 40%
Combined → 45 % (In PGI 12 option was given as 50%. So, it should be the answer)
Incidence of cleft → 1: 600-1000
Incidence of cleft in negroes (minimum) 1: 2000 [Q]

- Cleft Lip and palate surgery: *(AIIMS Nov 12)*

Cleft Lip surgery → millard's repair, Tennison–Randall repair, Veau 3 repair
Cleft palate surgery → Von Langerbeck repair, Veau Wardill V-Y push back palatoplasty

LAST 5-YEAR QUESTIONS FROM THIS TOPIC

1. **In patients with surgically corrected Cleft Lip and palate anomaly, what is the most common anomaly seen?** *(AIPG 12, AIIMS Nov 11)*

Ans. Unilateral/bilateral cross bite

2. **Lowest incidence of cleft palate is seen in:** *(AIPG 10, 07, AIIMS May 08, May 07)*

Ans. Negroes (Ref: OP Kharbanda 1/e p491)

3. **Alveolar bone grafting in a cleft palate patient is done:** *(AIPG 09)*

Ans. After maxillary expansion, cross bite correction and before canine eruption

4. **A 2 year old child presents with cleft of hard and soft palate which extends till the incisive foramen . according to Veau's classification this case comes under:** *(KCET 13, PGI Dec 11)*

Ans. Group 2

5. **The most important reason for placing an alveolar graft in cleft palate patient is:** *(KCET 12, 11)*

Ans. Make eruptive pathway for permanent canine (Ref: Profit p323-324)

DIAGNOSIS

- **Note:**

Chronic medical problems like DM/SABE/treated juvenile periodontitis etc. don't contraindicate orthodontic treatment if the medical problem is under control and if special precautions are followed.
In cases of recently diagnosed leukemia, orthodontic Rx should be avoided till remission of disease occurs. *(AIPG 04)*

- Orthodontic triage

Step 1: syndrome and developmental anomalies
Step 2: facial profile analysis
Step 3: dental development
Step 4: space problems
Step 5: other occlusal discrepancies

- Cephalic index = $\frac{\text{Maximum skull width}}{\text{Maximum skull length}}$

Dolicocephalic < 76
Mesocephalic 76–81
Brachycephalic > 81

- Jarback ratio = $\frac{\text{Posterior facial height}}{\text{Anterior facial height}} * 100$

This index is used to diagnose long face syndrome *(AIPG 04)*
Ratio < 62 % verical growers

- Facial index = $\frac{\text{Distance between nasion to gnathion}}{\text{Bizygomatic width}}$

Euryprosopic → 79–83
Mesoprosopic → 84–88
Leptoprosopic → 88–93 (Seen in long and narrow face as well As dental arches) *(KCET 09, 08)*
In AIPG 04 question asked was normal facial index and according to options given answer should be 80–90%

- Golden proportion:

During smile, a pleasure curve is formed following the curve of anterior teeth and some portion of mesial surfaces of each tooth is visible
This ratio is called golden proportion/esthetic rule which is equal to 62 % (AIIMS 06,PGI June 08), i.e. apparent width of lateral incisor should be 62 % of width of central incisor and so on
Height to width ratio of teeth (central incisor) is 80 % (PGI)

- Essential diagnostic tools:

Study model
3-basic radiograph (periapical, bitewing, OPG)
Facial photograph

- Hypotonic upper lip associated with

Class 2 div 1
Mouth breadthing
Note: In class 2 div 2 no straining of lips seen *(PGI Dec 08)*

- Upper facial height: lower facial height:

45: 55 [Q]
Lower facial height is reduced in growing children, skeletal Deep bite, class 2 div 2

- Position most important in diagnosis of anterior/posterior cross bite is the point of 1st contact in centric relation *(AIPG 05)*
- Normal interincisal distance → 40 to 45 mm
- Kinesiography:
  Records rest position of mandible 3-Dimensionally
- Orthometer is used to read ideal arch width in premolar and molar region directly
- Gnathostatic model:

It is orthodontic study model whose maxillary cast base is trimmed according to FH plane

- Kesling diagnostic set up:

Individual teeth and their associated alveolar process are sectioned off and replaced on model base on desired position
It helps in simulating various tooth movements that are planned for patients

- EMG:
- Detect abnormal muscular activity associated with malocclusion
- Edge and centroid:

Centroid is center of long axis of upper incisor root
Edge is incisal edge of lower incisors
Edge–centroid relationship measures distance between perpendicular Projections of lower incisal edge and centroid of upper incisor root onto Maxillary occlusal plane
Normally edge is 1 mm ahead of centroid
Overbite reduction is more stable if edge is in front of centroid

- Retrognathia means retruded mandible

- Esthetics:

Width of maxillary central incisor is 80% of the height
Gingival zenith: is the most apical point of gingival tissue. For maxillary central incisors and canine, it is distal to the long axis of tooth while for maxillary lateral incisors it coincides with long axis.

- Rotation of jaw: *(Very Important for PGI)*

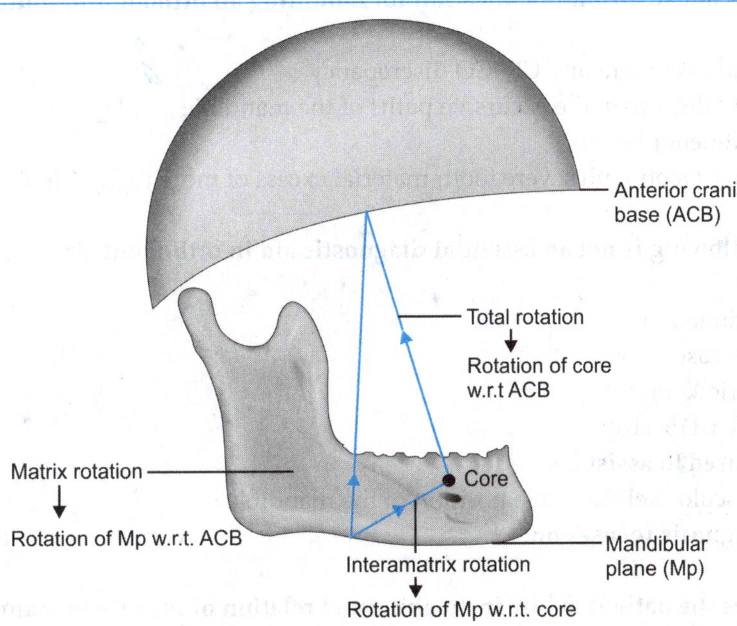

Fig. 7.15: Rotation of jaw

In addition to rotations in transverse, saggital and vertical planes, rotation around axis perpendicular to these planes should also be evaluated .these rotations are:

- Pitch–up, down around saggital plane
- Roll–up–down around transverse plane
- Yaw–left–right around vertical plane

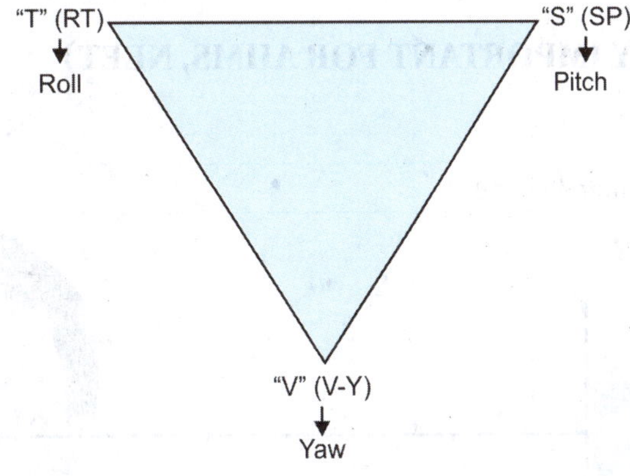

Fig. 7.16: TSV plane

- Down syndrome:

Anterior cross bite seen due to flaring of mandibular incisors
It is due to large protruded tongue

- Achondroplasia:

'Snub–nosed dwarf'
Due to failure of growth of Nasal septal Cartilage

LAST 5-YEAR QUESTIONS FROM THIS TOPIC

1. **The following is not an absolute indication for mounting an orthodontic study cast on an articulator:** *(KCET 12)*
   a. To record and document any CR–CO discrepancy
   b. To record and document the excursive paths of the mandible
   c. Surgical treatment planning
   d. Class 2 malocclusion with severe tooth material excess of more than 14 mm

Ans. d

2. **Which of the following is not an essential diagnostic aid in orthodontics:** *(KCET 11)*
   a Case history
   b. Clinical examination
   c. Plaster study cast
   d. Cephalometric X–rays

Ans. d (Ref: Balajhi 3/e p115-116)

3. **A leaf gauge is used to assist in:** *(KCET 10)*

Ans. Locating the musculo skeletal stable position of the mandible

4. **Orthodontic diagnosis focuses on:** *(COMEDK 13)*

Ans. Social smile

5. **Tooth loss causes the patient to bite in an abnormal relation of maxilla to mandible, in order to obtain:** *(COMEDK 12)*

Ans. Convenience bite

6. **What is the width to length ratio of incisors in a person with a good esthetic smile ? (PGI june 11)**

Ans. 8:10 (Esthetic Dentistry-An Artist's Science-by Dr Ratnadeep patil p65)

7. **According to farkass theory of 1981, what is the correct statement?** *(PGI Dec 10)*

Ans. Interpupillary distance = width of mouth (Ref: Essentials of orthognathic surgery by Johan P. Reynke p19, 30)

CEPHALOMETRY: (VERY IMPORTANT FOR AIIMS, NEET)

- Cephalostat:

Introduced by broadbent and hofrath in 1931	*(KCET 08)*

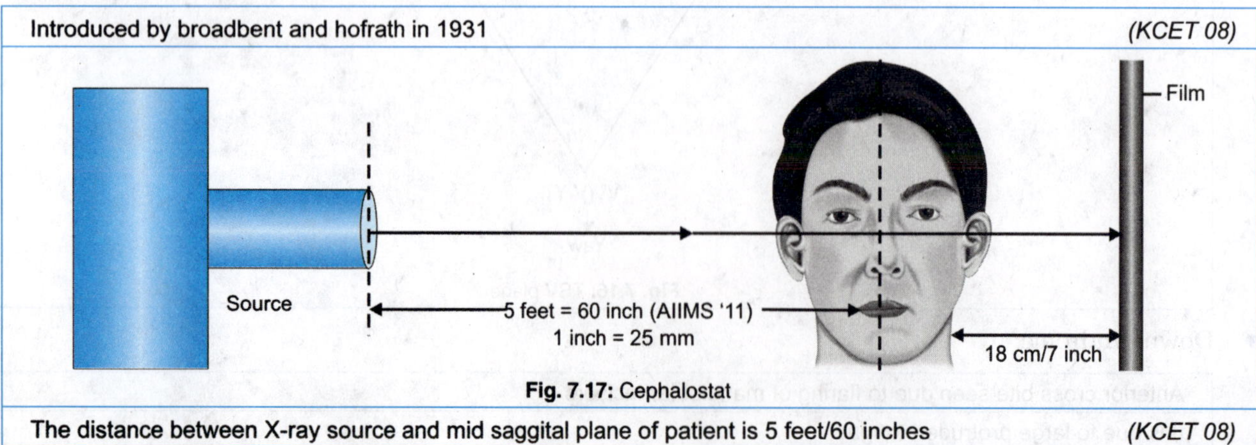

Fig. 7.17: Cephalostat

The distance between X-ray source and mid saggital plane of patient is 5 feet/60 inches	*(KCET 08)*

On cephalometry → Left side of face is towards cassette. So, viewed clearly
Cephalogram used to view discrepencies in A-P and vertical plane and not to visualize lateral asymmetry [Q]
In cephalogram, a magnification of 7-12 % (PGI 06) is considered normal
Some median points on cephalogram are: Sella, ANS, point A, point B, menton, nasion, pogonion, gnathion But Gonion is not a median point (AIPG 06),it is most posterior point on mandible *(PGI Dec 11, Dec 10, June 10)*

- Cephalometric analysis:

1st cephalometric analysis that emphasizes vertical and horizontal relationship is sasouni's analysis
Steiner's analysis is used in treatment planning
SN plane is the most stable plane as growth of anterior cranial base is completed most earliest *(AIIMS 05)*
FH plane is constructed by joining orbital to superior aspect of external auditory meatus *(AIPG 05)*
MPA in down's analysis = 17–30 degree

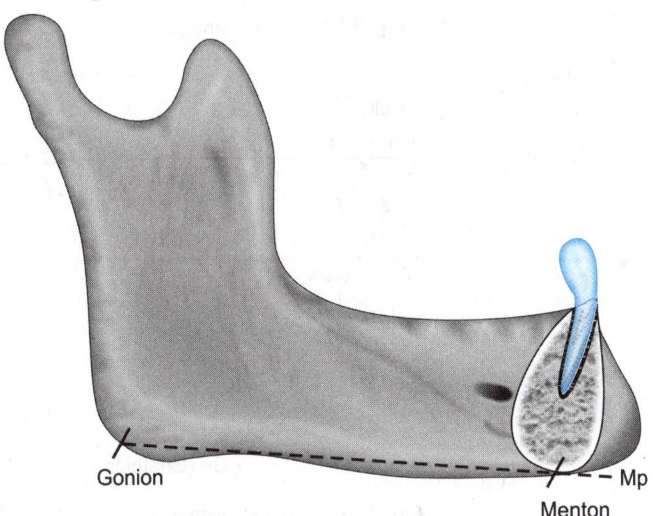

Fig. 7.18: MPA in Down's analysis

Steiner's analysis = 32 degree

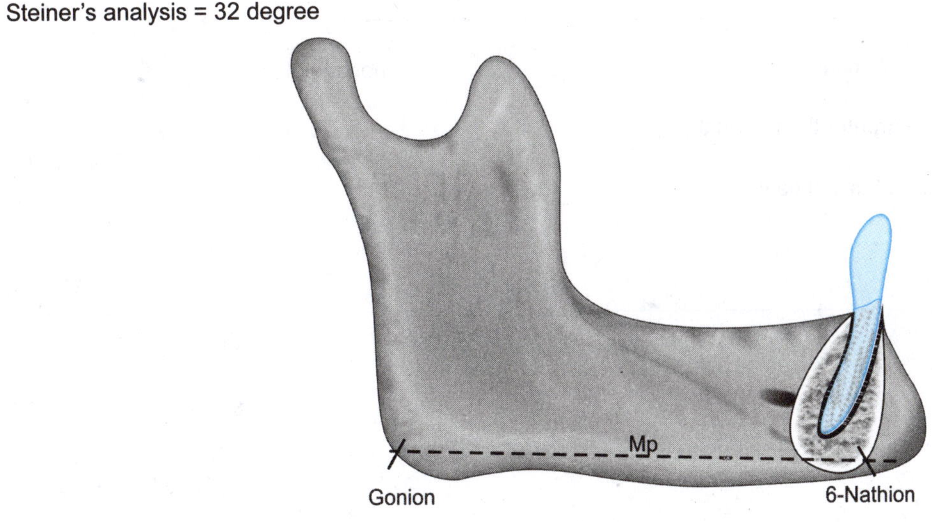

Fig. 7.19: Steiner's analysis

Tweed's analysis = 25 degree

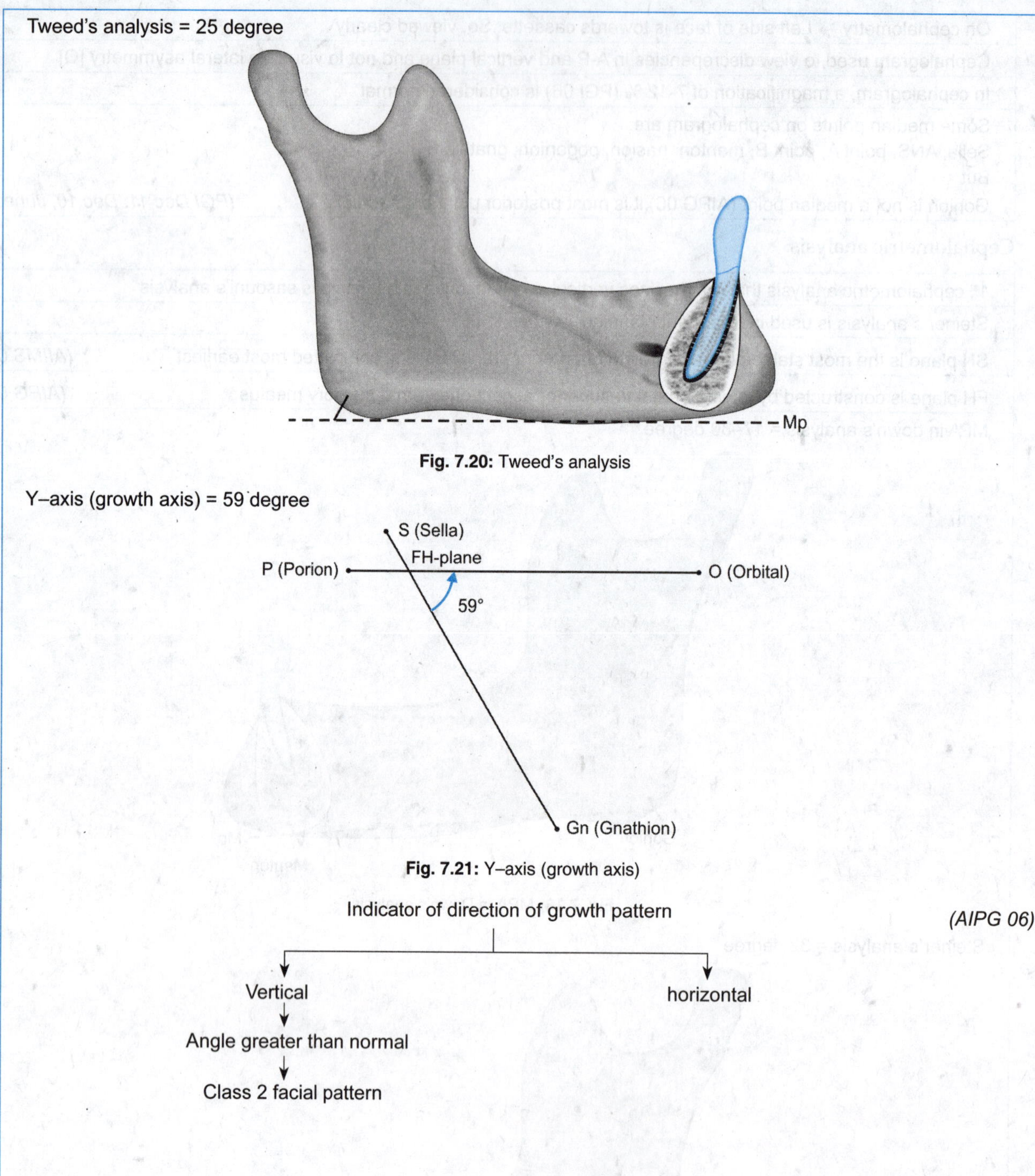

Fig. 7.20: Tweed's analysis

Y–axis (growth axis) = 59 degree

Fig. 7.21: Y–axis (growth axis)

(AIPG 06)

Angle of convexity:

In Down's analysis average value is 0 degree *(KCET 05)*

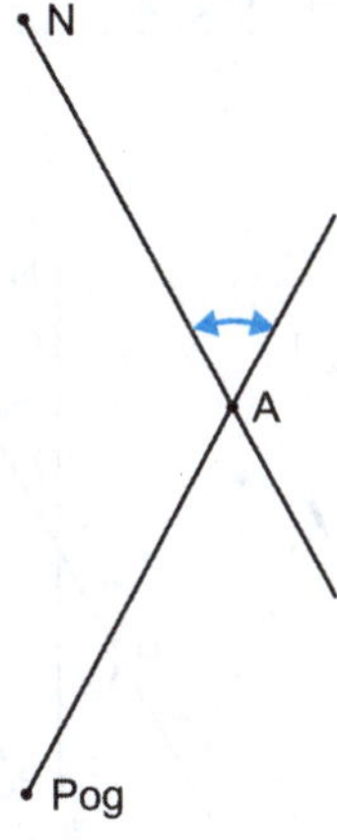

Fig. 7.22: Angle of convexity

Decreases with age

Positive value indicates prominent maxillary base w.r.t mandible

Negative value indicates prognathic mandible

Facial angle:

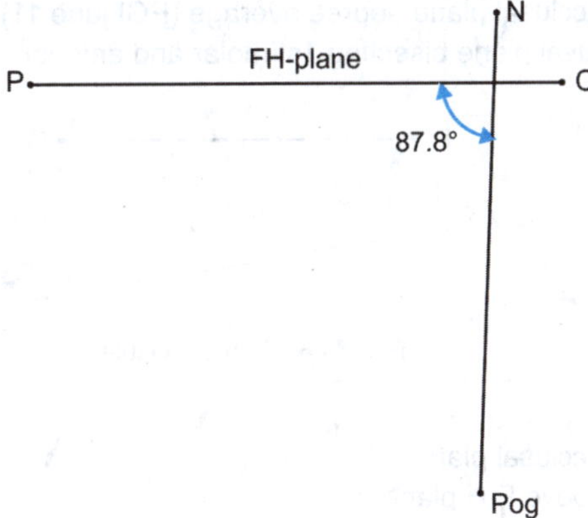

Fig. 7.23: Facial angle

Decreases with age

ANB angle: 2 degrees indicates the normal relationship of maxillary alveolar base to mandibular alveolar base *(AIIMS 07,06)*

A-P relation (like wits appraisal) (remember N → A and N → B)

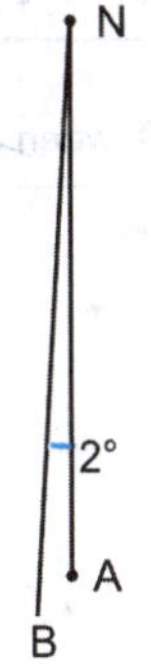

Fig. 7.24: ANB angle

Decreases with age
Increases in class 2 [Q] but decreases in class 3 [Q]

A-B plane angle: 9 to 0 degree (Mostrly –ve)
May be + ve in class 3 [Q]

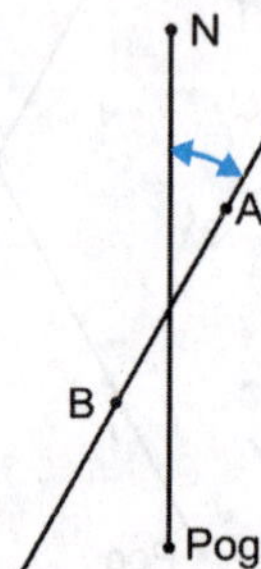

Fig. 7.25: A-B plane angle

Cant of occlusion:
Angle between F-H plane and occlusal plane degree average (PGI june 11)
Increases in class 2 as the occlusal plane bisecting 1st molar and anterior
Overbite is sloped downwards

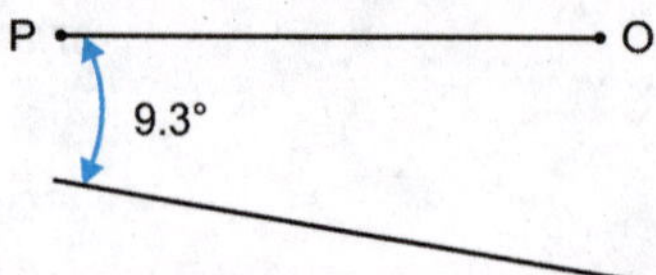

Fig. 7.26: Cant of occlusion

Angle between S-N plane and occlusal plane:
Note: S-N plane is 6-7 degree above F-H plane
So, the angle between S-N plane and occlusal plane is 15 degree
Decreases with age

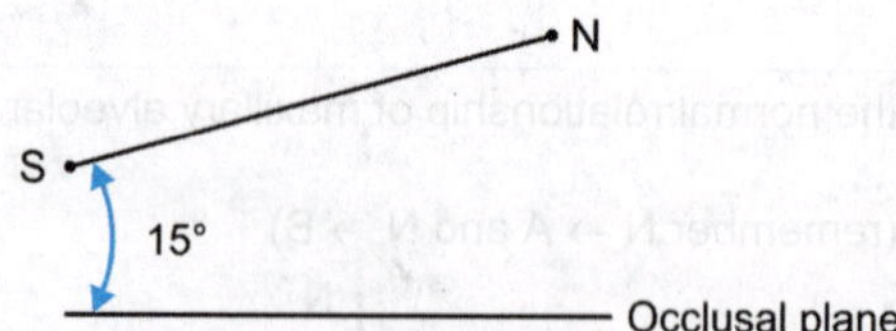

Fig. 7.27: Angle between S-N plane and occlusal plane

Innterincisal angle:
Normally 135 degree
Decreases in proclined cases so, decreases in class 2 div 1 and bimax. Protrusion (PGI Dec 08)

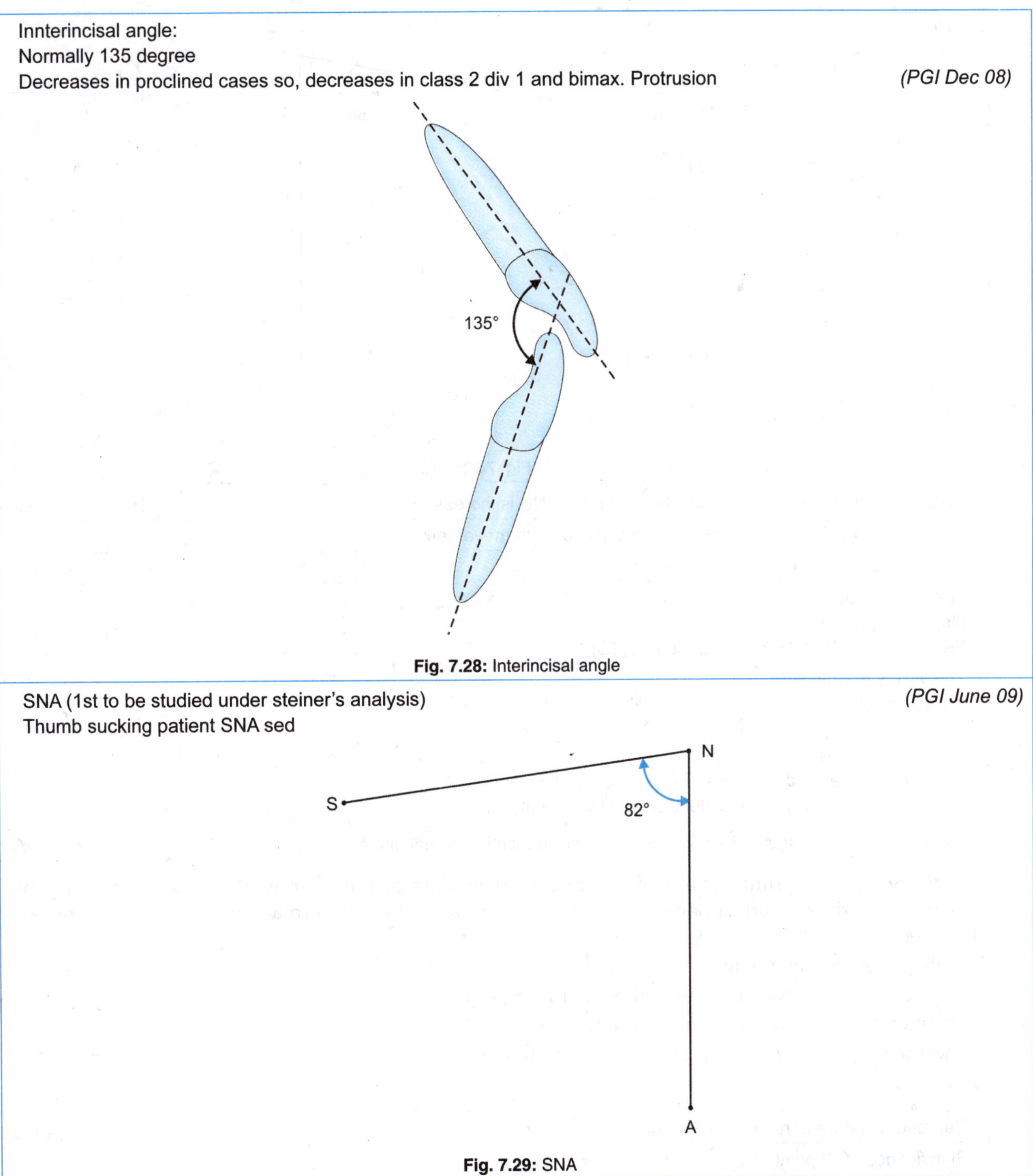

Fig. 7.28: Interincisal angle

SNA (1st to be studied under steiner's analysis) (PGI June 09)
Thumb sucking patient SNA sed

Fig. 7.29: SNA

SNB

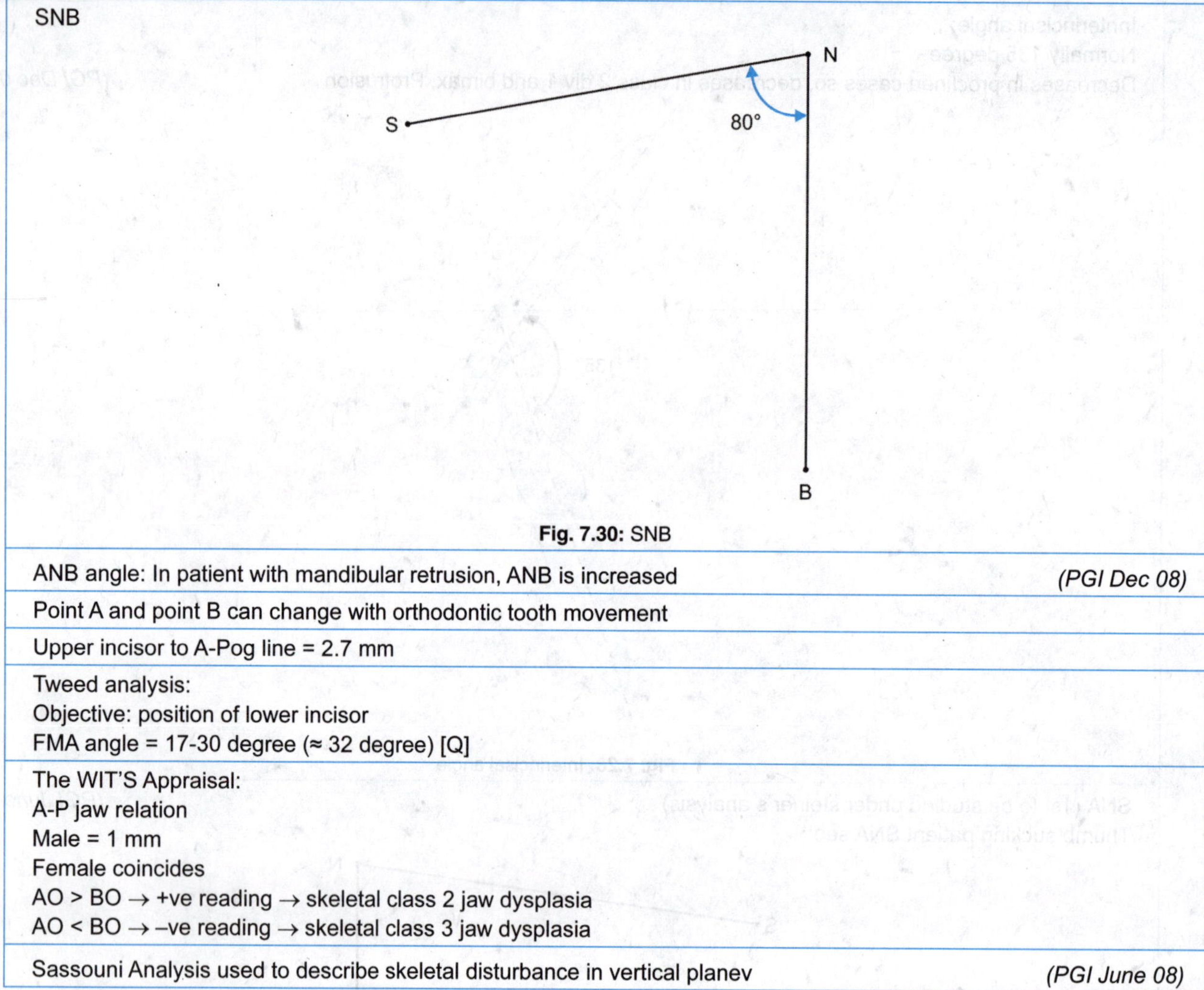

Fig. 7.30: SNB

ANB angle: In patient with mandibular retrusion, ANB is increased	*(PGI Dec 08)*
Point A and point B can change with orthodontic tooth movement	
Upper incisor to A-Pog line = 2.7 mm	
Tweed analysis: Objective: position of lower incisor FMA angle = 17-30 degree (≈ 32 degree) [Q]	
The WIT'S Appraisal: A-P jaw relation Male = 1 mm Female coincides AO > BO → +ve reading → skeletal class 2 jaw dysplasia AO < BO → –ve reading → skeletal class 3 jaw dysplasia	
Sassouni Analysis used to describe skeletal disturbance in vertical planev	*(PGI June 08)*

- Key ridge: lowest point on outline of zygoma/contour of anterior wall of infratemporal fossa in deciduous dentition. Corresponds to maxillary 2nd molar while in permanent dentition it corresponds to MB root of 1st molar
- Broadbent registration point:
- Demonstrates growth of structure farthest from the point *(AIIMS 06)*
- Point anterior to foramen Magnum = basion
- Highest point posterior to occipital condyle = Bolton's point
- Xi-Point:

Represents certre of ramus of mandible	*(AIPG 10)*
Significance of XI point: Is at the level of occlusal plane Corresponds to entrance of neurotropic bundle Is key landmark of ricket's analysis	

- PTM point:

Is the intersection of the inferior border of the foramen rotundum With the posterior wall of the pterygomaxillary fissure.

LAST 5-YEAR QUESTION FROM THIS TOPIC

1. **The highest point in the concavity present behind the occipital condyle is:** *(AIPG 10, 07, AIIMS May 10, May 08)*

Ans. Bolton's point (Ref: Bhalajhi 3/e p147)

2. **Centre of ramus is indicated by which of the following cephalometric point:** *(AIPG 10, 07)*

Ans. Xi-point (Ref: OP Kharbanda 1/e p181)

3. **The point which can be altered by orthodontic tooth movement** *(AIPG 10)*

Ans. Point A

4. **Cephalometrics is useful for assessing all of the following relationships except:** *(AIPG 08, 06)*
   a. Tooth to tooth
   b. Bone to bone
   c. Tooth to bone
   d. Soft palate to gingival

Ans. d

5. **Which is the most stable and most often used plane for the superimposition of lateral cephalogram for studying the growth of a child?** *(AIPG 08, 06)*

Ans. SN plane

6. **Superimposition in cephalometric studies is done from registration point . this demonstrates best:** *(AIPG 08, AIIMS 06)*

Ans. Growth of structures farthest from that point

7. **Long face syndrome patient with increased lower facial height, the palatal plane will be:**

Ans. Sloped posteriorly downward (Ref: Proffit 4/e p117)

8. **If the interincisal distance is 131 degree, it implicates** *(AIIMS May 11)*

Ans. Incisors are proclined (Ref: Singh 2/e p110)

9. **What is the normal mandibular plane angle?** *(AIIMS May 11,05)*

Ans. 17–30 degree (Ref: DiPietro and Moergeli. Significance of Frankfort mandibular plane angle to prosthodontics. J prosthet Dent Dec 1976 ; 36 (6): 624-35)

10. **In cephalometric analysis, the Y-axis is formed by:** *(AIIMS May 11)*

Ans. Angle formed by the plane joining sella to gnathion and FH plane (Ref: Singh 2/e p110)

11. **Which is the correct patient position for left lateral cephalogram?** *(AIIMS May 11)*

Ans. Mid–sagittal plane should be 5 feet from the tube (Ref: Ghom. Textbook of oral Radiology p256)

12. **The interincisal angle between deciduous incisors is:** *(KCET 13)*

Ans. 150 degree

13. **A 15 years old boy comes with a complaint of irregular teeth .on tracing his lateral cephalogram, steiner's analysis shows SNA of 82 degrees and SNB of 86 degrees . he would most probably have:** *(KCET 13)*

Ans. Class 3 malocclusion

14. **The projection of the points A and B to the occlusal plane is used in:** *(KCET 12)*

Ans. Wit's analysis

15. **The Broadbent–Bolton cephalometer was devised in:** *(KCET 10)*

Ans. 1931 (Ref: Dean shoe leather survey for fluorosis/mottling was also conducted in 1931)

16. **Which of the following is not a unilateral landmark on the lateral cephalogram?** *(KCET 10)*
   a. Nasion

b. Anterior nasal spine

c. Gnathion

d. Gonion

Ans. d

17. Not a landmark on mandible is: *(PGI Dec 12)*

Ans. Porion

18. The AO and BO in witt's appraisal is relationship of: *(PGI Dec 11, Dec 10, Dec 09)*

Ans. Maxilla to mandible (Ref: Bhalajhi 3/e p158)

19. While diagnosing an orthodontic case, 3/4th lateral view photograph is taken in order to ? *(PGI June 11)*

Ans. Check mandibular asymmetry, 1/3 middle face asymmetry (Ref: Singh 2/e p129)

20. According to tweed's analysis if FMA is 350 then what is the value of FMIA? *(PGI June 11)*

Ans. 650 (Ref: Singh 2/e p119)

21. In cephalometric analysis, the point which is most prominent on symphysis menti: *(PGI June 10)*

Ans. Gn point (Ref: Balajhi 3/e p148)

MODEL ANALYSIS:

- Carey 's arch perimeter analysis:

Discrepency	Inference
0–2.5 mm	Proximal stripping
2.5–5 mm	Extraction of 2nd premolar
> 5 mm	Extraction of 1st premolar

- Ashley howe's analysis:

Helps to find whether to expand/no extraction required [Q]
Arch width is more important than arch length [Q]
If basal arch width to premolar diameter < 37 % extract 1st premolar
If ______________ 37–44 % boderline case
If ______________ > 44 % non-extraction case

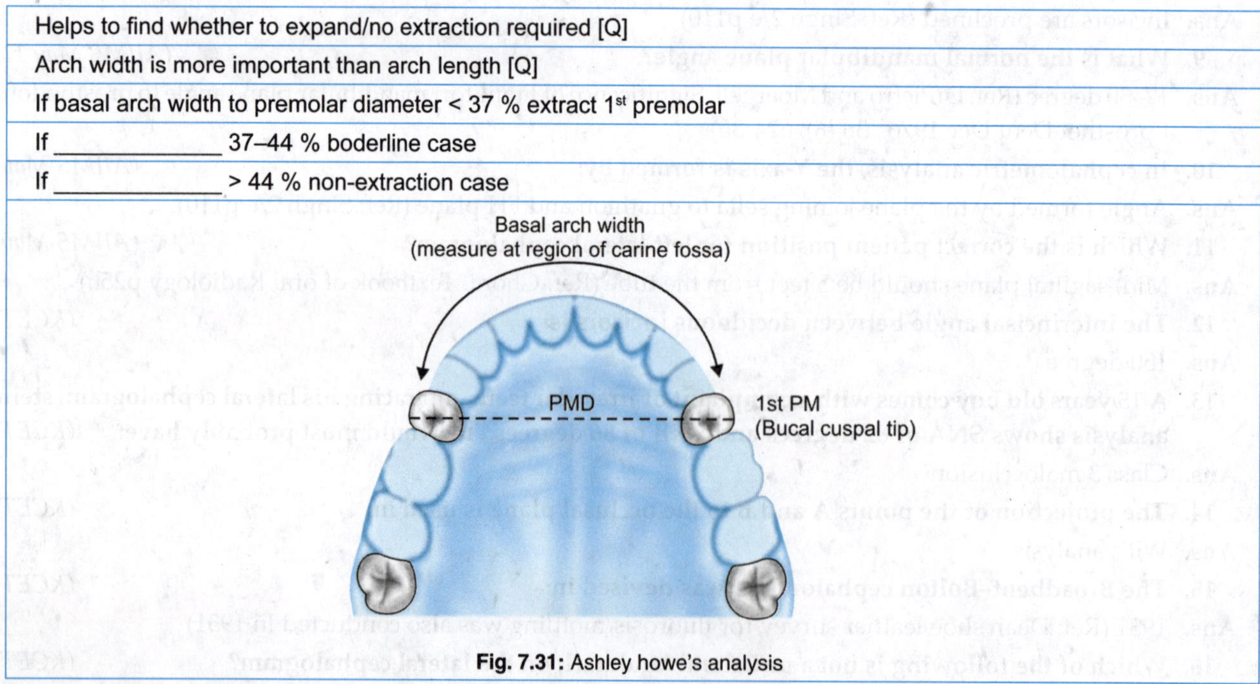

Fig. 7.31: Ashley howe's analysis

- Bolton's analysis:
- Helps to find out disproportion between size of maxillary and mandibular teeth *(KCET 12, 05)*

- Pont's analysis:

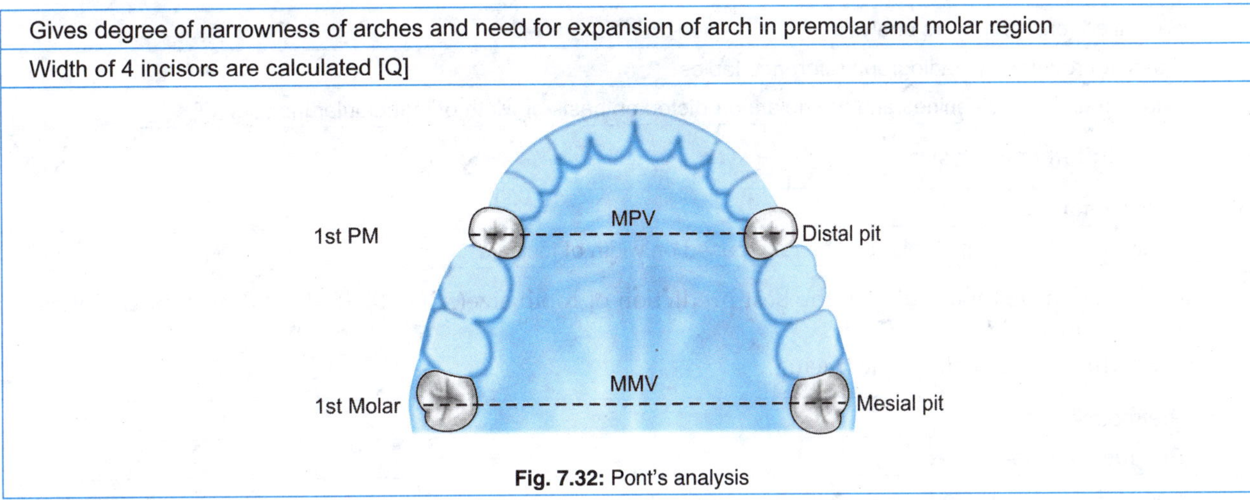

Fig. 7.32: Pont's analysis

- Korkhaus analysis:

Similar to pont's analysis Also tells proclined/retroclined incisors based on the line perpendicular to Line joining 2nd premolars Makes use of linder harth's formula	Tells incisors are proclined/Retroclined 2nd PM **Fig. 7.33:** Korkhaus analysis

- Peck's and pecks analysis:

For predicting mandibular incisor crowding *(PGI 05)*
Proportion = $\frac{\text{Mesio distal width}}{\text{Labio lingual width}} * 100$
Mean value of lower central incisor should be < 88 to 92 %
Mean value of lower lateral incisor should be < 90-95 %

- Moyer's mixed dentition analysis:

Used for both maxilla and mandible
Size of unerupted 3, 4 and 5(upper and lower both) can be predicted based on sum o the width of 4 lower permanent incisors *(AIPG 03)*
It makes use of probability table with 75 % reliability

- Tanaka and Johnson analysis:

Simplified form of moyers analysis
Does not require any radiograph/reference tables
Width of unerupted canines and premolars predicted on basis of width of Mandibular incisors [Q]

- Hixon–old father analysis:

Only for mandible
Width of canine and premolar can be read based on width of incisors

- Stanley–kerber method will give the best prediction of tooth size(AIPG 02) followed by Tanaka–Johnson and moyer's analysis
- Color coding for cephalometric tracing:

Pretreatment → black	
Progress → blue	
End of Rx/post → Rx red	*(COMEDK 05)*
Retention → green	

LAST 5-YEAR QUESTION FROM THIS TOPIC

1. **All of the following assumptions are considered true when doing space analysis for calculating space discrepancy except:** *(AIPG 12)*
   a. All permanent teeth will develop normally
   b. Correlation in size of mandibular incisors and succedaneous teeth
   c. Prediction tables are most valid for all populations
   d. Arch dimensions remain stable

Ans. c

2. **For class 2 div 1 malocclusion of 14 years old boy, which analysis is indicated to detect the tooth extraction?** *(AIIMS Nov 11)*

Ans. Ashley and Howe's analysis (Ref: bhalajhi 3/e p176-177)

3. **Which is a mixed dentitional analysis?** *(KCET 13)*

Ans. Moyer's analysis

4. **The term applied when it is doubtful, according to mixed dentition analysis whether there will be space for all the teeth:** *(KCET 12)*

Ans. Space supervision

5. **Bolton's analysis is used to determine the:** *(KCET 12, 11)*

Ans. Proportion of the mesiodistal width of the mandibular teeth to that of maxillary teeth (Ref: balajhi 3/e p178–179)

SKELETAL MATURITY INDICATOR

- Hassal and Farman used cervical vertebrae as SMI [Q]

C2, C3, and C4 shapes are used to assess skeletal maturation	
Stages involved:	
Stage 1 → Initiation	Stage 2 → Acceleration
Stage 3 → Transition	Stage 4 → Deceleration
Stage 5 → Maturation	Stage 6 → Completion

- Greulich and Pyle gave the radiological method of assessment and prediction of skeletal growth.

LAST 5-YEAR QUESTIONS FROM THIS TOPIC

1. **Fishman's smi is a method of evaluation of:** *(NEET 13, KCET 05)*

Ans. Skeletal maturity

2. **Which of the following bone is used for estimation of growth in an individual:** *(AIPG 10,07, AIIMS May 07)*

Ans. Cervical vertebra (Ref: bhalajhi 3/e p171-173)

3. **Hand wrist radiograph in orthodontics are used to accurately determine:** *(AIPG 08)*

Ans. Skeletal maturity (Ref: bhalajhi 3/e p162)

4. **The use of cervical vertebrae as skeletal maturity indicators was 1st done by:** *(KCET 13)*

Ans. Lamparski (According to the key given)

5. **Number of bones seen in a hand wrist radiograph is:** *(KCET 09, 08)*

Ans. Thirty

6. **Number of bones analysed in fishman's analysis:** *(PGI Dec 12)*

Ans. 4

PHONETICS (VERY IMPORTANT TOPIC LINK THIS TOPIC)

- With setting of teeth in CD patients)
- Labial/bilabial sounds:

'b, p, m'
First speech sound to develop
Insufficient lip support affects them

- Labiodental sound:

'f, v'
If anterior tooth are long then 'f' changes to 'v' (in case of CD patients)
Affected in class 3 malocclusion

- Linguodental/dental sounds:

'Th'
Produced by Tip of tongue extending between upper and lower anterior Teeth ↓ So, affected in anterior open bite *(PGI 12)*

- Linguoalveolar/alveolar sound:

't, d, s, z ,v'
'd' pronounced as 't' if teeth placed too far anteriorly or vice versa

- Sibilants are a type of alveolar sound:

e.g 's,z, sh, ch, j'
The upper and lower incisors approach but do not touch ↓ So, affected in anterior open bite
'sh, ch, j' are the silverman's closest speaking space
Note: when maxillary removable orthodontic appliance is first placed, the patient will have difficulty in pronouncing linguoalveolar consonants for a few days. *(AIIMS 07 ,06)*

- Linguopalatal:

A truly palatal sound
e.g 'year ,she, vision, onion'
Less problematic to denture wearer

- Velar sound:

'k, g, ng'
Have no affect on denture wearers (PGI June 12)
Vovels + velar sounds have no affect on denture wearer
Note: 's' and 't' cause most problem in denture wearers

- Speech difficulty related to malocclusion:

Speech sound	Problem	Related malocclusion
Sibilant	Lisp *(KCET 05)*	Anterior open bite, large gap between incisors
Linguoalveolar sounds	Difficulty in production	Irregular incisors especially lingual position of maxillary incisors
Labiodentals frecatives [Q]	Distortion	Skeletal class 3 *(PGI Dec 11, June 08)*
linguodental frecatives	Distortion	Anterior open bite

LAST 5-YEAR QUESTIONS FROM THIS TOPIC

1. **The 1st speech sounds produced by developing child is:** *(KCET 11, COMEDK 11)*

Ans. Bilabial (Ref: Profit p85)

2. **Distortion of labiodentals sounds occurs in:** *(KCET 09, PGI June 08)*

Ans. Skeletal class 3 (Ref: profit)

3. **'V' is used to determine:** *(PGI June 12)*

Ans. A-P relationship of maxillary and mandibular teeth

BIOLOGY AND MECHANICS OF TOOTH MOVEMENT

- Post emergent spurt: *(KCET 03)*
- The stage of relatively rapid eruption from the time of tooth 1st penetrating gingival until it reaches the occlusal level
- Uprighting:
- Mesio–Distal correction of root
- Accepted theories of tooth movement:

Pressure tension theory by schwarz
Fluid dynamic/blood flow theory by bien
Bone bending piezoelectric theory

- Hyalinized zone:

Is the histological section of tooth under orthodontic Forces.
It is an avascular layer in pdl. *(AIPG 06)*

- Physiologic response to sustained pressure against a tooth:

Time	Event
< 1 sec	Pdl fluid incompressible, alveolar bone bends, piezoelectric signal generated
1-2 sec	Pdl fluid expressed, tooth moves within pdl space
3-5 sec	Blood vessels within pdl partially compressed on pressure side (KCET 12), dilated on tension side (AIPG 06), pain is normally felt after application of heavy force *(COMEDK 06)*

- Controlled, uncontrolled tipping and torquing:

Controlled tipping	Uncontrolled tipping (AIPG 02, 01)	TORQUING
Center of rotation at apex [Q]	Center of rotation away from Apex near the center of resistance (PGI Dec. 11, Dec 10), i.e. middle 1/3rd	Reverse tipping Centre of rotation at incisal edge/in bracket slot
Minimal movement of root	Movement of crown in 1 direction while movement of root in other direction	Mainly root movement. Characterized by lingual movement of root
A couple of force required	Single force required	

- Both intrusion and bodily movement are difficult to accomplish
- In Translation/bodily movement centre of rotation is at infinity *(AIIMS 05)*
- Intermittent vs interrupted force: (Please read carefully as many students develop wrong concept during their UG level) (A very important topic in COMEDK and KCET)

Intermittent Forces	Interrupted Forces
Force level decline abruptly to 0 when appliance is taken out and resume when it is reinserted into mouth	Force level declines to 0 between activation but not abruptly
e.g all patient activated appliance(PGI Dec 10, Dec 08) such as removable plates, headgear, elastics	e.g. screw *(COMEDK 10)*

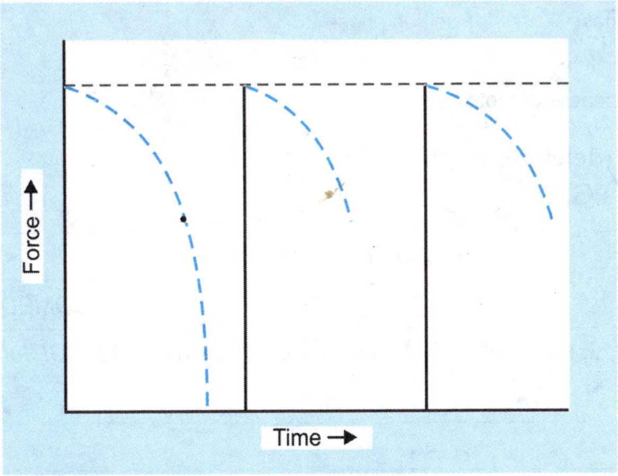

Fig. 7.34: Intermittent forces

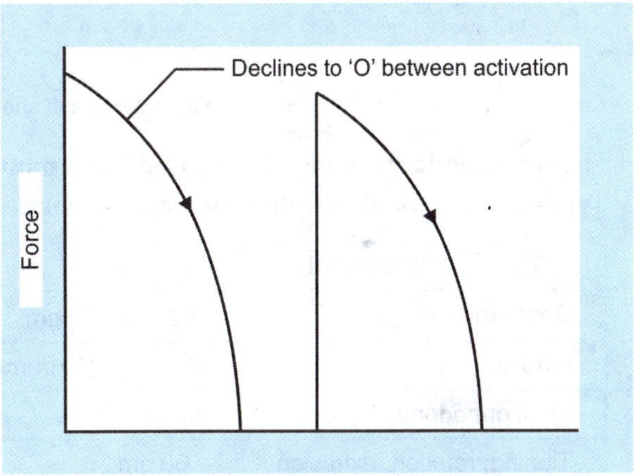

Fig. 7.35: Interrupted forces

- Removable appliance:

Bring about mostly tipping movement
While
Fixed appliance bring about mostly bodily movement .

- Ideally:

Light continuous forces produces most efficient tooth movement	*(AIPG 05, KCET 07)*
By causing frontal/direct resorption	*(COMEDK 05)*
Capillary blood pressure = 20–26/cm^2 In orthodontics to prevent damage to the tissue, force should not exceed capillary blood pressure	

- Intrusion is best produced by light continuous forces *(COMEDK 10)*
- Moment: force for bodily movement = 10:1 *(PGI Dec 08)*
- Moment: force for tipping movement = 1-7
- Elastics:

Class 2 malocclusion elastics used in Class 2
Class 3 malocclusion elastics used in Class 3
These elastics are, e.g. of stationary anchorage

- Graph showing phases of tooth movement:

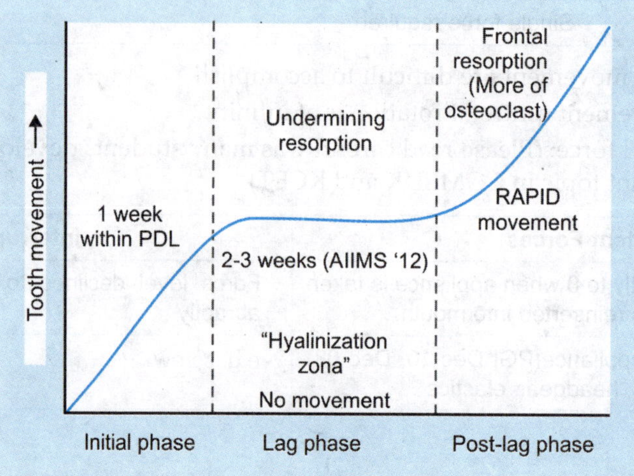

Fig. 7.36: Graph showing phases of tooth movement

- Higher orthodontic force → increased tooth mobility (deleterious effect), Pain
- Types of movement vs optimum force (Important for PGI):

Types of Movement	Optimum Force
Bodily movement	100 gm–150 gm *(COMEDK 07)*
Intrusion	10-20 gm (Extremely light, least amount of force required) *(KCET 08, PGI June 09)*
Ideal orthodontic force	20–25 gm
Tipping, rotation, extrusion	– 60 gm

- Root uprighting requires force > 100 gms *(PGI Dec 10)*
- Center of resistance: (Fixed point)

Single rooted tooth–middle 1/3rd
Multirooted tooth -1-2 mm Below furcation area

- Center of resistance is based on: *(AIIMS 05)*

Size and shape of crown and root
Pdl attachment
Level of alveolar bone

- Center of rotation (variable):

For tipping–apical 1/3rd of root	*(PGI Dec 11, June 10)*
Translation–infinity	
A single force acting through center of resistance will produce translation of tooth	*(AIPG 05)*
For extrusion/intrusion is outside the tooth	
At incisal edge for torquing	

- Center of resistance of Maxilla:

Located postero superior aspect of zygomatico–maxillary suture [Q]
Located between roots of the premolars [Q]

- Tooth movement is purely 'pdl' phenomenon
- The ratio of PDL area in the anchorage unit to PDL area in the tooth movement unit should be:

2: 1 Without friction
4: 1 With friction

- The 1st bone formed in response to orthodontic loading is woven bone *(COMEDK 07)*
- Anchorage types:

Anchorage type	Example
Simple anchorage	• Labial movement of lingually placed maxillary central incisor with Z–spring • Buccal movement of premolar with screw appliance • Retraction of anterior teeth with Hawley's appliance. Utilizes tipping movement. [Q]
Stationary anchorage	• Class 2 elastics use this anchorage Use 1st resistance of bodily movement [Q] of molars to retract maxillary anteriors by tipping them *(AIIMS 05, COMED 10)*
Reciprocal anchorage	Resistance units of equal size pull against each other • Closure of midline diastema • Use of cross bite elastics • Arch expansion using fixed/removable appliance, e.g. using hyrax *(KCET 07,05)*
Reinforced anchorage	
Muscular anchorage	

- Anchorage obtained from nape of neck represents cervical anchorage *(AIPG 06)*
- Baker's anchorage refers to the use of cross elastics *(KCET 07)*
- Micro/mini implant:

They provide excellent anchorage and are called skeletal/absolute anchorage.
They are also called temporary anchorage devices (TAD).
Bicortical titanium screw most frequently used in orthodontics
Diameter = 0.9 to 1.6 mm
Retention = mechanical

- Most common tooth movement: Tipping
- Most easiest tooth movement: Extrusion
- Optimal orthodontic force should not exceed capillary pressure (i.e. 20- 26 gm/cm2) *(AIIMS May 12, KCET 07)* average root length changes during orthodontic Rx:

Central/lateral incisors - 2 to 2.5 mm
Canine and premolars -1.5 mm (PGI 08)

LAST 5-YEAR QUESTION FROM THIS TOPIC

1. **If the centre of rotation is at the apex of the root, then the orthodontic movement which results is:** *(AIPG 10,07, AIIMS May 10, May 08, May 07)*

Ans. Controlled tipping (Ref: Bhalajhi 3/e p198)

2. **If the center of rotation is present at the center of bracket slot, orthodontic movement which occurs is:** *(AIPG 10, 07, AIIMS May 10, May 08, May 07)*

Ans. Torquing (Ref: Bhalajhi 3/e p198)

3. **One of the greatest advantages of using extra oral anchorage is that:** *(AIPG 08, 06)*

Ans. It permits the posterior movement of teeth in one arch without adversely disturbing the opposite arch

4. **The LAG phase for tooth movement usually lasts for:** *(AIIMS Nov 12)*

Ans. 2-3 weeks (Ref: Bhalajhi 3/e p188)

5. **Baker's anchorage is a type of:** *(AIIMS Nov 12)*

Ans. Inter maxillary anchorage (Ref: Bhalajhi 4/e p225)

6. **Light orthodontic forces produces:** *(KCET 12)*

Ans. Compression of blood vessel within 3-5 secs on the pressure side

7. **Intermittent forces are applied with the help of:** *(KCET 11)*

Ans. Elastics, headgear, removable plates (Ref: Contemporary orthodontics by profit p341)

8. **What is the optimum force required for the intrusion of a tooth?** *(KCET 10)*

Ans. 10–20 gm

9. **Hyalinization is a frequent complication of:** *(KCET 10)*

Ans. Excessive force application

10. **Which of the following is not an example of reciprocal anchorage?** *(KCET 10)*
    a. Closure of midline diastema
    b. Buccal movement of palatally placed premolar
    c. Correction of a single tooth posterior crossbite
    d. Expansion of the maxillary arch with jackscrew

Ans. b.

11. **The type of force exerted by headgears/facemasks is:** *(KCET 09)*

Ans. Intermittent force

12. **Optimum pressure which should be used is:** *(COMEDK 12)*

Ans. 20 to 26 gms/sq. cm

13. **On application of very light forces to teeth, the axis of rotation is located at:** *(COMEDK 12)*

Ans. At/close to Apex of root

PREVENTIVE AND INTERCEPTIVE ORTHODONTICS

- Preventive and interceptive orthodontics cannot be carried Out after eruption of 2nd molar
- Chances of successful opening of palatal suture is nearly 100 % before age of 15 years. *(AIPG 05)*
- After rapid expansion, it takes 3 months for bone to fill the suture

- SME vs RME:

SME	RME
Activation–0.5 to 1 mm/week for 2-3 month	Activation–0.2 to 0.5 mm/day (Option given in *COMEDK 07* was 0.5 to 1 mm/day) for 1-2 week
Skeletal: dental expansion = 1:1	Skeletal: dental expansion = 1:1 *(COMEDK 07)*
Mainly causes dental type expansion	Mainly causes skeletal type expansion
e.g: jack screw coffin spring quad helix Ni Ti expander (newer type) Schwarz appliance (used in mandible)	e. g: • Removable appliance incorporating jack screw *(AIPG 04)* • Fixed tooth and tissue borne appliance like derichsweiler hass type • Fixed tooth borne appliance like Hyrax type (have a heavy gauze wire extension, made of 0.036 inch stainless steel) *(AIPG 04)* Isaacson type (MINI expander, a spring loaded screw) [Q]

- Hyrax is used in RME *(COMEDK 10, PGI Dec 08)*
- In improvement of nasal breadthing RME is universally accepted
- Pitch of screw = 0.8 mm of expansion (90 degree turn produces 0.18 mm expansion)
- SME compared to RME can be done at "Any Age " and gives stable result, i.e. less chance to relapse
- RME causes maximum opening of midpalatal suture occurs in maxillary central incisor region *(AIPG 03)*
- Midline diastema created after successful RME (KCET 08) will be closed in 3-5 month because of trans septal fiber traction
- Concept:

RME not done in class 1 as skeletal abnormality, as no skeletal abnormality present and normal musculature also present
In class 2 there is definitive change in muscular balance. So, change in position of teeth by arch expansion may be a more valid Rx

- Coffin spring is W shaped = 1.25 mm [Q]
- Quad helix:

Is of 0.038 inch [Q]
Quad helix has 4 helix used for SME and bringing about rotation of molar applies reciprocal force *(PGI Dec 10)*

- Pendulum appliance:

0.032 inch TMA wire *(PGI 12)*
It is used for distalisation of molar in class 2 molar relation *(PGI June 11)*

- Concept:

If in early mixed dentition phase there is insufficient space in anterior segment for erupting permanent lateral incisor, then some Rx is necessary to prevent ectopic eruption of lateral incisor. Extraction of deciduous cuspid may lead to mesial movement of primary molars and lingual movement of incisors, which may further aggrevate the condition. More over it can also lead to impaction of permanent canine. So, best option in early stages is to DISC the deciduous cuspids *(AIPG 02)*

- Serial extraction/guidance of occlusion/guidance of eruption:

Kjellgren	1st used the term serial extraction
Nance	Termed planned and progressive extraction
Hotz	Active supervision of teeth by extraction

Treatment objective	Is to intercept a developing arch–length deficiency and to reduce/eliminate the need for extensive appliance therapy *(COMEDK 08)*
Time to start serial extraction	Is early mixed dentition
Indication:	• Class 1 malocclusion with arch length discrepancy > 5 mm/quadrant with no skeletal abnormality (No class 2 and class 3 or open bite and deep bite)
Methods utilized:	• Dewel's CD4 (most accepted) *(PGI Dec 11, Dec 09)* – Tweeds → DC4 – Nancy → D4C

- Force required for headgear to restrain maxillary growth = 250 to 500 gm/side
- Case:

Q.1.	A dentist performed restorative procedure in an 11 year old child and found that the primary molars were in various stages of exfoliation with slight anterior crowding present . when should his next appointment be scheduled? *(AIIMS 07, 06)*
Ans:	After 3 months for observation because in such a child there is a good chance that anterior crowding will resolve on it's own by partial utilization of leeway space of Nance. This leeway space provides an excellent opportunity for natural/orthodontic adjustment of occlusal relationships at the end of dental transition. 77 % of cases of crowding upto 4.5 mm could be resolved by this process

- Arch length preservation is best carried out by restoring carious teeth *(AIPG 05)*
- Space maintainer for premature loss of deciduous 2nd molar:

• In case of unilateral loss: band and loop space maintainer
• In case of bilateral loss: – Band and loop – Nance palatal holding arch – Transpalatal arch
• Space maintainer for pre mature loss of deciduous 2nd Molar BUT prior to eruption of permanent 1st molar to guide eruption of 1st molar *(KCET 07)* Distal shoe space maintainer and rochet's appliance Willet's distal shoe was the 1st version of distal shoe *(AIPG 06)* ↓ Bar type gingival extension Rochet → 'V 'shaped gingival extension
• Lingual arch used for multiple loss of primary molars bilaterally in same arch *(KCET 07)* Most effective 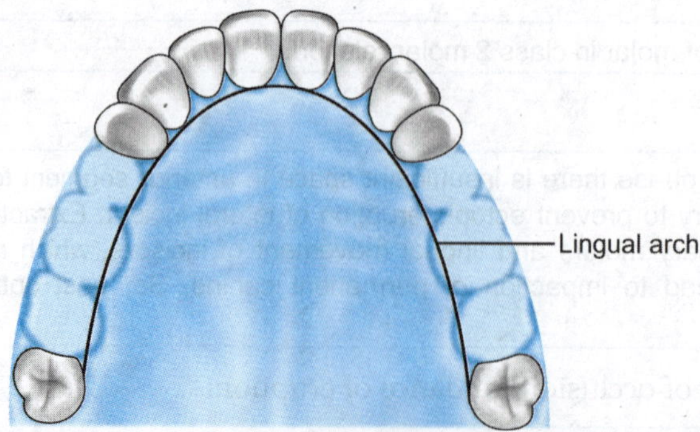 **Fig. 7.37:** Lingual arch
• Lingual arch with U-loops on mesial of each molar used to regain space Disadvantage: Flaring of mandibular incisors

- Band and loop:
  For unilateral and "Single loss" of tooth
  Facio–lingual dimension of loop = 8 mm [Q]\

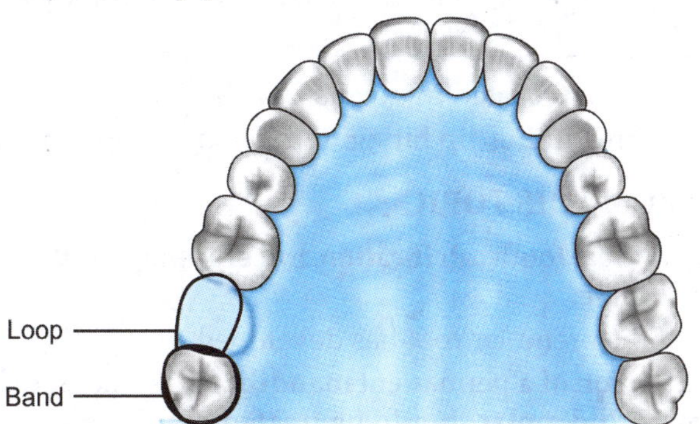

Fig. 7.38: Band and loop

- Crown and loop is similar to band and loop except crown is used
- Best indication of transpalatal arch:
  Unilateral loss of multiple deciduous teeth while other side of arch is intact

Pin and tube is a space maintainer for loss of upper primary incisor . It is best because it allows lateral growth of bone [Q]

- Space maintainer is least indicated in maxillary primary incisors

- Wilkinson advised extraction of all 4 1st permanent molar *(COMEDK 08)*
- Balancing extraction:

When 1 deciduous canine is lost prematurely, it is important
To prevent midline shift by extracting canine of opposite side of same arch

- Compensating extraction:

Sometimes extraction of teeth in opposite arch is carried out
To preserve buccal occlusal relationship

- 1st premolar is most commonly extracted teeth
- Space regainer:

Under Distalisation of Molar	
• Pendulum appliance • Buccal coil spring • Head gear	Both have nance button for anchorage

- Myofunctional appliance used in Developing cross bite Rx by tongue blade 1-2 hrs/day for 2 week
- Myofunctional appliance used only before adolescent growth spurt

While

- Orthognathic surgery done after growth ceases
- Space maintainer for deciduous and permanent incisor area:

- Deciduous teeth:
  - RPD with replacement disadvantage is that it cannot be used for children who do not show a degree of cooperation and interest, e.g. a 3 year old child
  - Fixed appliance with replacement for small child, e.g. 3 year old

• Permanent teeth: – The loss of anterior permanent teeth require immediate Rx if intra arch changes are to be prevented
To prevent mesial migration of permanent 1st molar, immediately after extraction space maintainer should be given in case of premature loss of 1° 2nd molar *(PGI Dec 08)*

- Myofunctional exercises were 1st advocated by rogers in 1918 *(KCET 06)*
- Oral screen is used for mouth breadthing, lip biting, retraction of upper protruded teeth. *(COMEDK 07)*

LAST 5-YEAR QUESTIONS FROM THIS TOPIC

1. An 8 year old child with normal tooth calcification and eruption has the primary lower 2nd molar extracted. The resulting space should be: *(AIPG 08, 06)*

Ans. Maintained until 2/3rd of the premolar root has developed

2. Mesioangular ectopic eruption of a permanent mandibular 1st molar causing resorption of distal surfaces of the roots of the primary 2nd molar should be treated by: *(AIPG 08)*

Ans. Use of a brass wire to move the permanent molar distally (NBDE Q)

3. Force generated by 90 degree rotation of finger spring in "Pendulum appliance" while distalisation: *(AIIMS Nov 11, PGI Dec 12)*

Ans. 250 gm (Ref: Profit 4/e p580)

4. 5 years and 4 month child having smaller chin, he clinically presents distal step 2nd molar relation and narrow width of maxilla, having normal SNA angle, decreased SNB angle, with low FMA angle, then treatment should be: *(AIIMS Nov 12, Repeated 2 Times in Exam)*

Ans. Wait and Watch for 6 years (as treatment is done in late mixed dentition phase and not before)

5. Which of the following is not a space maintainer?

a. Distal shoe
b. Lingual holding arch
c. Transpalatal arch
d. E-arch

Ans. d.

6. Which among the following about removable space maintainer are wrong: *(KCET 12)*

a. Being tissue borne, they impose less stress on the remaining teeth
a. By virtue of tissue stimulation they often accelerate the eruption of teeth beneath them
b. They can be functional in the truest sense, hence better patient co-operation is to be expected
c. Easier to fabricate, requiring less chair–side time

Ans. c

7. Space regaining is indicated in all of the following except: *(KCET 12)*

a. One/more permanent teeth have been lost prematurely
b. Some space in the arch has been lost due to mesial drift of 1st permanent molar
c. Mixed dentition analysis shows that, once the lost space is gained back, there will not be any arch length–tooth material discrepancy
d. 1st molars are in end–to–end relation due to class 2 skeletal base and prognathic maxilla

Ans. d

8. A lingually erupting maxillary lateral incisor: *(KCET 12)*

Ans. Can be corrected by using a tongue blade if sufficient space exists in the arch

9. Best indication for a trans- palatal arch: *(KCET 12)*

Ans. When one side of arch is intact, with several primary teeth missing on the other side

10. Serial extractions are indicated when there is: *(KCET 09)*

Ans. No skeletal discrepancy with dental crowding > 10 mm

11. **Following the premature loss of a deciduous tooth, space closure:** *(COMEDK 13)*
    a. Occurs predominantly from the anterior in the maxillary arch and predominantly from the posterior in the mandibular arch
    b. Is more rapid 6 months after the loss of the tooth
    c. Occurs more rapidly in the maxillary arch than in the mandibular arch
    d. Inversely proportional to the time the deciduous tooth has been missing

Ans. According to the key given ans is "c."But both "b and c" are correct

12. **As a general rule in borderline crowding cases of a broad facial type:** *(COMEDK 13)*

Ans. An expansion Rx should be carried out

13. **Rate of activation with slow expansion is:** *(COMEDK 12)*

Ans. 1 mm for a month (According to the key given)

14. **When 1 primary canine is lost prematurely, it is imperative to maintain the:** *(COMEDK 12, 10)*

Ans. Midline

15. **2nd molars that get locked under the distal cusps of 1st molars during eruption are best:** *(COMEDK 12)*

Ans. Disimpacted with "Disimpaction springs"

16. **What is the chief disadvantage of a nonfunctional fixed space maintainer?** *(COMEDK 12)*

Ans. Continued eruption of opposing teeth

17. **During fabrication of band for band and loop space maintainer, where should be the band biter be placed for finalpositioning of the band:** *(COMEDK 12)*

Ans. Disto lingual aspect of the maxillary teeth and disto facial aspect of the mandibular teeth (ACCORDING to the official key given)

18. **Space maintainers are usually not necessary in which region?** *(COMEDK 12, 08)*

Ans. Maxillary anteriors

19. **A 12 year old boy reported with a class 2 div 1 malocclusion with proclined upper incisor and deep bite. Extraoral examination revealed a bilaterally symmetrical face, convex profile, potentially competent lips with normal incisor display during rest and smile. Cephalometric finding showed that the patient had a horizontal growth direction with CVMI stage 3, increased overjet and normal lower incisor inclination:** *(COMEDK 12)*

    Q.1. What would be the appliance of choice for this patient?

    Ans. Twin block

    Q.2. What is the right time to start deep bite correction with Twin block appliance:

    Ans. 1 week

    Q.3. What is the best method to prevent proclination of lower incisors while treating a case with Twin block appliance:

    Ans. Incisor capping

20. **Quad helix is used to correct:** *(COMEDK 11)*

Ans. Posterior cross bite (Ref: textbook of orthodontics by gowri Shankar 1/e p487)

21. **What is the important factor when space maintenance is considered after untimely loss of primary teeth?** *(COMEDK 10)*

Ans. Dental age of patient

22. **In case with premature loss of 2nd deciduous molar before eruption of 1st permanent molar, which space maintainer is indicated:** *(COMEDK 10)*

Ans. Cantilever type (according to key given

23. **In mixed dentition diastema of how much mm is considered normal, and closes on its own:***(PGI Dec 11)*

Ans. 1.5 mm (Profit 4/e p569) {In PGI June 10 both 1.5 and 2 mm was given in option. So, 2 mm >> 1.5 mm}

TREATMENT OPTIONS

- Chart on scientist:

Scientist	Appliance and contribution
Belcheir E.H. Angle, father of modern orthodontics Introduced the 1st typical fixed orthodontic appliance	Used vital stain • Classified malocclusion • E-arch appliance (1st contribution of angle) • Ribbon arch appliance *(COMEDK 05)* • Pin and tube appliance • Edge wise appliance (Last contribution) [Q]
E.C Angell(don't confuse with angle)	Father of R.M.E
BEGG	Begg's technique/modified ribbon arch technique/light wire differential force technique
Andrews	Straight wire/preadjusted edgewise appliance
Kurz	Lingual technique
Pierre Fauchard	Bandelette, the first orthodontic appliance [Q]
Bunocore	Acid etch technique
Anderson	Activator
Dewey	Modified angle's classification of class 1 and class 3 malocclusion
Lischer	Substitution of class 1, 2 and 3 with neutron occlusion, disto occlusion, mesio occlusion
Bennet (PGI 12)	Classification on basis of local causes
William Clark	Twin block appliance
Rickets	Visual treatment objective (VTO)
Dunlop	B–hypothesis to break oral habits
Schwartz	Split plate for maxillary expansion
Oppenheim	Chin cap
Le Felon	Coined term orthodontics
Tweed	Cephalometric analysis Classification of anchorage preparation Serial extraction procedure Mandibular incisor school of retention

- Removable appliances most readily accomplish tipping movement *(COMEDK 05)*
- Stainless steel discovered by brearley (don't confuse with stainless steel crown humphrey)
- Roughness and frictional resistance of wire:

• β-TMA has maximum friction resistance [Q]
• Roughness order: NiTi > β-TMA > stainless steel *(KCET 11)*

- Critical surface tension is maximum for stainless steel bracket
- β–Ti:

Was given by Goldberg and Burston
Has a good formability → so, bands and loops can be incorporated → So, used for final finishing

- NiTi alloy:

Given by 'Buchler'
Introduced as orthodontic wire by 'Anderson'
NiTi wires are available at following temperatures: 15, 27, 35, 40 degree Celsius [Q]

- Elgiloy (Co-Cr) can be heat treated
- Wire materials and their application:

Wire Material	Application
Nitinol	• Used for initial alignment • It has 2 properties: superelasticity (COMEDK 05) and shape memory (AIPG 03) • Disadvantage: resistant to taking bend, helices/loop. Cannot be soldered/welded as it lacks formability (Neet 13) (This property is improved in TMA wires
TMA wire/β–titanium wires	• Used for space closure and finishing • Used for final adjustment in torquing movement • Has high formability

- In spring role of helix is for activation (AIPG 06) but in arch wire (Robert's retractor) increases flexibility
- The most important disadvantage of removable appliance is that they are dependent on patient cooperation *(KCET 05)*
- Springs:

• Z spring/double cantilever spring: Used for labial movement of incisors and MINOR rotation of incisors Ideal for anterior tooth cross bite where - ve overbite/overlap < freeway space and teeth are mildly rotated Z-spring used along with posterior bite plane if overbite > 2 mm OR Opposing teeth are periodontally compromised
• T spring: Used for buccal movement of premolars and sometimes canine
• Coffin spring: Is removable type of expansion spring
• Canine retractor: It is a spring used to move canine Distally.

- Canine retractor:

• U-loop canine retractor: Least effective Used when minimal retraction of 1-2 mm required
• Helical canine retractor/reverse loop canine retractor: Indicated in patients with shallow sulcus and mandibular arch
• Palatal canine retractor: Indication for retraction of palatally placed canines
• Buccal canine retractor: Indicated for retraction of buccaly placed canines

- Bows:

Is the active component that is activated by bending towards the teeth.
Short and long labial bow lack flexibility. So, used for anterior space closure and minor overjet reduction
Other modifications are: • High labial bow: Used to carry apron springs Indicated for retraction of anteriors with large overjet • Robert's retractor: Indicated in patients having severe anterior proclination With an overjet of 4 mm High flexiblity due to incorporation of coil and thin wire 0.5 mm Fig: • Mills retractor/extended labial bow: Indicated in patients with large overjet Fitted labial bow: • Used as retainer

- Component and diameter of wire:

Component	Diameter of Wire
Adam's clasp	0.7 mm (KCET 07)/28 mil/22 gauze wire
Low labial bow	0.7 mm/0.8 mm
High labial bow	0.9 mm/1 mm (apron wire = 0.4 mm)
Labial bow in Anderson appliance/activator	0.9 mm
Lip bumper	0.9 mm
Robert's retractor	0.5 mm
Springs	> 0.5 mm
Coffin spring	1.25 mm

- Southend clasp by Stephens is more effective on upper central incisors
- Supernumerary teeth and cross bite should be corrected as early as possible [Q]
- Anterior cross bite: basic requirement for correction

Spaces should be available anteriorly to move the maxillary teeth
Sufficient vertical overlap [Q] to maintain the correction after tipping movement

- Bite planes and inclined plane
- **Note:** Bite planes act by disengaging the occlusion

Appliance	Description
Anterior bite plane	• Used for deep bite correction (COMEDK 08) by causing selective eruption of posterior teeth • Should provide a clearance of 2-3 mm between upper and lower posterior teeth to provide space for supra eruption
Posterior bite plane	• When combined with Z spring used in Rx of anterior cross bite by removing interferences [Q] • Used in antertior open bite cases
Upper anterior inclined plane	• Provides reinforced/multiple anchorage • Constructed at an angle of 60 degree to occlusal plane • It can reinforce maxillary anchorage • Used for deep bite correction

SVED appliance	• A modification of upper anterior inclined plane • Has an additional upper incisor capping • Prevents the incisors from being forced labially
Catlans appliance/ lower anterior inclined plane	• Used to treat maxillary anterior teeth in cross bite *(AIIMS 09,05)* • Has a 45 degree inclination to occlusal plane *(KCET 06)* • Catalan's shouldn't be worn for more than 6 week as causes supraeruption of posterior

- Canine retractor:
  - They move the canine distally (don't confuse with buccal/palatal canine retractor. They move the canine buccaly/palatally with distal movement)
- Maximum amount of incisors retraction obtained is '7 mm'

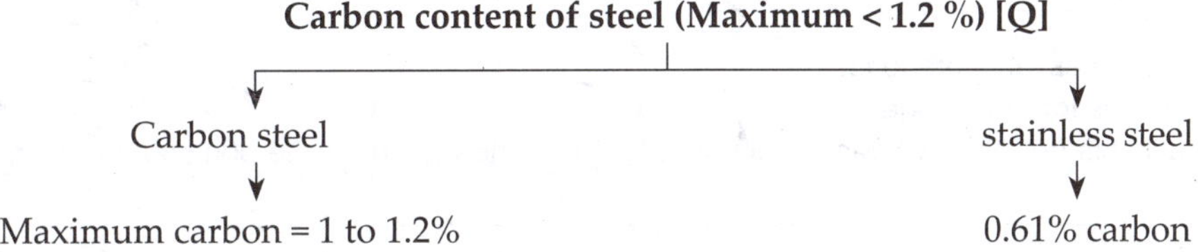

- For brackets mechanical bonding is preferred
- Ceramic bracket has higher friction than metal bracket
- Direct bonded orthodontic stainless steel brackets derive retention with composite due to mechanical interlock with mesh at bracket base [Q]
- Respond is an Adhesive–precoated (APC) self ligating bracket *(KCET 06)*
- Formulas:

Strength D ^ 3
Springiness
Force applied by spring *(AIIMS May 12, KCET 05,COMEDK 05)*
Flexion = $\left\{\frac{\text{Length}}{\text{Occluso-Gingival Height}}\right\}$ ^ 3

- Clasp:

  C-clasp/three quarter clasp
  U–clasp/Jackson's clasp } Inadequate retention is partially erupted teeth

- Adam's clasp:

Liverpool clasp/universal clasp/modified arrow head clasp
Provides maximum retention
Can be used in partially erupted teeth (Single arrow head) and in both deciduous and permanent dentition

- Concept: Chemical bonding for temporary restoration and brackets is not done
- Straight wire appliance was given by andrews
- Width of bracket commonly used: *0.028 inch and 0.018 * 0.025 inch *(PGI June 10)*
- Copper NiTi wires are available in temperature range of 27, 35, 40 degree celcius

- Edgewise Appliance:

<table>
<tr><td colspan="3">The unique feature is having a rectangular arch wire in a rectangular slot enable control of tooth movement in all 3 planes. This rectangular wire helps to correct crown root position. (AIIMS 07, 06)</td></tr>
<tr><td colspan="3">For this purpose angle described the use of an ideal arch wire that incorporated certain BENDS:</td></tr>
<tr><th>1st order bend</th><th>2nd order bend</th><th>3rd order bend</th></tr>
<tr><td>In and out bend to compensate for B-L prominence of teeth</td><td>To correct M-D inclination</td><td>To correct B-L root movement</td></tr>
<tr><td>In horizontal direction</td><td>In vertical direction</td><td>Twisting/torquing</td></tr>
<tr><td colspan="3">USE: Edgewise appliance is primarily meant for correction of crown–Root position (AIIMS 07)
With edgewise appliance excellent root control is possible</td></tr>
<tr><td colspan="3">Disadvantage:
Need to apply 'Heavy forces' anchorage loss
Need for extra oral forces for anchorage
IF an edgewise bracket is not pressed completely on a tooth on mesial side while bonding, the side effect would be rotation of tooth [Q]</td></tr>
</table>

- Begg appliance:

Light wire differential force technique
Light force is used (Unlike edgewise)
This appliance uses the concept of differential force and tipping of teeth rather than bodily movement (In edgewise)
Stages: The treatment using BEGG appliance is carried out in 3 stages Correction of alignment, crowding, rotation ,spaces and achieving edge to edge anterior bite, bite opening *(KCET 05) [Q]* Extraction spaces are closed Uprighting and torquing is carried out [Q]
Advantage: Light force, no need for extroral anchorage (Continuous)

- Straight wire appliance:

Given by 'Andrews' [Q]
No need of bending .So, also called preadjusted edgewise appliance

- Rx procedure and disadvantage

Treatment Procedure	Disadvantage
Milwaukee braces	Class 2 malocclusion is the result of retarded mandibular growth
Up righting 1st molar with loop lingual arch	Flaring of mandibular incisors
Use of buccal coil spring to regain space for mandibular 2nd premolar	Tendency of 1st premolars to rotate *(AIIMS 07,06)*
Laminated arch wire	Abruptness in response to adjustment *(AIPG 03)*
Cervical head gear therapy	Extrusion of molar *(KCET 13)*

- Orthopedic appliance:

• Head gear Causes movement of maxillary molar in all 3 planes Bodily movement of molar(when force passes through center of rotation), distal root tipping, distal crown tipping. Used for correction of deep bite, restrict growth of maxilla [Q] Distalisation of molar – High pull/parietal headgear: By causing intrusion of maxillary incisors Used for vertical growers, class 2 div 1 malocclusion *(PGI Dec 08)* – Cervical headgear: By causing extrusion of molar Harizontal growers

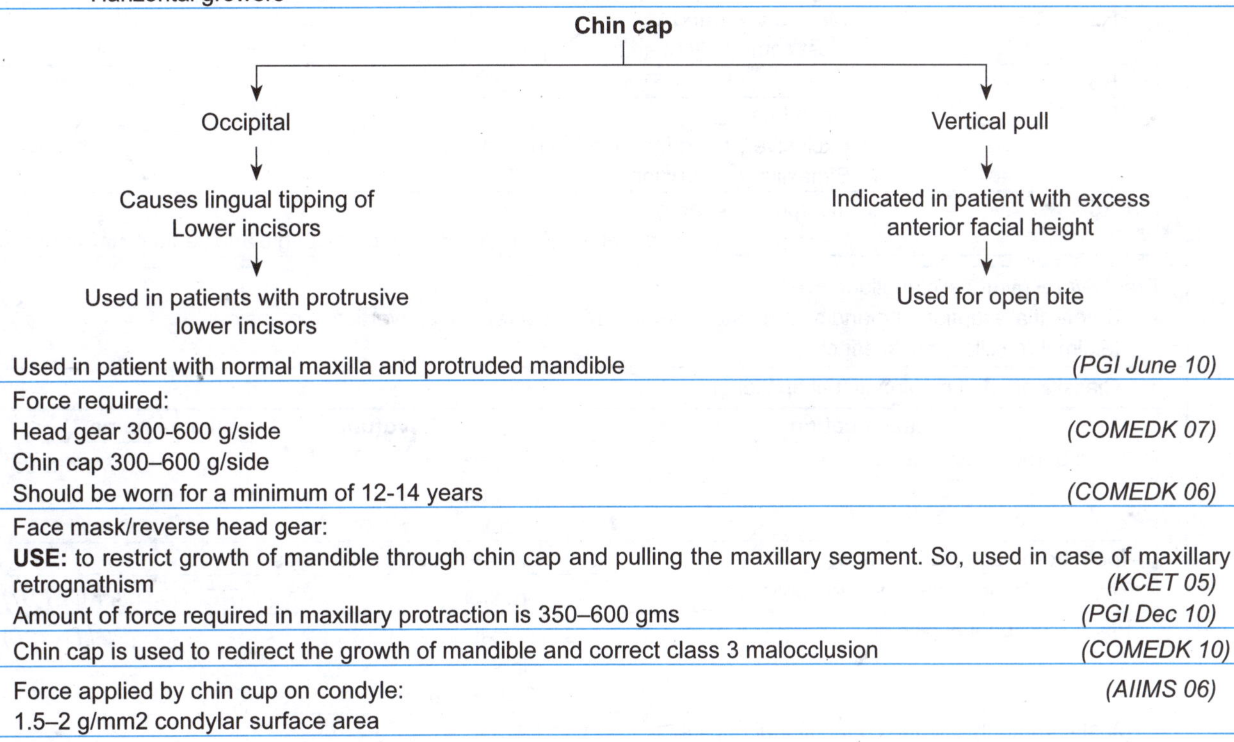

Used in patient with normal maxilla and protruded mandible	*(PGI June 10)*
Force required: Head gear 300-600 g/side Chin cap 300–600 g/side Should be worn for a minimum of 12-14 years	 *(COMEDK 07)* *(COMEDK 06)*
Face mask/reverse head gear: **USE:** to restrict growth of mandible through chin cap and pulling the maxillary segment. So, used in case of maxillary retrognathism Amount of force required in maxillary protraction is 350–600 gms	 *(KCET 05)* *(PGI Dec 10)*
Chin cap is used to redirect the growth of mandible and correct class 3 malocclusion	*(COMEDK 10)*
Force applied by chin cup on condyle: 1.5–2 g/mm2 condylar surface area	*(AIIMS 06)*

- Concept:

Rx of class 2 malocclusion may NOT be done in Pre-school and mixed dentition phase because in these phases it may be transient and growth spurt may change the relation to class 1 with time

- Stages in Rx followed nowadays:

• Leveling and allingment (Rotations are also corrected)
• Overbite reduction
• Overjet reduction
• Final tooth positioning

- Concept: Growth modification by means of functionaland orthodontic appliance elicit better response during growth spurt, i.e. late mixed dentition. Only Surgical procedure is carried out after cessation of growth spurt
- Myofunctional/functional appliance:

Loose fitting/passive appliance [Q]	
Myofunctional appliances act by changing the direction of growth	*(AIPG 05)*

Term myofunctional therapy was given by lischer

VTO:
An important diagnostic test undertaken before making a decision to use a Myofunctional appliance

The main AIM of frankel appliance is to influence outer neuromuscular envelop *(KCET 06)*

Classification of frankel appliance:

Frankel type	Use
FR1 A	Class 1 + crowding + deep bite
FR1 B	Class 2 div 1 + overjet < 5 mm
FR1 C	Class 2 div 1 + overjet > 7 mm
FR2	Class 2 div 1 and 2 Most commonly used frankel [Q]
FR3	Class 3
FR4	Open bite Exclusively used for mixed dentition period Bimaxillary protrusion [Q]
FR5	Incorporate head gear Used in long face patient with high mandibular plane angle and vertical maxillary excess

Frankel/oral gymnastic appliance/vestibular appliance:

- Differential eruption of mandibular posteriors to correct discrepancy in vertical dimension
- Minimal maxillary basal effect
- Classification of myofunctional appliance:

Classification	Myofunctional appliance name
Tooth borne passive appliance	Activator *(AIIMS 05)* Bionator Herbst
Tooth borne active appliance	Expansion screws/springs
The only tissue borne passive appliance	Frankel *(PGI Dec 08, KCET 07)*
Fixed functional appliance	Herbst *(PGI Dec 10)* Mars Jasper jumper
Most commonly used fixed functional appliance	Herbst
Removable functional appliance	Activator Bionator Frankel
Most commonly used functional appliance OR Most commonly used removable functional appliance	Activator
Most accepted functional appliance	Twin block
Group 1 appliance (transmits muscle force to the teeth)	Oral screen Inclined plane
Group 2 appliance (repositioning of mandible)	Activator Bionator
Group 3 appliance (repositioning of mandible But there area of operation is vestibule)	Frankel Vestibular screen
Semi-fixed functional appliance OR Removable fixed functional appliance	Lip bumper/ Lip plumber

- **Note:** Class 3 growers are best treated surgically as other appliances do not provide stable treatment. [Q]
- A major indication for orthognathic surgery before puberty is ankylosis of mandible *(KCET 12)*
- Functional appliance work on 2 principles:

• Force of elimination
• Force application

- All functional appliance consists of 3 basic components:

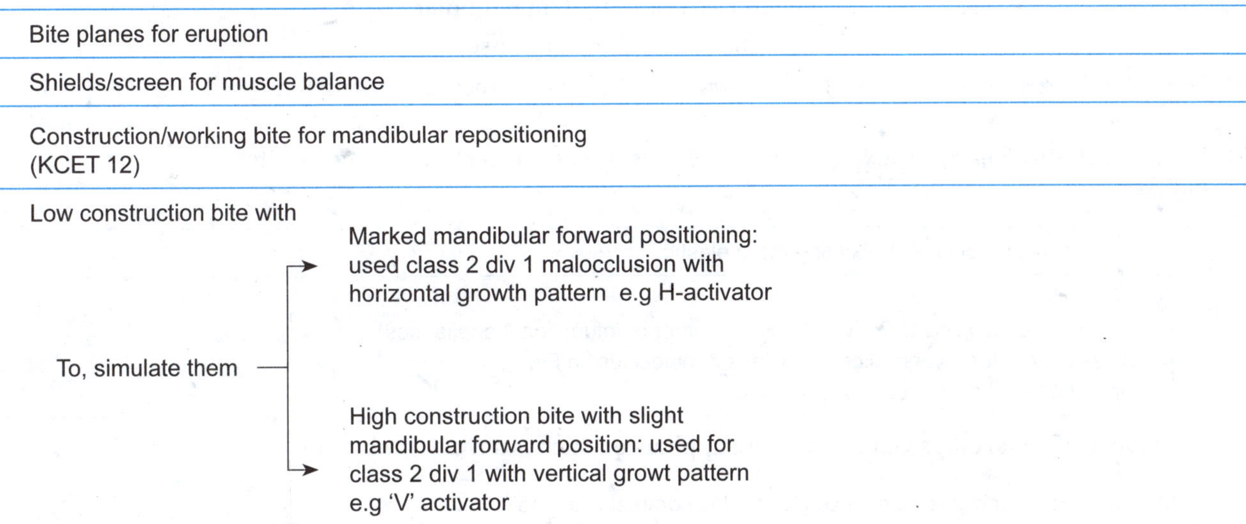

Bite planes for eruption
Shields/screen for muscle balance
Construction/working bite for mandibular repositioning (KCET 12)
Low construction bite with To, simulate them → Marked mandibular forward positioning: used class 2 div 1 malocclusion with horizontal growth pattern e.g H-activator High construction bite with slight mandibular forward position: used for class 2 div 1 with vertical growt pattern e.g 'V' activator

- Activator/Anderson appliance:

Introduced by Anderson *(KCET 07)*
Activator induces musculoskeletal adaptation by inducing new pattern of mandibular closure. Patient has to move the mandible forward to engage the appliance. This leads to stretching of elevator muscles of mastication Which starts contracting .the therapy sets a 'myotactic reflex' which causes: • Prevents further forward growth of maxilla • Distal movement of maxilla • Reciprocal forward growth of mandible In addition to 'myotactic reflex' also causes condylar adaptation by backward and upward growth (Favourable changes in TMJ region)
Indication: all cases
C/I: Maxillary and mandibular teeth should be well aligned .so, not used in class 1 with crowded teeth (this is applicable for all myofunctional appliances) Vertical growers (Excessive vertical growers) Causes mandibular rotation anteriorly downwards (Again this is for all myofunctional appliances)
Labial bow for activator made with 0.8–0.9 mm wire *(COMEDK 06)*

- Concept:

Case selection for myofunctional appliance including activator and frankel: best suited for class 2 div 1 with horizontal growers, i.e. normal maxilla and retrognathic mandible [Q]
For orthopedic appliance: Protrusive maxilla and normal mandible

- Rx of:

Anterior open bite
- → High FMA cases with mandibular Retrognathism: activator/ Myofunctional appliance should be used with high pull headgear (For maxilla)
- → High FMA cases with mandibular Prognathism: Chin cup is used

- Single tooth cross bite is mostly of dental origin and can be corrected by using removable/fixed appliance *(AIPG 02)*
- Extraoral elastics/head gear/expansion appliance is used to correct skeletal cross bite
- Bionator:

Similar to activator but less bulky and more elastic .
Types: • Standard: used in class 2 div 1 (Similar to other myofunctional appliances) • Class 3 bionator/reverse bionator: Class 3 malocclusion Fig • Open bite appliance: used for open bite

- Twin block: (Don't confuse with twin wire appliance which is a fixed appliance)

Most accepted functional appliance (Today it is commonly in use)
It is basically upper and lower hawley's with upper and lower inclined bite plane (interlock at 45 degree) (this angle should vary between 45–70 degree depending on patients comfort. But 70 degree is most common *(AIPG 04, KCET 06)* If patient fails to bite then it is reduced to 45 degree)
It induces favorably directed occlusal forces by causing mandibular displacement
Upper block runs from 2nd premolar to last molar of 2nd premolar (lower molar is kept free to help in eruption of if needed)

- Herbst appliance:

Fixed functional appliance. *(KCET 05)*
It's like an artificial joint working between maxilla and mandible . keeps the mandible in continuous anterior position
Indication: Same as other functional appliance + used as anterior repositioning splint in patient having TMJ disorder. Pecifically indicated in post adolescent patient (Above 20 years) [Q]

- Jasper jumper:

Fixed functional appliance like herbts but is flexible
Produces both skeletal and dentoalveolar changes in the ratio of 40: 60 (dental > skeletal) (Important than KCET)
Indication: same as other myofunctional appliances

- Lip bumper:

In maxillary arch it is called 'denholtz appliance'
It is a 'combined' removable fixed appliance (Semifixed appliance)

- Surgical management of malocclusion:

Malocclusion	Surgical rx
Skeletal class 2 with mandibular retrognathism	BSSO with mandibular advancement
Class 2 due to maxillary protrusion	Anterior maxillary segmental set back
Class 3 due to mandibular prognathism	BSSO with mandibular set back
Class 3 due to maxillary retrusion	Lefort 1 osteotomy with maxillary advancement
Class 2 with skeletal open bite	• Lefort 1 with maxillary impaction to correct open bite • BSSO for mandibular advancement
Bimaxillary protrusion	Maxillary and mandibular segmental Osteotomy with set back of anterior maxilla and mandible
Long face due to maxillary excess	Lefort 1 with maxillary impaction

- Decompensation:
- Most severe jaw discrepancy are partly compensated by change in axial inclination of the anterior teeth
- Concept: PDL problems and fixed appliance therapy:

Elimination of gingivitis prior to placing orthodontic appliance to prevent development of periodontitis.

- Camoflage Rx:
- Skeletal class 2 can often be camouflaged .skeletal class 3 and long face don't camouflage well and even make it worse
- Lingual orthodontic technique:

Kruz developed this technique
Fujita developed light wire lingual appliance known as MUSHROOM appliance
Can be based on both edgewise and begg's technique

- Edgewise bracket vs Ribbon arch bracket

Edgewise bracket	Ribbon arch bracket
Horizontal slot	Vertical slot
Rectangular wire used	Round wire used
Performs bodily movement	Causes tipping movement
Used in edgewise and straight wire technique	Used in BEGG'S appliance

- Rotation correction > 45 degree can be Hazardous
- Twin wire appliance:

Fixed appliance (COMEDK 08) given by Johnson
To obtain a better combination of springiness and strength, 2/more strands
Of small and springy wire are combined

- Concept: midline diastema

The most important factor to be considered before attempting to close a midline diastema using a removable appliance is age of the patient. *(AIPG 06)*
But midline diastema > 2 mm rarely closes spontaneously with further development BUT still wait for permanent canine to erupt.
If midline diastema is due to fibrous frenum, then frenectomy before orthodontic Rx is C/I .post treatment frenectomy should be attempted to prevent delay in treatment due to scar formation. *(AIPG 02)*

- Frenectomy:

Rx usually done if eruption of permanent lateral incisor and canine fails to close the diastema	*(COMEDK 07)*
"Z" or "V-Y" Plasty is done to correct abnormal frenum attachment	*(COMEDK 08)*

- Relapse:

Is primarily because of gingival fibers (AIPG 03) (Supralveolar/supracrestal) which are removed by gingivectomy	*(KCET 07)*
It is due to relapse tendency of the stretched gingival (AIPG 05) fibers The trans-septal and alveolar crestal group of gingival fibers remain stretched and don't readily adapt to the new tooth position	
Principle fibers of pdl reorganizes in 3-4 month	
Supra alveolar gingival fibers take 40 week nearly 1 year to re arrange so, it suggests that gingival fibers are more sluggish to readaptation and mainly responsible for relapse	
Relapse most commonly seen with rotation	*(KCET 05)*
Pericision can be done to prevent relapse following correction of rotation	*(COMEDK 07)*
Treatment of rotation is the least stable orthodontic correction	*(AIPG 05, 04)*

- Indication for active retainer:

Realignment of irregular incisors with spring retainer
Class 2, 3 relapse with modified functional appliance
Correct relapse

- Theories of retention:

• Malocclusion should be over corrected as safety factor
• Correction carried out during period of growth are less Likely to relapse as active growth period allow the tissue System to adapt well
• Arch form particularly mandibular arch shouldn't be altered As increased risk of relapse Mandibular intercanine and intermolar width are uncompromising

- Retention:

• No retention required Anterior and posterior cross bite Serial extraction Extrusion of teeth	*(AIIMS 05)*
• Limited retention Corrected deep bites Class 2 div 2 Ectopic eruption/supernumerary teeth Class 1 and 2 extraction cases	*(AIIMS 05)*
• Permanent/semipermanent retention [Q] (Important as generally it is asked in exams) Midline diastema Severe rotations Patient exhibiting abnormal musculature/tongue habits Cleft Lip and palate Generalized spacing	
Active retainer indicated in realignment of irregular lower incisorsand to correct relapse	*(PGI June 10)*

- Retainers (classification):

<table>
<tr><td>

- Removable retainers:
  - Hawley's appliance: most commonly used
  - Begg retainer
  - Clip–on retainer/spring aligner also brings correction of rotation commonly seen in lower anterior region
  - Wrap around retainer extended version of spring aligner. Covers all teeth. not commonly used in orthodontic practice BUT used in stabilizing periodontally weakened dentition
  - Kesling tooth positioned made of thermoplastic rubber like material . does not require regular activation at regular interval disadvantage: speech difficulty and risk of TMJ problem
  - Invisible esthetic retainer made from biostar machine

</td></tr>
<tr><td>Bonded retainer
Popular in lower anterior region</td></tr>
<tr><td>

- Fixed retainer
  - Banded canine to canine retainer commonly used in lower anterior region [Q]
  - Bonded lingual retainer canine to canine. is the best retainer
  - Band and spur retainer used in cases where single tooth has been treated for rotation/labio- lingual displacement

</td></tr>
</table>

LAST 5-YEAR QUESTIONS FROM THIS TOPIC

1. **Orthodontic tooth movement in a patient with concussion, subluxation, Extrusion and simple crown/root fracture should be postponed by:** *(AIPG 12)*

Ans. 3 months (Ref: Kindelan SA, Day PF, kindelan JD, Spencer JR, Duggal MS. Dental trauma: an overview of its influence on the management of orthodontic treatment. Part 1. J Orthod. 2008 June: 35 (2): 68–78

2. **Teeth with root fracture cannot be moved orthodontically for:** *(AIPG 12)*

Ans. 1 year (Ref: Kindelan SA, Day PF, kindelan JD, Spencer JR, Duggal MS. Dental trauma: an overview of its influence on the management of orthodontic treatment .part 1. J Orthod . 2008 June: 35 (2): 68–78)

3. **The undesirable side effect most commonly associated with the use of finger spring to tip the crown of a tooth is:** *(AIIMS Nov 12)*

Ans. Tendency of the root apex to move in the direction opposite from the crown (Ref: NBDE Q)

4. **The most stable orthognathic procedure for anterior open bite correction is:** *(AIIMS Nov 09)*

Ans. Le Fort 1 osteotomy (Ref: Proffit et al. Long term stability of surgical openbite correction by Le Fort 1 osteotomy. Angle Orthod 2000; 70: 112- 17)

5. **Catlan's appliance is used:** *(AIIMS May 09)*

Ans. To correct anterior crossbite (Ref: Singh. Textbook of Orthodontics 2/e p660)

6. **The edgewise appliance was developed by:** *(KCET 13)*

Ans. E.H. Angle

7. **A 10 year old boy comes to the clinic presenting with a distal step molar relation in the mixed dentitional stage. He would most probably need which of the following appliance:** *(KCET 13)*

Ans. Functional regulator

8. **Which of the following is a myofunctional appliance?** *(KCET 13)*
   a. Catalan's appliance
   b. Hawley's appliance
   c. Expansion screw
   d. Derichsweiler appliance

Ans. a.

9. **The line passing through the cingulated of the anterior teeth and central fossa of the posterior teeth is:** *(KCET 13)*
   a. Angles line of occlusion

b. Andrew's line of occlusion
c. Catenary curve
d. All of the above

Q was deleted in the exam but answer should be both 'a and c'(Ref: Profit)

10. The angulation of the bite blocks in a standard twin block is: *(KCET 13)*

Ans. 70 degree

11. Which of the following myofunctional appliance can be used in uncooperative patients with class 2 malocclusion *(KCET 13)*

a. Activator
b. Frankel 2
c. Bionator
d. Herbst

Ans. d.

12. A major disadvantage of Rx using cervical head gear is: *(KCET 13)*

Ans. Extrusion of incisors

13. A major indication for orthognathic surgery before puberty is: *(KCET 12)*

Ans. Ankylosis of mandible

14. The wax "Working bite" prior to functional appliance construction is made primarily with the intention of: *(KCET 12)*

Ans. Registering desired mandible position

15. Retention in orthodontic Rx means: *(KCET 12)*

Ans. Maintaining newly moved teeth in new position till it stabilizes

16. Myofunctional appliances are indicated in cases with: *(KCET 11)*

Ans. A class 2 skeletal malocclusion with a faulty mandible (Ref: Balajhi 3/e p333)

17. Concept of lingual orthodontic appliance was introduced by: *(KCET 11)*

Ans. Kurz (Ref: Textbook of Orthodontics by Gowri Shankar 1/e p1)

18. Catlan's appliance is given for a period not more than 6 weeks because it: *(KCET 11, 12)*

Ans. Causes overerupiton of posterior teeth and anterior open bite (Ref: Balajhi 3/e p429)

19. Rotation correction of tooth can be a hazardous process if correction is required over more than degrees *(KCET 11)*

Ans. 45

20. Which of the following statement(s) regarding the adjustment of Adam's clasp for a proper fit is true? *(KCET 10)*

A. Bending the arrowheads very slightly towards the tooth
B. Bending at appoint buccally to where the tag makes contact with the teeth at the contact point
C. Bending the tag where they emerge from the base plate

a. A and B | b. B and C | c. A and C | d. All the above

Ans. a.

21. Treatment of which type of malocclusion requires no post treatment retention: *(KCET 10)*

Ans. Anterior cross bite (Difficult to treat but easy to retain)

22. A maxillary anterior bite plane appliance is used to correct: *(KCET 09)*

Ans. Increased anterior overbite/deep bite

23. Appliance of choice in cases with anteroposterior maxillary deficiency: *(KCET 09)*

Ans. Reverse pull headgear

24. Camouflage Rx is best avoided in: *(KCET 09)*

Ans. Severe skeletal class 3 malocclusion

25. The choice of retention for lower incisors following orthodontic correction is: *(COMEDK 13, 08)*

Ans. Bonded canine to canine retainer

26. In adults seeking orthodontic Rx with esthetic appliances the following may be choices except: *(COMEDK 13)*

a. Lingual orthodontics
b. Ceramic brackets
c. Clear aligner therapy
d. Titanium brackets

Ans. d.

27. Adjunctive orthodontics refers to: *(COMEDK 13)*

Ans. Mild–Moderate orthodontic corrections in patients with periodontal and/or restorative needs

28. Andreason Appliance is known as: *(COMEDK 13)*

Ans. Activator

29. Case study: A 21 year old male healthy patient reported with a prognathic mandible, intraoral he has anterior cross bite and class 3 molar relationship, cephalometrically has an SNA of 78 degrees, SNB of 89 degrees: *(COMEDK 13)*

Q.1. What would be the Rx of choice for the adult class 3 skeletal malocclusion with a prominent chin?

Ans. Surgical orthodontics

Q.2. The presurgical orthodontic procedures involves:

Ans. Decompensation

Q.3. The surgical procedure of choice for correction of mandibular excessive prognathism is: *(COMEDK 13)*

Ans. Bilateral sagittal split osteotomy

30. An upper anterior inclined plane provides: *(COMEDK 12)*

Ans. Reinforced anchorage

31. Fibrotomy to prevent rotational relapse was advocated 1st by: *(COMEDK 12)*

Ans. Edwards

32. Which of the following surgical procedures aids in prevention of relapse: *(COMEDK 11)*

Ans. Circumferential supracrestal fibrotomy (Ref: Textbook of orthodontics by gowri Shankar 1/e p677)

33. Whip spring is used for the correction of: *(COMEDK 10)*

Ans. Rotation (Ref: Orthodontic appliances by lohakare 1/e p47)

34. The time during which Pdl fibers realign themselves after orthodontic Rx is: *(COMEDK 10)*

Ans. 280 days

35. The greatest disadvantage of removable appliance is dependence on: *(COMEDK 10)*

Ans. Patient cooperation

36. Spring used for buccal movement of premolar is: *(COMEDK 10)*

Ans. T-spring

37. Appliances which make use of forces exerted by muscles of tongue, face ,neck and mastication are: *(COMEDK 10)*

Ans. Functional appliances

38. In gnathosurgical procedure for normal occlusion how much space should be there between incisors? *(PGI Dec 11)*

Ans. 0.005 Inch

MISCELLANEOUS

- The major force producing part of fixed appliance is the arch wire *(COMEDK 08)*
- Device used to measure force generated by orthodontic elastics, springs, loops etc. is dontrix gauge (AIPG) and corex gauge
- Strength of wire is so, if diameter of spring is doubled strength will become 8 times *(AIIMS 05)*
- Ceranic bracket has highest friction with arch wire. do not confuse with highest critical surface tension which is for stainless steel bracket. This results in greatest accumulation of plaque
- Par index: (AIPG 04) (2 Q had been asked from the same topic in the same year. So, read the topic completely)

Stands for Peer Assessment Rating
Developed to measure success of orthodontic Rx *(AIPG 04)*
Features and their weightings are

Feature	Rating
Crowding	1
Buccal segment relationship–in AP, vertical and transverse plane	1
Overjet	6
Overbite	2
Centrelines	4

- High success of Rx is indicated by a mean % reduction greater than 70%
- Scan index
- Standarized Continum of Aesthetic Need
- Has AC (Aesthetic Component)
- IOTN index
- Index of Orthodontic Treatment Needs
- Has 2 components
- DHC (Dental Health Component) SCA index *(KCET 07)*
- (Aesthetic Component)
- Loss of tooth length of premolar in case of orthodontic Rx is 1.5 mm *(PGI Dec 08)*
- Treatment protocol for tooth with dental injury:

Type of injury	Observation period
Crown and crown/root fracture without/ with pupal involvement	3 months
Root fractures	1-2 years
Minor damage to periodontium Concussion/subluxation/extrusion/ Lateral luxation	3 months
Moderate to severe injury to periodontium like moderate/severe lateral luxation/ intrusion/avulsion/replantation	1 year if no ankylosis can be detected. Orthodontic tooth movement is not recommended before complete healing has occurred (6 months)
Immature traumatized teeth	Await radiographic evidence of continued root development .clinical and radiographic controls should be carried out after 6 months, 1 year, and 2 years.

Teeth requiring endodontic treatment due to caries	Immediate orthodontic movement provided no periapical pathosis is evident.
Teeth requiring endodontic treatment due to inflammatory resorption	Allow to heal atleast for 1 year before orthodontic treatment. Such teeth when moved orthodontically show greater degree of resorption.
Auto transplanted teeth	3-9 months i.e. after PDL healing (8 weeks) and before complete alveolar bone repair

- Laser welding stronger than solder joint:

Lesser heat generation
Can be done with Ti *(COMEDK 08)*
Choice of laser → CO_2 and Nd: YAG laser

- Drugs and orthodontic Rx:

Promoter drugs (enhances bone resoption) Prostaglandins (PGI Dec 09), leucotriens, cytokines (All these are example of chemotactic factors in inflammation) Vitamin D, osteocalcin, corticosteroids These agents when applied locally near moving unit i.e. anteriors Reduces duration of treatment
Suppressor agents (reduce bone resorption) NSAIDS, bisphosphonates(Used in Rx of osteoporosis [Q] and cancer) These agents when applied locally near anchor unit e.g molars Enhances anchorage and retention Aspirin and ibuprofen affect orthodontic treatment But acetaminophen, selective cox 2 inhibitor (e.g. celecoxib and parecoxib) does not affect orthodontic Rx

LAST 5-YEAR QUESTIONS FROM THIS TOPIC

1. **Dontrix gauze is used to:** *(AIPG 10, AIIMS May 10, May 08, May 07)*

Ans. Measure force

2. **Which of the following soft tissue response may occur as a response to orthodontic bands:** *(AIPG 08, 06)*

Ans. Marginal gingivitis

3. **Which of the following metals shows the property of twinning:** *(AIIMS Nov 12)*

Ans. Nickle–titanium alloy (Ref: Orthodontics–Current principles and techniques. Grabber, vanasdall and Vig 4/e p351)

4. **The highest critical surface tension is for which of the orthodontic brackets:** *(AIIMS Nov 12)*

Ans. Stainless steel (Ref: Orthodontic materials: scientific and clinical aspects. Brantley 1st p14)

5. **Surface of NiTi wire is:** *(KCET 11)*

Ans. Rougher than β titanium wire and rougher than stainless steel wire *(Ref: Profit p378)*

6. **Which form of stainless steel is used for the manufacturing of orthodontic wire?** *(KCET 11)*

Ans. Austenite (Ref: Phillips science of dental materials 11/e p639)

7. **What is the effect of doubling the diameter of a cantilever spring?** *(KCET 10)*

Ans. Strength increases by 8 times, springiness decreases by 16 times

8. **Which of the following wires possess 'shape memory' characteristic?** *(KCET 09, 06, 05)*

Ans. Nickel–Titanium

9. **When the diameter of the wire is doubled, the flexibility of the spring:** *(KCET 09)*

Ans. Decrease by sixteen times (springiness/flexibility)

10. Hook's law applies to all wires except: *(PGI June 12)*

a. TMA
b. Nitinol
c. A-NiTi
d. M-NiTi

Ans. c (Ref: profit 4/e p365

11. Which wire can be heat treated: (PGI dec 11,june 08)

Ans. Elgiloy (Ref: Profit 4/e p361)

12. NiTi wire exhibit super elasticity due to/can flex without fracture? *(PGI June 11)*

Ans. Stress induced change from austenite to martensitic.

CHAPTER

8

Oral Pathology

Topic

- Developmental Disorders
- Diseases of Bones and Joints
- Skin and Vesiculobullous Lesion
- Salivary Gland
- Infection
- Oral and Metabolic Diseases
- Cyst and Tumor
- Periapical and Pulpal Infection
- Blood
- Caries
- Miscellaneous

DEVELOPMENTAL DISORDERS

- Most common Superumerary teeth → Conical

- Odontome is also a supernumerary teeth

- False anodontia: Trick: Fame

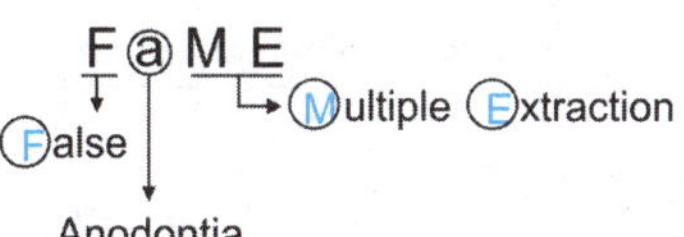

Fig. 8.1: False anodontia

- In Severe illness teeth affected:
- Below 1 year → Centrals + Laterals + 1 st molar + tip of cuspid[Q]
- After 3 years → Premolars, 2 and 3rd molars

- Supernumerary teeth associated with:

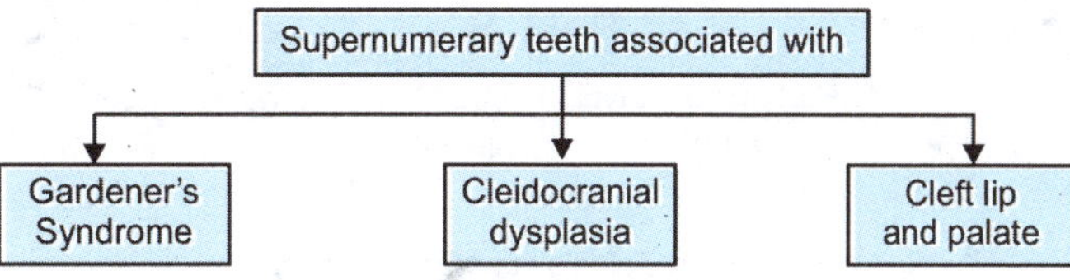

Fig. 8.2: Supernumerary teeth associated with

- Natal teeth seen in:
  1. Ellis–Van-Crevelod/Chondroectodermal dysplasia
  2. Soto syndrome
  3. Cleft Palate
  4. Pierre Robin
  5. Pachonychia congenita

  Not seen "Van der Woud Syndrome" *(AIIMS 11)*

- Glossoptosis:

  Airway obstruction caused by power Posterior displacement of tongue

  Aglossia: Microglossia with extreme glossoptosis

  ↓

  Lack of muscular stimulus for the growth of the arches

  ↓

  Retarded growth of mandibular arches

  ↓

  Severe dentoskeletal malocclusion

- Palpebral fissure:

  - Palpebral fissure
    - Mongoloid → Upward slant → Down syndrome
    - Anti mongoloid → Treacher collin's syndrome → Reverse and mongoloid

  Fig. 8.3: Palpebral fissure

- Taurodontism:[Q]/Bull's teeth

  Highest incidence in mandibular 1st Molar

  seen in:

  Trichodentosseous syndrome

  Klinefilter's syndrome[Q] *(AIPG 10)*

  AI type IV

  Note: Trichodentosseous syndrome is associated with AI type IV *(KCET 12)*

- Talon's cusp/Eagle's cusp:

  Trick = **R M S**

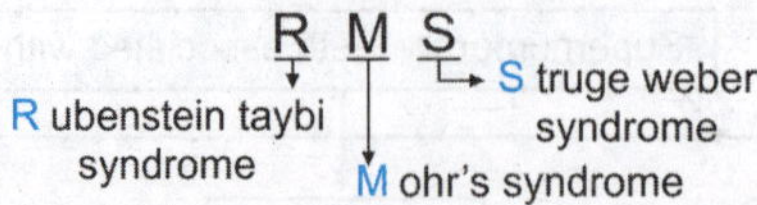

Fig. 8.4: Talon's cusp/Eagle's cusp

Enamel Pearl/Leong's PM when PM affected

- Proteins syndrome
  Beckwith Widman Syndrome
  Mc Cune Albright
  Neurofibromatosis
  } [Q]Hemifacial hypertrophy

- Macroglossia:
  Seen in Beckwith Widman syndrome (Most common cause)[Q] Amyloidosis *(PGI 06)*

- Cheilitis granulomatosa: Seen in
  Melkarson Rosenthal syndrome
  Sarcoidosis
  Crohn's

Note: Melkerson Rosenthal characterized by:
- Upper lip and facial oedema
- Fissured tongue *(KCET 07)*
- Bell's palsy
- Parotid hyperplasia

- Turner's hypoplasia/Turner's teeth: Premolars >> Maxillary incisor

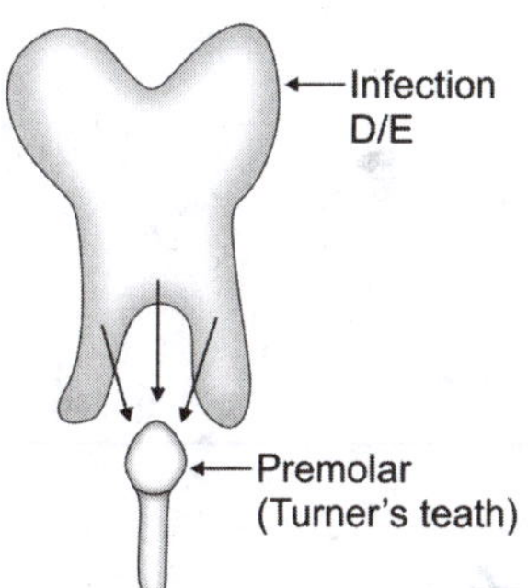

Fig. 8.5: Turner's hypoplasia

- Ankylosis of deciduous teeth
  ↓
  "Submerged teeth"
  ↓
  Most commonly seen in Deciduous Mandibular 2nd molar *(AIPG 12, PGI 08)*
  ↓
  So, Permanent 2nd premolar is most commonly missing

- **Most common:**

• Most common supernumerary teeth	Mesiodens anterior maxilla
• 2nd most common supernumerary teeth	Maxillary 4th molars followed by mandibular 4th molars
• Most commonly ankylosed/submerged tooth	Deciduous mandibular 2nd molar
• Most commonly missing deciduous teeth	Maxillary and mandibular lateral incisors
• Most commonly missing permanent teeth	3rd molars > maxillary laterals
• Supernumerary roots	Mandibular canine and Premolars
• Teeth commonly involved in Turner's hypoplasia	Permanent PMs>> permanent maxillary incisors
• Teeth commonly affected with microdontia	Max Lateral incisor >> 3rd molars
• Regional Odontoplasia	Incisor > Lateral incisors canine

- Monro abscess seen in:

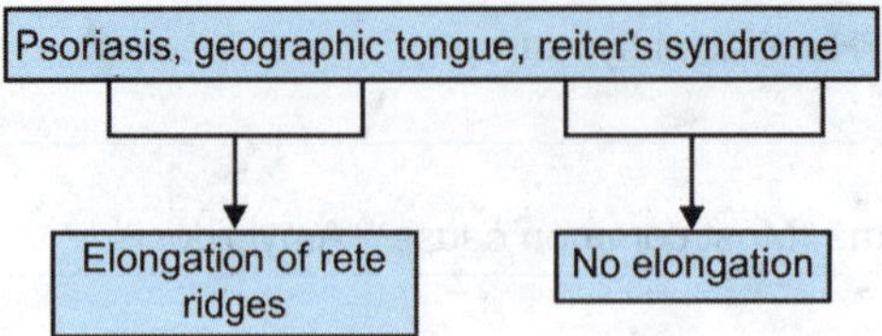

Fig. 8.6: Monro abscess

In Psoriasis → "Test tube" shaped rete ridges.

- Names and diseases
  1. Congenital epulis → Neuman's tumour
  2. Hemifacial atrophy → Parry Rhomberg syndrome
  3. Posterior Atrophic candidiasis
     ↓
     Median Rhomboid glossitis/Kissing lesion
  4. Patterson – Kelly syndrome
     ↓
     Plummer Wilson syndrome
     ↓
     ↑sed risk of SCC

- Transposed teeth:
  Canine ⇌ Premolar (Most commonly)
  Canine ⇌ Lateral incisor (2nd most common)

- Concrescence:
  Most commonly seen in maxillary molars

- In Cleidocranial Dysplasia/Dysostosis
  Enamel hypoplasia is not seen[Q]

- Various conditions associated with delayed eruption:

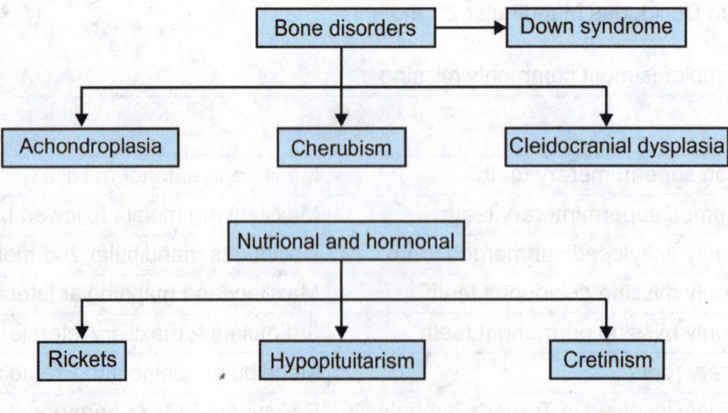

Fig. 8.7: Delayed eruption

3. Fibromatosis gingiva

- Supernumerary teeth more common in:

  ↓

  Anterior Maxilla

  ↑

  Ghost Teeth more common in

- Serum alkaline phosphatase elevated in:

  Paget's disease

  Fibrous dysplasia

  Hyper parathyroidism (Brown's tumour)

  Note: Serum alkaline Phosphatase level is normal in multiple myeloma [Q]

- Parulis = Pus pocket

  ↓

  Inflammation at end of sinus tract

- Down syndrome:
- (Oral manifestation)

  1. Maxillary hypoplasia
  2. Small mouth
  3. Tongue – Macroglossia and fissured tongue
  4. Juvenile Periodontitis
  5. Anodontia, Delayed eruption, enamel Hypoplasia, Microdontia, conical teeth
  6. Small mouth + large tongue

     ↓

     Drooling of saliva

     ↓

     Angular chelitis
  7. Hypotonic with hypermobility *(AIPG 04)*

- Order of missing teeth:
- Mandibular 3rd molar > Maxillary lateral Incisor = Mandibular 2nd Premolar

- Order of impaction:

  Mandibular 3rd molar > Maxillary 3rd molar > Maxillary canine

- Gemination → Number of teeth remains same

  Fusion → Number of teeth reduces

  Twinning → Number ↑ses (1 tooth divides)

  ↓ ↓

  1 normal tooth 1 supernumerary tooth

- Type I DI → Tulip shaped
- Type I dentinal dysplasia → Radicular dentinal dysplasia Obliterated pulp chamber

  } **Obliterated pulp chamber**

  Type II DI → Shell teeth

  Type II dentinal dysplasia → coronal dentinal dysplasia

  } **Abnormally large pulp chamber**

  ↓

  Thistle tube appearance

- Revised Shield's classification of Dentinogenesis imperfecta

  Type I: (Shield's type II)

  - AD trait
  - Dentinogenesis imperfect without Osteogenesis imperfect

    Mutation of Dentine sialophosphoprotein (DSSP)

    ↓

  Mapped on chromosome 4

  - Defects:

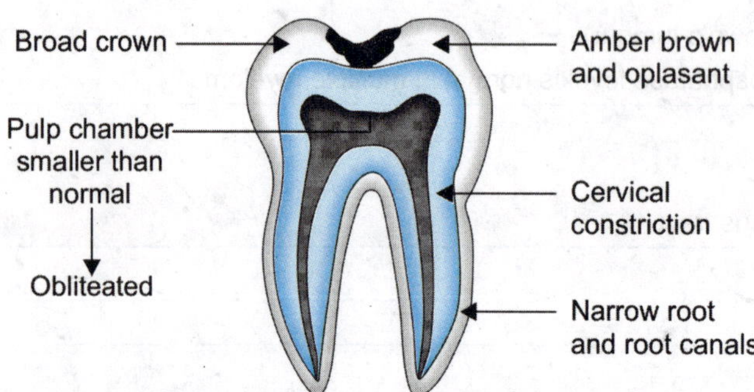

Fig. 8.8: Dentinogenesis imperfecta

'TULIP' shaped

- ↑sed 2° dentine formation/calcification irregular dentinal tubules with larger diameter, less in number.
- H_2O content sed 60% of normal
- Micro Hardness of Dentine ~ cementum

Type II: (Shield type III)/Brandywine/shell teeth

- DSSP + DMP1 + 1 BSP + SPPI genes affected

  Defects:

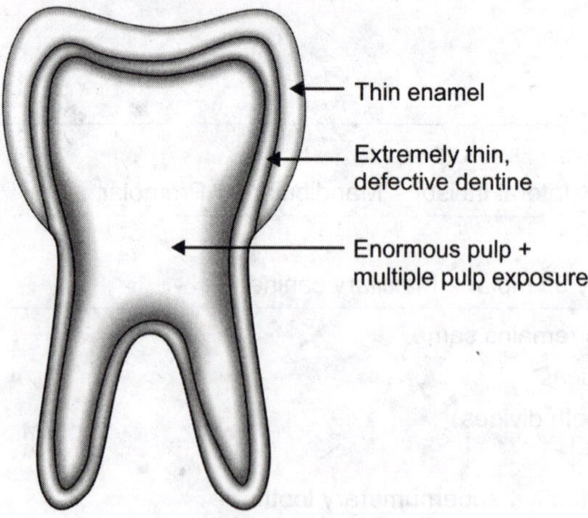

Fig. 8.9: Brandywine/shell teeth

Note: Dentine is opalescent and translucent DEJ absent → enamel lost early

↓

Early attrition of enamel and occlusal wear

- Ascher's syndrome: (features)
  Trick: NBD

(N)→(N)on toxic thyroid enlargement

(B)→(B)lepherochalasia (edema and upper eye lid)

(D)→(D)ouble lip

Fig. 8.10: Ascher's syndrome

- Vander Woude's syndrome
  ↓
  Congenital lip pits and fissures
  ↓
  Lower lip commonly affected

- Fusion of teeth: Common in deciduous teeth
  while supernumerary teeth common in maxillary permanent teeth (Mesiodens)

- Globulo maxillary cyst: Arises from medial nasal process[Q]
- Nasoalveolar cyst ® No radiographic features

- Non odontogenic developmental cyst:

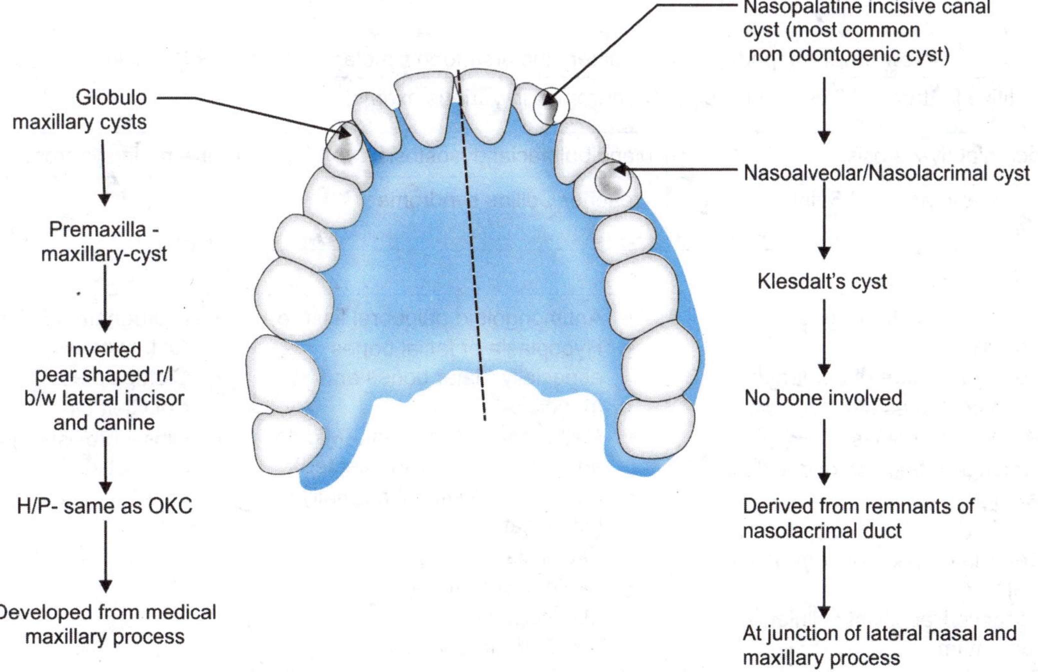

Fig. 8.11: Non odontogenic developmental cyst

- **Note:** Fissural/Inclusion cyst includes Globulomexillary cyst, Nasoalveolar cyst, Median palatal cyst, Nasoalveolar cyst, median mandibular cyst.

- All these cysts have keratin filled "onion ring" appearance

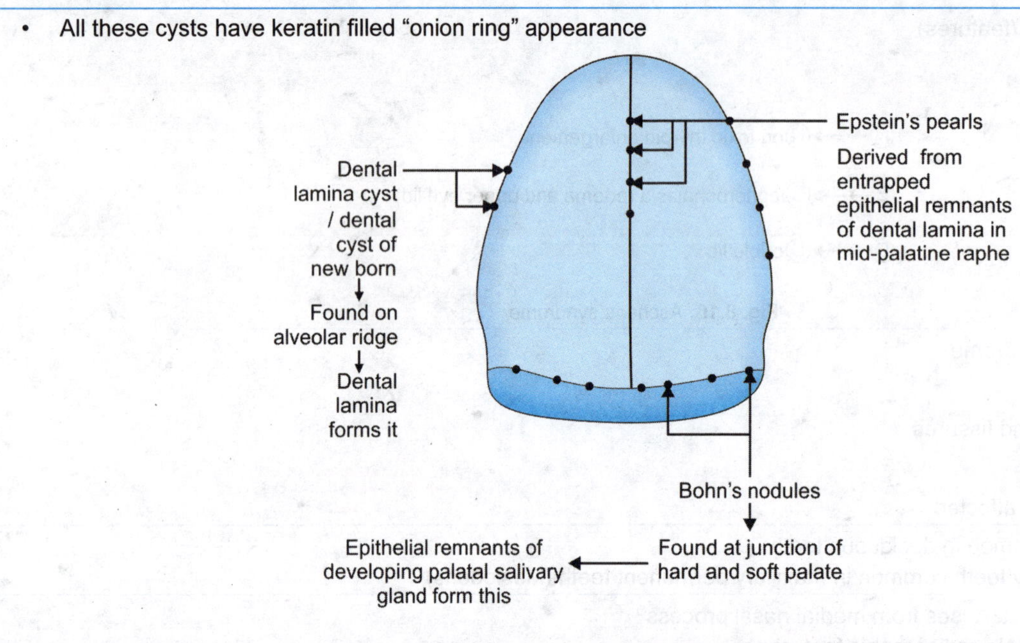

Fig. 8.12: Non odontogenic developmental cyst

- Congenital syphillis

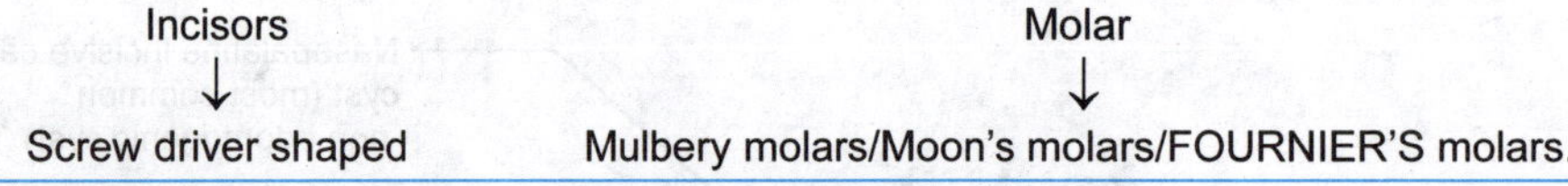

- Compartitive features of 3 commonly asked syndromes in various exams:

Cleidocranial dysostosis	Mandibulofacial dysostosis	Pierre robin syndrome
Other names-marie and Sainton's disease	Treacher Collins syndrome	
Features:		
• Partial/complete absence of clavicles • Delayed closure of Fontanels • Wormian bones seen • Maxillary Hypoplasia • Prolonged retention of deciduous teeth ↓ • Delay in eruption of permanent teeth • Absence/Paucity of cellular cementum • Then short root • Numerous unerupted supernumer-ary teeth	• Antimongoloid palpebral fissure • Hypoplasia of facial bones especially Malar bones and mandible • Malformed external ear, (Middle and Internal ear also affected) • Macrostomia with abnormally high palate • Facial cleft • Skeletal deformities • Malocclusion • Bird/Fish like face.	• Micrognathia/Retrognathia (of Lower jaw) • Cleft palate • Not Cleft Lip • Glossoptosis + airway obstruction

- Features of Peutz – Jehger's syndrome

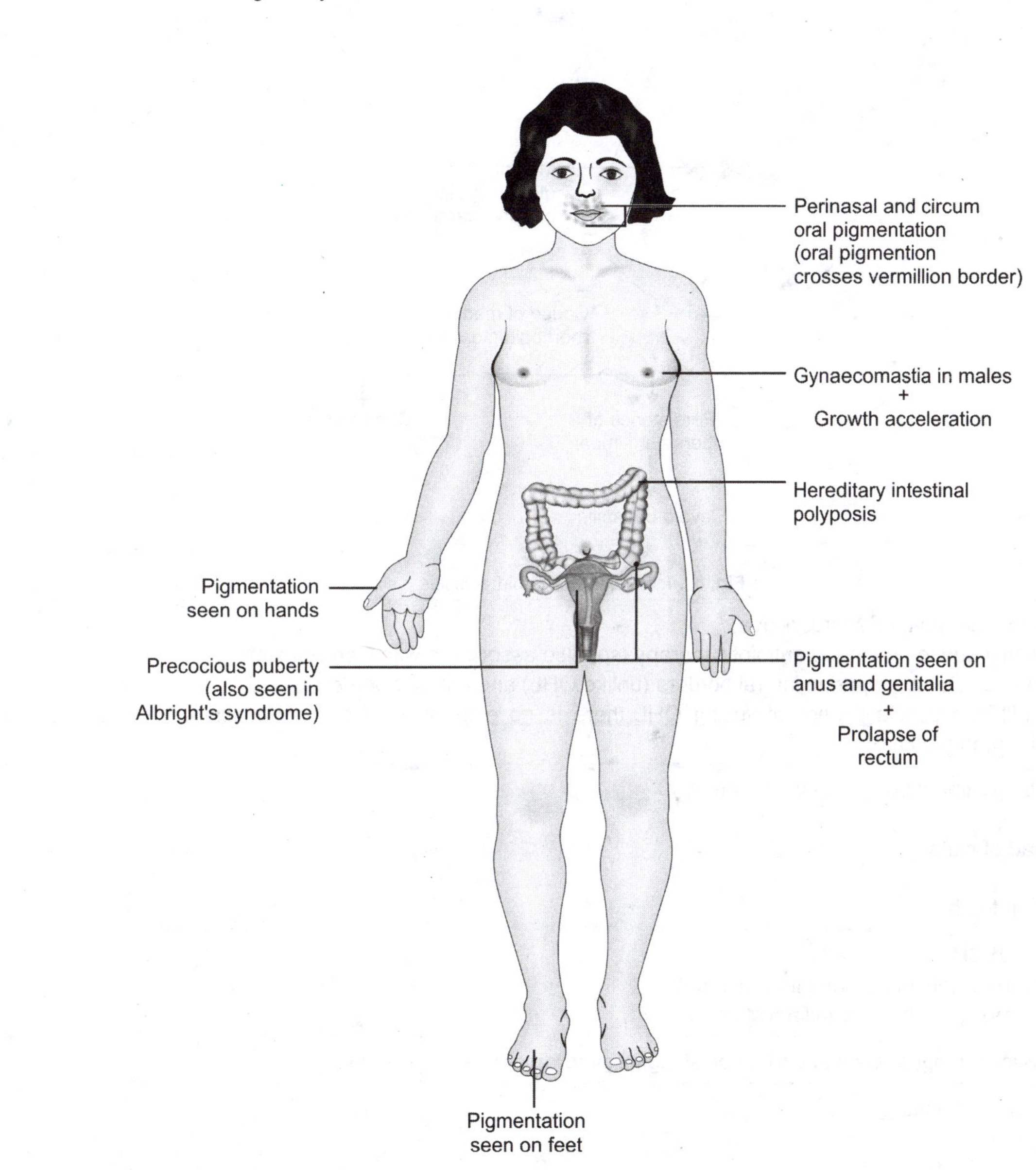

Fig. 8.13: Peutz – Jehger's syndrome

- Heredity of diseases:
- Trick: whatever diseases you know are "AD"

except

- X-linked: Ectodermal dysplasia + Wiskott Aldrich + Papillon Lefever +
- AR → Chediak Hegaski + Acrodermatitis enteropathica
- Non-Hereditary → Stage Weber + Fibrous dysplasia + Regional odontodysplasia

- Median rhomboid glossitis ~ M: F = 3: 1

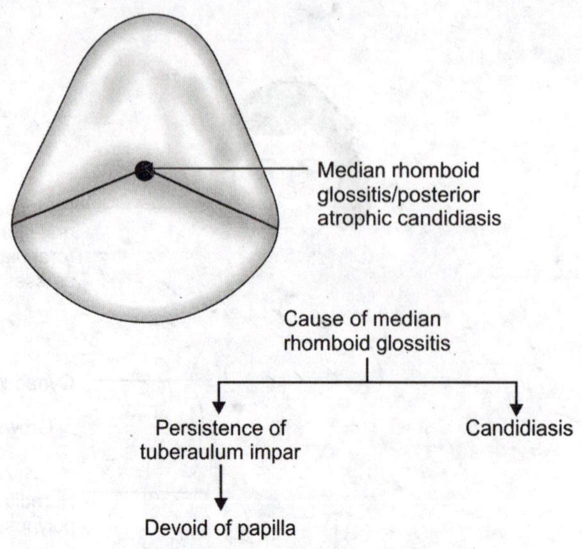

Fig. 8.14: Median rhomboid glossitis

- Black hairy tongue: (Lingua Nigra/Villosa)
  Most commonly due to prolonged antibiotic therapy (so, also associated with Candidiasis)
  Most common on Dorsum sparing lateral borders (unlike OHL) and anterior borders.
  Elongated Filliform papilla [Donot confusing OHL there is no elongation of filliform papilla but Hyperkeratosis on lateral border of the tongue]

- Teeth with large amount of globular dentine
  ↓
  Rapid spread of caries
  ↓
  Malocotic/soft tooth

- **ANKYLOGLOSSIA**
  True – union between tongue and floor of mouth
  False – Tip of tongue attached to lingval frenum

- Bifid Tongue/cleft tongue: seen in Oro – Facial digital syndrome

- Etiology of Dilacerations
  ↓
  Trauma

- Crenated tongue:
  When lateral border of tongue consists of indentation of teeth.

- Transitory papilla of tongue
  ↓
  Fungiform filliform

- Generalized Microdontia seen in pituitary dwarfism

- Hemifacial microsomia/occulo auricular vertebral dysplasia/GOLDENHAR syndrome. Origin and migration of NEURAL Crest cell (also seen in Treacher Collin syndrome)
  (PGI 11)

LAST 5-YEAR QUESTIONS FROM THIS TOPIC

1. The other name of Premaxilla-premaxillary cyst is:

Ans. Globulomaxillary cyst (Ref: Shafer's 6/e p64) *(AIPG 12)*

2. Marked reduction in the amount of dentine, widening of predentine layer, presence of large areas of interglobular dentine and irregular pattern of dentine is seen in: *(AIIMS May 11, 12)*

Ans. Regional odontodysplasia (Ref: Shafer 6/e p57)

3. The most common developmental cyst is:

Ans. Nasopataline cyst (Ref: Nevilli, 2nd)

4. Which of these is NOT associated with an abnormal cusp on central incisor? *(AIIMS Nov 09)*

a. Mohr syndrome
b. Struge Weber
c. Rubinstein Taybi syndrome
d. Proteus syndrome

Ans. d (Ref: Shafer 6/e p41)

5. The deficiency of which of the following affects tooth development? *(AIPG 11)*

Ans. Vit.A (Also Vit. C and D)

Vit.A ↓ Epithelial cell growth; Vit. C ↓ Collagen formation; Vit. D ↓ Calcification

6. Teeth that erupts within 30 days of birth are: *(AIPG 11)*

Ans. Neonatal (Ref: McDonalds 8/e p183)

7. Turner's hypoplasia is caused by:

Ans. Hypoplasia due to local trauma *(Shafer 5/e p72-73)*

8. Hutchinson's triad is? *(AIPG 10)*

Ans. Interstitial keratitis, mulberry molars, 8th nerve deafness.

9. Lowest incidence of cleft lip and palate is found in? *(AIPG 10)*

Ans. Negroes (Ref: Bhalaji 3/e)

10. An Angulation, sharp bend/curve in a root is called: *(AIPG 10)*

Ans. Dilaceration (Ref: Shafer 4/e p56)

11. Taurodontism is associated with: *(AIPG 10)*

Ans. Klinefelter syndrome.

12. True about primary teeth is: *(AIPG 09)*

a. Furcation is close to the cervical line
b. Pulp chambers are large
c. Roots are narrowed and thin
d. All of the above

Ans. d.

13. A patient with severely discoloured teeth, fractured enamel, undefined DEJ and severe attrition has: *(AIPG 09)*

Ans. Amelogenesis imperfect (Ref: Shafer 4/e p58, 59)

14. Turner's tooth is seen in: *(AIPG 09)*

Ans. Permanent maxillary incisors.

Note: Most commonly turner's tooth is seen in maxillary/mandibular premolar and permanent maxillary incisors)

15. Teeth present in the oral cavity on the date of first birthday of a child are? *(PGI Dec 11)*

Ans. Neo-Natal teeth (Ref: Shafer 5/e p81)

16. Fordyces spots are: *(PGI June 11)*

Ans. Ectopic sebaceous glands (Ref: Shafer's oral pathology 5/e p31)

17. Goldenhar syndrome includes: *(PGI June 11)*

Ans. Epibulbardermoid auditory appendics, vertebral involvement (Ref: Shafer's 5/e p4)

18. Characteristic thistle-tube-shaped appearance of pulp chambers of single rooted teeth are seen in: *(COMEDK 12)*

Ans. Type II dentine dysplasia.

19. Failure of descent of thyroid analage can be seen in the tongue: *(COMEDK 12)*

Ans. Near the base of tongue close to foramen caecum.

20. The following genetic syndromes are associated with supernumerary teeth, except? *(KCET 12)*

a. Grinspan's syndrome
b. Gardner's syndrome
c. Cleidocranialdysostosis
d. Fabry's disease

Ans. a

21. All of the following are seen on attached gingiva of children, except: *(KCET 12)*

a. Retrocuspid papilla
b. Fordyce's granules
c. Interdental clefts
d. Stippling

Ans. d

22. One of the following is seen in tricho-dentosseous syndrome: *(KCET 12)*

Ans. Amelogenesis imperfecta.

23. Fissured tongue is a component of: *(KCET 09)*

Ans. Melkersson-Rosenthal syndrome.

24. Which of the following is NOT a clinical feature of Pierre Robin syndrome? *(KCET 09)*

Ans. Coloboma of lower eyelid (**Note:** Micrognathia + Retrognathic + Glossoptosis)

25. Fordyce granules are: *(COMEDK 10)*

Ans. Ectopic sebaceous glands.

26. The lip Swelling, fissured tongue and unilateral facial palsy is seen in: *(COMEDK 10)*

Ans. Melkerson-Rosenthal syndrome.

27. Benign migratory glossitis is also known as: *(KCET 10)*

a. Geographic tongue
b. Wandering rash
c. Erythema migrans
d. All of the above

Ans. d

28. Eagle syndrome is associated with: *(KCET 10)*

Ans. Elongation of stylohyoid ligament.

29. Morphological types of supernumery teeth is/are: *(KCET 10)*

a. Conical
b. Supplemental
c. Odontome
d. All of the above

Ans. d

30. Neonatal teeth erupt: *(COMEDK 11)*

Ans. In first 30 days

31. A developmental alteration where a single tooth bud divides incompletely resulting in the formation of a tooth with a bifid crown and a single pulp chamber is called: *(KCET 11)*

Ans. Gemination (Ref: Shafer's 5/e p54)

32. The percentage of supernumerary teeth found in maxillary region: *(PGI June 09)*

Ans. 90% (Ref: Nevilli 2/e p71)

33. Most common cleft lip defect is: *(PGI Dec 09)*

Ans. Isolated left unilateral deformities (Ref: Shafer's 5/e p15, 21)

34. Which of the following has polygenic inheritance? *(PGI June 10)*

a. Cleft tongue *(PGI June 10)*
b. Cleft palate
c. Both of the above
d. Note known

Ans. b (Ref: Shafer 6/ep23)

35. A patient with familial dysartonomia (rib day syndrome) will show the absence of: *(PGI June 10)*

Ans. Fungiform papillae (Ref: Khurana medical physiology 1/e p337)

36. Developmental enamel defects are most commonly seen in: *(PGI June 10)*

Ans. Permanent incisors (Ref: Shafer's 4/e p51-58)

37. Atrophic red areas seen in geographic tongue due to? *(PGI June 11)*

Ans. Increased neutrophillic infillteration (Ref: Shafer's 5/e p41)

38. True anodontia is considered to be a failure of: *(COMEDK 12)*

Ans. Initiation.

DISEASES OF BONES AND JOINTS

• Fibrous dysplasia: – Non-Hereditary[Q] – Mutation GNAS 1 – Camp *(AIIMS 11)* – Coarse Woven bone seen – Ostoblastic differentiation and maturation defective
• Pagets → AD → Abnormal persistence of woven bone
• Ground glass appearance: Fibrous dysplasia (Monostotic form) + Hyperparathyroidism (Brown's tumour) + cherubism
• Orange peel appearance: • Fibrous dysplasia
• Acid phosphatase → "Osteopetrosis" released from "Defective Osteoclasts"[Q]
• Mandibular Retrognathism → seen in "Treacher Collin", "Pierre robin"
• Pagets[Q] and Polyostotic fibrous dysplasia transform into Osteosarcoma
• Osteoclastoma = central giant cell granuloma → "Pulsatile lesion" • Odontoclastoma = Internal resorption

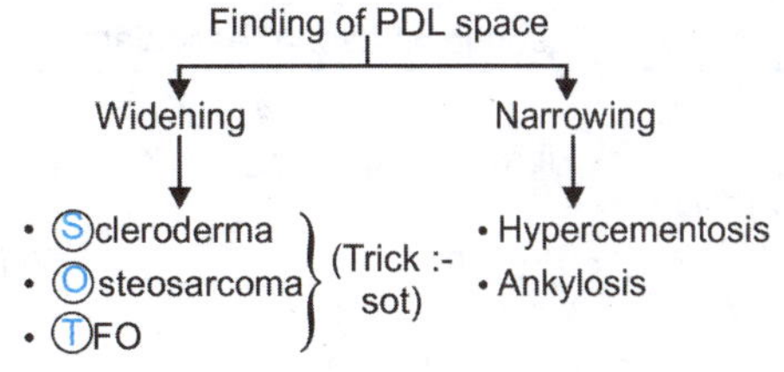

Fig. 8.15: Finding of pdl space

- Osteitis Fibrosa cystica (Q) = Hyper parathyroidism (1°)
- Development of osteosarcoma is most important complication of Pagets
- Rind sign: seen in Fibrous dysplasia
- In MPDS muscle exhibiting tenderness
- Lateral pterygoid >> Masseter
- Rheumatoid arthritis in children called as "Stills disease"
  ↓
- Results in class II Div 1 with anterior open bite.
- In Cleidocranial dysplasia
  ↓
- Maxillary hypoplasia seen
  ↓
- Not enamel hypoplasia
- Rugger Jersy sign
  ↓
  Osteopetrosis (↑sed acid phosphatase)
  Note: Rugger jersey Spine seen in Renal osteodystrophy
- Osteopetrosis = Marble bone disease = Albert Schonberg disease
- Achondroplasia: Mentally alert, disproportionate body (Endochondral ossification affected while intra membranous ossification normal)
- Rx of Fibrous dysplasia: Surgical curettage + grafting[Q] Cosmetic recontouring[Q]
- Enamel hypoplasia → Rickets + Hypoparathyroidism
- Hans Schuller disease ~ Advanced pdl disease
- Mazabraud syndrome: Fibrous dysplasia associated with Intramuscular myxoma
  ↓
  Greater risk of Sarcomatous transformation seen
- Sclerodactyly/claw hands → Scleroderma + Hurler syndrome
  ↓
- (Ulnar nerve involved) *(NEET 13)*
- Arachnodactyly → Marfan syndrome
- **Note:** In Huler syndrome rest all features similar to Acromegaly
- BLUE sclera seen in: associated with **O**I + **R**ickets + **M**arfan + **E**lhers Danlos Syndrome + Ostio**p**etrosis + **N**ormal infants [TRICK = NREM Post Office]

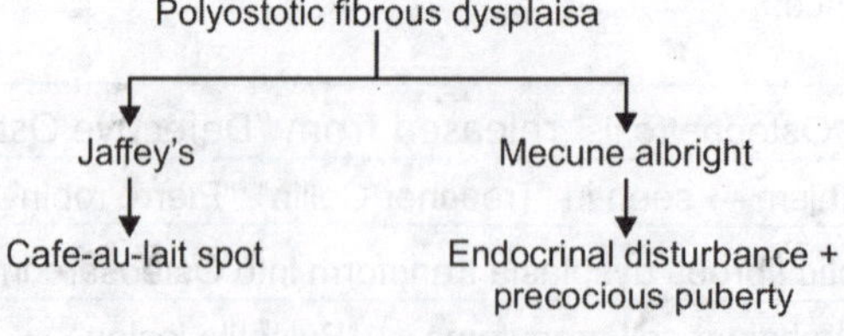

Fig. 8.16: Elhers Danlos syndrome

- Monostotic fibrous dysplasia: term "Leontiasis ossea" associated
- Laboratory findings

		Fibrous dysplasia	Pagets
I.	Serum calcium + PO_4^{3-}	N	N
II.	ALP	↑	↑
III.	NTX + CTX		
IV.	Urinary hydroxyl proline sed		

Note: H/P most similar to ossifying fibroma

- OI: the basic defect is failure of Foetal collagen to transform to Mature collagen
- TMJ involvement in Rheumatoid arthritis is common in Marie–Strumpell type of Rheumatoid arthritis
- "Apert syndrome" ®associated with Syndactyly otherwise similar to Crouzon disease
  ↓
  The main dermatological manifestation of Crouzon is Acanthosis Nigricans
  ↓
  Insulin Resistance + obesity + Hyperpigmentation
- Rx for Pagets:
  Calcitonin – promising result
  Bisphosphonate – has been used with some success
- Concept:
- In cementoma Radio opacity attached to tooth while in condensing osteitis it is not (but is around root)
- Earlist R/f of Osteomyelitis:
  Trabeculae become Fuzzy
- Vit. D resistant rickets
  - Pulp horn reaching DEJ
  - ↑sed interglobular dentine

  Elhers Danlos
  - Lack of Normal Scalloping of DEJ
  - Dentinal tubules reaching Enamel
- Aneurysmal Bone cyst (ABC)
  ↓
  Radiographic feature
  ↓
  Eccentric Expansile lesion[Q]
- Eccentric lytic lesion: ABC, giant cell tumour, fibrous cortical defect.
- Simple bone cyst → is central lytic lesion.
- Cleidocranial dysplasia: Marie and Sainton's disease.
- Precocious puberty ~ McCune Albright + Peutz Jerger's syndrome.
- H/P of multipe Myeloma is cartwheel/checker board pattern
- Jaw abnormality and associated disease

	Jaw abnormality	Disease
1	Underdeveloped maxilla ↓ Class III malocclusion	Cleidocranial dysplasia Craniofacial dysostosis Achondroplasia Down syndrome Ostiogenesis imperfect
2	Underdeveloped mandible ↓ Class II malocclusion	Treacher Collins syndrome Pierre Robin syndrome[Q]
3	Under developed maxilla + mandible	Hypopituitarism
4	Enlargement of maxilla	Monostotic fibrous dysplasia
5	Enlargement of mandible	Acromegaly
6	Enlargement of both maxilla + mandible	Pagets disease (Maxilla >>> Mandible)
7	Residual asymmetric deformity of mandible (due to cortical thickening)	Caffey's disease[Q]
8	Unusual prominence of Premaxilla	Thalassemia
9	Underdeveloped premaxilla	Congenital syphilis

- Laboratory finding Vs. disease

	Laboratory finding	Disease
1	↑sed serum alkaline phosphatase	Pagets Caffey's disease Hyperparathyroidism fibrous dysplasia
2	↓sed serum ALP	Scurvy Hypophosphatasia Hypothyroidism
3	↑sed ALP, sed LDH ↓sed G6PD, ↓Acid phosphatase	Odontogenic myxoma
4	↑sed serum acid phosphatase	Ostiopetrosis
5	↑sed phosphorylase enzyme	OI
6	(N) Serum Ca and phosphorus (N) ALP Trick: All normal	Cherubism

Note: (N) ALP seen in Multiple myeloma + cherubism

- Features vs Disease

	Features	Disease
1	Mosaic bone Jigsaw-Puzzle bone cotton wool bone Abnormal Persistence of Woven bone	Pagets/Osteitis deformans **Note:** Jig saw puzzle also seen in membranous type of Basal cell Adenoma by h/p
2	"Orange Peaud" or ground glass/orange peel appearance of bone with C-Shaped/Chinese character shaped trabeculae	Monostotic Fibrous dysplasia
3	Salt and pepper bone on X-ray	"Thalassemia" **Note:** On MRI these features will be seen in Sjogren's syndrome
4	Total disappearance of bone	Massive osteolysis/phantom vanishing bone/Gorham syndrome
5	Drill bone[Q]/Riders bone/Exercise bone (seen in young Athletes)	Traumatic myositis ossificans *(PGI 12)*
6	Brittle bone	OI
7	Wormian bones	Cleidocranial dysplasia[Q]
8	Coarse woven bone	Fibrous dysplasia

- 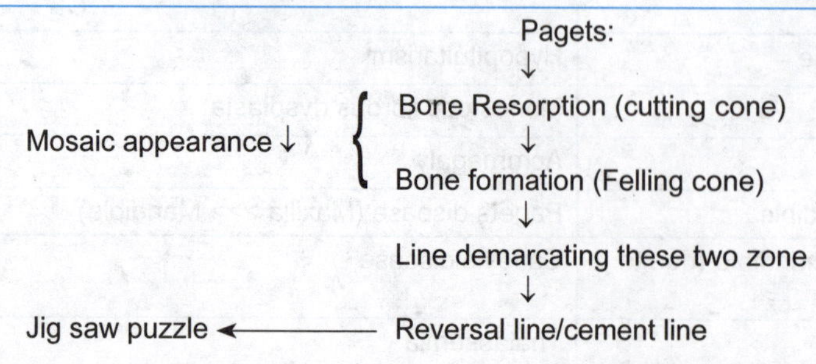

Apert syndrome:

1. Craniostenosis resulting in acrocephaly, brachycephaly, large late–closing fontanels,
2. Hypertelorism
3. Depressed nasal bridge
4. Parrot-beaked appearance
5. Poly dactyly, syndactyly with fusion of 2nd, 3rd, 4th digits (Mitten hands and Sock feet)
6. Prominent mandible
7. High arched palate
8. Bifid uvula
9. Cleft palate
10. Anterior crowding, malocclusion, delayed and ectopic eruption
11. Shovel-shaped incisor, supernumerary teeth

LAST 5-YEAR QUESTIONS FROM THIS TOPIC

1. Bilateral mandibular involvement is seen in: *(AIPG 12)*

Ans. Cherubism (Ref: Neville 3/e p629)

2. Which of the following is not part of Crest syndrome:

a. Syndactyly
b. Endocrinopathies
c. Calcinosis
d. Raynauds Phenomenon

Ans. b (Ref: Neville 3/e p801)

3. Multiple punched out lesions on seen in: *(AIIMS May 10)*

Ans. Multiple myeloma: (Ref: Shafer 5/e p259, 261, 262)

4. The human malformation which associated with anomaly with HOX gene is? *(AIIMS Nov 09)*

Ans. Poly syndactyly (Ref: Malcolm. Genotype 2nd p211)

5. Mosaic pattern of bone is seen in: *(AIPG 11)*

Ans. Osteitis deformans (Ref: Shafer's Textbook of Oral Pathology 5/e p1005)

6. Which of the following is seen with acromegaly?

a. Large tongue
b. Micrognathia
c. Crowding
d. Hypoglycemia

Ans. a (**Note:** Hyperglycemia is seen with acromegaly)

7. The disorder characterized by craniosynostosis, craniofacial anomalies, severe, symmetrical syndactyly (Cutaneus and bony fusion) of the hands and feet along with preaxial polysyndactyly and variable soft tissue syndactyly is: *(AIPG 11) [This is the complete questions]*

Ans. Carpenter syndrome (Ref: Nelson Textbook of Pediatrics, 16/e p1813)

8. Osteitis fibrosa is due to: *(AIPG 10)*

Ans. Hyperparathyroidism (Ref: Shafer 5/e p893)

9. Enamel hypoplasia is NOT seen in: *(AIIMS May 09)*

Ans. Cleidocranial dysostosis (Ref: Shafer 4/e p53)

10. A patient aged 50 years presented with history of jaw expansion and increased size of maxilla. The diagnosis is? *(PGI Dec 11)*

Ans. Paget's Disease (Ref: Shafer 5/e p1002)

11. HLA-B27 histocompatibility antigen is seen in:

Ans. Ankylosing spondilitis

12. A non-neoplastic hereditary bone lesion, histologically similar to central giant cell granuloma, affects the children and shows a bilateral involvement of the jaws with eye to heaven appearance clinically *(KCET 09)*

Ans. Cherubism

13. A histologic evidence of widespread formation of globular hypocalcified dentin and high pulp horns reaching the DEJ, absence of lamina dura around the teeth in radiograph are the characteristic features of: *(KCET 09)*

Ans. Vitamin D-resistant rickets

14. Still's disease is a form of: *(COMEDK 09)*

Ans. Rheumatoid arthritis

15. Reiter syndrome is a tetrad of:

Ans. Arthritis, bleeding, pyelonephritis, recurrent apthous ulcers.

16. Polyarthritis, urethritis, conjunctivitis is characteristically seen in:

Ans. Reiter's

17. Blue Sclera is a feature of: *(KCET 10)*

Ans. O I

Other syndromes are:

a. Turner's syndrome
b. Cherubism
c. Marfan's syndrome
d. Paget's disease

18. Patient with Down syndrome normally have:

Ans. Brachycephalic skull

19. Serum alkaline phosphatase levels is found to increase in: *(KCET 10)*

Ans. Paget is disease

20. A form of fibrous dysplasia occurring in children is termed as: *(KCET 11)*

Ans. Cherubism (Ref: Shafer's 5/e p979)

SKIN AND VESICULOBULLOUS LESION

- Ehlers Danlos – 'AD'[Q]
  Ectodermal dysplasia – X-recessive[Q]
  Pemphigus, pemphigoid, lichen planus – Auto immune
  Steven – Johnson syndrome
  \+
  Erythema multiform
  } Type III hypersensitivity reaction

- COUP de Sabre – Facial hemiatrophy + Scleroderma[Q] *(KCET 10)*

- Psoriasis: "Koebner's phenomena"
  ↓
  Generation of new lesion at the site of trauma
  ↓
  Suggesting a role of EXOGENOUS Stimuli[Q]

- Tzanck smear test →
  Pemphigus, HZ, HS
  ↓
  Tzank cell
  ↓
  Intra nuclear inclusion bodies
  ↓
  "Lipchutz body"

- Intra Epithelial bulla vs Sub Epithelial Bulla
  ↓
  1. Pemphigus (Only → other pemphigoid types have)
     ↓
     Subepithelial bulla
  2. Viral diseases HS
     HZ
     Chicken Pox

- Immunofluorescence test:

Disease		Type of Flourescence
1.	Pemphigus	"Granular" intercellular space fluorescence IgGand C_3 deposits on Inter cellular space ↓ Fish net appearance[Q]
2.	Lichen planes	Fluorescence along the basement membrane zone with extensions into lamina propria
3.	Pemphigoid Erythema multiformae	"Patchy Linear" pattern along the basement membrane[Q]
4.	Lupus Erythematosus	"Speckled"/ "Particulate" pattern at basement membrane

- White sponge nevus/Cannon's disease
  ↓
  'AD' trait[Q]

- Pseudo epitheliomatous Proliferation: Seen in granular cell myeloblastoma
  (AIIMS 04)
  Candidiasis, EpulisFissuratum, Median Rhomboid Glossitis (Posterior atropic candidiasis→ kissing lesion), Blastomycosis, Wegners Granulomatosis)

- Tuberous sclerosis[Q]:
  Epilepsy + mental deficiency + Angiofibroma

- Bloom's syndrome: (DNA repair Defect)
  Café – au – lait spot +Leukaemia + Rash

- Multiple pulp stones[Q]
  Ehler Danlos + Type II/coronal dentinal dysplasia

- Ehler's Danlos syndrome: Hypermobility of TMJ
  ↓
  Associated with repeated TMJ dislocation
  Loss of normal scalloping of DEJ

"Acanthosis Nigrican" = Dermatosis of Hypermigmentation of Tongue and lips (most commonly involved) + Obesity + insulin resistance + Pseudohorn cyst seen. *(AIPG 10)*

- Crohn → Recurrent aphtous ulcer
  + Cobble stone mucosal stratification
  + minor salivary gland duct pathology
  Ulcerative colitis → *Pyostomatitis Vegetans*
  ↓
  Hall mark of Crohn's disease

SLE causes fibrinoid thickening of glomerular capillaries
↓
Produced characteristic "Wire loop"
↓
Results in renal insufficiency

Cicatricial pemphigoid: (Bening mucous membrane pemphigoid)
Pathogenesis: IgG directed against antigens on
Epidermal side of salt–split skin
↓
It is BP 180/XVII[Q] collagen

Antigen present on Dermal side
↓
Epiligrin/laminin 5
c/f:
> ♂ :: 2: 1
Bleeding from gingiva
Ocular blindness ®So, also called (Ocular pemphigus)

- "Bullous pemhigoid":
  Most common "Sub epithelial blister"[Q]
  In contrast to Cicatricial pemphigoid, basement membrane remains attached to the connective tissue

- Oral lesion → for less than Cicatricial pemphigoid

- PUVA therapy used for:
  Pemphigus + Psoriasis
  Trick: ['P' for puva; 'P' for pemphigus + psoriasis]

- In psoriasis oral manifestation is rare

- Celiac sprue:
  Steatorrhea,
  Oral changes – Similar to pernicious anemia + Recurrent apthous ulcer

- Absent rete ridges:
  OKC + Primodial cyst

- Saw tooth appearance of rete pegs:

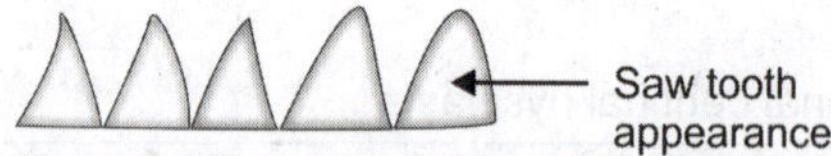

Fig. 8.17: Saw tooth appearance of rete pegs

  Seen in Lichen planus.

- In Darrier disease:
  Characteristic Corps, Rounds and Grains
  T/t → Vit. A (as caused due Vit. A deficiency)

- Epidermolysis bullosa occurs due to defect in structure of Type VII Collagen *(KCET 09)*

- Lichen Planus: *(PGI 12)*
  Skin lesion more common on "Flexural Surface" of Forearm; Inner aspect of Kneesand thighs. Severe pruritis is the 1° Symptom.
  F: M = 1.4: 1 / 3: 2

• Erythema multiformae: (Etiology) (EM) ↓ Minor ↓ HSV 1, HSV 2 ↓ Major ↓ Drugs (systemic)
• Toxic epidermal necrolysis: (Lyell's disease) Most severe form of EM ↓ Peeling of skin Almost always drug induced
• Nikolsky sign: 1. If lateral pressure is applied, bulla on gingiva peels off Or 2. If lateral pressure applied ↓ Bullae formed on normal appearing skin
• Non Erosive Arthritis: SLE + Reiter syndrome
• Penicillin is not associated with SLE / Lichenoid like reaction
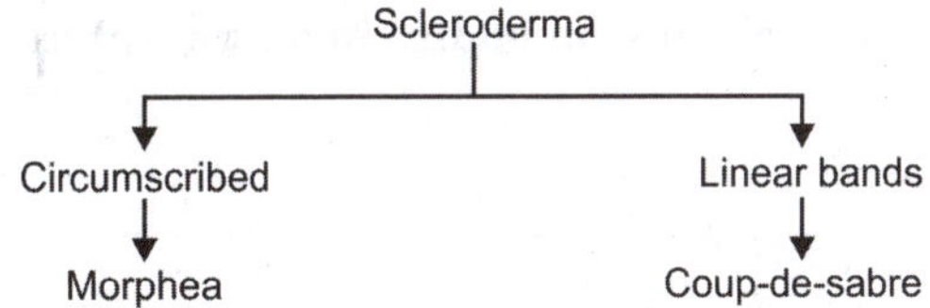 **Fig. 8.18:** Scleroderma
• Behcet's disease: Magic (**m**outh **a**nd **g**enital ulcer with **i**nflamed **c**artilage) Triad of Recurrent oral ulcer + recurrent genital ulcer + eye involvement (Hypopyon) **Note:** Behcet's syndrome should have at least 2 of the findings of Behcet's disease +ve Pathergy test seen in Behcet's disease.
• Recurrent apthous ulcer = Cancer sore
• Crohn's: Associated with Chelitis Granulomatosa Indurated polypoid tag like lesion seen in vestibule and Retro-molar pad.
• Melasma/Chloasma: Pigmentary change associated with pregnancy/OCP estrogen + Progesterone in combination induces the pigment (not alone)
• White lesion with defined precancerous potential: Leukoplakia, OSMF, DLE[Q], Hyperplastic candidiasis, Actinic Keratosis, Lichenoid reaction erosive lichen planes[Q]
• Erythema Multiformae: – Young patient – Crusted lip – Bleeding mucosal ulcer (+ Target lesion)
• Lichen planus is associated with severe pruritis
• Scleroderma = Hide bound disease

- 'DLE' rash:
  ↓
  Forceful removal of scale
  ↓
  Carpet track extension[Q]
  Peripheral growth
  ↓
  Periphery pink

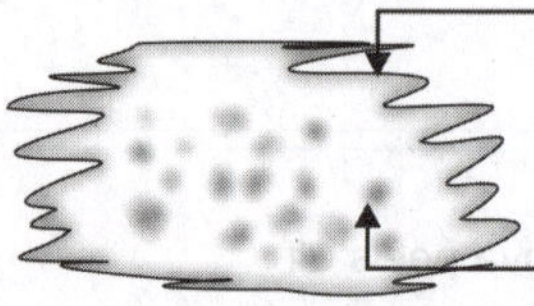

Fig. 8.19: DLE rash

Centre atrophic/Scarred

- "Cancer sore" = Recurrent apthous ulcer

LAST 5-YEAR QUESTIONS FROM THIS TOPIC

1. **Eosinophillic ovoid intranuclear inclusion bodies in herpes infection is called as:** *(KCET 12)*

Ans. Lipschutz bodies

2. **Acantholysis is pathogenic of:** *(KCET 09)*

Ans. Pemphigus

3. **Histological clefts in lichen planus are:** *(COMEDK 09)*

Ans. Max-Joseph spaces

4. **Scarring on healing of oral ulcers are seen in:** *(COMEDK 10), (AIPG 05)*

Ans. Recurrent aphthous ulcer

5. **Oral lesion associated with ulcerative colitis:**

Ans. Pyostomatitis vegetans (Ref: Shafer 5/e p1126)

6. **Autoantibodies are directed against type VII collagen seen in:** *(COMEDK 10)*

Ans. Epidermolysis bullosa acquisita (Ref: Autoantibodies by Yehuda Shoenfeld, 2/763)

7. **Multiple pulp stones are seen in:** *(COMEDK 10)*

Ans. Ehlers-Danlos syndrome

8. **Behcet's syndrome is characterized by:** *(KCET 10)*
   a. Recurrent oral aphthous and genital ulcers
   b. Eye and Skin lesions
   c. All of the above
   d. None of the above

Ans. c.

9. **Pin point haemorrhages on skin are known as:** *(KCET 10)*

Ans. Petichial

10. **Butterfly rash is typically seen in:** *(KCET 10)*

Ans. SLE

11. **A 40 year-old woman reposts with the complaint of burning sensation in the mouth clinical examination reveals lesions consisting of radiating white striations in a retiform arrangement affecting buccal mucosa, tongue, lips and gingiva bilaterally. An incisional biopsy is suggestive of Lichen planus.**

1. **The whitish striations in Lichen Planus are called:**

Ans. Wickham's striations (Ref: Shafer's 5/e p1103-1105)

2. **The following are different clinical forms of Lichen Planus, except:**

Ans. Verrucous Lichen Planus

3. **One of the following syndromes is associated with Lichen Planus:**

Ans. Grinspan's syndrome (Ref: Shafer's 5/e p1103-1105)

12. Case study: A 10 year-old female patient diagnosed as a case of Down's syndrome having: *(COMEDK 11)*

1. **A mosaicism variety which type of head shape is commonly seen:**

Ans. Brachycephaly

2. **Often IQ of the patient will be:**

Ans. 25-50

3. **Following dental problems are usually association with it, except:**
   a. Retarded eruption
   b. Late shedding of deciduous teeth
   c. Hypodontia
   d. Microdontia

Ans. b.

4. **The syndrome is usually associated with (a 10 year old female patient diagnosed as a case of Down's syndrome having a mosaicism variety)**

Ans. Congenital heart lesions

13. Coup-de Sabre is commonly associated with: *(KCET 11)*

Ans. Systemic Sclerosis (Ref: Shafer's 5/e p1146)

14. Hydropic degeneration of the basal cell of the stratum germinativum is a feature of ? *(PGI June 10, PGI Dec 11)*

Ans. Lichen planus (Ref: Shafer 6/e p802, 848)

15. Disuse atrophy of periodontium occurs in all, except: *(PGI Dec 10, 09)*

a. Erythema multiform
b. Lupus lrythematosus
c. Herpangina
d. Chicken pox

Ans. c.

16. Radiographic examination of a child revealed several missing primary and permanent teeth. No teeth had been extracted. The history indicated practically no perspiration during hot summer months. These factors would lead to a preliminary diagnosis of: *(AIIMS May 09)*

Ans. Ectodermal dysplasia (Ref: White and Pharaoh 5/e p333, 334, 646)

17. Degeneration of basement membrane and loss of rete pegs is seen in: *(AIPG 11)*

Ans. Lichen planes (Ref: Shafer, 6/e p802)

18. Ehlen's Danlos syndrome is: *(AIIMS Nov 10)*

Ans. AD (Ref: Shafer 5/e p1146)

19. Saw tooth rete pegs are seen in:

Ans. Lichen Planus

20. White radiating lines on the buccal mucosa are seen in: *(AIPG 09, 12)*

Ans. Lichen planus (Ref: Shafer 5/e p130, 1104, 1121)

21. All are present in Bechets syndrome, except: *(AIPG 12) P@ssword123*

a. Arthritis
b. Hepato-splenic involvement

c. Mucocutaneous involvement
d. Neuro-ocular involvement

Ans. b (Ref: Neville 3/e p290-291) *(AIPG 12)*

22. Which of the following is not part of Crest syndrome:

a. Syndactyly
b. Endocrinopathies
c. Calcinosis
d. Raynauds Phenomenon

Ans. b (Ref: Neville 3/e p801)

SALIVARY GLAND

- Sialodochitis → Dilatation of salivary duct due to Repeated inflammation/Infection secondary to epithelial atrophy. *(KCET 11)*

- Stimulated salivary flow rate (Lashley cup test)[Q]
  Normal → 5 ml/min (2-5 ml/min)
  Sjogren syndrome → < 0.5 ml/min [Comes near to unstimulated flow rate]
  Unstimulated flow rate of whole saliva
  ↓
  0.2 – 0.4 ml/min *(PGI 05)*

- Pleomorphic adenoma andAmeloblastoma
  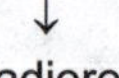
  Radioresistant[Q]

- Caries associated with Xerostomia affect gingival 1/3rd andincisal/cusp tips

  Seen 3 month after exposure of X-ray

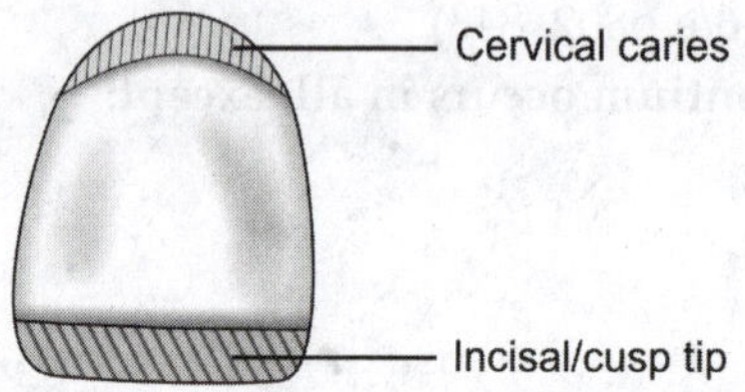

Fig. 8.20: Caries associated with xerostomia

- Sialosis/Sialadenosis:
  Non-inflammatory non-neoplastic asymptomatic enlargement due to Hormonal/Alcoholic/Malnutrition

- Parotid tumour → facial palsy
  Adenoid cystic Ca → multiple nerve lesion due to perineural involvement

- Chocolate colour fluid seen in space of Warthin's tumor[Q]

- Arthritis is an integral part of 2° Sjogren's syndrome

- Honey comb/Swiss cheese patter: Adenoid cystic Ca [other patterns are tubular and solid pattern which has 100% recurrence]

- Salivary gland Aplasia seen in LADD syndrome + Hemifacial microsomia + Trencher Choline
  L → Lacrimal
  A → Airicular
  D → Dental
  D → Digital

- Spindle cell carcinoma is a variant SCC[Q]

- In Xerostomia salivary pH ↓ses
  (↑sed bacteria → sed acid production ↑ced ↓pH)
- Sialolith → is cystaline in nature and made of Hydroxyapatite
- Tubular/Canallicular adenoma
  ↓
  Occurs maximally on upper lip
  ↓
  It is an adenoma of accessory salivary gland
- Most salivary gland tumour involves Female except Warthin (which is the disease of men)
- Most salivary gland tumour involves PAROTID and less of Minor salivary gland Except Necrotising S. Ialometaplasia
  ↓
  It involves Minor salivary gland on PALATE
  ↓
  Forms Crateriform ulcer
- Warthin tumour → 2nd Most common salivary gland tumour
- No accessory gland involvement
- Pleomorphic adenoma arises from Myoepithelial cells + Ductal cells
- Chemical mumps = Iodine mumps
  ↓
  It is an idiosyncrasy reaction

Concept: Parotid enlargement is more common in 1° Sjogren syndrome than 2° Sjogren syndrome where Rheumatoid Arthritis is an integral part.

- Mikulicz's disease = Benign lymphoepithelial lesion
  ↓
  B/L enlargement of lacrimal + Salivary gland[Q]
  H/P → shows epimyoepithelial islands.
  Sial orchitis → inflammatory enlargement of duct
- Atresia → congenital occlusion/absence of one/more major salivary gland
- Anti silagogues:
  Anticholinergic ~ Atropine
  Sympathomimetics
  Anti histamines
  Anti depressants
  Anti hypertensives
- Mumps = epidemic parotitis + orchitis/oophoritis + pancriatitis
- Jan Diego criteria for Sjogren's syndrome:

1°Sjogren	• Occular dryness → Schermer's test (< 8 mm writing) + but (Break up time) + Rose Bengal dye test
	• Dry mouth → Lashly cup test + Biopsy of minor salivary gland
	• Serological ↑sed R.F/anti SSA (Ro)/Anti SSB (La)/ANA

- 2° Sjogren→ 1° Sjogren + (RA/SLE/Polymyositis/Scleroderma/Biliary cirrhosis)
- Central mucoepidermoid carcinoma – seen mostly in Mandible in PM and M region
- Etiology of necrotising sialometaplasia: Local ischemia
  ↓
  Coagulative necrosis
- Pleomorphic Adenoma:
  One of the characteristic is the microscopic presentation of tumour outside the Incomplete Capsule. So, the recurrence of pleomorphic adenoma is due to Incomplete Capsule[Q]

• Adenoid cystic carcinoma = Cylindroma
• Spindle cell carcinoma: H/P → Proliferation + Dropping off basal cells to spindle cell
• Mumps is associated with Xerostomia
• Lymphoepithelioma → extremely malignant, metastasizes widely and causes early death
• Fatty change of parotid: associated with chronic liver cirrhosis, chronic alcoholism, malnutrition, ↑sed age, hormonal
• Malignant tumour of salivary gland ↓ Shows Late metastasis

LAST 5-YEAR QUESTONS FROM THIS TOPIC

1. **The most common site of sialolith is in:**

Ans. Submandibular duct (Ref: white and Pharaoh 5/e p603)

2. **The break up time test is performed to evaluate the function of:** *(KCET 11)*

Ans. Lacrimal gland

INFECTION

• **B**lastomycosis (Gilchrist disease) ↓ **D**oubly refractile capsule + Pseudoepithelial hyperplasia Trick = **BiDi** **Bi** = lastomycosis **Di** = **D**oubly refractile capsule **Note:** Features are similar to Actincmycosis
• Cryptococcus: Thick gelatinous capsule Tissue microcyst
• Mucormycosis: Diabetes mellitus + cellulitis + Thrombus[Q] Non-Septal hyphae with branching at obtuse angle/90°
• Aspergillosis: – Septate hyphae with Dichomatous branching at 45°[Q] – Respiratory infection – Fleeting Radio Opacity (R/o)
• Commonest Opportunistic infection in Aids cases World: Pneumocystic Carinii India: TB
• In Herpes 1° lesion is vesiclular In OLP (Oral Lichen Planus)lesion is Papular
• 1° Herpetic gingivostomatitis is subclinical infection mainly.
• Organism causing Acute Osteomyelitis (if nothing is mentioned) = Staphylococcus In jaw it is Streptococcus (because abunndant Normal flora of oral cavity)
• End arteritis obliterans is also seen in Lues Glossitis leading to Malignant transformation **Note:** endarteritis obliterans is also seen in Osteuradionecrosi
• Leprosy is not seen in Gingiva. It is common on lip, palate, tongue.

- TB: Pulmonary TB → BActerial smear of Sputum
  ↓
  Is Gold standard
  Lupus vulgaris → Biopsy[Q]

- Botromycosis:
  Is a bacterial infection[Q]
  Sulphur granules seen

- Jarish Heshaemer Reaction:
  Seen in lepra/Syphillis
  ↓
  Seen after vigorous antibiotic therapy
  ↓
  Etiology: Due to Release of Lytic products
  ↓
  Rx: Symptomatic (Antihistamines and NSAIDS)

- Schick's test, ELEK test used to detect Diptheria

- Syphillis:
  1. 1° stage → chancre seen
     ↓
     Painless [painful only when 2° infection seen]
     ↓
     Oral Chancre is most common site → lip[Q]
  2. 2° stage/ ®develops 6 weeks after 1° stage
     ↓
     Mucous patches
     Highly infectious
     Split papules
  (PGI 03, 05)
     Condyloma Latum
     ↓
     Painless
     ↓
     Serological test + ve Snail – Track
     ↓
     In immunocompromised patient LUES MALIGNA seen
  3. 3° stage → CNS + CVS involvement Gumma on *palate* and tongue
     └→More commonly
     Leutic glossitis More common them 1° and 2°[Q]
     Causes perforation of Palate[Q]
  4. Quateranary → late syphilis seen 1 to 2 decades after 1° syphilis
     ↓
     CVS sphillis (Aortic Aneurysm)
     +
     Neurosyphllis
  5. Congenital syphilis:

- Lupus vulgaris → 1° TB of skin[Q]
  Pottis disease → TB spine[Q] (Kyphosis)
  Scrofula → TB cervical andsubmaxillary lymph nodes[Q] *(AIIMS 09)*
  Miliary TB → blood borne TB

• Most common site: [Very Important] TB → tongue Hemangioma→ lip Necrotising sialometaplasia→ Palate BCC → upper lip Mucocels → lower lip Melanoma → Malar region Ectopic salivary gland tumour → Palate Peripheral giant cell granuloma → Gingiva
• Kviem – Slitzbach (KS test) ↓ Used for diagnosis of Sarcoidosis **Note:** syphillitic+ Trophic ulcer ⇓ Painless
• 2° TB most commonly seen on Tongue [Q]
• Location of Tongue disorder: 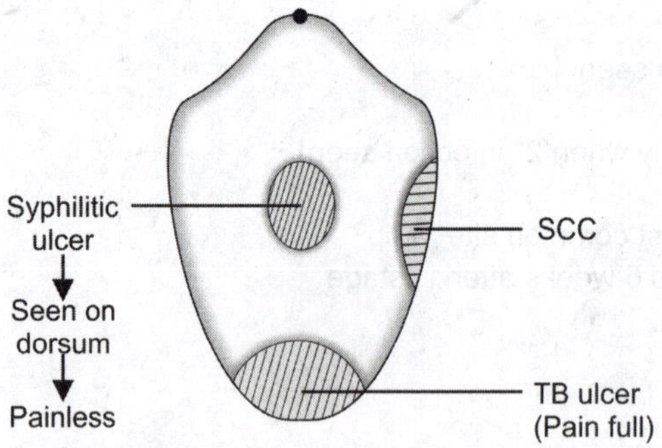 **Fig. 8.21:** Location of tongue disorder
• Oncogenic virus: EBV, HBC, HPV (POX virus) HCV, CMV (but less), HTLV, simian 40 HSV 1 and 2
• Fever blister = Cold sore → 1° HSV (Recurrent Herpes Labialis)
• VZ most commonly latent in Dorsal root ganglion of spinal chord. Other ganglions involved → Trigeminal nerve and geniculate ganglion
• Flask shaped ulcer seen in Amoebiasis
• Congenital syphilis → Early manifestation similar to severe 2° Syphillis (Lymphadenopathy + hepatosplenomegaly + highly infections condyloma lata) **Note:** ÷ Condylomalata are enlarged papules seen in moist area
• "Canker sore" – Recurrent apthous ulcer
Rubeolla OR Measles + Mumps → caused by PARAMYXO Virus Rubella caused by TOGA virus Trick: **MMR** viruses **M**easles + **M**umps = Paramyxo virus **R**ubella = Toga
• Lip Schutz bodies seen in Herpes simplex
• HS and HZ Intranuclear inclusion bodies seen in both

- Botromycosis:
  Caused by S. aureus
  Chronic granulomatous infection like Blastomy Cosis
- Cryptococcus Neoformans→ "Melanin production"
- Oral finding in Infectious Mononucleosis gingivitis and stomatitis
- HSV binds to epithelium using Heparan sulphate
- Salivary Peroxidase system → Active against Lactobacillus.
- Cat scratch disease:/Perinaud's oculoglandular syndrome
  Caused by Bartonella Henselae
  Carrier → Cat bite

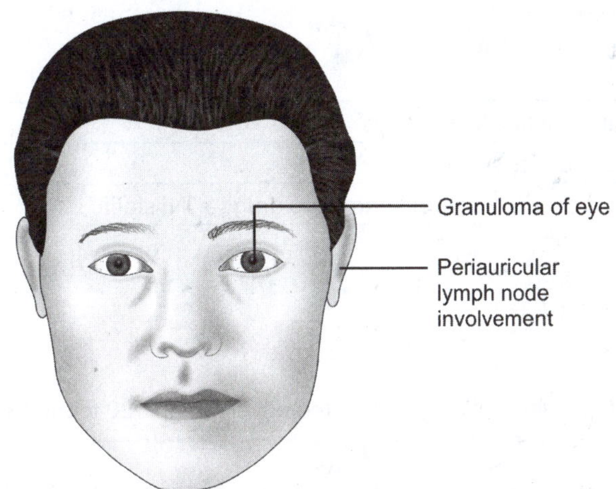

Fig. 8.22: Cat scratch disease

- Organism detected by "Warthin Starry Ag stain"
- In late syphilis → External Rectus muscle paralysis leads to Strabismus due to paralysis of 6th CN [LR6]
- Epulis Fissuratum/Inflammatory fibrous hyperplasia/Denture injury TUMOR: more common on MANDIBULAR anterior region.

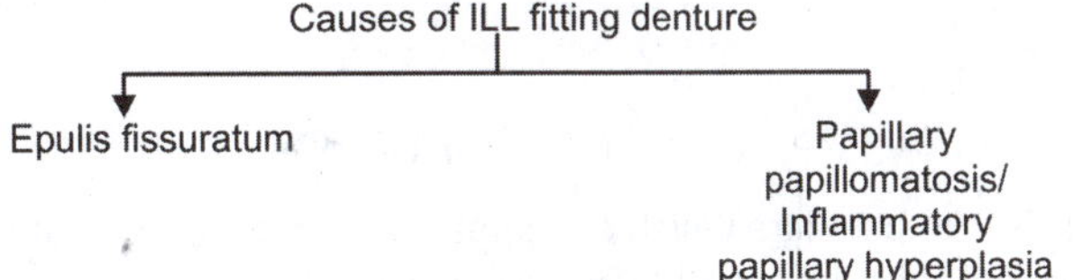

Fig. 8.23: Epulis fissuratum

- Koilocyte: HPV altered epithelial cells with nuclear Pyknosis and perinuclear space.
- Mumps → Pancreatitis ®sed serum lipase
- S.mutans converts Glucose →Glucans (Dextran is more important)
  and
  Fructose → Fructans (Levans)
  Glucan is insoluble and causes adherence of S. mutans. So, more important
  Levan → highly soluble
- Infectious mononucleosis: Kissing Disease/Glandular fever pin point petechial on plate[Q] + acute gingivitis and stomatitis + ulcers which bruise easily[Q]

- Dengu: Incubation period → 2 – 7 days
  Note → Measles this period is 1-2 weeks for others it is 2-3 weeks
  Diagnosis → confirmed by 4 fold rise in Ig G titer
- Candidiasis: Gram + ve fungi
  Acute → pseudo membranous Thrush[Q]
  Acute atrophic → Antibiotic stomatitis[Q] Painful
  Cronic hyperplastic → Leukoplakic type of candidiasis
  Premalignent condition
  Chronic atrophic → Denture stomatitis/sore mouth
- Angular Chelitis: is Chronic B/L ulcer at corner of mouth due to:
  1. Chronic atrophic candidiasis
  2. Riboflavin deficiency
  3. Iron Deficiency anaemia (IDA)
  4. Folate deficiency
- Oral thrush → seen in infants 6 to 10th days[Q]
- Penicillin is Drug of choice for syphillis
- Candidiasis → Drug of choice "Azoles" Alternative drug → "Nystatin"
- HIV: 1st reported case 1981
  – Virus detected in 1983 *(AIIMS Nov. 12)*
  – 2 main TARGET of HIV →
    1. Immune system
    2. CNS
  – The 1st step in virus infection is binding of the envelope gp 120 to the CD_4 surface protein of T-helper cell[Q]

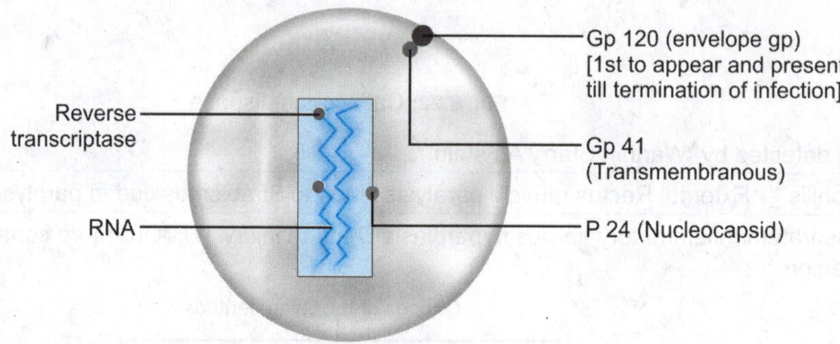

Fig. 8.24: HIV

  – Viral load parallels with p 24 titre which disappears after appearance of IgM
  – Most common Neoplastic disease of Aids – Kaposi sarcoma
  – Most rapidly sing malignancy of Aids: Non-Hodgnin's lymphoma
- Measles: Warthin – Frinkeldey giant cells pathognomic H/P feature
- Ramsay Hunt syndrome:
  Chicken pox → 1° infection by VZ
  ↓ 2° infection

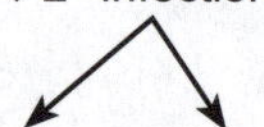

  HZ (Shingles) Ramsay Hunt syndrome
- Herepes Gladiataram: Seen in wrestlers special form of Hz
- Herpangina → Apthous pharyngitis Posterior part of oral cavity involved seen in children causative organism:
  COX A → Herpangina[Q]
  COX A10 → Acute lymphonodular pharyngitis *(KCET 06)*
  COX A16 → Hand – foot mouth disease

• TB → 1° Oral TB seldom occurs most common site → Tongue
• Leproma → Oral lesion of leprosy. Seen on Tongue/lip/hard palate
• Tetanus: Risus Sarcodinus (Lock jaw due to rigidity of Masseter) + opisthotonus (rigidity of back muscle resulting in arched back)
• Congenital/prental syphilis: Both Higomi Naski sign (irregular thickening of Sternoclavicular portion of clavidi) + Rhagades (Fissures radiating from lips) are seen: 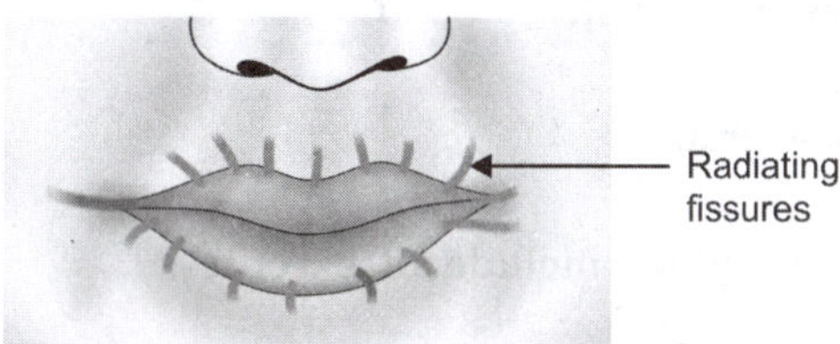 **Fig. 8.25:** Congenital/prental syphilis
• Perleche is called angular chelitis
• Id rk^n is associated with Candidiasis
• Rubella → Teratogenic Rubeolla is not teratogenic
• HSV is not epidemic **Note:** epidemic viral diseases are: ↓ Hand foot and mouth + Herpangina ↓ Caused by Cokasaki virus
• Tzank smear is nothing but Giemsa stain → for pemphigus, HZ, HS
• Histoplasmiosis = Darling disease[Q] South American Blastomycosis = Lutz's disease [**Note:** Lues = Syphillis][Q] North American Blastomycosis = Gilchrist[Q] Coccydomycosis = Valley fever Candidiasis = Monialiasis
• Types of Phycomycosis ↓ ↓ Mucormycosis Zygomycosis

LAST 5-YEAR'S QUESTIONS FROM THIS TOPIC

1. **Focal Epithelial hyperplasia caused by HPV 13 and 32 are also termed as:** *(COMEDK 12)*

Ans. Hecks disease

2. **A 20 year male complains of recurrent attacks of sore throat since 2 years the total leucocyte count was 1000/ul. A differential count revealed severe neutropenia. The diagnosis is:** *(COMEDK 12)*

Ans. Agranulocytosis.

3. **Otomycosis is caused by:** *(COMEDK 12)*

Ans. Aspergillus niger

4. **General paresis in Neurosyphilis is a feature of:** *(KCET 12)*

Ans. 3° stage of syphilis

5. **Papulovesicular oral lesions are seen in:** *(KCET 12)*

Ans. Herpangina

6. **Saint Antony's fire is a description given for:** *(KCET 12)*

Ans. Erysipela's

7. **Actinomycosis is a:** *(KCET 12)*

Ans. Anaerobic bacterial disease

8. **Mumps is caused by which of the following viruses?**

Ans. Paramyxo virus

9. **Higoumenaki's sign is seen in which of the following disease?**

Ans. Syphilis

10. **Kissing Lesion" is representative of:**

Ans. Candidiasis

11. **The cell wall deficient bacteria:** *(KCET 09)*

Ans. Mycoplasma

12. **Oral lesions of secondary syphilis include all, except:** *(KCET 09)*
    a. Snail track ulcers
    b. Mucous patches
    c. Chancre of tongue
    d. Hutchinson's wart

Ans. c.

13. **Sulpher granules is a characteristic feature of:** *(COMEDK 10)*

Ans. Actinomycosis

14. **The virus which causes HZ is same as that which causes:** *(COMEDK 10)*

Ans. Chickenpox

15. **Which of the following infections can produce unilateral facial pain:** *(COMEDK 09)*

Ans. HZ

16. **Which type of candidiasis is associated with leukoplakia:** *(COMEDK 09)*

Ans. Chronic hyperplastic candidiasis

17. **Ramsay Hunt syndrome is a feature of:** *(KCET 10)*

Ans. Herpes Zoster

18. **Following are the characteristics of vincent's angina, except:**
    a. Ulcerative gingivostomatitis
    b. Caused due to malnutrition
    c. A symbiotic infection
    d. Caused by Leptospira interrogans

Ans. d.

19. **Agglutination test for the diagnosis of infectious mononucleosis:**

Ans. Paul Bunnel test

20. **Botryomycosis is a _______ disease:**

Ans. Bacterial

21. **The first sign of tetanus is:** *(KCET 10)*

Ans. Trismus

22. **Lupus vulgaris is:** *(KCET 10)*

Ans. Tuberculous lesion (Skin) on face

23. **Which of the following is a Virus induced epithelial hyperplasia:** *(KCET 10)*
    a. Molluscum contagiosum
    b. Focal epithelial hyperplasia
    c. Squamous papilloma
    d. All of the above

Ans. d. All of the above

24. Herpetic whitlow is seen in: *(KCET 10)*

Ans. Fingers

25. Snail track ulcer are seen in: *(KCET 10)*

Ans. 2° syphilis

26. Following are the characteristics of Cryptococcus neoformans, except: *(KCET 10)*

a. Non capsulated fungus infecting man
b. Causes meningitis
c. Melanin production related to virulence
d. Basidiomycetes yeast

Ans. a.

27. Dentine sore mouth is a _______ type of candidiasis: *(KCET 10)*

Ans. Chronic atrophic

28. Case study: A 55-year-old female patient with denture wearer reported to the dentist. Her chief complaint was pain in the denture-bearing area. On examination, revealed inflammation of the denture, bearing area, erythematous in nature more diffuse involving entire denture bearing area.

1. **What is this clinical called.**

Ans. Denture stomatitis

2. **Among the different types of denture stomatitis diagnosis of candida - associated denture stomatitis is confirmed by:** *(COMEDK 11)*

Ans. By finding myclellia/pseudohyphae in a direct smear/isolation of candida in high numbers

3. **One of the systemic factors predisposing to candida-associated denture stomatitis is:**

Ans. Nutritional deficiencies

4. **In the management of candida-denture stomatitis the following is used:**

Ans. Local therapy with nystatin/AMB

29. General paresis is Neurosyphilis is a feature of: *(KCET 11)*

Ans. Tertiary stage of syphilis (Ref: Shafer's 5/e p452)

30. Warthin – Finkeldey multinucleated giant cell is diagnostic of: *(COMEDK 11)*

Ans. Measles

31. Pathogenesis of diphtheria is attributed to: *(COMEDK 11)*

Ans. Exotoxin (Ref: Anantanarayan 6/e p215)

32. Kissing disease is also known as: *(KCET 11, 12)*

Ans. Glandular fever (Ref: Shafer's 5/e p1065)

33. Shingles is caused by: *(KCET 11, 12)*

Ans. Varicella Zoster (Ref: Shafer's 5/e p480)

34. The causative agent for occuloglandular syndrome of Parinaud is: *(KCET 11)*

Ans. Bartonella hensilae (Ref: Shafer's 5/ep468)

35. Herpes simplex virus binds to epithelium using: *(KCET 11)*

Ans. Heparan sulphate

36. Small round superficial erosions in the mouth which coalesce to form the so-called snail track ulcers are seen in: *(KCET 11)*

Ans. Secondary syphilis (Ref: S. Das 4/e p586)

37. Koplik's spots are commonly seen in: *(KCET 11)*

Ans. Measles (Ref: Shafer's 5/e p476)

38. Acute infection of bacteria which affects the nervous system: *(KCET 11)*

Ans. Tetanus (Ref: Shafer's 5/e p449)

39. True about syphilis is: *(PGI Dec. 09)*

Ans. Oral lesions are seen at any stage (Ref: Oral and Maxillofacial pathology by Robert Marx and Diane stern/ Pg 72-76)

40. Acute pseudomembranous candidiasis is, all except? *(PGI June 09)*

a. Known as oral thrush
b. Mot commonly over in immunocompromised patients
c. May be associated with denture stomatitis
d. None

Ans. c. Ref: Shafers 5/e p743

41. The incubation period of measles is: *(PGI June 09)*

Ans. 7-14 days (Ref: Shafer's 4/e p476)

42. Feature that distinguishes Herpes Zoster from other vesiculobullous eruptions is: *(PGI June 10)*

Ans. Unilateral occurrence (Ref: Shafer 6/e p345)

43. Group of lymph nodes involved maximally in tubercular lymphadenitis is: *(PGI Dec. 10)*

Ans. Cervical

44. Koplik spots are seen in? *(PGI Dec 11)*

Ans. Measles (Ref: Shafer 5/e p476)

45. Hand foot and mouth disease caused by: *(PGI June 11)*

Ans. Coxsackie A16 (Ref: Shafer's oral pathology 5/e)

46. True about syphilis is? *(PGI Dec 11)*

a. Oral lesion are seen at any STAGE
b. Clinical manifestations occurs after few months of exposure
c. VDRL test is positive in early stages of 1° syphilis
d. Penicillinase is ineffective

Ans. a.

47. A 7 year-old child presents with generalized ulceration of mouth, malaise and fever. Treatment is: *(AIPG 11)*

Ans. Gently debride the ulcers and symptomatic treatment only (Ref: Burkitt 11th p46)

48. The lesion which is erythematous and shows recurrent vesicles that are distributed along the sensory nerve trunk is: *(AIIMS May 10)*

Ans. Herpes zoster (Ref: Shafer 5/ep481)

49. In HIV infection, the blood cells that are infected the most are: *(AIPG 10)*

Ans. CD4

50. Viral load detection is done through: *(AIPG 10)*

Ans. RT-PCR (Ref: Shafer 5/e p495)

51. Herpangina is caused by: *(AIPG 11)*

Ans. Coxsacke's Virus (Ref: Shafer 4/e p181, 191, 5/e p276)

52. Hutchinson's triad is? *(AIPG 10)*

Ans. Interstitial keratitis, mulberry molars, 8th nerve deafness

53. The lesion which is erythematous and shows recurrent vesicle that are distributed along the sensory nerve trunk is: *(AIIMS May 10)*

Ans. Herpes zoster (Ref: Shafer 5/e p481)

54. Infections mononucleosis is caused by: *(AIIMS May 10)*

Ans. EBV (Ref: Shafer 5/e p1065, 1068)

55. Incubation period of herpes zoster is: *(AIPG 12)*

Ans. 7-14 days (Ref: Pediatrics: A concise Text)

56. What is the cell count of CD_4 cells in HIV below which it is considered as full blown HIV: *(PGI June 11)*

Ans. 200 Ref: Shafer's 5/ep490)

57. Which of the following is not a feature of Hutchinson's triad? *(KCET 11)*

a. Facial nerve paralysis
b. Mulberry molars
c. Ocular interstitial keratitis
d. Vestibulocochlear nerve paralysis

Ans. a.

ORAL AND METABOLIC DISEASES

• Hypophosphotasia: ↓sed ALP[Q] ↓ Defective Bone mineralisation + No cementogenesis ↓ Premature loss of dentition Characterised by sed excretion of phosphorethanolamine in urine
• Delayed eruption of teeth: Rickets (Hypovitaminosis D) Hypothyroidism Hypoparathyroidism Trick = ALL "Hypo" conditions
• Hyper Parat Hyroidism → No effect on teeth only effects Bone
• Enamel Hypoplasia[Q] Seen in Rickets (Both adult and child type) + Hypoparathyroidism Pulp horn reaching DEJ
• Lamina dura Lost in: Pagets + Fibrous dysplasia (FD) + Vit. D resistant rickets + Hyperparathyroidism + Osteoporosis + Osteomalacia Trick = All important and common bone disorders you know Thickening of lamina dura – TFO, Osteopetrosis
• Cu deficiency causes → Wilson/Hepatolenticular degeneration OR Menke Syndrome (Steelykinky hair syndrome)
• Cu required for normal Erythropdesis and Fe absorption Cu deficiency ↓ Fe deficiency anaemia ↓ Microcytic hypochromic anaemia
• Vit. C is not produced/stored by body.
• Café – au – lait spot seen in: – NeurofibromatosisQ – Mc Cune Albright syndromeQ – Blooms syndromeQ

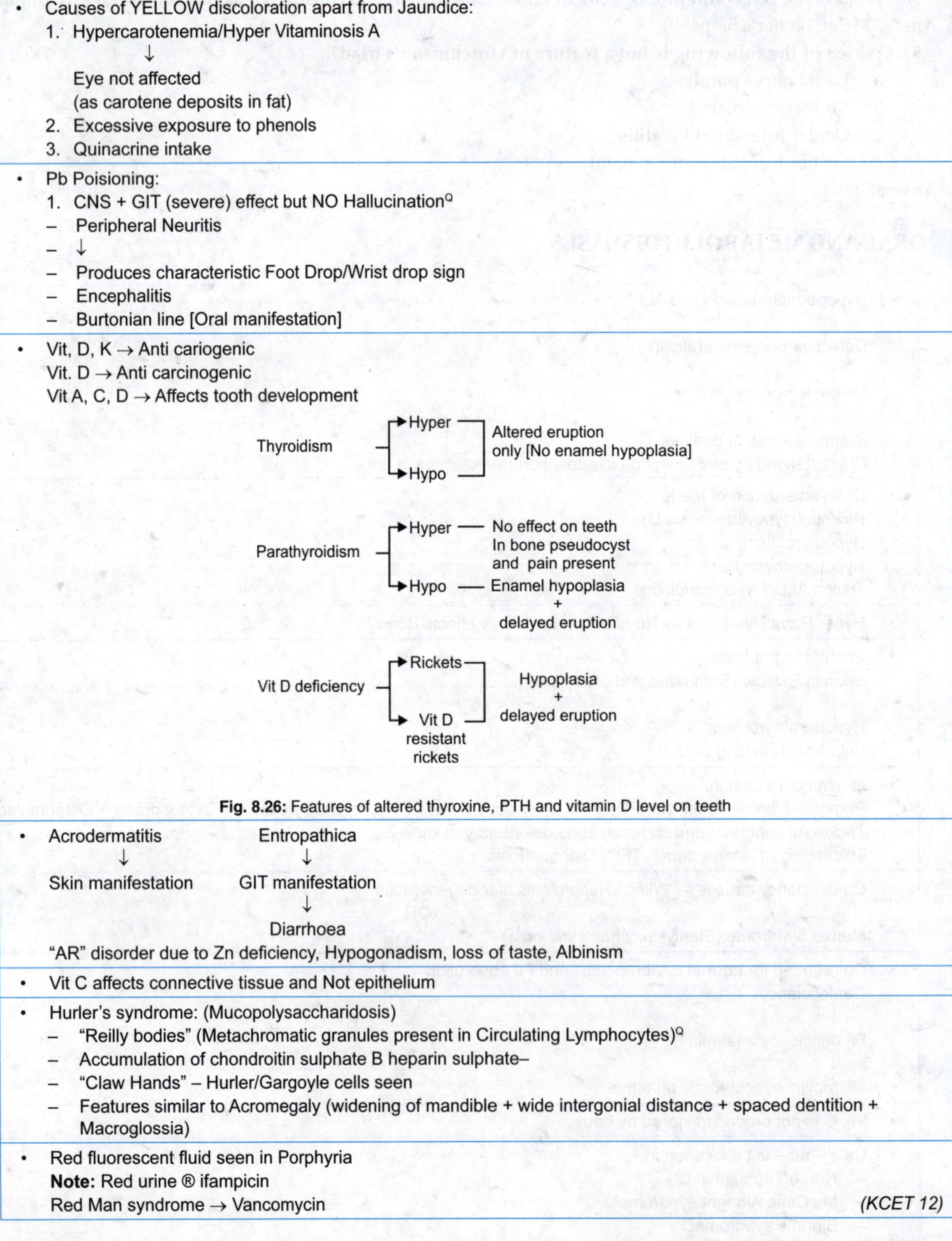

- Causes of YELLOW discoloration apart from Jaundice:
  1. Hypercarotenemia/Hyper Vitaminosis A
     ↓
     Eye not affected
     (as carotene deposits in fat)
  2. Excessive exposure to phenols
  3. Quinacrine intake

- Pb Poisioning:
  1. CNS + GIT (severe) effect but NO Hallucination[Q]
  – Peripheral Neuritis
  – ↓
  – Produces characteristic Foot Drop/Wrist drop sign
  – Encephalitis
  – Burtonian line [Oral manifestation]

- Vit, D, K → Anti cariogenic
  Vit. D → Anti carcinogenic
  Vit A, C, D → Affects tooth development

Fig. 8.26: Features of altered thyroxine, PTH and vitamin D level on teeth

- Acrodermatitis Entropathica
  Acrodermatitis ↓ Skin manifestation
  Entropathica ↓ GIT manifestation ↓ Diarrhoea
  "AR" disorder due to Zn deficiency, Hypogonadism, loss of taste, Albinism

- Vit C affects connective tissue and Not epithelium

- Hurler's syndrome: (Mucopolysaccharidosis)
  – "Reilly bodies" (Metachromatic granules present in Circulating Lymphocytes)[Q]
  – Accumulation of chondroitin sulphate B heparin sulphate–
  – "Claw Hands" – Hurler/Gargoyle cells seen
  – Features similar to Acromegaly (widening of mandible + wide intergonial distance + spaced dentition + Macroglossia)

- Red fluorescent fluid seen in Porphyria
  Note: Red urine ® ifampicin
  Red Man syndrome → Vancomycin *(KCET 12)*

• Amylodidosis: – 1° Amyloidosis/ → Multiple myeloma Type B/AL amyloid – 2° Amyloidosis/ →Chronic infection (Osteomyelitis, TB, syphillis) AA type Non infectious chronic infection (RA + malignancy [R.C.C; Hodgkin's lymphoma]) Type "C" →Ageing/pheochromocytoma
• C/f of Acrodynia: (seen in children) – Severe sweating (constant finding) – Skin peels off frequently – Patchy hair loss
• Hg Toxicity: – GIT + CNS – Oral: Ptyalism Also seen with Vit C deficiency ← [Destruction of alveolar bone (loosening of teeth)
• Melasma/Chloasma: Pigmentary change associated with pregnancy/Oral contraceptive pills (OCP), Estrogen + Progesterone in combination induces the pigmentation (Not alone)
• Vit D resistant resistant ricket Vs Ectodermal dysplasia – Pulp horn reaching DEJ – Lack of Normal scalloping of DEJ – ↑sed interglobular dentine – dentinal tubules reaching Enamel
• 1° Nutritional deficiency is due to failure of ingestion Conditioned nutritional deficiency is due to lack of Absorption: 2° Hyperparathyroidism → Brown Tumor[Q] ↓ Most commonly 2° to Renal failure ↓ ↓ced Vit D synthesis ↓ ↓ced Ca absorption from get ↓ ↑sed PTH secretion
• Vit A deficiency: earliest sign is loss of sensation to green light > dim light >Nyctalopia[Q] Xeropthalmia > Keratomalacia ↓ Abnormal dryness and thickening of cornea and conjunctiva
• Glycogen storage disorder: Von Gierke's → Glucose – 6- phosphatase (type I) deficient Pompe's disease → lysosomal glucosidase (type II) deficient Gaucher's disease → Glucocerebrosidase deficient ↓ Glucocerebroside stored Nieman pick disease → sphengomyelin

LAST 5-YEAR'S QUESTIONS FROM THIS TOPIC

1. **Which one of the following features is NOT associated with 1° hyperparathyroidism?** *(KCET 09)*
   a. Giant cell tumour
   b. Sharply defined radiolucencies of maxilla and mandible
   c. Partial loss of lamina dura
   d. Hypercementosis

Ans. d.

2. **Sicca complex is associated with:** *(KCET 10)*

Ans. 1° Sjogren's syndrome

3. **Oral ulceration resembling apthae are encountered in:** *(COMEDK 11)*

Ans. Gluten enteropathy

4. **Sarcoidosis is:** *(COMEDK 11)*

Ans. Less common in smokers + seen in temperate climate

5. **Kveimsiltzbach test is useful in the diagnosis of:** *(COMEDK 11)*

Ans. Sarcoidosis (Ref: Shafer's 5/e p924)

6. **Kevin test is done for:** *(KCET 11)*

Ans. Sarcoidosis (Ref: Shafer's 5/e p924)

7. **False regarding hypophosphatasia:**
   a. Loss of cementum
   b. Precocious exfoliation of primary teeth
   c. Craniostenosis stenosis
   d. Increased level of alkaline phosphatase

Ans. d Ref: Shafer's 6/e p639

8. **Hyperthyroidism in children is not associated with:** *(PGI June 10)*
   a. Periodontal destruction
   b. Precocious eruption of teeth
   c. Mandibular retrognathism
   d. Osteoporosis

Ans. c (Ref: Shafer 5/e p898)

9. **A disease which only affects the formation and eruption of tooth but does not cause hypoplasia is:** *(PGI June 10)*

Ans. Hyperthyroidism (Ref: Shafer's 6/e p81, 650)

10. **Enlarged tongue is associated with:** *(PGI Dec 10)*

Ans. Amyloidosis (Ref: Shafer's 6/e p649)

11. **A 2 and a half year old child with horizontal bone loss but cementum appears normal. What is the disease?** *(PGI June 11)*

Ans. Hypophosphatasia (Ref: Carranza 10/e p407)

12. **Increase in the height of the mandible and appearance of interdental spaces in an elderly man are due to:** *(AIIMS Nov. 11, 09)*

Ans. Hyperpituitarism (Ref: Becker. Principles and Practice of Endocrinology and Metabolism 3rd p1984)

13. **Alder-Reilly bodies are present in:** *(AIPG 10)*

Ans. **Lymphocytes**
[**Note:** Alder-Reilly bodies are also seen in monocytes, neutrophils]

14. **Osteitisfebrosa is due to:** *(AIPG 10)*

Ans. Hyperparathyroidism (Ref: Shafer 5/e p893)

15. **Which of the following is seen with acromegaly?**
   a. Large tongue
   b. Micrognathia
   c. Crowding

d. Hypoglycimia

Ans. a (**Note:** Hyperglycemia is seen with acromegaly)

16. A 9 year-old child has increased horizontal anterior bone loss, less cementum and on test shows excretion of phosphor ethanol amine in the urine. The child is suffering from: *(AIIMS Nov. 10)*

Ans. Hypophosphatasia (Ref: Shafer 4/e p645)

17. Hyperbilirubinemia associated tooth discoloration is called:

Ans. Chlordontia (Ref: Neville 3/e p71, 72) *(AIPG 12)*

CYST AND TUMOR

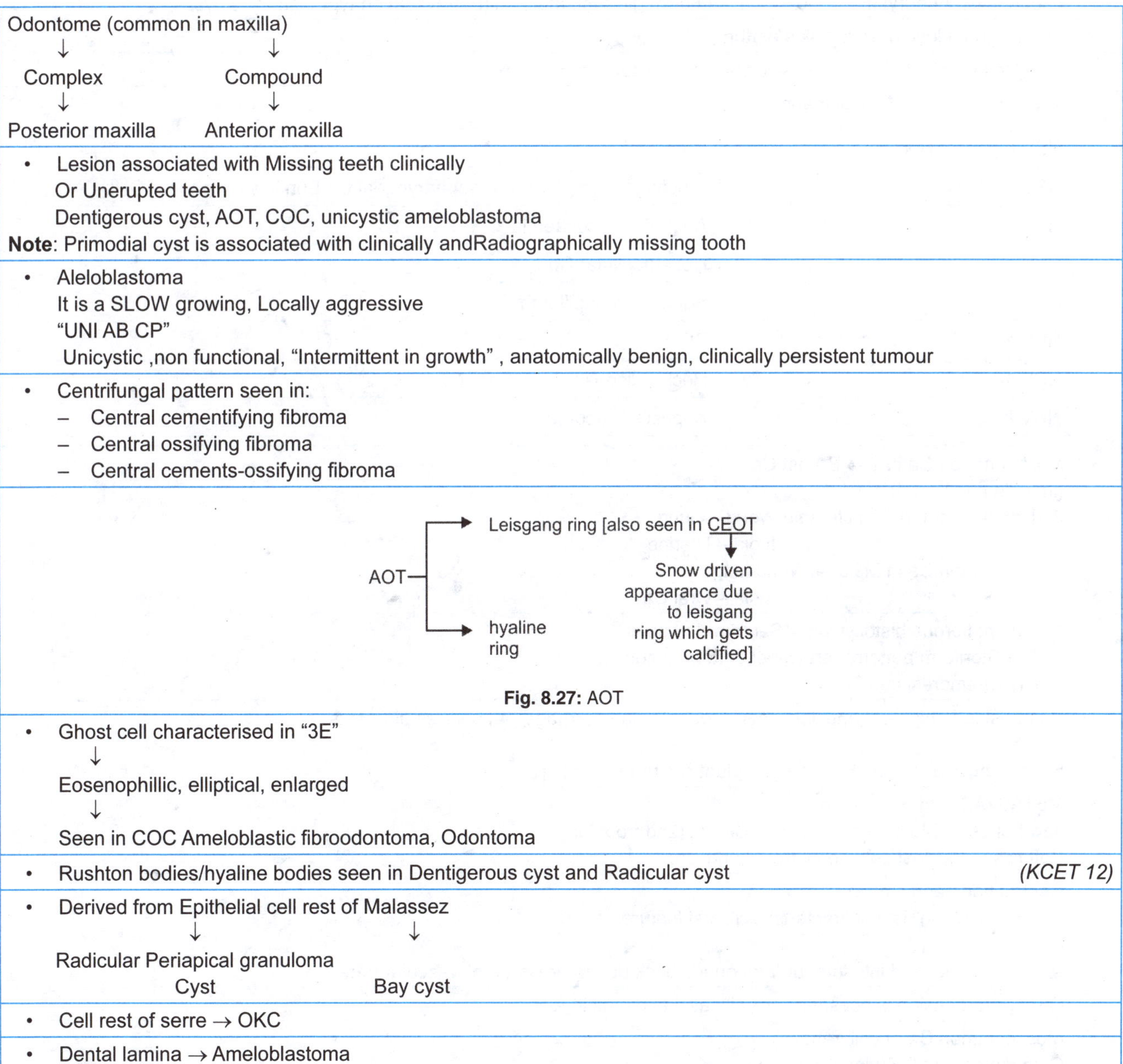

Odontome (common in maxilla)
↓ Complex → ↓ Posterior maxilla
↓ Compound → ↓ Anterior maxilla

- Lesion associated with Missing teeth clinically
  Or Unerupted teeth
  Dentigerous cyst, AOT, COC, unicystic ameloblastoma

Note: Primodial cyst is associated with clinically andRadiographically missing tooth

- Aleloblastoma
  It is a SLOW growing, Locally aggressive
  "UNI AB CP"
  Unicystic ,non functional, "Intermittent in growth" , anatomically benign, clinically persistent tumour

- Centrifungal pattern seen in:
  - Central cementifying fibroma
  - Central ossifying fibroma
  - Central cements-ossifying fibroma

Fig. 8.27: AOT

- Ghost cell characterised in "3E"
  ↓
  Eosenophillic, elliptical, enlarged
  ↓
  Seen in COC Ameloblastic fibroodontoma, Odontoma

- Rushton bodies/hyaline bodies seen in Dentigerous cyst and Radicular cyst *(KCET 12)*

- Derived from Epithelial cell rest of Malassez
  ↓ Radicular Cyst
  ↓ Periapical granuloma Bay cyst

- Cell rest of serre → OKC

- Dental lamina → Ameloblastoma

- Stratum Intermedium
  ↓
  CEOT
- Ree → Dentigerous cyst + Eruption cyst
- Hemorrhagic bone cyst/solitary bone cyst/simple bone cyst/idiopathic bone cavity/traumatic bone cyst: R/t → scalloping r/l between roots of teeth
- Stafne cyst/static bone cavity/lingual mandibular bone cavity
- OKC: P-keratinized form more invasive and shows more recurrence than O-Keratinized (this form **not** associated with Basal cell nevus syndrome)
  Picket fence/tomb stone appearance of Basal layer[Q]
- Pseudocyst: Aneurysmal bone cyst, Haemorrhagic cyst, mucocel(Extravasation type), stafne's cyst
- Premalignant lesion:leukoplakia/erythroplakia
- Satellite lesion with locally invasive character is seen in Haemangioma
- Virus associated with malignancy:

HSV II/genital Herpes	Ca cervix
HSV – IV/EBV	African jaw lymphoma Nasopharyngeal Ca Burkitt's lymphoma OHL
HTLV	Adult T-cell leukaemia
HBV	Hepatocellular Ca
HPV 6, 11	Squamous papilloma
HPV 16	SCC
HPV 13, 32	Heck's disease
HHV 8	Kaposi's Sarcoma

- Most common Ca in ♀ → Breast Ca
  (in India and World)
  2nd most common Ca in female World → lung
  India – Uterine
  Most common Ca in Male → World-lung
  India – Oral Ca
- Malignant fibrous histocytoma: "Sarcoma" of adult
  H/P → Storiform pattern/Cart wheel pattern of spindle cells[Q]
  Highly Chemoresistant[Q]
- Haemosiderin pigment (multiple capillaries with haemorrhage → liberates pigments)
  ↓
  Seen in **both** Peripheral and central giant cell granuloma
- METASTASIS to oral region:
  Jaw bones → Most commonly from Breast (2nd from lung)
  Soft tissue → Most commonly from Lung Ca.
- Central haemangicma:
  "Pumping action" is a characteristic clinical feature
  ↓
  When tooth pushed into tumour it rebounds back due to pressure of Vascular network.
- OKC → Expansion is not seen clinically as it expands in A-P
- Most common Ca of children:
- Osteosarcoma >3 Euring's sarcoma
- Phlebolith seen in cavernous Haemangioma

- CLEAR cells seen in:
  ↓ Clear cell Ca
  ↓ Chondro-sarcoma
  ↓ Muco-epidermoid Ca
- OHL also called Greenspan Lesion
- BCC also called benign carcinoma
- Lymphangioma[Q]
  ⇓
  Macroglossia + Papillomatosis
- Malignant melanoma:
  Xeroderma Pigmentosum associated with Malignant Melanoma

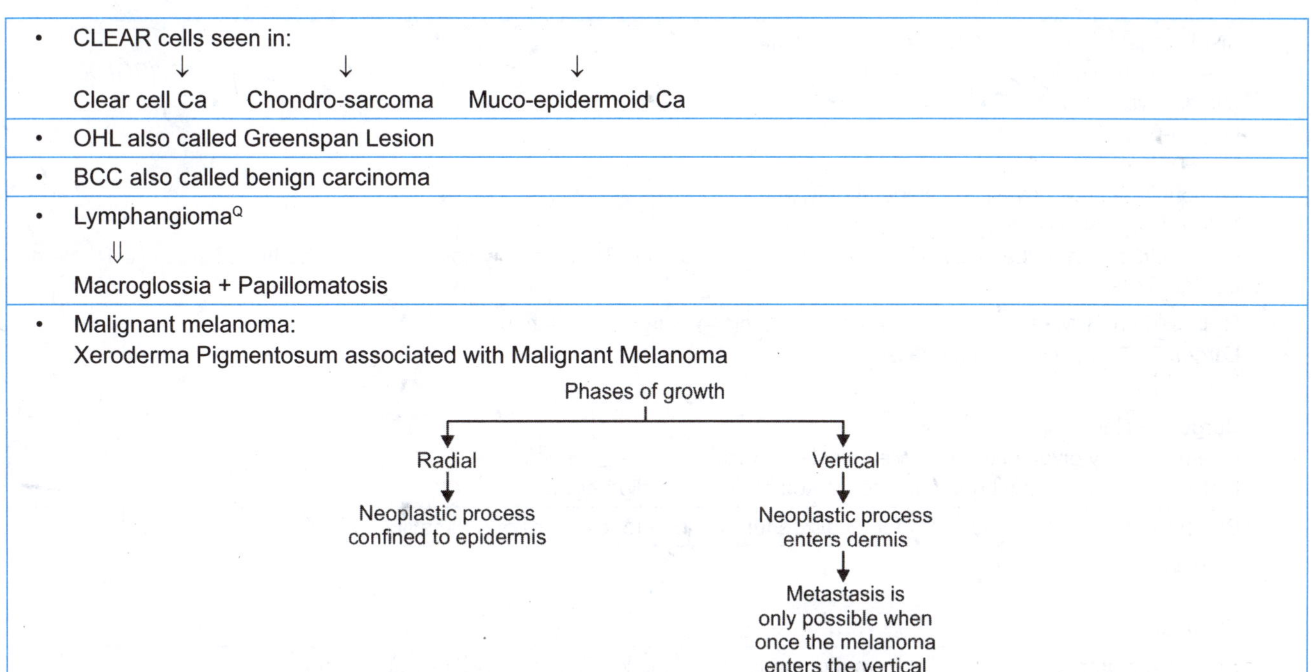

Fig. 8.28: Malignant melanoma

Types:

1. Superficial spreading → 65%, most common[Q]
2. Nodular → most malignant, Invasive
   Note: This form is Most common type of BCC[Q]
3. Lentigo Maligna/Melanotic freckle of Hutchin son

Clinical diagnosis:

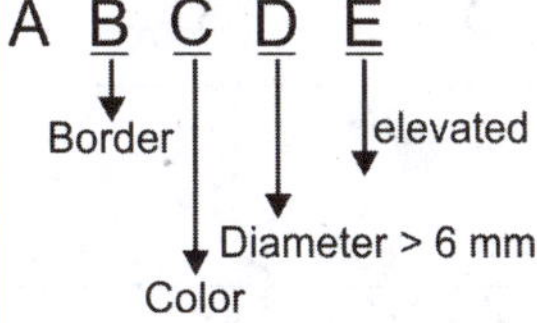

Tumor < 0.75 mm rarely metastasises (Q)
H/P: epitheloid melanocyte distributed in "Pagetoid manner"

- Clark system:
  Level 1 → Epidermis
  Level 2 → Papillary dermis
  Level 3 → Through out papillary dermis and impinging on reticular dermis
  Level 4 → Reticular dermis
  Level 5 → Sub Cutaneus fat
  T/t: Surgery (main t/t)
  Tumours located in BANS (Back, arm, Neck, Scalp)

- TNM staging: T_1< 2 cm T_2> 2 < 4 cm T_3> 4 cm
  T_4→ "When invades" (No size value) *(PGI 08)*
  (No size value)
  N_2→ 3-6 cm
  N_3→ >6 cm
  Without T_4→ N_1 always gives stage III only with T_4, N_1gives stage IV
  N_2/N_3 always gives stage IV
  Key points to remember. Rest stages are easy to remember. There is only confusion in stage III and stage IV. Remember this Trick.

- R_x based on TNM staging T_1/T_2 without metastasis → Surgery/Radiation
  Larger T_2, T_3, T_4 without metastases
  ↓
  Surgery + Radiation
  Chemotherapy given only when Metastasis occurs.
  Note: Cancer involving bone can't be treated alone by Radiotherapy

- Brachy Thrapy → 1° R_x modality for localized tumour in anterior 2/3 rd of oral cavity

- Leukoplakia in Floor of mouth
  ↓
  Worst prognosis

- Staghorn patter is H/P feature of Hemangiopericytoma and lesion resembles Glomus tumor

Concept: All sarcomas metastasizes by Blood except Rhabdoyosarcoma
All carcinomas metastasized by Lymph Nodes except → RCC

- Leimyoma → Smooth muscle tumour
  Rhabdomyoma → Skeletal muscle tumour

- Following flap is used for repair of LIP of Large lip defect:
  1. LIP switch/Abbe-Estlander flap
  2. Karapandzic
  3. Webster/Bernard repair

- Marginal Mandibulectomy is C/I in patients who are edentulous and have SCC involving alveolar ridge as this ↓ces bone height of already edentulous patient

- ↑sed incidence for Malignant transformation among Leukoplakia
  ↓
  Nodular/speckled variant[Q]

- Keratoacan Thoma/self healing Ca
  ↓
  Clinically and H/P similar to SCC

- Most common cyst → Radicular
  Most common developmental cyst → Dentigerous
  Most common Non-odontogenic cyst → Nasopalatine
  ↓
  Develops from respiratory epithelium

- R_x of Tumors:
  Partsch I → Marsupalisation/Decompression
  Partsch II/ ®marsupalisation + enucleation for a large cyst[Q]
  Waldron technique

- Odontogenic Myxoma:
  Benign tumour with aggressive nature and INFLTRATION. So, excision of lesion done
  ↓
  Enbloc Resection
  Note: with curettage recurrence seen

- R_x of Langerhan's Histocytoma: Aggression curettage/resection with 5 mm margin *(AIIMS 09)*
  Radiotherapy for Multifocal Hans Schuller disease and Unifocal eosenophilic granuloma in less accessible areas.
  Acute/Chronic disseminated letter sure disease treated with Chemotherapy
- "AOT": is Benign non-aggressive lesion so, treated with Curretage/Enucleation
- Mucocele/ranula:
  Mucocele is of 2 types:
  1. Mucous extravasation (pseudocyst type)
     ↓
     More common
  2. Mucous retention cyst/sialocyst (true cyst type)
     Ranula is an extravasation type of mucocele both are not a true cyst → As no true epithelial lining (Both mucocele and Ranula)
- Salivary duct cyst/sialocyst → True cyst
- Method to differentiate Cyst and Granuloma:
  1. Injection of R/O dyes
  2. Page – cyst shows intense albumin pattern white granuloma shows Faint to moderate pattern.
  3. Aspiration of Straw coloured fluid indicates presence of cyst.
  4. Biopsy is Gold standard.
- Piezoelectric Lithotripsy: Is a non-invasive method of disintegrating Sialocith
- Substance filled in bone cavity after incubation of cyst ÷ Autogenous medullary bone graft (graft with greatest Osteogenic potential)
- Posterior Illiac crest graft is often used in oral and maxillofacial surgery
- Carnoys solution: used in R_x of "OKC" incubation and curettage followed by 3 min application of Carnoys solution ($FeCl_3$ + Alcohol + chloroform + glacial acetic acid)
  [Peripheral Ostectomy can also be followed instead of chemical cautery] *(PGI)*
- R_x of Mucocoele:
  Excision with removal of associated acini → This reduces chances of recurrence *(AIPG)*
- Lateral pdl cyst + OKC + dentigerous cyst: Exclusively associated with "Vital Tooth"
- Teratoma → All 3 germ layers involved
  Choriostoma → Ectopic (this the difference KEY word from Hamartoma)
- Traumatic bone cyst:
  Bone cavity filled with air. So, R/o
- Ossifying fibroma has R/f:
  Unilocular R/L (Best Answer)
- AOT = Adeno ameloblastoma
  Ameloblastoma = Admantinoma
- **Note:** Midline lymph nodes are IPS'Lateral
- Hibernoma: Benign soft tissue tumour arising from "Brown Fat" *(KCET 07)*
- Glomangioma: Glomus tumour commonly seen on nail bid[Q]
  In surgery of lip carcinoma ½ to 2/3rd of lip is removed.

Classical Radical neck dissection (RND)	→	Modified RND	→	Selective neck dissection
↓		↓		↓
Sacrifice every thing		Preserve any of the 3:		Sacrifice only few lymph nodes
		Spinal accessory nerve, SCM, IJV		
		↓		
		Also called functional neck dissection		

- Men III → Multiple mucosal neuroma of oral region. *(NBDE + KCET)*
  Blubbery[Q]/Blumpy lips
- Malignant transformation for OSME: 4 to 13%
- In all Langerhan cell histocytosis: teeth floating in air seen R/f
  Note: Floating teeth also seen in Cherubism
- Irregular pink gray nodule + Macroglossia = Pathognomic of lymphangioma
- Most common odontogenic tumour → Odontoma
  2nd most common odontogenic tumour → Ameloblastoma
- Dentigerous cyst → Central variety is most common
  Concept:
  Any small harmless appearing area that don of respond to usual therapeutic measures should be considered Malignant and do the Biopsy
- Traumatic neuroma:Reactive lesion NOT a true neoplasm. Failure of peripheral nerves to regenerate
  Note: In case of metastasis there is no anatomical continuity between 1° and 2° neoplasm.
- Hemangioma: When pressure applied BALNCHING occurs
- Prognosis of different Cancer: Lung Ca < oral Ca < colon Ca < uterine Ca < Breast Ca
- Osteoid osteoma Vs Osteoma:

Osteoid osteoma	Osteoma
→C/f: severe pain (merciless sharp) Classicaly pain relieved by Aspirin *(AIIMS 11)*	→ C/f: associated with compact/cancellous bone. Either endosteal/periosteal → Soft tissue osteoma of oral cavity ↓ Most commonly Tongue then oral mucosa → There is seldom any pain

- Irritational fibroma = Traumatic fibroma least likely to recur after excision
- Lymphoepithelioma: extremely malignant, metastasizes widely causing very early death occurs chiefly in Nasopharynx[Q]
- Keratoacanthoma: Self healing Ca clinically and pathologically similar to SCC. A variant of SCC.
  Origin → Pilosebaceous gland
  O → M: F = 2: 1
  Sun exposed areas affected
  Lip vermillion border of upper and lower lip are affected with equal frequency
- Floor of mouth and Lateral border of tongue
  High risk site for malignant transformation
- White lesion with defined precancerous potential:
  Leukoplakia, OSME, DLE[Q], Hyperplastic candidiasis, Actinic Keratosis, Lichenoid reaction
  Erosive Lichen planus[Q]
- Eccentric Lytic Lesion: ABC[Q], Giant cell tumour, fibrous vertical defect
  Note: Simple bone cyst → is central lytic lesion
- In OSTEOSARCOMA cumulus cloud densities formed within the intra medullary and soft tissue.
- Kaposi sarcoma – is a painless slow growing tumour
- Neurofibroma and Neurilemmoma
  ↓
- Both are common in tongue
- Verocay bodies (hyaline structures)
- Cowden syndrome: Multiple hamartoma and Neoplasia syndrome [It's a marker of Breast Ca]

- LIP Carcinoma:
  Most common on Lower lip
  Metastasis → late → so, good prognosis
- Neurofibroma: Schwann cells → Origin
  Non-encapsulated + High Malignant transformation
- Starry sky appearance in Burkit's lymphoma: Due scattered macrophages.
- Bence Jones (BJ) protein: seen in Multiple myeloma, Leukaemia, Polycythemia
- Poikilokaryosis: Division of nucleus without division of cytoplasm
- Abtropfung/drooping off effect: seen in Junctional nevus, i.e. Growing down into connective tissue [+ also seen in spindle cell CA]
  ↓
  A variant of SCC
- Microcherry and venous lake in Haemangioma
- Carcinoma in site:
  Intra epithelial CA
  A premalignant condition
  1. Bulbous Rete ridges
  2. Bowen disease (associated with this in patient on Arsenic therapy)

  No invasive malignant property
  ↓
  So, Metastasis is Impossible in CA in site
- AOT is most commonly associated with Unerupted maxillary Cuspid
  H/P tubular duct like/microcyst lined by losenophillic Hyaline ring
  OKC + COC
- Dentigerous cyst transforms into Mural type of Ameloblastoma (epithelium of cyst proliferates into connective tissue capsule)
- Term Ameloblastoma was given by Churchill nodular growth pattern = Centrifugal growth pattern
  (e.g. central ossifying/cementifying/cement-ossifying fibroma)
- Dental Cyst = Radicular cyst
- Struge Weber: Non-Hereditary (EncephaloTrigeminal Haemangiomatosis)
  ↓
  Also called Mother Spot disease/Phako Matoses
  ↓
  1. Post wine stain/Naevus flammeus-confined exclusively to Trigeminal nerve supply of face
  2. Intra cranial/Leptomeningial/Tram line calcification
  3. Unilateral distribution of angiomatous malformation which never arises midline [Pathognomic]
- Osler-Weber-Randeu. Syndrome/Osler's disease:

Hereditary	Hemorrhagic	Telangiectasia
↓	↓	↓
Hereditary	Recurrent Epistaxis	Telangiectasia present

- Tongue Ca: (Painless)
  Most common on postero lateral (2/3rd cases)
  20% → Antero lateral/ventral
  4% → on Dorsum (Rare) *(AIIMS 12)*
  Tongue is the only site where oral Congenital SCC reported
- Plummer Vinson Syndrome: Triad of IDA + Koilonychia (also seen in IDA) + Predisposition for Post Cricoid carcinoma
- Dental cyst = Radicular cyst
- Periapical granuloma → predominant cell is Lymphocyte

• In cementoma R/o attached to tooth while in condensing osteitis, it is not (is around Tooth)
• Nodular growth pattern = Centrifugal growth pattern (e.g. central ossifying/cementifying/cement ossifying fibroma)
• Term ameloblastoma was given by Churchill
• Dentigerous cyst transforms into Mural type of ameloblastoma (epithelium of cyst proliferates into connective tissue capsule)
• Classic Basal cell feature seen in OKC + COC
• AOT most common associated with unerupted maxillary Cuspid • H/P → Tubular duct like/microcyst lined by Eosinophilic hyaline ring
• ABC: R/f → eccentric EXPANSILE lesion[Q]

LAST 5-YEAR QUESTIONS FROM THIS TOPIC

1. Cyst arising from dental lamina: *(COMEDK 12)*
Ans. Glandular odontogenic cyst

2. Benign tumour which shows metastasis: *(COMEDK 12)*
Ans. Ameloblastoma

3. Syndrome associated with increased risk of Leukemia is: *(COMEDK 12)*
Ans. Plummer Vinson syndrome

4. The most common odontogenic cyst is: *(KCET 12)*
Ans. Radicular cyst

5. Perineural invasion is a characteristic feature of which of the following tumours? *(KCET 12)*
Ans. Adenoid cystic carcinoma

6. Sturge weber syndrome is associated with? *(KCET 12)*
Ans. Hemangioma

7. Causes for 1° hyperparathyroidism: *(KCET 12)*
Ans. Parathyroid carcinoma

8. Presence of Bence Jones Proteins is characteristic of: *(KCET 12,11)*
Ans. Multiple Myeloma(Shafer's 5/e p261)

9. Pel-Ebstein fever is a feature of: *(KCT 12)*
Ans. Hodgkn's disease

10. Apical cysts having a direct connection with apical foramen have been termed as: *(KCET 09)*
Ans. Bay

11. Squamous papilloma is induced by: *(KCET 09)*
Ans. HPV

12. Developmental cyst associated with impacted tooth: *(KCET 09)*
Ans. Dentigerous cyst

13. "Ghost cells are characteristically seen in the epithelial linings of: *(KCET 09)*
Ans. COC (Also seen in Ameloblastic fibro odontoma + odontoma)

14. Rushton bodies are sometimes seen in: *(COMEDK 09,11)*
Ans. Gingival cyst of newborn(Ref: Shafer's 5/e p369, 674)

15. Adenolymphoma refers to: *(COMEDK 09)*
Ans. Warthin'stumor

16. The growth of odontogenickeratocyst mainly takes place in the direction of: *(COMEDK 10)*
Ans. Anterior Posterior

17. Adematoidodontogenic tumour is characterized histologically by: *(COMEDK 10)*
Ans. Tubular/duct like cells

18. Histological appearance of "Abtrofung"/"dropping off" is commonly seen in: *(KCET 11)*

Ans. Junctional nevus (Ref: Shafer's 5/e p120)

19. The most common clinical pattern of BCC is: *(COMEDK 10)*

Ans. Nodular (**Note:** Morpheaform is most aggressive

20. The most common reported oral malignancy in HIV infection is: *(COMEDK 10), (AIPG 09)*

Ans. Kaposi Sarcoma

21. A patient with carcinoma check has tumour of 2.5 cm located close to and involving the lower alveolus. A single mobile homolateral node measuring 6 cm is palpable.

Based on these clinical findings TNM stage of tumour is: *(COMEDK 10)*

Ans. $T_2 N_2$ Mo

22. Which is the most common cyst in mandibular PM region?

Ans. Lateral periodontal cyst

23. The presence of Leisegang ring type of calcification is a feature of: *(KCET 10)*

a. CEOT

b. Pindborg tumour

c. Both a and b

d. None of the above

Ans. c

24. Which of the following is potentially malignant disorder?

Ans. Leukoplakia

25. OKC is currently known as: *(KCET 10)*

Ans. Keratocystic odontogenic tumour *(PGI June 11)*

26. Rodent ulcer is: *(KCET 10)*

Ans. BCC

27. The sunray appearance is seen in: *(KCET 10)*

Ans. Osteosarcoma

28. Which is NOT a feature of chondrosarcoma? *(KCET 10)*

a. Most common primary malignant tumour

b. Most common site is anterior part of maxilla

c. Connective tissue origin

d. Drifting and mobility of teeth

Ans. a

29. CASE STUDY: *(COMEDK 11)*

A 25 year old male patient reports with a bony expansile swelling of the right body of the mandible and mild Paresthesia of the right IDN OPG shows a multilocular radiolucency without root resorption.

1. **What would be your choice of next investigation.**

Ans. Aspiration cytology

2. **A dirty white aspirate with a protein estimation of $< 4g\%$ is suggestive of:**

Ans. Odontogenic Keratocyst

3. **Odontogenic Keratocyst is noted for its:**

Ans. Daughter cysts and high rate of recurrence

4. **Management of OKC involves:**

Ans. Enucleation with peripheral osteotomy

30. Most common salivary gland tumour arising in the jaw? *(COMED 11)*

Ans. Micoepidermoid (carcinoma)

31. Mucocutaneous lesion associated with neoplasia is: *(COMEDK 11)*
Ans. Paraneoplastic pemphigus (Ref: Shafer's 5/e p1131)

32. The cyst which is associated with a non-vital tooth is: *(KCET 11)*
Ans. Radicular cyst (Ref: Shafer's 5/e p376)

33. Cylindroma is another name for: *(KCET 11)*
Ans. Adenoidcystic carcinoma (Ref: Shafer's 5/ep330)

34. Periapical cement-osseous dysplasia occurs frequently in the:
Ans. Mandibular anterior region (Ref: Nevilli 3/e p641)

35. Small palpable mass elevated above the epithelial surface is: *(KCET 11)*
Ans. Papule (Ref: Burkitt oral medicine 10/e p51)

36. Papule is: *(PGI June 09)*
Ans. Solid elevation greater than 5 mm in diameter (Ref: Burkitt's 10/e p216)

37. Goltz and Gorlin syndrome is associated with: *(PGI June 09)*
Ans. Multiple papillomas (Ref: Shafers 3/e p273)

38. Rhabdomyoma is the tumour: *(PGI Dec. 09)*
Ans. Benign tumour of skeletal muscles

39. According to malignant melanoma classification fo the tumour invasion, the level 3 is: *(PGI June 09)*
Ans. Tumour cells found throughout papillary dermis and impingement on reticular dermis and is in a vertical growth phase (Ref: Shafer's 5/e p178)

40. The most common cyst found in the midline of the neck of 3 year old child is: *(PGI June 09)*
Ans. Thyroglossal cyst (Ref: S. Das 3/e p617)

41. Teratoma is best described as: *(PGI June 10)*
Ans. Hamartous development manifestation consisting of 3 different layers (Ref: Shafer 4/e p312)

42. Type of carcinoma developed in Marjolin ulcer is: *(PGI June 10)*
Ans. SCC (Ref: S.Das surgery 3/e p108)

43. Most commonly used fixative after biopsy is: *(PGI Dec 10)*
Ans. 10% Formalin (Ref: Shafer's 4/e p599)

44. Giant cell lesions of the gingiva are best considered as: *(PGI Dec 10)*
Ans. Reactive lesions (Ref: Shafer's 6/e p130)

45. The new name of OKC is?
Ans. Keratoodontogenic tumour (Shafer's 6/e p258)

46. TNM staging does not include which of the following?
Ans. a. Tumour size
b. Tumour site
c. Nodal involvement
d. Metastasis

Ans. a (Ref: Baily and Love's 23/e p154-155)

47. Reed sternbery cells are seen in? *(PGI June 11)*
Ans. Hodgkin's disease

48. Classification of Leukoplakia does not include: *(PGI June 11)*
a. Speckled
b. Bullous
c. Homogeneous
d. Ulcerative

Ans. b (Ref: Shafer's 6/e p90)

49. Most common benign, neoplasia of oral cavity is? *(PGI Dec, 11)*

Ans. Fibroma (Ref: Shafer 5/e p178)

50. The most common clinical pattern of basal cell carcinoma is: *(PGI Dec 11)*

Ans. Nodular

Note: Superficial form is most common in Malignant melanoma

51. Teratoma is: *(PGI Dec 11)*

Ans. Hamartomous developmental manifestation consisting of 3 different layers.

52. Dermal and oral manifestations are most commonly seen in which type of Leukaemia. *(AIPG 12)*

Ans. Monocytic (Ref: Shafer's 6/e p777)

53. Facial nerve paralysis is common in which tumour:

Ans. Epidermoid carcinoma of parotid gland (Ref: Shafer's 6/e p232)

54. Most potentially aggressive and destructive cyst is: *(AIPG 12)*

Ans. Dentigerous cyst (Ref: shafer's 6/e p257)

55. Best technique to differentiate between periapical cemental dysplasia and periapical granuloma in a woman with a history of cardiac valve replacement is:

Ans. Tooth vitality (Ref: Cohen 8/e) *(AIPG 12)*

56. Self-healing carcinoma among the following is: *(AIIMS May 11)*

Ans. Keratoacanthoma (Ref: Shafer 5/e p116)

57. The most common developmental cyst is:

Ans. Nasopataline cyst (Ref: Nevilli, 2nd)

58. Which of the following is most commonly associated with malignant transformation *(AIIMS May 11)*

Ans. Junctional nevus (Ref: Shafer 6/e p83-85)

59. A patient comes with pain in the pharyngeal region and is having carcinoma of nasopharynx. The most probable diagnosis is: *(AIIMS Nov 10)*

Ans. Trotter's syndrome (Ref: Shafer, 4/e p855)

60. Out of syphilitic glossitis, Plummer-Vinson syndrome, Hepatitis A and Mikulicz'sdiseae, scc can occur in: *(AIIMS Nov. 09)*

Ans. Syphilliticglossitis and plummer-Vinson syndrome (Ref: Pedlar, Oral Maxillofacial surgery, 2001, p130)

61. DNA repair defect is associated with: *(AIPG 10, 11)*

Ans. Xerodermapigmentosa (Ref: Robbins 8/ep103, 302)

TRICK for Defective DNA repair associated cancers: *[Big FAX]*

B – Bloom syndrome

F – Fanconi anaemia

A – Ataxia telangiectasia

X – Xeroderma pigmentosa

62. The most common tumour of parotid gland is:

Ans. Pleomorphic adenoma

63. Which of the following is a T-cell neoplasm? *(AIPG 10)*

Ans. Mycosis fungoides (Ref: Shafer 5/e p247)

64. An Ann Arbour classification stage III corresponds to: *(AIPG 10)*

Ans. Involvement of lymph node regions/lymphoid structures on both sides of the diaphragm (Ref: Shafer 5/e p256)

65. **Which is the most common site of Keratoacanthoma?** *(AIPG 09)*

Ans. Lip (Ref: Shafer 5/e p116-117)

66. **Rhabdomyosarcoma is a disorder of** *(AIPG 09)*

Ans. Striated muscle (Ref: Shager 5/e p266)

67. **Staghorn pattern is sun in:** *(AIPG 09)*

Ans. Hemangiopericytoma (Ref: Shafer 5/e p230, 233, 243)

68. **The epithelial lining of radicular cyst is** *(AIPG 09)*

Ans. Non-Keratinized (Ref: Shafer, 5/e p377)

69. **Excisional biopsy is done by:** *(AIPG 09)*

Ans. Complete excision of the tumour along with some part of normal tissue (Ref: Shafer 5/e p615)

70. **Non vital tooth is associated with:** *(AIIMS May 09)*

Ans. Radicular cyst (Ref: Shafer 5/e)

71. **Café-au-lait macules are seen in:** *(KCET 10)*

Ans. Von Recklinghausen's neurofibromatosis + Bloom syndrome + Albrifht syndrome

PERIAPICAL AND PULPAL INFECTION

- "Internal" resorption = odontoclastoma
- Streptococcus → Cellulitis
  Staphylococcus → Abscess (as No Hyaluronidase)
  ↓
  It is not proteoglycan but GAG
  S. Aureus → causes osteomyelitis
- Periapical granuloma = H/P consists of both granulation tissue and granuloma
  Majority of cases donot show antibody production
  It is "Sterile".
- Condensing osteitis/focal sclerosing osteitis can be seen with pulpitis/pulpal necrosis, i.e. can be associated with both vital and Non-vital tooth
- Ostietis seen around APEX not periosteitis
- Periostitis seen in Grave's OM
- Ludwig angina caused by aerobic streptococci

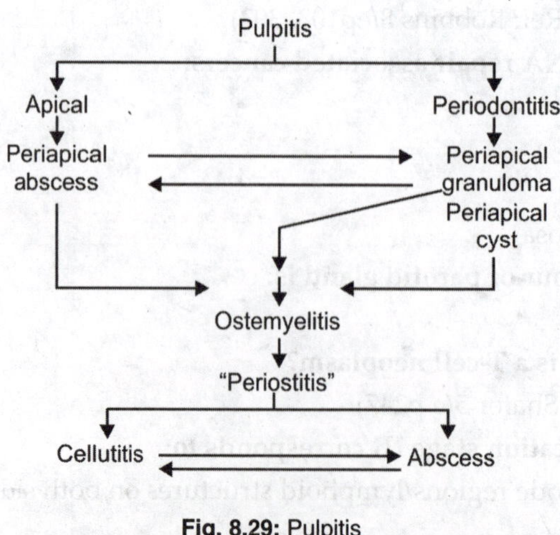

Fig. 8.29: Pulpitis

- Pariapical granuloma → Predominant cell is Lymphocytes
- Ludwig's Angina → 2nd and 3rd M are chief source of infection
  [**Note:** Hyaluronic acid is universal intercellular substance]

LAST 5-YEAR QUESTIONS FROM THIS TOPIC

1. "Punched out" crater-like necrosis involving the interdental papillae is a diagnostic feature of: *(KCET 09)*

Ans. NUG

2. Pulp polyp is a feature of: *(KCET 10)*

Ans. Chronic hyperplastic pulpitis

3. Gare's sclerosing Osteomyelitis is also known as: *(KCET 11)*

Ans. Proliferative Periostitis (Ref: Shafer's 5/e p691)

4. Complications of osteomyelitis include: *(PGI Dec 10)*

a. Ludwig's angia
b. Cavernous sinus thrombosis
c. Parotid gland involvement
d. All of the above

Ans. d (Ref: Shafer 5/e p341)

5. Periapical and periodontal abscess can be differentiated by: *(AIPG 09)*

Ans. Pulp vitality (Ref: Shafer 5/e p559, 682)

6. An 8 year old boy is suffering from ANUG which of the following systemic antibiotic would be the drug of choice for him? *(AIPG 12)*

Ans: Penicillin + metronidazole

BLOOD

- Crew at/Hair on end appearance on skull radiograph → Thalassemia + SCA (sickle cell anaemia)
- Salt and Pepper effect on X-ray
  ↓
  Thalassemia
- Safety Pin cell on Peripheral smear

  ↓
  Thalassemia
- TTP/ITP → B.t. ↑sed
  → Clot retraction time ↑sed
  T/t → Plasmapharesis
- Tear drop/pear shaped cells
  ↓
  "Pernicious anemia"
- Hallmark of chediak Higaski syndrome
  ↓
  P.S. has abnormal granules in leukocytes Neuropathy
  Hypopigmentation Calbinism) ®occulo Cutaneus
- Patterson-Kelly syndrome is another name of Plummer Wilson syndrome
  Associated with IDA + sed predilection for SCC (oral and pharyngeal Ca)
- Tranexamic acid + Aminocaprioc acid are antifibrinolytic used in post operative care of haemophilia

- Red fluorescent fluid seen in porphyria
  Red urine → Rifampicin
  Red Man syndrome seen with Vancomycin

- DIC → BT, CT, PT, aPTT (Al are ↑sed) FDP ↑sed
  Most common site → Brain (for thrombus formation)

- In all Langerhan cell Histocytosis: Teeth floating in air seen on Radiograph.
  [Also floating teeth are seen in Cherubism]

- BT → "1 to 4 min" (under 5 min Duke's method)
- CT. → 2 to 8 min
- Concept: any small harmless appearing area that donot respond to usual therapeutic measures should be considered malignant and do the BIOPSY.

- Hemangioma → when pressure applied
  ↓
  Blanching seen

- Plumbism→ RBC tends to be fragile
  +
  Basophilic Stipling of RBC

- Glanzman thrombosthaenia (Familial Thrombasthenia)
  Qualitative defect in platelets → ↑sed BT without ↓se in platelet count.

- Antischow cell: Seen in All anaemia + Apthous ulcer + Behcat.

- Agranulocytosis: WBC < 2,000
  Ragged necrotic ulcer covered by grey/black membrane. No inflammation

- Erythroblastosis foetalis: Rh-ve mothers are given anti-Dr globulin to prevent immunisation. It binds to antigenic receptor sites on fetal cells, making them non immunogenic

- Thala semia: (Rodent facies)
  - Cooley's anaemia/Mediterranean disease/Erythroblastic anemia
  - AD pattern
  - Exhibits racial pattern α Thallasemia Major

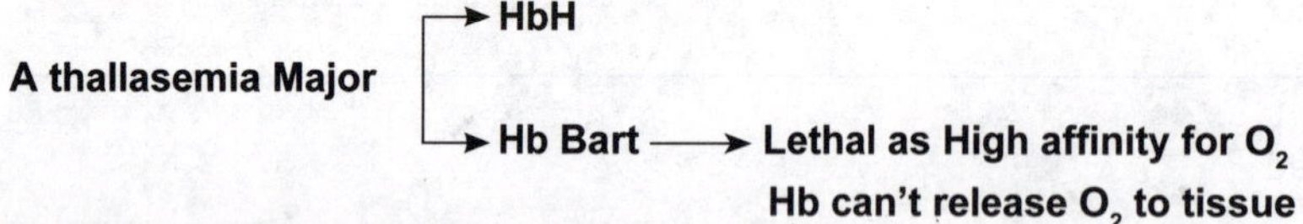

  - Hb Bart →Hydropsfetalis→ still born
  - Hetrozygotes→ Thalassemia minor
  - C/f;
    Splenomegaly
    Hepatomegaly
    Rodent facies
  - Unusual prominence of premaxilla
  - Lab. Finding: c cellular hyperplasia → ↑RBC + ↑WBC
  - R/f: Rib within Rib appearance crew cut/hair-on-end appearance

- Different names of anemia:
  1. Pernicious anemia → Biemr anaemia
     Addisonian anaemia
     Lederar anaemia
     B_{12} deficiency anaemia
  2. Thalassemia → Coley's anaemia
     Mediterranean anaemia
     Erythroblastic anaemia
  3. Plummer Vinson syndrome → Patterson-Brown Kelly syndrome

Condition	Neutrophil abnormality	Chromosomal abnormality	PdL manifestation
Neutropenia, agranulocytosis	↓sed No. of neutrophil		Aggressive periodontitis
Chediak–Higashi syndrome	– ↓sed neutrophil Chemotaxis – Mega bodies seen	AR Chr-1 defect of LYST gene ↓ Lysosome can't fuse with phagosome to form "Phagolysosome	Aggressive periodontitis + Oral ulceration
Papillon-Lefever syndrome	– Multiple neutrophil defect – Myeloperoxidase deficiency	Chr 11 AR	Aggressive periodontitis
LAD 1	– Impaired migration and phagocytosis – CD18 defect	Chri-21	Aggressive periodontitis
LAD 2	Neutrophil fail to express CD15	Chr 11	Aggressive periodontitis

LAST 5-YEAR QUESTIONS FROM THIS TOPIC

1. **Rh hump is commonly associated with:** *(KCET 11)*

Ans. Erythroblastosis fetalis (Ref: Shafer's 5/e p1053)

2. **An example of a sex-related disease more commonly seen in males is:** *(KCET 11)*

Ans. Haemophillia (Ref: Shafer's 5/e p1081)

3. **Von-Willebrand's disease is due to the:**

Ans. Deficiency of factor VIII and decreased platelet adhesion

CARIES

- Incipient caries → Demineralization begins with inter rod substance
  ↓
  So, ↑sed prominence of rods[Q]
- V and Mo → cariostatic [opposite for Se, Cd, As]

Zone of cries

Enamel caries

Zone 4 (surface zone)

Zone 3 (body of lesion) (5-25% pore volume)

Zone 2 → Dark zone (3-4% pore volume)

Zone 1 (Translucent zone) 1 % pore volume

Fig. 8.30: Enamel caries

Zone 4 →↑sed prominence of STRIAE of RETZIUS *(AIPG 09)*

Zone 3 → Body of lesion is MOST demineralized zone *(BHU 07)*

↓

Extend 10-15 um from surface foci of miller

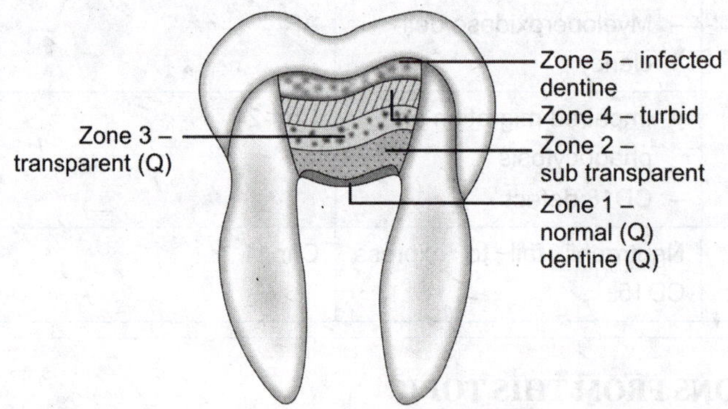

Fig. 8.31: Dentinal caries

- S.Sanguis after S. Mutans (2nd most common) cause of caries
- Spread of pit and fissure caries → from lateral surface of pit → fissure
- Most selective medium for S. mutans is, MSA (Mitis salivarius bacitracin Agar)
- Initiation of caries is by production of Insoluble dextran[Q] andglucosyl transferase[Q]
- Vit.D, K → Anti cariogenic
  Vit A → Anti carcinogenic
  Vit A, C, D → Tooth development
  ↓
  Defect causes enamel hypoplasia
- S. mutans converts Glucose → Glucan (Dextran) (More important)
  ↓
  Fructose to → Fructose (Levans)
  Glucan is insoluble and causes adherence of S. mutans. So, more important
  Levan → highly soluble

• Teeth with large amount of globular dentine ↓ Rapid spread of caries → called MALACOTIC or soft tooth
• In caries B A I has no work ↓ ↳ Al Iron Barium
• Buffering capacity of saliva α caries resistant person.
• NH_4 compounds and Urea have anticarogenic properties. Urea $\xrightarrow{\text{urease}}$ $NH_3\uparrow$. Now NH_3 neutralizes the acid produced by micro organism and thus interfering bacterial growth.
• In early stage of caries ↓ Initial bacteria penetrating tubules ↓ Pioneer bacteria

LAST 5-YEAR QUESTIONS FROM THIS TOPIC

1. **The caries on enamel surface leads to accentuation of:** *(AIIMS May 11)*

Ans. Incremental lines of Retzuis (Ref: Shafer 5/e p617)

2. **The most caries forming sugar is:** *(AIIMS May 11)*

Ans. Sucrose (Pals, Leme, et al The role of sucrose in cariogenic dental biofilm formation new insight J Dent Res, 2006 Oct, 85 (10), pg 878-87)

3. **Dental caries is associated with?** *(AIIMS Nov 09)*

Ans. S. rattus (Ref: lamont. Oral Microbiology at a Glance, 1/st p2010, p7)

4. **Dental plaque adheres to the tooth surface by:** *(AIIMS Nov 11, 09)*

Ans. Dextran (Ref: Shafer 6/e p420)

5. **False regarding S.mutans is:** *(AIPG 10)*
   a. Acidogenic and aciduric
   b. Unable to multiply easily
   c. Main causative organism in dental caries
   d. First colonizer

Ans. b (Ref: Shafer 6/e p415)

6. **Radiation induced xerostomia, would cause dental caries in:** *(PGI Dec 11)*

Ans. 3 months (Ref: sturdevant 5/e p94)

7. **The enzyme glucosyl transferase secreted by S. mutans synthesizes glucans from:** *(COMEDK 09)*

Ans. Sucrose

8. **Xylitol is a low caloric sweetener, inhibits the growth of:** *(KCET 10)*

Ans. S. mutans

9. **Sorbitol acts in the prevention of dental caries by:** *(COMEDK 11)*

Ans. Microorganisms lack the enzyme to metabolize

10. **Salviary protein which prevents transmission of HIV via saliva is:** *(COMED 11)*

Ans. Salivary leukocyte proteinase inhibitor

11. **Salivary peroxidase system is known to be effective against:** *(KCET 11)*

Ans. Lactobacillus acidophilus (Ref: Shafer's 5/e p594)

12. **In reflected light, dead tracts are seen as:** *(KCET 11)*

Ans. White zones (Ref: Orban's 11/e p125)

MISCELLANEOUS

- Multiple intestinal Polyposis associated with Peutz Zeigler syndrome andGardners.

- Myositis Ossificans: *(PGI 12)*
  - Often preceded by Trauma[Q]
  - Usually develop in athletes and young adult
  - Often develop in skeletal muscle of proximal extremity
  - Painless, hard, well demarcated swelling
  - Distinguished from other fibroblastic proliferation by presence of Metaplastic Bone
  - R_x: Simple excision is curative
  - Most commonly – Masseter involved

    ↓

    Fixation of face and jaw occurs

    ↓

    Pt. transformed to "Petryfied man"

- Ca, Al, Pb → cause Constipation

- Vitamins: (Deficiency)

Vitamins	General manifestation	Oral manifestation
1. Vit A	Night blindness Xeropthalmia, Bitot spots, Keratomalacia	• Keratinising metaplasia • Occlusion of s.g. duct with keratin • Enamel hypoplasia[Q] • Atypical dentine
2. Vit B1 (Anti Beri-Beri/anti Neuritic vitamin) ↓ Seen in population eating polished rice	– Dry beriberi ↓ Peripheral neuritis – Wet beriberi ↓ Cardiac manifestation – Cerebral/wernickesencelopathy *(AIPG 10)* + Korsakoffis psychosis	
3. Vit B_2 (Riboflavin) ↓ Dairy source	– Vascularisation of cornea	– Glossitis (Magenta tongue) – Cheilosis – Ocular lesion
4. Vit B3 (Niacin)	– Pellagra (4D) Dermatitis + diarrhoea + dementia + death – Casal's necklace	– Bald tongue of sandwith – Raw beefy tongue *(AIPG 10)* – Neonatal seizures – Fiery red, painful mucosa
5. Vit B6 (pyridoxine)	– Peripheral neuropathy – INZ is Vit B6 antagonist	
6. Vit B7/H/Biotin/antie-egg white injury factor		
7. Vit B10 Folic acid ↓ Required for normal synthesis of DNA	– Macrocytic anemia	– Glossitis (fiery red tongue)

Vitamins	General manifestation	Oral manifestation
8. Vit B12 (Extrinsic factor of castle)	– Pernicious anemia – Neurological degeneration of postero-lateral tract of spinal chord	– Moeller's glossitis – Hunter'sglossitis – Beefy red tongue
9. Vit C (Ascorbic acid) ↓ Not produced/stored by body[Q]	– Scurvy (spongly gums, loose teeth, anemia, swollen joints) – "BOWING of legs"[Q] – Defective collagen synthesis[Q] – "cork-screw" hair pattern – "Woody legs" – Trimmer field zone/zone of complete disintegration seen in h/p of bone	– Interdental papilla swollen called "Scurvy buds"

Note: If dose of Vit. C ↑sed then ↑sed incidence of kidney stone
Vit C affects only connective tissue NOT epithelium[Q]

Vit D	– Rickets – Osteomalacia – Pigeon chest – Renal osteodystrophy – Calcitriol (plasma) ↓ced alkaline phosphatase activity ↑sed	– Delayed eruption – Wide predentine with much interglobular dentine – Multiple dental abscess – Pulp horn extending to DEJ

- Note: **Oral manifestation same in Rickets and Vit. D resistance rickets except Rickets → enamel hypoplasia + delayed eruption**

Vit D resistant rickets → loss of lamina dura
Vit E (Anti sterility vitamin) – ↑sed male fertility
– nutritional muscular dystrophy

• Recurrent apthous ulcer with GIT disorder ↓ Crohn's celiac sprue
• Recurrent Apthous ulcer (Bacterial cause of Apthous ulcer)
• Trigeminal Neuralgia/Tic douloureux/Fothergils' disease – Right side of face affected commonly – Stabbing/lancinating pain – Trigger zone present
• Trotter's syndrome: *(AIPG 09)* – Pharyngeal pain – Nasopharyngeal carcinoma seen
• HZ/Shingles: ophthalmic division of TN affected
• Ramsay Hunt syndrome: – HZ affecting geniculate ganglia – External ear/oral mucosa affected + Facial paralysis
• Reader's syndrome: Ocular sympathetic paralysis + severe headache + pain in area of trigeminal nerve
• Orofacial pains of vascular origin *(AIPG 11)* – Chronic paroxysmal hemicrania – Temporal arteritis – Cluster headache

- Causalgia: seen after "traumatic nerve injury" during difficult extraction
  +
  Burning pain
  +
  Allodynia
- Hyperpathia → ↑sed reaction to a stimulus
  +
  ↑sed threashold
  +
  Faulty identification and localization of stimulus
- Dysesthesia → Unpleasant abnormal sensation *(PGI 12)*
- Paraesthesia → Abnormal sensation [NOT unpleasant]
- Hyperaesthesia → ↑sed sensitivity
- Hypoesthesia → ↑sed sensitivity to stimuli
- Hyperalgesia→ ↑sed painful response to stimuli
- Allodynia → Non-painful stimuli produces pain
- Anesthesia dolorosa → sensory loss following injury to cranial nerve (mostly TN)
- Sphenopalatine neuralgia/cluster headache/Horton's syndrome/sluder's headache
  - Dilatation of Internal maxillary artery[Q]
  - Vidian nerve/Nerve of pterygoid canal (Deep + greater petrosal nerve) involved
  - No Trigger zone[Q]
  - Unilateral pain in[Q] (Fig. 8.32)

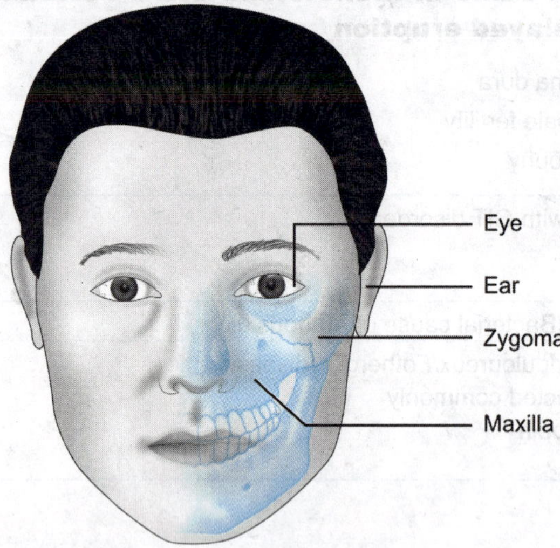

Fig. 8.32: Sphenopalatine neuralgia

  - Pain aggravated by emotional stress and alcohol
  - Alarm clock headache[Q]
- Frey syndrome/Gustatory sweating/Auriculo temporal syndrome
  - Parasympathetic innvervation of sweat glands
  - Ach secretion seen
- Horner's syndrome = Triad of Miosis + ptosis + anhidrosis
  +
  Enopthalmus[Q]
- Glossopharyngeal neuralgia:
  - Trigger zone in posterior oropharynx

- Eagle's syndrome: (Elongated styloid process)
  - Dull pain in oropharynx and posterior auricular region.
  - Dysphagia
  - Limited range of neck motion
  - Pain relived by styloidectomy

- Lead line/Burtonian line
  - Bluish linear Pigmentation of marginal gingiva

- Argyria → violet marginal line

- Bismuth, arsenic and mercury:
  - Black marginal line
  - Blue-black line seen bismuth pigmentation

- Mesentric line:

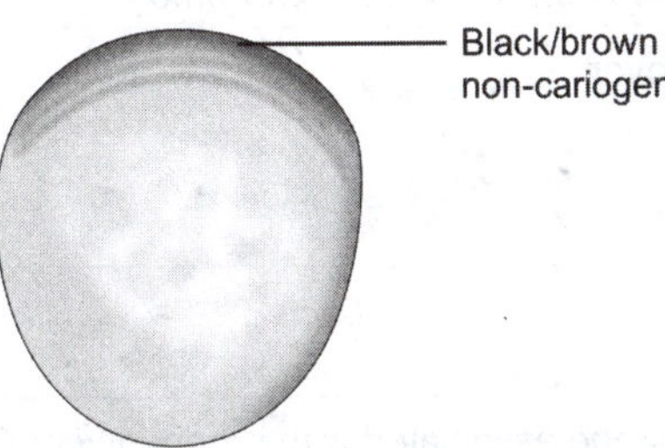

Fig. 8.33: Mesentric line

- ANGULAR chelitis = Perleche

- Intrinsic cause dental erosion is Perimolysis

- Facial paralysis → tested by Whistiling

- Carmazipine: complications are *Aplastic anaemia* + leucopenia
  ↓
  BUT rare

- 100% O2 is abortive medicine for CLUSTER headache

- Marcus jaw Winking syndrome/Trigemino Occulomotor synkinesis

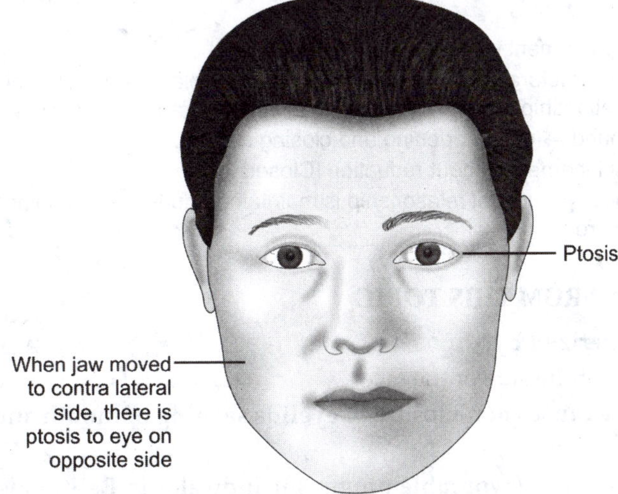

Fig. 8.34: Marcus jaw Winking syndrome

- Most common manifestation of Vit. K deficiency of gingival bleeding

- Macroglossia seen in:
  - Beckewith-Weidman syndrome (97.5% cases)
  - Lymphangioma
  - Hemangioma
  - Cretinism
  - Acromegaly
  - Hurler's syndrome
  - Amyloidosis
  - Scurvy
  - Down's Syndrome
  - Neurofibromatosis

- Cu deficiency → Menke's syndrome/steely/kinky hair syndrome

- Strawbery tongue seen in Scarlet fever
- Glossodynia → Painful tongue
- Glossopyrosis → Burning tongue
- Glossoplegia → paralysed tongue

- Tetracyclin stain:
  Dentine >>> Stained than enamel

- Melasma/chloasma: Pigmentary change associated with pregnancy or OCP

- Estrogen + Progesteron in combination induces the pigmentation (Not alone)

- ^{99m}Tc – MDP is most widely used ligand for skeletal imaging

- Cheiloscopy → examination of LIP Prints
  Ankyloglossia → True → union b/w tongue and floor of mouth
  → Partial → Tip of tongue attached to lingual frenum

- Fissured tongue → In down's syndrome + Melkerson Rosenthal syndrome

- Bifid tongue/ Cleft tongue: seen in Qrofacial digital syndrome

- Crenated tongue: When lateral borders of tongue consists of indentation

- DISC displacement:
  1. Anterior disc displacement with reduction "Clicking joint"
     → Alternation of structural relationship of condyle-disc relationship. The misaligned disc improves its structural relationship with condyle when mandibular translation occurs with mouth opening.
     → Joint/click sound → during opening and closing mouth.
  2. Anterior disc displacement without reduction [Closed lock]
     Altered disc condyle structural relationship is maintained during mandibular translation, i.e. altered relationship does Not improve.

LAST 5-YEAR QUESTIONS FROM THIS TOPIC

1. Bell's palsy is characterized by? *(COMEDK 12)*

Ans. Bilateral involvement of the side of the face

2. Injury to which nerve causes non-closure of eyelids sagging of mouth and dribbling of saliva: *(KCET 12)*

Ans. Facial nerve

3. Which of the following is a favourable prognostic indicator in Bell's palsy? *(KCET 12)*

a. Hyperacusis
b. Severe taste impairment
c. Persistence of the stapedial reflex
d. Complete paralysis within a week.

Ans. c

4. **Frey's syndrome results from surgery of the:** *(COMEDK 09)*

Ans. Parotid gland

5. **The most common site of mucocele is:** *(COMEDK 09)*

Ans. Lower lip

6. **Burning mouth syndrome describes pain associated with:** *(COMEDK 10)*

Ans. No Detectable oral disease

7. **Deficiency of which vitamin causes megaloblastic anaemia:** *(KCET 10)*

Ans. Vitamin B12

8. **Anticonvulsants "frequently" used in management of trigeminal neuralgia:** *(KCET 10)*

Ans. Phonytoin + Gabapentin + Baclofen

9. **The characteristic alarm clock headache is a feature of:** *(KCET 10)*

Ans. Sphenopalatine neuralgia

10. **A pathologic condition caused due to over-extension of borders is called as:** *(KCET 10)*

Ans. EpulisFissuratum

11. **Frey's syndrome is caused due to the injury of:** *(COMEDK 11)*

Ans. Auriculotemporal nerve

12. **Which of these is NOT a premalignant condition for oral cancers** *(COMEDK 11)*

Ans. Aphtous ulcer

13. **Thrombocytopenia due to increased platelet destruction is seen in:** *(COMEDK 11)*

Ans. SLE (Ref: Shafer's 5/e p1142)

14. **Sinuisitis may cause referred pain in:** *(COMEDK 11)*

Ans. Maxillary posterior teeth

15. **Which of the following is most common feature of trigeminal neuralgia?** *(COMEDK 11)*

Ans. Pain usually crossing the midline of the face (Ref: Shafer's 5/e p845)

16. **Intake of which of the following leads to increased incidence of dry socket** *(COMEDK 11)*

Ans. Oral contraceptives (Ref: Shafer's 6/e p601)

17. **Which of the following is not true regarding PapillonLefever syndrome?** *(PGI June 10)*
    a. Autosomal recessive
    b. Quantitative defect of neutrophil
    c. ELISH is reliable
    d. There is exfoliation of 1° teeth before eruption of permanent teeth

Ans. b (Ref: Shafer 5/e p560-561)

18. **Apthous like oral lesions are seen in children in:** *(PGI Dec 11)*
    a. Bechet's disease
    b. PFAPA syndrome
    c. Sweet syndrome
    d. All of the above

Ans. d

Note: PFAPA = periodic fever, aphtous stomatitis, pharyngitis, and cervical adenitis syndrome in children
sweet syndrome → neutrophilic dermatoses

19. **The most common cause of Xerostomia in adults is:** *(AIPG 09)*

Ans. Antihistaminics (Ref: Myers and Ferris. Salivary Gland Disorders)

20. **A patient is suffering from sever facial pain and a nasopharyngeal tumour is present on the lateral wall of larynx. The patient is suffering from:** *(AIPG 09)*

Ans. Trotter's syndrome

21. **All are true for geniculate neuralgia, except:** *(AIPG 09)*
    a. Pain in ear, soft plate
    b. Follows herpes zoster infection
    c. Follows traumatic surgery/procedure
    d. Treatment is by acyclovir and corticosteroid

Ans. c

22. **Drug used in the treatment of TN is:** *(AIPG 09)*

Ans. Carbamazepine

23. **Geniculate neuralgia is associated with which cranial nerve?** *(AIIMS Nov. 10)*

Ans. Facial (Ref: Burkitt 10/e p329)

24. **In jaw winking syndrome, there is:** *(AIPG 09)*

Ans. Unilateral ptosis (Ref: Shafer 5/e p1177)

25. **Raw beefy tongue is seen in deficiency of:** *(AIPG 10)*

Ans. Niacin

26. **Melanin pigmentation of seen-exposed skin of face and neck, which is strongly associated with pregnancy and use of oral contraception, is called:**

Ans. Melasma (Ref: Lanigan, Zohra, Zaidi p311)

27. **The deficiency of which of the following affects tooth development?** *(AIPG 11)*

Ans. Vitamin A (Also Vitamin C and Vitamin D)

Vitamin A	Vitamin C	Vitamin D
↓	↓	↓
Epithelial cell growth	Collagen formation	Calcification

28. **Burning tongue might NOT be associated with?** *(AIIMS Nov 09)*
    a. Ranula
    b. Diabetes mellitus
    c. Local irritation
    d. Pernicious anaemia

Ans. a (Ref: Shafer 5/e p1168)

29. **A patient had a tooth reimplanted following trauma few years back X-ray analysis reveals roots fused to alveolar bone. When the tooth is percussed, a high pitched sound is heard. The tooth involved is showing signs of:** *(AIPG 12)*

Ans. Ankylosis (Ref: Cohen 8/e p624)

30. **A 9 year-old child's mother comes to a dental clinic with the complaint of oral ulceration, fever and shedding of skin of palm and soles. She is giving a history of premature exfoliation of teeth, increased sweating and breathing. Also, she gave a history of using a new teething gel for past one month the child is suffering from:** *(AIIMS Nov 10)*

Ans. Acrodynia (Ref: Shafer 4/e p578-579)

31. **Acrodynia occurs due to:** *(PGI June 10)*

Ans. Exposure of minute amount of Hg (Ref: Shafer 6/e p556)

32. **During parotid gland surgery, injury to auriculotemporal nerve leads to:** *(PGI June 10)*

Ans. Frey's syndrome (Ref: BD Chaurasia Vol. 3; 4/e p137)

CHAPTER

Radiology

Topic

- General Radiology
- Diagnosis

GENERAL RADIOLOGY

- Production of X-ray:

Brehmstalung	Characteristic Radiation
(Major)	
Direct hit / near miss	

- Interaction of X-ray with matter (KCET 05):

Comptom scattering	Photo electric emission	Coherent
(62%) (KCET 12)	(30%)	(8%)

- Pb apron us 98% of total gonadal exposure
- Particulate radiation have high LET so, more damaging biologically .
- X-ray has low LET – So, less damaging
- Maximum exposure to natural radiation is by RADON [Q]
- Radiation Exposure:

Bone scan > CT scan > X–ray (But MRI given in option, then it is the answer) *(AIIMS May 10)*

- Thyroid dose form OPG = 0.074 mGy [Q]
- Comparison of Deterministic and Stochastic effects of radiation (Very important and conceptual topic):

	Deterministic effects	**Stochastic effects**
Examples	• Mucositis (radiation induced) • Radiation induced cataract	• Radiation induced Cancer (Somatic effect) • Heritable effects
Caused by	Killing of many cells	Sublethal damage to DNA

Threshold dose?	Yes Sufficient cell killing required to cause a clinical response	No even 1 photon could cause a change in DNA ↙ ↘ Cancer Heritable changes
Security of clinical effects and dose	directly to dose(COMEDK-11)	Independent of Dose "All / None law" ↓ Patient either has / does Not have it.
Probability of having effect and dose	Independent of dose dose > Threshold All individuals show effect	Directly to dose ↑sed Dose ↓ ↑sed chance of having disease

- Cells are most sensitive to radiation in G_1 and Early 'S' Phase (KCET 09-12)
- Both arms of chromosome are affected
- Most radio resistant in S-Phase
- Effects of Radiation on oral tissue:

Mucositis – Developes after "2 weeks" of radiation therapy • Healing completed after "2 months" of therapy • Later the oral mucous membrane becomes Atrophic (COMEDK 09)
Salivary Gland • 60 mGy Xerostomia develops [Q] • Taste Loss – Reversible – recovery 60 to 120 days
Alopecia: develops when 3–4 weeks on 4Gy on scalp
Life Long threat: Hyposalivation • Radiation caries Occurs 3 months after expose (PG1) • Trismus • Osteoradionecrosis > 70 Gy
Acute radiation syndrome 2–7Gy – Haematopoetic injury [Q] 7–15 Gy – Injury > 50 Gy – CVS / CNS
Effect of radiation on Dental pulp – Fibro atrophic change [Q] Not Necrotic

- **Osteoradionecrosis:**

Caused by endarteritis of blood vessels (AIIMS Nov. 11)
Note: lues glossitis/syphilitic glossitis is also caused by same etiology

- Prevention of radiation caries – Apply 1% neutral NaF
- In radiotherapy Dose of radiation should be in fraction Dose:

2–10–64–70 Gy
2Gy is delivered daily, for a weekly exposure of 10 gy . this continues typically for 6-7 weeks until a total dose of 64 to 70 Gy is administered

- Brachytherapy:
- Rd, Id – 125, Cs, Ir, Au used
- P-32, Strontium -89, Samarium-153, (NOT iridium -192) are used in systermic radionucluide (AIPG-06)
- P-32 emits B-rays (AIPG -06)
- Average of X-ray used in dentistry – 0.6 to 1A°
- Average of photon used in dental radiography – 0.1 to 10^{-3}nm
- Al fitter – 1.5 mm for 70 KVP (for Total filtration)
  (Average of 0.5 to 2 mm) – Inherent filtration
- Collimation (Pb used) – to a circle of 7 cm / 2.75 inches
- Density of radiograph:

$\frac{mA \times KVP}{Fsfb \times filtration \times collimation}$
$= (Fsfd)^2$

- T (Exposure time):

$\frac{(Fsfd)^{\wedge}2}{KVp \times mA}$

- Useful range of Dental X-ray – 0.3 to 2
- **Units** (Dosimetry) (Very important):

1st	exposure	SI unit	conventional
		C/kg or Air kerma	Roentgen
2nd	Absorption	Absorption *(COMEDK 09)*	Rad
3rd	Equivalent / Effective dose **Note:** effective dose is used to compare effects of Different Types of radiation on tissue [Q]	Sv *(PGI june)*	Rem *(KCET 11)*
	Radioactivity	Bacqueral (SI) *(AIPG 07)*	Curie (Conventional)

- 1 Gy = 100 rads
- 1 Sv = 100 rem
- Quantity of X–ray (Dose) $(KVp)^2$
- Defination and Detail

Describe Image "Sharpness"
Increases as focal spot size reduces

- Optical density:

Greatest diagnostic value of film – 0.6–3
Gross fog / Base plus fog (minimal density of an unexposed film)
Inherent – 0.2 –0.3

- Concept:

• For better detection of an early lesion (Incipient carries lording surface of cortex) use: • Low KVp • Low mA • Low exposure time

- "CT Scan" – CT number ranges from – 1000 to +1000:

– 1000 = air
0 = water
+ 1000 = bone (Dense)
CT number is called "Housefield number"

- Collimation dose not se density but improves image quality by reducing 2° radiation reaching the film. It ↓ ces size of X-ray and ↓ ces exposure [Q]
- Filteration – ↓ ces patient exposure without loss of any information
- In children exposure 50% of adult
- Film Badges should be worm by dental technician "Every month"
- In comparison to 'E' film Rectangular collimation ces the risk of exposure.
- 3 inherent qualities of radiograph are:

• Definition
• Contrast
• Density *(AIPG 08)*

- KVp has direct relation with contrast i.e.
- High KVp *(AIIMS May 12)*
  ↓
- Low contrast
- to view a thick hyper calcified bone – se KVP [Q]
- An ideal radiograph should have optimal density and Contrast and minimum Distortion *(AIIMS 05)*
- Density / Overall darkening of a radiograph depends on: *(AIIMS 06)*

• Thickness of object
• The quality and Quantity of X-rays
• Velocity of e^- emitted from the cathode

- **Note:**

Consistent radiograph requires constant mA and KVp
But is maintained by automatic processing *(AIIMS 07)*

- Contrast on a radiograph demonstrates range of densities *(AIIMS 07)*
- Exposure and Film (NBDE Q):

Film–	A	B	C	D	E
Exposure–	1R	½	¼	1/8	1/16

- **Film:**

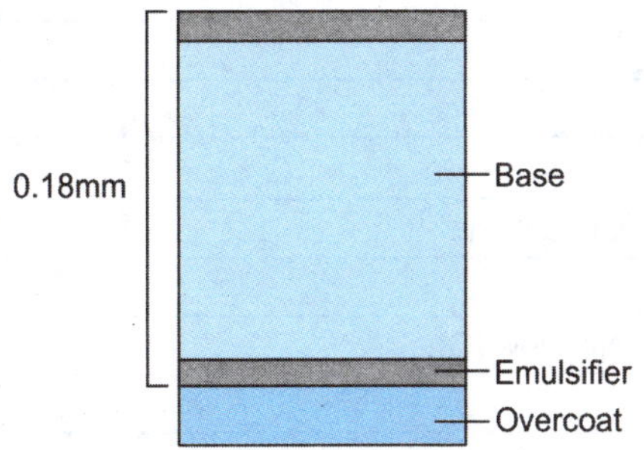

Fig. 9.1: Film

- Iodide crystals added to Ultraspeed (D–films) films Not insight:

• It has tabular large crystal requires only ½ exposure of ultraspeed
• E and F films are insight films

- Intensifying Screen: (↓ ses patient exposure) *(AIIMS 06) (AIPG 08)*

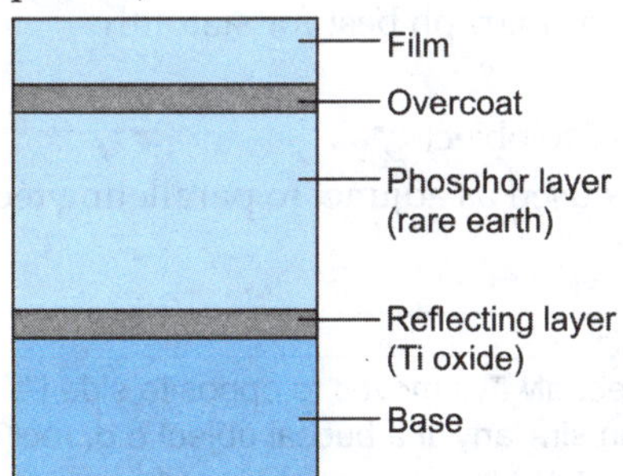

Fig. 9.2: Intensifying screen

- **Radiation induced caries:** 3 types

• Most common type – Superficial lesion involving all tooth surfaces *(COMEDK 09)*
• Cervical lesion
• Dark pigmentation of entire crown

- Radiation exposure (DOSE LIMIT):

Occupational – 5 rem / yr
Non – occupational – 0.5 rem/yr Or (10 mR /week)

- IOPA with minimum SKIN exposure of 100–600 mR (NBDE Q)
- Compared to round collimation, rectangular collimation ↓ces exposure by 60% *(COMEDK 10)*
- Grid is kept between patient and film to ↓ce scattered radiation
- Grid has a disadvantage of increased exposure time *(AIIMS 07, 05, KCET 10)*
- **FILMS of choice:**

Routinely used for caries detection – "E" Recommended for caries detection – "F"
Best for caries detection – "D"

- **Size of films:**

Size 0 – 22 x 35 – 1° dentition
Size 1 – 24 x 40 – Anterior
Size 2 – 31 x 41 – Adult *(KCET 10)*
Note: Size 1 and 2 is used transitional dentition
57 x 76 mm film – occlusal view
8 x10 inch – lateral cephalograms, PNS view [Q]
6 x12 inch – OPG [Q]
1.5 x 7 inch – TMJ + lateral oblique view

- X-ray films are insensitive to yellow/Red Light
- Focal spot:

Actual 1x 3 mm
Effective 1x 1 mm

- Reversal of lead foil on X-ray film: Herring bone / Embossed Tram track pattern
- Cross sectional mandibular occlusal radiograph best for sialolith
- Fore shortening occurs when:
- X-ray perpendicular to film but NOT to object
- Long cone open cylinder technique is used as adjunct to paralleling technique to prevent Elongation of image / Magnification (NBDE Q) *(AIIMS 07, 05, AIPG 10, 08, 07)*
- **Concept:**

According to SLOB rule BUCCAL object always moves to opposite side i.e. if on mesial projection object moves distally vice versa with distal projection similarly, if a buccal object e.g. root of a tooth moves to distal side on projection, then it is projected form mesial side. *(AIIMS Nov. 11) (AIPE 09 , 08)*

- In OPG patient cross infection is prevented by using Disposable bite block while Digital sensor is covered by Impervious barrier
- OPG:

Nearer to focal trough

- Reduced and blurred.
- Interaction of photon with matter:

• Direct effect	• Indirect effect
Contributes to 1/3rd of effect	Contributes to 2/3rd of effect as 70% of body weight is H2O
Target action theory	Poison chemical theory.

- Discovery:

Xeroradiography:- Discovered by Carlson [Q]
OPG– Hudson, Dickson, Kampula

- Gray Scale:

Long gray scale	Short gray scale
Low contrast	High contrast

- Fixing time = 2x developing time
- ↑ sing order of λ:

Cosmic ray < x-ray < γ-ray < UV ray < VR < IR < Microwave < Radio wave ↓ Ionizing radiation – used in "COLD" sterilization
Particulate radiation – α, β, Cathode rays
MRI is non ionizing in nature *(AIIMS 07)*

- Ionizing power (Damaging Power):

α/He > β-Particle > X-ray > r-ray *(AIPG 06)*
Penetration power – Reverse order of Ionizing power

- Methods of heat dissipation from target:

• Keeping target inclined at 20°
• Rotating anode.

- Dosimeter:

• Film badges
• Thermolluminiscent dosimetry
• Ionization chamber – Best method *(COMEDK 08) (KCET 09)*

- During production of X-ray, 90% electron energy is converted into heat *(COMEDK 09)*
- Long Wavelength of X-ray most likely to cause harm to patient's body *(AIIMS Nov. 11)*
- Sensitivity of different cells to radiation:

Cells of spermatogenic, erythoblastic and basal cells of oral mucous membrane are most Radiosensitive
Note: RBC, muscle cells and nerve cells are least sensitive *(AIPG 10, 12, COMEDK 11)*

- Vegetative intermitotic cells – most radio sensitive
  ↓
  spermatogenic cell, erythroblast
- Fixed post mitotic cells – Most radio resistant
  ↓
- Muscle, nerve, RBC, Optic lens
- Radio sensitivity of organs:

High – Lymphoid organs, Bone marrow, testis, Intestine, mucous membrane

- Foreshortening and elongation of image:

If +ve angle ↑ sed (Vertical) ↓ Fore shortening of image
If –ve angle ↑ sed (vertical) ↓ Elongation of image

- Susceptibility of different organ to radiation induced cancer:

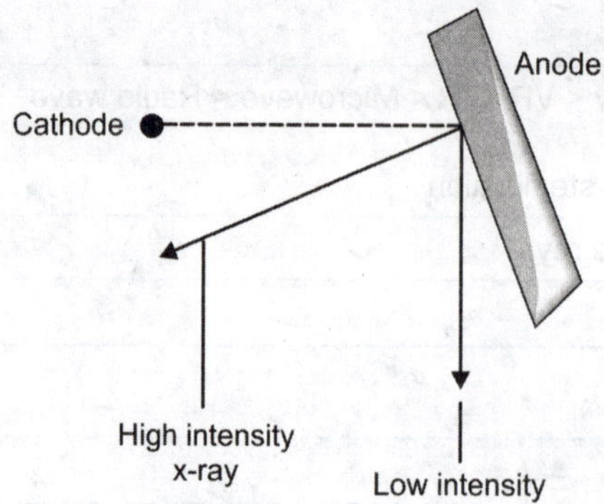

Fig. 9.3: Half valve layer (HVL)

• Measures the quality of X-ray (NBDE)
• It is the thickness of absorber like Al required of reduce X-ray photon of half.
• At tube voltage of 30 to 70 Kvp HVL is 1.5 mm of Al.

- Most radiosensitive organs of body heel effect:

When cathode ray strikes anode target X-rays with high intensity are found towards cathode side of central ray. While low intensity X-ray are found towards anode.

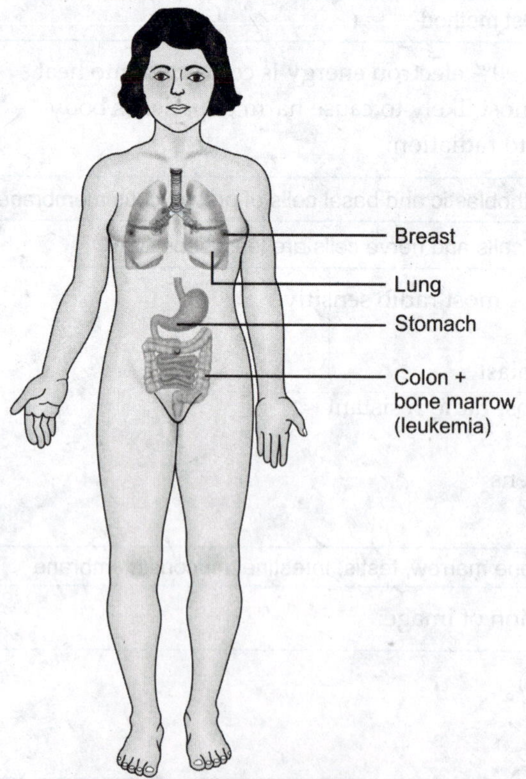

Fig. 9.4: Most radiosensitive organs of body

So, No more than 20° angulations of target anode should be present

- **Best method for radiation protection of OPERATOR Stand behind lead barrier** *(COMEDK 09)*

If not available then next best is "Position distance rule"

- **According to ICRP occupational radiation dose units (yearly limits) are:**

50 msv / year and 100 msv in 5 year	*(COMEDK 10)*

- Developer: used at 72°F for 4 min. for every rise of 2°F developing time is use by ½ min washing is running water for 10 min.
- Components of Developer: (Trick = DAPR)

Developer →	Phenidione, Hydroquinone "ENOL" ↓ Ist e^- donor (initiator) [Q] Amplifeis latent image converts Ag X crystals to metallic Ag.
Activator/Alkalizer →	Sodium/Potassium Hydroxide maintain alkaline pH also cause gelatin to swell for developer to diffuse.
Preservative →	Sodium sulfite prevents oxidation of developer
Restrainer →	Sodium / Potassium Bromide Reduces unexposed Ag X crystals ANTI FOG Agent [Q]

- Components of Fixer:

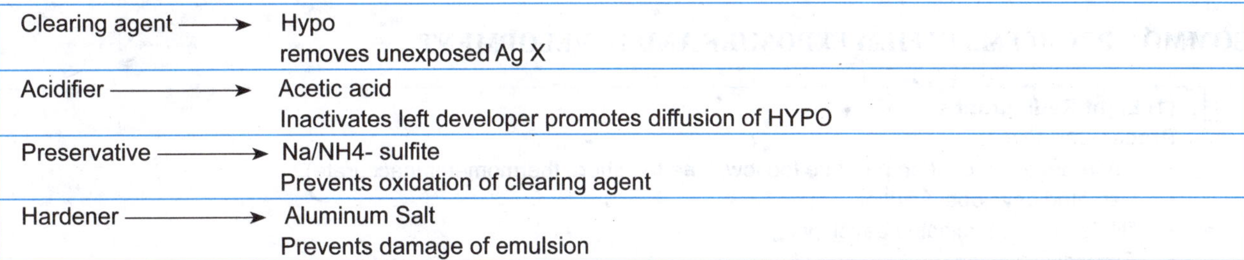

Clearing agent →	Hypo removes unexposed Ag X
Acidifier →	Acetic acid Inactivates left developer promotes diffusion of HYPO
Preservative →	Na/NH4- sulfite Prevents oxidation of clearing agent
Hardener →	Aluminum Salt Prevents damage of emulsion

- Angulations of PID in bisecting angle technique:

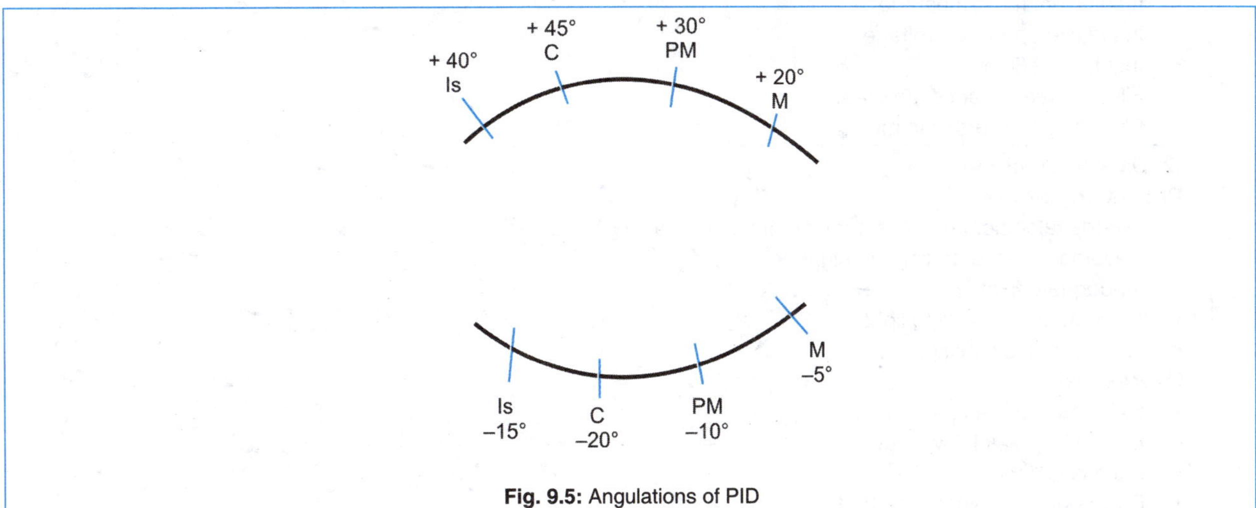

Fig. 9.5: Angulations of PID

(Trick – Start from molars and remember both U and L arch has canine with maximum value)

- In bitewing – Angulation is +10° i.e. 10 degree below horizontal [Q] (AIIMS may 10, 07, AIPG 10)
- Parallex / SLOB technique gives range of densities on a radiograph (AIIMS 07)
- RVG does not produce finer details than X-ray films (AIIMS 06)
- Safe light:

Dark room should have safe light with low intensity and long wavelength (red light)
safe light should be mounted in work area on wall behind the processing tank.
GBX-2 filter are recommended safe light should be mounted at least 4 feet above the processing tank *(AIPG 07)*

- OPG: Most Panaromic machine now use a continuously moving center of rotation rather than a multiple fixed location.
- Occlusal projection:

	Maxillary	**Mandibular**
Anterior occlusal	Tip of nose vertical angle – +45° Horizontal angle – 0°	Tip of chin
Cross sectional occlusal	Bridge of the nose Below nasion Vertical angle – +65°	3 cm below the tip of the chin Horizontal angle – 0°

- Nutrient Canal are commonly seen is mandibular anterior region
- Y line of Yennis:

In maxillary canine region floor of nasal fossa and maxillary sinus may cross over leading to an inverted Y shaped R/o line called Y-line of yennis.

COMMON PROBLEMS IN FILM EXPOSURE AND DEVELOPMENT

(1) Light Radiographs **Processing Errors** • Underdevelopment (temperature too low, time too short, thermometer inaccurate) • Depleted developer solution • Diluted or contaminated developer • Excessive fixation **Underexposure** • Insufficient milli amperage • Insufficient peak kilovoltage • Insufficient time • Film-source distance too great • Film packet reversed in mouth
(2) Dark Radiographs **Processing Errors** • Overdevelopment (temperature too high, time to long) • Developer concentration too high • Inadequate fixation • Accidental exposure to light • improper safe lighting **Overexposure** • Excessive milli amperage • Excessive peak kilovoltage • Excessive time • Film-source distance too short

(3) **Insufficient contrast** • Underdevelopment • Underexposure • Excessive peak kilovoltage • Excessive film fog
(4) **Film Fog** • Improper safe lighting (Improper filter, excessive bulb wattage inadequate distance between safelight and work surface, prolonged exposure to safelight) • Light leaks (cracked safelight filters, light form doors, vents, or other sources) • Over development • Contaminated solutions • Deteriorated film (stored at high temperature, stored at high humidity, exposed to radiation, outdated)
(5) **Dark spots or lines** • Fingerprint contamination • Black wrapping paper sticking to film surface • Film in contact with tank or another film during fixation • Film contaminated with developer before processing • Excessive bending of film • Static discharge to film before processing • Excessive roller pressure during automatic processing dirty rollers in automatic processing.
(6) **Light Spots** • Film contaminated with fixer before processing • Film in contact with tank or another film during development • Excessive bending of film
(7) **Yellow or Brown Stains** • Depleted developer • Depleted fixer • Insufficient washing • Contaminated solutions
(8) **Blurring** • Movement of patient • Movement of X-ray tube head • Double exposure
(9) **Partial images** • Top of film not immersed in developing solution • Misalignment of X-ray tube head ("Cone cut")
(10) **Emulsion peel** • Abrasion of image during processing • Excessive time in wash water

LAST 5-YEAR QUESTIONS FROM THIS TOPIC

1. **As compared to the conventional method by using RVG, the exposure time:** *(AIIMS May 11)*

Ans. Is reduced to 1/5th at least (Ref: Ghom, Textbook of oral radiology I/e p82-84)

2. **Bisecting angle technique is based on:** *(AIPG 09, AIIMS 11, KCET 11)*

Ans. Cieszynski's rule of isometry (Ref: white and pharoh 5/e p125)

3. **Moth eaten appearance is seen in all except:** *(AIIMS Nov. 10)*
   a. Osteomyelitis
   b. Haemorrhageic cyst
   c. Osteosarcoma

d. OKC

Ans. d (Ref: White and Pharaoch 5/e p405)

4. In OPG, cross infection is bests prevented by? *(AIIMS Nov. 09)*

Ans. Disposable bite block (Ref: White and Pharoh 5/e)

5. Difference between digital and conventional radiograph is that: *(AIIMS May 09)*

Ans. A sensor is used in digital radiography (Ref: white and Pharaoh 5/e p57, 282)

6. In radiology, the latent period is the time period between: *(AIPG 10)*

Ans. Exposure to radiation and development of radiation induced pathology

Note: If latent image period is asked then it is exposure of film and development of image.

7. Following exposure, the X-rays interact with patient tissues within: *(KCET 11)*

Ans. 10^{-13} sec (Ref: Oral Radiology principles and interpretation white and Pharoach p25)

8. "Penny test" is the quality assurance test to detect: *(KCET 11)*

Ans. Unsafe illumination (Ref: Oral radiology Principles and Interpretation white and Pharoah, p112)

9. Compared with calcium tungstate screens, rare earth screens decrease patient exposure by about: *(COMEDK 11)*

Ans. 55% (Oral radiology by white and Pharoh 5/e p57)

10. Which of the following interactions does not cause film fog? *(COMEDK 11)*

a. Coherent scattering

b. Transient scattering

c. Photoelectric absorption

d. Compton scattering

Ans. c (Ref: Textbook oral radiology by white and Pharoh 5/e p17)

11. Cervical burnout is a phenomenon caused by decreased X-ray absorption region of: *(COMEDK 09)*

Ans. Normal teeth (Ref: Oral radiology by white and pharoh 5/e p166)

12. Which of the following is false? *(COMEDK 10)*

a. Tungsten target is set in a copper block

b. Dental X-ray tube is self rectified

c. Filtration reduces the exposure time

d. Grid reduces the secondary radiation reaching the film

Ans. c

13. Brachytherapy means? *(COMEDK 10)*

Ans. Radiation administered interstially through catheters

14. Which of the following does have no effect on response of cells to irradiation? *(COMEDK 10)*

a. LET

b. O_2

c. Image receptor used

d. Dose rate

Ans. c

15. Radiation induced Xerostomia would cause dental caries inL *(PGI Dec. 11)*

Ans. 3 months (Ref: Sturdvent 5/e p94)

16. Best X-ray view to see impacted right maxillary canine is: *(PGI Dec. 11)*

Ans. IOPA X-ray with tube shift (Ref: Samir bishara impacted, canines and textbook of oral radiology by GHOM P185)

17. In maxillary 2nd molar, radiograph, the radiopaque structure that obliterate the PDL is:

Ans. Zygomatic process (Ref: Endodontics by Ingles 5/e p363)

18. Cathode in X-ray tube is made up of:

Ans. Mo (Ref: White and Pharoah 5/e p12)

19. Radiation exposure in digital RVG is reduced by? *(PGI June 11)*

Ans. 80% of normal (Ref: White and pharaoh 5/e p233)

20. What is the method of calculating mineral density of a tooth? *(PGI June 11)*

Ans. Autoradiography (Ref: Harrison 17/e p211)

21. If the amount of X-rays measured at a distance 2meters from X-ray source are 1 Gys, then the amount at a distance of 1 meters from source is?

Ans. 4 (Ref: white and pharaoh 5/e p16)

Note: $I_1 / I_2 = D_2^2 / D_1^2$

22. Most penetrating rays are: *(PGI Dec 09)*

Ans. Hard X-rays (Ref: White and Pharaoh 5/e p15, 16, 56-58, 60 and 149)

23. Which of the following is not a contrast radiography? *(PGI Dec. 09)*

a. Sialography
b. Single photon emission computer technology
c. Tomogram
d. Arthrogram

Ans. c (Ref: Vinod kapoor 2/e p368)

24. Pantograph is used to measure: *(PGI June 09)*

Ans. Jaw movements

25. Pantographic style uses how many style: *(PGI June 09)*

Ans. 6 (Ref: Nallaswamy 1/e p150)

DIAGNOSIS

- Osteoclastoma = Central giant cell Granuloma
- Odontoclastoma = pink tooth of mummery
- In fibrous dysplasia Inferior Alveolar canal is displaced Superiorly (UNIQUE)
- Cementoma= Periapical Osteofibroses
- Ossifying fibroma manifests as unilocular R/L (best answer) *(AIIMS 07, AIPG 10, 07)*

Normal follicular space → 3–4 mm
Cyst when > 5 mm / 1 cm
Granuloma when < 5 mm

- Non–vital teeth → periapical abscess, periapical cyst, periapical Granuloma, osteomyelitis
- Soap Bubble appearance:

Trick: AA CC OO

A → Ameloblastoma → A → ABC, C → Cherubism, C → Central giant cell granuloma, O → OKC, O → Odontogenic myxoma

- Ground glass appearance:

Brown tumor / hyper parathyroidism *(AIPG 11, 09)*
Monostotic fibrous dysplasia
cherubism

- Moth eaten appearance: *(AIPG 09, 07)*

Osteomyelitis (AIIMS 07), Osteoradionecrosis, Osteosarcoma, Burkett lymphoma, Regional odontodysplasia

- Hemangioma (Central) – Honey comb appearance of Ameloblastoma + Sun Burst appearance of Osteosarcoma
- Hypercementosis:

"Generalized" → seen in pagets disease [Q] and Hyperpituitarism Note: In trauma Hypercementosis present But not generalized		
Hypercementosis	**Cementoblastoma**	**Cementoma**
	• Periapical Osteofibroses • True cementoma	• Periapical cemental dysplasia (PCD)
Old age	Younger age <25 yrs.	30-50 yrs
	No FEMALE predilection	FEMALE > > > male(AIIMS 07) (9: 1) Like Sjogren syndrome Like sjogren syndrome
	Mandibular posterior	Mandibular anterior
	Causes root resorption	least likely to cause root Resorption
	R/f.: R/L R/O **Fig. 9.6:** Cementoblastoma Similar R/F seen in Odontoma	
Note: All 3 are associated with vital tooth but Cementoma is more common than cementoblastoma		

- Central giant cell granuloma.:

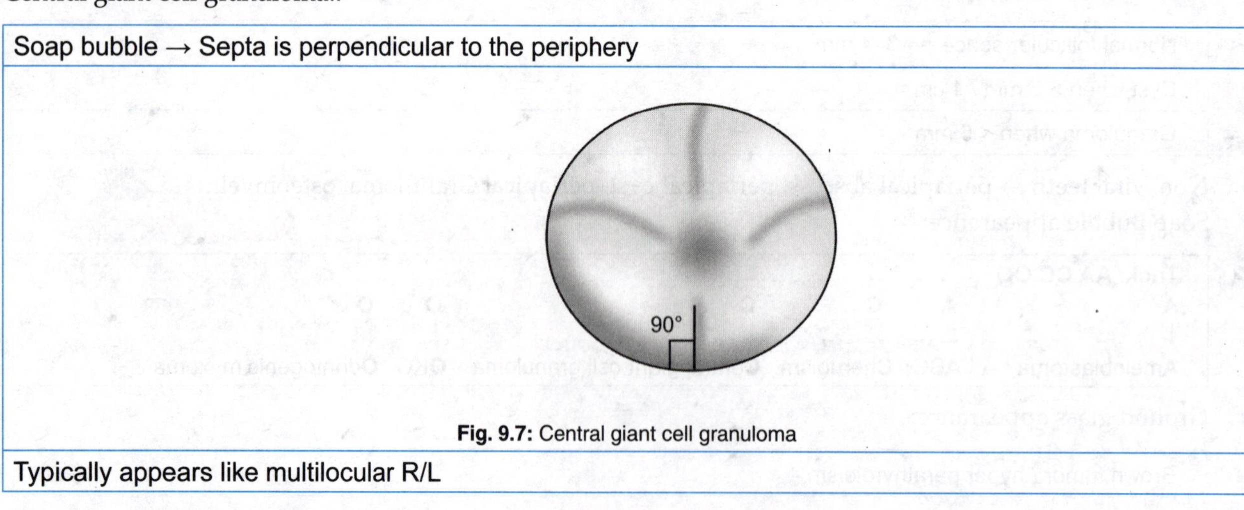

Soap bubble → Septa is perpendicular to the periphery

Fig. 9.7: Central giant cell granuloma

Typically appears like multilocular R/L

- Cherubism: R/F (Very important):

Bilateral Multilocular [Q]
↓
Mandibular Swelling *(AIIMS Nov. 09, Nov. 12)*

- Tennis Racket R/L:

Odontogenic myxoma [Q]

- Minimal dentinal destruction to get evident on radiography = 40 μ [Q]
- Cystein is the only R/O Stones
- Xanthine, Allopurinol, Orotic acid →R/L Stone
- **Osteoarthritis VS Rheumatoid Arthritis**

Osteoarthritis	Rheumatoid Arthritis
Joint deterioration and new bone Formation (Osteophyte [Q]	Sharpened pencil (erosive) [Q]
In severe cases Osteophyte break off and lies free in joint space (Joint MICE/Mouse) [Q]	"PANNUS formation" Inflammatory process results in abnormal proliferation of synovial tissue
	Pannus **Fig. 9.8:** Rheumatoid arthritis

R/O restoration	R/L restoration
Amalgam	Silicate
Gold	Composite
Stainless steel pins	Ca $(OH)_2$ (Note: Ca $(OH)_2$ with Ba salts is R/O)
ZnOE cement	Porcelain not fused with metal
$Zn_3(PO_4)_2$ cement	

- Fluoroscopy: [Q]

Real time radiography
Used to view dynamic movements

- **γ–camera + Respiratory gating**

γ–camera → used to measure radioactivity [Q] having large crystal detector called → "Scintillation Crystals"
Respiratory gating→ Used during radiotherapy to counter act the effect of tumor motion due to breathing. *(AIPG 05)*

- **Investigation of choice:**

Bone metastasis → Bone Scan
Spine metastasis → MRI (Also best for fibrous ankylosis)
Acute head injury → "CT"scan → Also best for bony ankylosis

- MRI:

T_2 weighted – Demonstrates pathological condition like inflammation of TMJ
T_1 Weighted – Shows normal osseous and discal tissues

- "Scintigraphy"→ 99 m T_c

Bone scintigraphy	Salivary gland scintigraphy
Osteomyelitis, Avascular necrosis, metastatic bone Lesion, condylar hyperplasia seen	Advantageous for condition in which sialography is contra indicated like acute salivary gland infection, During thyroid function test / Allergic to iodine
Functional defect	
Disadvantage–can't differentiate benign and malignant lesion	

- Sialography:

Best when sialolith is R/L
Various appearances: • Normally → Leafless tree [Q] limbs with bloom *(COMEDK 07)* • Sialodochitis (dilated obstructed duct due to recurrent infection) → Sausage link • Sialadenitis → pruning of tree • Tumor of Acini → Ball-in-hand

- USG:

Used in the head and neck region for evaluation of neoplasm of thyroid parathyroid, salivary gland (Sialolith + Sjogren Syndrome), vessels of neck including carotid artery
1° application of USG is differentiating between solid and cystic lesion

- Sialolith in Wharton's duct is viewed on "Gross sectional mandibular occlusal projection" *(AIPG 08)*
- Lateral cephalometry: has "Wider Latitude" low contrast film → so, both soft and hard tissue seen
- MRI best for articular disc. BUT in case of disc perforation and physiologic information of TMJ – Arthrography is the best
- CT scan gives more definitive picture of bone (e.g. as in osteomyelitis)
- Lateral skull is the best view for multiple myeloma
- Reverse town (Open mouth) → Improves visualization of condyles
- SMV → underexposed → View improves the zygomatic arches
- Transpharyngeal/ PARMA / Intracranial:

Used to view condylar # / Erosive changes
Depicts medial aspect of TMJ
Central ray directed through sigmoid notch [Q]

- Transcranial:

used to detect TMJ ankylosis + [Q] Gross osseous changes [Q] *(KCET 11)*
Depicts lateral aspect of TMJ

- Transorbital:

Zimmer projection
Very useful in viewing condylar neck #
depicts anteromedio-lateral aspect of TMJ

- Difference between cyst/benign and malignant lesion:

Cyst / benign odontogenic tumor	**Malignant odontogenic tumor**
Causes bodily displacement of tooth Not mobility	Causes bone destruction around teeth → Mobility (Trick **'M'** for **m**alignant **'M'** for **M**obility)
	In developing teeth it disrupts the crypt and displaces tooth in an occlusal direction → so, does not cause unerupted tooth

- **Note:** Both lesions cause root resorption
- **Grenz:**

Ultra soft X-ray
Used in treatment of Bowen's disease (Carcinoma in situ), Actinic keratosis, psoriasis, Eczema, Lichen planus, Histo-cytosis
Note: Hard X-ray used in diagnosis
Soft X-ray used for therapeutic purpose.

- Hypo plastic defect of enamel: thickness of enamel ced – R/L appearance on radiograph
- Digital image in computerized radiography is made up of pixels *(COMEDK 11, 09)*
- Actual size of a carious lesion is Deeper as compared to that seen on a radiograph *(AIPG 08)*
- Advantage of digital radiography over conventional radiography is that image can be stored in computer *(AIIMS 08)*
- R/O of zygoma superimposes on roots of Ist and 2nd molar Not 3rd Molar [Q]
- Technical aspects of extra oral radiographic projection:

1. Lateral ceph

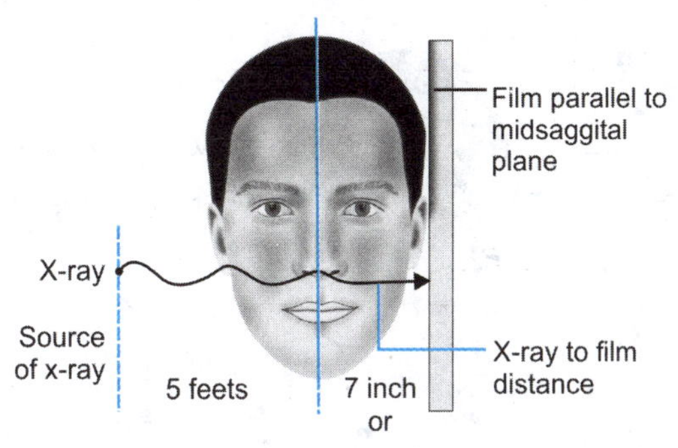

Fig. 9.9: Lateral ceph

Best view for: Nasal bone *(# Seen AIIMS May 10, 08, AIPG 07, 10)*
Frontal sinus
Sphenoidal sinus + gonial angle *(PGI-09, AIIMS-06, AIPG-08)*

7-12% enlargement / magnification considered normal

Note: Frontal sinus is best visualized by "Caldwell's view" [Q] i.e. Occipito-Frontal view

2. SMV / JUG handle view:

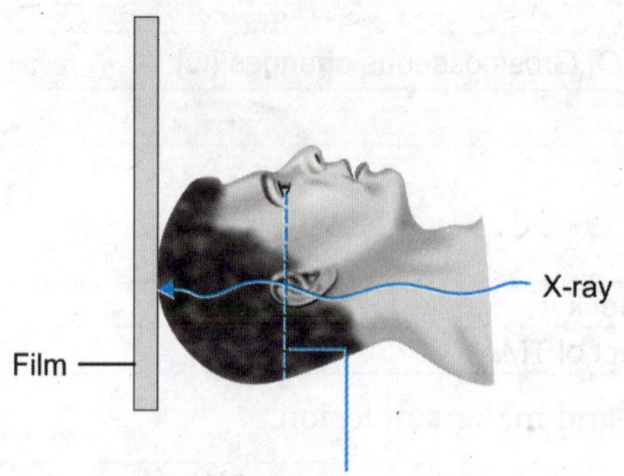

Fig. 9.10: SMV/JUG handle view

Best view for: Zygomatic arch, Sphenoidal sinus

Also used to show: Base of skull position and orientation of condyle *(AIPG 08, AIIMS May 09)*

3. Water's view / occipitomental view:

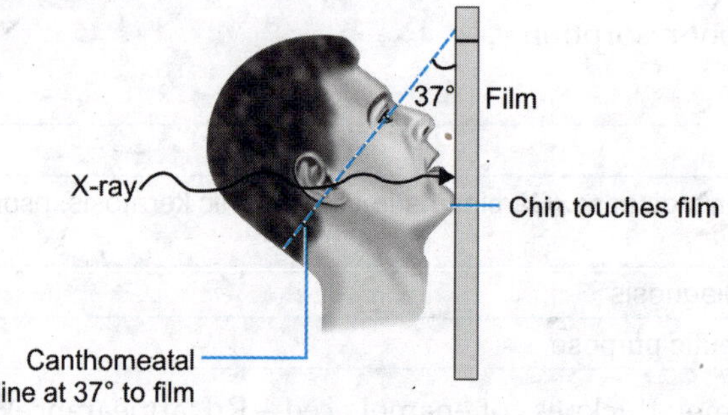

Fig. 9.11: Water's view/occipitomental view

Best view for: Maxillary #
Coronoid process *(PGI 12)*
Orbit
Zygoma
Maxillary sinus
Also useful in Nasal bone view

4. PA ceph:

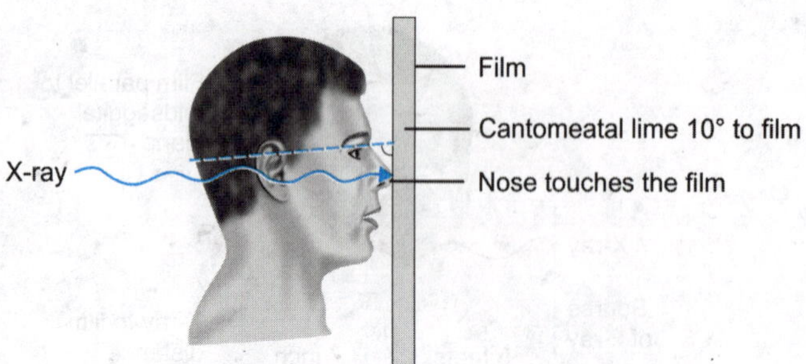

Fig. 9.12: PA ceph

Best view for: Orbit
Nasal cavity
Frontal sinus
Also used for coronoid process (Next but after waters view)\ Reverse town:

5. Reverse town:

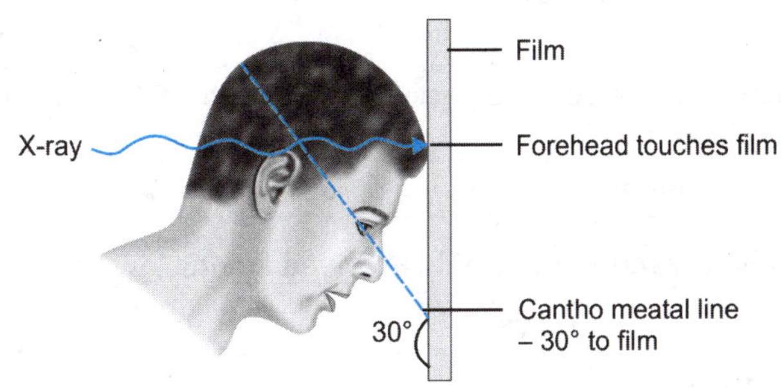

Fig. 9.13: Reverse town

Best view for: condylar neck condylar head

6. Oblique lateral (Body)

- Film touches check at molar region
- Central x-ray beam aims at molar-premolar region
- Best for mandibular body
- Used to view horizontally favorable and unfavorable # *(AIIMS 08, AIPG 10, 07)*

7. Oblique lateral ramus:

- Film touches cheek at Ramus area
- central beam aims the ramus area
- Best view for: Ramus, Coronoid process, Condylar neck

8. OPG:

- Used for all larger views best view for mandibular body, ramus, posterior maxilla

- Campbell line:

Seen on occipitomental /view *(AIIMS Nov. 10, May 10, 07, AIPG 10, 09, 07)*

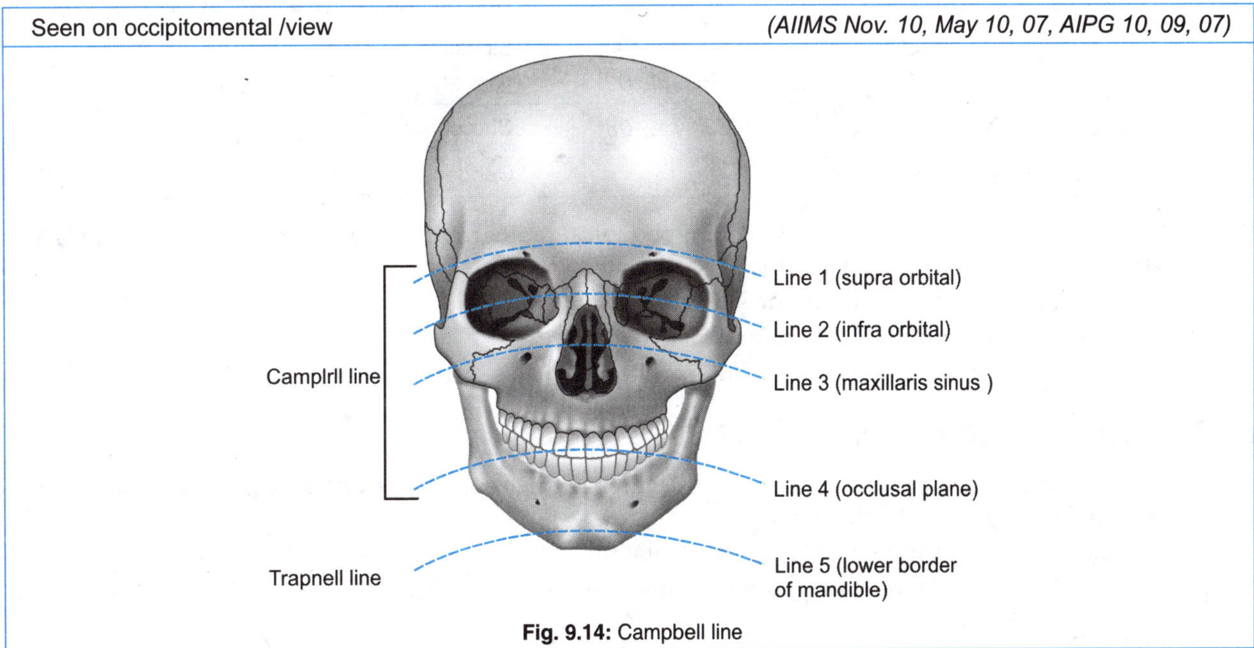

Fig. 9.14: Campbell line

- Tram line calcification of skull seen in Struge Weber syndrome / Trigeminal encephalo angiomatosis
- Occlusal radiography:

Used for locating supernumerary, unerupted, impacted teeth, foreign bodies, salivary duct stones, mesio lateral extent of disease #
Especially useful in patient with trismus

- In multiple myeloma mandible is more commonly involved among jaw bone but vertebrae are more commonly involved.

Radiographic feature	Condition
• Mirror image arch shaped Vertical bone loss	• LJP
• Regular periapical R/L < 1 cm	• Periapical granuloma
• Regular periapical R/L > 1cm	• Periapical cyst
• Irregular periapical R/L	• Periapical abscess
• Regular bordered multiple punched Out lesion *(AIIMS May 10, 07, 06, AIPG 07)*	• Multiple myeloma
• Irregular bordered multiple punched out lesion	• Eosinophilic granuloma
• Bulls eye R/f • Note: Bulls eye lesion seen in erythema multiformae *(AIIMS May 12)*	• Lingual impacted 3rd M
• Hollowing out of entire ramus up to condyle and Coronoid process	• Dentigerous cyst
• Driven snow appearance *(AIIMS 07)*	• CEOT / Pindborg tumor
• Crew cut / Hair on End appearance *(KCET 11)*	• Thalassaemia Sickle cell anemia *(AIIMS May 12, Nov. 08)* (go for this answer even if SCA is given)
• Fluid level and clouding *(AIIMS Nov. 08, AIPG 11, 09)*	• Sinusitis
• Floating teeth *(AIIMS Nov. 08)*	• Cherubism
• R/O at apex of carious molar	• Condensing osteitis

- Lingual developmental groove on an intra oral periapical radiograph is seen as small pulp chamber size, with constriction of the canal as compared to the contra lateral tooth. *(AIIMS 06)*
- Chloromas → Leukemic cells infiltrating skin etc
- Pumping action → typical feature of central Hemangioma
- Radiant faces (Chipmunk faces) + Intracellular inclusion bodies seen in thalassaemia

LAST 5-YEAR QUESTIONS FROM THIS TOPIC

1. If a histological slide of the tooth and the content of its canal space could be obtained, the most likely finding in the region of R/L would be: *(AIIMS May 11)*

Ans. Normal pulp (Ref: Frommer radiology in dental practice, 2004, p243, 248, 253)

2. On x-ray, which of the following can be found most accurately? *(AIIMS May 11, AIPG 11, 09)*

a. Acute pulpitis
b. Periapical granuloma

c. Mental foramen

d. Cementoma

Ans. c (Ref: White and pharaoh 6/e p166, 326, 433)

3. Suitable technique used for diagnosis of posterior interproximal caries in children is: *(AIIMS Nov. 10)*

Ans. Bitewing with RVG

4. What percentage of enamel demineralization should be present for early detection on a radiograph? *(AIIMS Nov. 10, COMEDK 11, 10)*

Ans. 40% (Ref: Ongole and Praveen, Oral diagnosis and radiology p108)

5. Radiological appearance seen in paget's disease is? *(AIIMS May 10, 07)*

Ans. Cotton wool appearance (Ref: Shafer 5/e p1005)

6. Investigation of choice for a lesion of the temporal bone is: *(AIIMS May 09)*

Ans. CT scan (Ref: Burkets, oral medicine 10th ed. P40)

7. Intra oral sensor of RVG is kept infection free by (AIIMS may 09)

Ans. Using an impervious barrier (Ref: white and pharaoh 5/e p118)

8. Fibrous dysplasia is associated with: *(AIIMS May 09)*

Ans. Ground glass appearance (Ref: white and pharaoh 5/e p290-91, 533, 520)

9. Radiographic examination of a child revealed several missing 1° and permanent teeth no teeth had been extracted. The history indicated practically no perspiration during hot summer months. These factors would lead to a preliminary diagnosis of: *(AIIMS May 09)*

Ans. Ectodermal dysplasia (Ref: White and Pharaoh 5/e p333, 334, 646)

10. Vertical R/L line seen between maxillary left central incisor and lateral incisor is: *(AIIMS Nov. 08)*

Ans. A nutrient canal (incomplete question from NBDE)

11. Radio graphically, a tooth of a young patient shows periapical R/O. The tooth also has deep carious lesion. The diagnosis is: *(AIIMS Nov. 08)*

Ans. Apical condensing osteitis (Ref: Burket's oral medicine. Diagnosis and Treatment 10/e.)

12. R/O is least seen in: *(AIIMS Nov. 08)*

a. Odontoma

b. Periodontal abscess

c. Chronic periodontitis

d. Cementoma

Ans. b (Ref: White and Pharaoh 5/e p322, 424, 425)

13. In a 18 yr old patient, multiseptate radiolucencies seen from 36 to 44, teeth are vital then the diagnosis is: *(AIIMS Nov. 11)*

Ans. Central giant cell granuloma (Ref: Shafer's 5/e p187-188)

14. Effect of X-ray on living cell by: *(AIIMS Nov.11)*

Ans. Ionization (Ref: White and Pharoh 6th ed. P18)

15. Radiation effect blood supply because of: *(AIIMS Nov. 11)*

Ans. Endarteritis of small blood vessels (Ref-white and Pharoh 6th ed. P25-26)

16. A dye injected into space to see the joint is known as: *(AIIMS Nov. 11, Nov. 12)*

Ans. Arthrography (Ref: Oral and Maxillofacial surgery by SM bhalaji P459)

17. CBCT is most useful is diagnosis and treatment planning of which malocclusion? *(AIIMS Nov. 11)*

Ans. B/L impacted maxillary canine (Ref: Different diagnostic tools for the localization of impacted maxillary canines: Clinical consideration by: Rossella maverna, Antonio Gracco) (Department of orthodontics, university of Ferrara director: Prof. G. Sicilliani) p28 to 37)

18. In a 35 year old man there is a recently developing class III malocclusion, there is a bony mass seen protruding towards lateral pterygoid on panorex, condition is: *(AIIMS Nov. 12, 11)*

Ans. Osteochondroma (Ref: White and Pharoh 5/e p550, 443, 444)

19. Radiographically level of normal alveolar crest is related to: *(AIPG 09)*
Ans. CEJ
20. On radiograph, irregularities were found on the roots of lower incisors. It may be: *(AIPG 09)*
Ans. Subgingival calculus
22. Radiograph alone can diagnose: *(AIPG 09)*
a. Periodontal pocket
b. Periodontal abscess
c. Anatomic root length
d. Bifurcation involvement
Ans. c
23. On the radiograph, the mesial site of mandibular Ist M revealed bone loss of 2-3 mm. One probing 6 mm pocket was revealed. The discrepancy could be due to: *(AIPG 09)*
Ans. Superimposition of bone remaining on facial and lingual surfaces (Ref: Dental radiography by haring–Jansen 2nd ed. P490)
24. CBCT, the latest diagnostic aid, stands for: *(AIPG 12)*
Ans. Cone bone CT
25. Hanging drop appearance in maxillary sinus when viewed on a radiograph is suggestive of: *(AIPG 12)*
Ans. Blow out of orbit (Ref: Brit J. opthal. (1970, 54, 90)
26. Osteoradionecrosis is: *(AIPG 12)*
Ans. Radiation trauma infection
27. Which of the following is considered as best imaging modality for detecting sequestra in osteomyelitis: *(COMEDK 10)*
Ans. CT
28. Which one of the following associated with periodontal disease may not be imaged on radiograph? *(COMEDK 09)*
a. Open contacts
b. Calculus
c. Bacterial plaque
d. Overhanging restorative
Ans. c
29. The Articular disc of TMJ can be best visualized through: *(PGI June 09)*
Ans. MRI (Ref: white and pharoh 5/e p549)
30. Cervical burn out phenomenon which occur in relation to the mandibular 2nd molar is due to: *(PGI June 09)*
Ans. Less thickness of enamel (Ref: White and Pharoh 5/e p166)
31. The most radiopaque out of the following is: *(PGI June 09)*
a. Enamel
b. dentine
c. Cementum
d. Amalgam
Ans. d
32. The exposure time in case of digital radiography the total dose of radiation is: *(PGI June 09)*
Ans. Less than ordinary X-ray (Ref: white and pharoh 5/e p225)
33. Appearance of a semicircular white area on radiograph is termed as: *(PGI June 09)*
Ans. Cone cutting (Ref. white and pharoh 5/e p107)

CHAPTER

10 Oral and General Surgery

Topic

- Local and General Anesthesia
- Emergency and It's Management
- Trauma and It's Management
- Exodontia
- Infection
- Cyst and Tumor
- TMJ
- Miscellaneous

- Words of wisdom: [*One of the most important subject in any MDS entrance exam*]

LOCAL AND GENERAL ANESTHESIA

- They are acidic salts of weak bases (can also be mentioned as WEAK BASES in the question)
- RNH+ ⟷ RN + H+

  RNH+ ↓ LA exists in this form; RN + H+ ↓ Active form
- LA does not act in acidic medium due to sed concentration of cationic form. *(AIPG 2011/2009 Q)*
- Structure of nerve and site of action of LA [Q]:

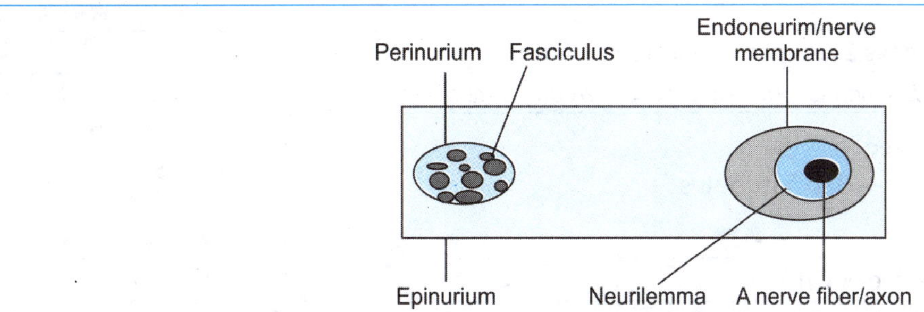

Fig. 10.1: Structure of a nerve

The actual site of action of LA is at endoneurium/nerve membrane[Q]
The most outer covering of nerve fibres is- perineurium *(AIIMS NOV 2006)*
IF the questn asks about the outer covering of A NERVE FIBRE – Ans should be neurilemma or, endoneurium.

- NaIon channel and action of LA:

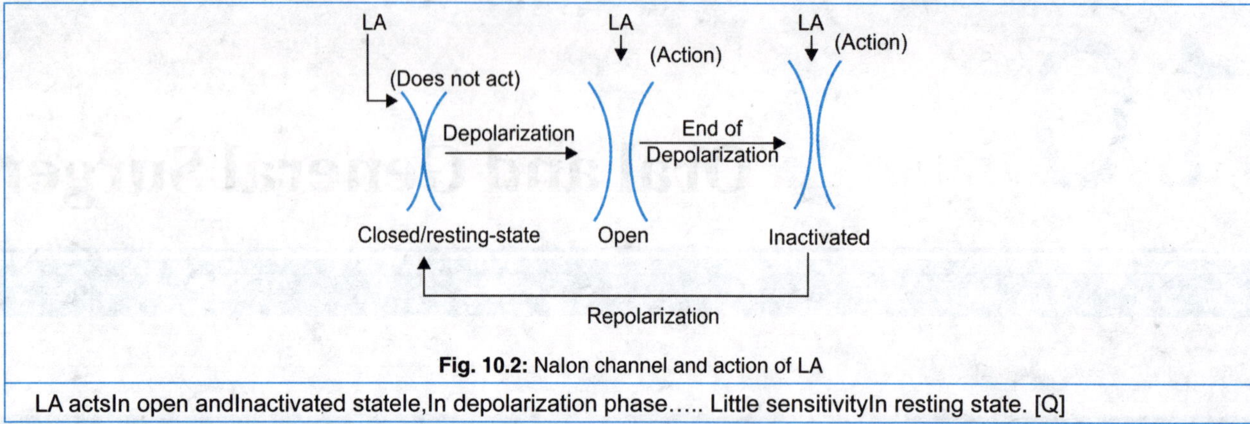

Fig. 10.2: NaIon channel and action of LA

LA actsIn open andInactivated statele,In depolarization phase….. Little sensitivityIn resting state. [Q]

- Order of duration of action of LA:

Etidocaine > Bupivacaine [Q] > tetracaine
Bupivacaine is preferredIn prolonged surgical procedure. *(KCET 2013)*

- Requirement of LA:

• LA without vasoconstrictorIn adult- 300 mg OR 4.4 mg/kgwt
• LA without adrenalineIn children- 1.4 mg/kgwt *(KCET 2012 ques)*
• LA with adrenalineIn adult – 500 mg OR 7 mg/kgwt *(AIIMS May 2012 med.)*
• LA with adrenalineIn children- 4.4 mg/kgwt

- requirement adrenaline with LA:

For normal patient 0.2 mg
For patient with heart problem 0.04mg [Q]
(Requirement of adrenalineIn ANAPHYLAXIS is 0.5 mgIn 1: 1000I.m) *(KCET and COMEDK 2013 Q)*

- Numerical on LA: (Points to remember)

• 2% lignocaine solution means 2 gm lignocaineIn 100 ml of solution
• 1: 2,00,000 adrenalineIn LA means 1 gm adrenalineIn 2,00,000 ml of LA solution

- Rate of LAInjection --- 0.1 ml/sec
- Onset of action of LIDOCAINE--- 3 to 5 minutes
- In haemophillics: W

Both field block and Nerve block C/I
Preferred LA for HAEMOPHILLICS:Intraligamentry

- Intrapulpal LA is the last resort. *(AIPG 2010 Q)*
- Nerve fibers and LA. *(A Very important topicIn NEET)*

• A –α is the largest diameter, myelinated fiber with fastest nerve conduction velocity. It providesInervation of motor function of skeletal muscle. *(AIIMS 2010 Q)*

- Pain is carried ONLY by "C and Aδ "fibers. Thus,If question is asked "fastest pain conductance among Aα, Aβ, Aγ and Aδ then answer will be "Aδ ".
- If question is asked just about "fastestImpulse conducting fiber" (NOT mentioning PAIN) answer will be "Aα ".
- MAXIMUM sensitivity to
  ↓
- PRESSURE "A fiber"   LA "C fiber"
  ↓
  - Due to high surface area to volume ratio [Q]
  - 80% nerves of pulp are unmyelinated C fibers [Q]
- Order of sensitivity to LA:
  B (preganglionic) fiber = C fiber > A fiber (NBDE Q)
- Order of sensation loss by LA
  PAIN > TEMPRATURE > TOUCH > PRESSURE
  Reversal takes placeIn opposite order

- MOST ACCEPTED theory of conduction of pain – MELZACK and WALL GATE CONTROLL THEORY [Q]
- Pain is modulated by "substantia gelatinosa *(AIPG 2012)*
- VARIOUS TECHNIQUES EMPLOYEDIN LA:

EXTRAORAL NERVE BLOCK

↓ MAXILLARY "needle is directed Anterior to lateral pterygoid plate"

↓ MANDIBULAR "needle is directed Posterior to lateral pterygoid plate"

Mental Nerve Block	Incisive Nerve Block
Mental nerve is anaesthetized anterior to mental foramen. LA not depositedInto mental foramen	GivenIn mental foramen.
Tooth not anaesthetised	Both teeth and soft tissue anaesthesized
UsedIn biopsy/suturing	UsedIn both exodontia and soft tissue management

IAN BLOCK:

<5YRS-5mm below occlussal plane *(KCET 2013)*
6yrs - at occlussal plane
>6YRS-above occlussal plane

IAN BLOCK COMPLICATION:
- Bells palsy-if needle positioned too posteriorly [Q]
- Trismus-if placed too medialy
- Sphenomandibular ligament damaged.

In PSA haematoma is most common because of penetrationInto pterygoid venous plexus *(Favourite Q of AIIMS and NEET)*

Direction of needle- upward,inward and backward [Q]
LANDMARK for administration are mucobuccal fold, occlusal plane,Coronoid process and anterior border of ramus *(AIPG 2007)*

Maxillary 1st molar is difficult to anaesthetize byInfiltration because of thick zygomatic bone over root
Bilateral mandibular nerve block: should be rarely performed except bilateral mandibular surgery.
GOW GATES: Technique requiring extra oral landmarks *(KCET 2013)* LANDMARKS are corner of mouth andIntertragic Notch *(KCET2013)* Target area is neck of condyle
VAZIRANI AKINOSI technique also called "tuberosity technique"/ closed mouth techqnique UsedIn trismus patient *(AIPG 2010)* BlocksIAN,incisive, mental,lingual and mylohyoid nerve

- REGIONAL LA is C\IIn SCA (sickle cell anemia) *(NEET 2013, AIPGMEE 2012)*
- OBSTETRIC and EPIDURAL anesthesia:

All LA can be except PROCAINE and TETRACAINE due to long onset of action.

- SOMEIMPORTANT LA AGENTS:

TRICK for amide LA agent = the agent will have 2 "i "inIt's name
ALL LA readily cross BBB and placenta Amide LA are more likely to cross placenta than esteric LA. *(NEET 2013)*
DIBUCAINE: Most potent,most toxic,longest acting LA. [Q] (direct Pick from line of KDT pharmacology) Don't confuse with Bupivacaine-It is poent, long acting, and cardiotoxic (NOT MOST TOXIC).
ARTICAINE: Amine based LA. Fast acting, metabolizedIn liver Half life is 20 min. infiltration produces adequate anesthesiaIn Primary molar so need for BLOCK anesthesia is eliminated. Rapid metabolism and rapid excretion is responsible for less toxicity *(AIPG 2012)*
Bupivacaine usedIn LA as 0.5% Very potent, highly cardiotoxic *(PGI; AIIMS 05 ques)*
Topical lidocaine available as 2%, 4 % (maximum concentration available) *(AIPG 2007 Q)*
LA are vasodilators EXCEPT ROPIVACAINE {It is a cutaneous vasoconstrictor [Q] usedIn epidural anesthesia [Q]}
In EPIDURAL anesthesia all LA can be used except PROCAINE and TETRACAINE
MEPIVACAINE: is least vasodilating LA.so, usedIn hyperthyroidism,heart patients where vasoconstrictor are contraindicated Also safeIn pediatric and geriatric patients
LIDOCAINE has a half life of 90 min. causes lesserIncidence of allergy.so, more commonly usedIn dentistry
When patient is allergic to both ester and amide antihistamine like DIPHENHYDRAMINE can be used
CENTBUCRIDINE: newer anesthetic agent. 5 TO 8 times potent than lidocaine.does NOT affect CNS and CVS adversely
BIOTOXIN: e.g tetrodotoxin and saxitoxin. They are ultra long acting anesthetic
ARTICANE: is the only anesthetic of amide type with thiophene Ring Only LA C/IIn patients with allergy to SULPHA drugs
in young patients, mentally/physically challenged short acting LA Like 2- chlorprocaine/ mepivacaine/4 % prilocaine recommended as they might bite/chew their lips/tongue

EMLA = eutectic mix of lidocaine and prilocaine c/IIn children below 6 months b\c metabolite of prilocaine MightInduce methaemoglobinemia. EMLA should be applied atleast 1 hr b\f procedure for theIntact skin *(AIPG 2011)*
PRILOCAINE is less toxic than lidocaine asIt is rapidly metabolized systemically (thoughIt causes methaemoglobinaemia)
Paraesthesia is more common with PRILOCAINE and ARTICAINE

- Methaemoglobinaemia: (Iron presentIn Fe 3+ form)

• Caused by LA: (trick = TAP) Topical benzocaine, Articaine, Prilocaine [Q]
• Most commonly due to o- toluidine metabolite of PRILOCAINE
• Methaemoglobinaemia < 20% does not produce any clinical sign
• Rx: Reversed within 15 min by administration of 1 to 2 mg/kg body wt. of 1 % methylene blue solution (AIPG 2012)I.v over a period of 5 min. Vit. C can also be used asIt stimulates production of Fe 2+In body

- Discovery:

LIDOCAINE	LOFGREN
COCAINE(1st LA agent)	ALBERT NIEMAN
N_2O	Name given by HUMPRY DAVY,1st prepared by JOSEPH PRIESTLY
ADRENALINE	ALBEL

- LA contaminated with alcohol

  ↓

  Causes NEUROLYSIS

  May resultIn paresthesia/permanent anesthesia

- DrugInteractionIn LA:

• CIMETIDINE ↑ ses plasma half life of circulating lidocaine. So this combination is relatively C/IIn CHF patient
• Esters such as PROCAINE and TETRACAINE produce PABA asIt's metabolite and mayInhibit the bacteriostatic action of sulfonamide
• The administration of adrenalineIn patients being treated with non- selective β- blocker (e.g propanolol, tinolol, atenolol)Increases the likelihood of serious elevation of b.p
• β – blocker retards lignocaine metabolism by reducing hepatic flow
TCA s (e.gImipramine) and MAO –Inhibitors (e.g isocarbaxazid) → ses CVS actions of exogenously administered vasopressors. SO, both adrenaline and noradrenaline absolutely C/IIn patients on TCA
• COCAINE stimulates norepinephrine release andInhibitsIts reuptakeIn adrenergic nerve terminals, thus producing a state of catecholamine hypersensitivity.
• Tachycardia and hypertension are frequently observed with cocaine administration.COCAINE abusers can also se risk of LA overdose reaction (**NOTE:** Due to same reason epinephrineImpregnated gingival retraction cord is absolutely C/I)

- Tachyphylaxis:

Defination: Increasing tolerance to a drug due to repeated reinjection of LA.
Cause: Edema, localized hemorrhage, clot formation, transduation Hypernatremia, decreased pH of tissue (result of secondInfection).

- Parasis =Incomplete paralysis [q]
- Paraesthesia = Persistant anesthesia caused by direct trauma to nerve by tip of needle.
- Toxicity of la: cns, cvs, respiratory depression

CNS - 4- 7 µg ---- CNS stimulation >7 µg ----- tonic clonic seizure
CVS - > 5µg ------ CVS depression and ECG changes start >10 µg ----- CVS collapse
(**NOTE:**In CVS the effect are only depression. Never stimulatory)
Lidocaine more frequently than procaine producesInitial mild depression and sedation [Q]

- Most common cause of death due to LA overdose- APNEA.

A patient can be best protected from the toxic effect of LA by using ASPIRATING technique (NBDE Q).This preventa LA from entering blood

- Rx of LA toxicity:

Drugs: diazepam/pentobarbital Na
Severe convulsion: Succinylcholine (Sch)
For depression: artificial ventilation

- Malignant Hyperthemia:

Abnormal seIn body temperature due to sustained muscle contraction (se release ofIntracellular Ca).
Mainly non- esteric LA causes and occursIn response to halothane and otherInhalational anesthetics or to Sch [Q]
Rx: dantrolene Na is the drug of choice [Q]
BARBITURATES and PROPOFOL (among GA can be given safelyIn these Patients)

- Topica LA commonly used: (trick = LBT)

Lidocaine, Benzocaine, Tetracaine NOT procaine *(KCET 2013 Q)*
SURFACE anesthetic is NOT much helpfulInINCISION and EXCISION *(KCET 2012)*

- Topical anesthesia effective upto- 2-3mm. *(PGI Q)*
- Allergic reactionIn LA is most likely due to preservative methyl paraben, SOIn such patients cardiac lidocaine should be used which is free of methyl paraben.
- VASOCONSTRICTORS used with LA:

Main aim of adding vasoconstrictor to LA is to prevent LA toxicity/ ↓ se LA toxicity
Vasoconstrictor Concentration: In LA higher concentration only provides se HEMOSTASISI.e less capillary **bleeding.** There is NO effect of concentration change on TOXICITY as only minimal concentration is required to prevent toxicity
N2 gas and sodium Metabisulphite – prevents oxidation of VASOCONSTRICTOR [Q]In LA solution.
Phenylephrine: - α 1 agonistIs the most stable and weakest vasoconstrictorIn dentistry
Noradrenaline not usedIn LA/dental practice because of α receptor action due to whichIt causesIntense VASOCONSTRICTION leading to NECROSIS

Adrenaline is absolutely contraindicatedIn HYPERTHYROIDISM
TCA + COCAINE + RESERPINE **All are adrenaline reuptakeInhibitor. so, ses adrenaline concentration**
Adrenaline: discovered by "ALBEL "(TRICK = A for "adrenaline" A for "ALBEL")
The action of Adr. is potentiated by all halogenated compounds. NOT only halothane(ex- cyclopropane, ethyl chloride) [Q]
Felypressin: **A synthetic analogue of ADH [Q].** It's a vasoconstrictor with minimal effect on artery so, usedIn CVS r isk patients,hyperthyroid and ASAlii andIv NOT recommended for use when haemostasis is necessary because of their predominant action on venous rather than on arterial circulation C/IIn pregnancy because of oxytocic action

- Alkanization of LA:

$NaHCO_3$ + CO_2 when added to LA causes • Rapid onset of action • IncreaseIts clinical effectiveness • MakeIt comfortable
Na bisulphateIn LA acts as a reducing agent *(AIPG 2007)*

- Metabolism of LA:

Ester	Amide
PrimarilyIn plasma	OnlyIn liver
SecondarilyIn liver	

- Trauma to Nerve: *(PGI 2009)*

NEUROPRAXIA	Characterized by conduction block where complete return of sensation is there and NO degeneration of axon occurs.
AXONTEMESIS	Axonal degeneration and subsequent regeneration is there.
NEURONTEMESIS	Severe disruption of nerve trunk with compromised sensory and functional recovery.

TRICK- "NAN "(in order ofIncreasing severity of damage)

General anaesthetics:

- O2 cylinder used is BLACK cylinder with WHITE collar [Q]
- N2 cylinder ——→ BLUEIn color (NBDE Q)
- 4 Stages of Anaesthesia

Stage 1.	Stage of analgesia	Stage of conscious sedation [Q]
Stage 2.	Stage of delirium	Associated with excitement [Q]
Stage 3.	Stage of surgical anaesthesia	
Plane 1.	Uncontrolled movement of eye ball	
Plane 2.	Loss of laryngeal reflex	
Plane 3.	Loss of light and corneal reflex,pupil start dilating	Preferred for surgery [Q]
Plane 4.	Starting of respiratory paralysis	
Stage 4.	Stage of respiratory paralysis	Cessation of breathing and failure of circulation leading to death.

- Sensation depressed last by GA – hearing.
- The last vital function depressed when pt. progressesInto deeper stage of anaesthesia – CVS COLLAPSE. [Q]
- Drugs:

• **ETHER:** Safe anaesthetic. [Q] Good anesthetic Good analgesic. Good muscle relaxation BUT slowInduction and recovery.
• **N_2O(LAUGHING GAS):** 70 % N2O is one of the safest anesthetic Potent analgesic but weak anaesthetic. A mix of 70% N2O +25-30% O2+ 0.2-2% another potent anaesthetic is employed for most surgical anaesthesia. **Has been used for dental and obstetric analgesia.so NOT C/IIn** PREGNANCY [Q] **Does not combine with Hb. is carriedIn physical solution.It does not decomposeIn the body. it is exhaled UNALTERED by the** LUNGS Specific gravity = 1.5 (AIPG) ↑2nd gas effect seen [Q] -when given with otherInhalation agent,it Ses the alveolar concentration of the other agent CONCENTRATION effect - alsoIt ↑ sesIt's OWN concentration Most common s\e- nausea Most common complication with N2O sedation ↓ BEHAVORIAL PROBLEM Complication- diffusion hypoxia, methaemoglobinemia.
• **HALOTHANE:** (features Opposite of N_2O). Potent anaesthetic, weak analgesic. Causes myocardial depression Sensitizes heart to adr. [Q] C\IIn liver failure [Q] M.C s\e is hepatitis.
• **KETAMINE:** Produces dissociative anaesthesia. [Q] IS the only which stimulates SNS soInduction agent of choiceIn shock.[Q] MarkedInc.In cerebral blood flow-Inc.Intracranial pressure. So C/IIn hypertensive patients. SafeIn asthmatics as relieves bronchospasm. [Also Halothane]
• **THIOPENTONE:** Ultra short acting barbiturates – quickestInduction, mainly used forInduction anesthesia. Highly lipophillic -Its loading dose depends on volume of distribution. [Q] UsedIn the treatment of status epilepticus. Complication –InjectingInto an artery leads to pain, necrosis [Q] Precipitate bronchospasm.

- **PROPOFOL:**
  Oil based preparation → so, Injection is painful
  MOST SUITABLEI. v anesthetic currently available
  Has ANTIEMETIC property [Q]
  I.v agent of choice for DAY CARE anesthesia [Q] (has favourable recovery characteristic)
  {DRUG usedIn DAY CARE anesthesia: TRICK = Manmohan

Singh A Prime Minister.
  M → Midazolam S → Sevoflurane (isoflurane)
  A → Alfentanyl (fentanyl) P → Propofol M → Mivacurium}
  along with opiods e.g fentanylIs agent of choice for TIVA
  (TotalI.V Anesthesia)
  Also used for sedationInI.C.U
  Can be given safelyIn patients with CONGENITAL PORPHYRIA
  Absolute C/IIn AIRWAY OBSTRUCTION and HYPERSENSITIVITY

- Halothane vs Fluranes: (AIPG)

Halothane	Flurane
Decreases HR and CO	All fluranes compared to halothane does not cause myocardial depression.

- Physiochemical Properties of Anesthesia (Induction and Recovery + Potency)
- Most Common for GA:

• Most common complication of GA = VOMITING
• Most common cause of death during GA = RESPIRATORY OBSTRUCTION
• Most common complication 24 hrs post operative = ATELACTASIS

- Order of Depression of CNS by GA:

CORTICAL → SPINAL → MEDULLARY

- GA C/IIn:

• Hemoglobinopathies
• Acute respiratory obstruction

- E.g of Inducing Agent (Faster Action):

• Thiopentone
• Propofol

Cerebral steal phenomenon	Reverse steal/robbinhood phenomenon
• Movement of blood AWAY from is chemic area to normal area due to vasodilation of adjacent normal areaI.e STEALING OF BLOOD from is CHEMIC AREA	• Barbiturates cause vasoconstrictionIn adjacent normal area. So, redistribution of blood to is chemic area ↓ PROTECTS BRAIN
	• E.g barbiturates (THIOPENTANE Na)

- Coronary Steal Phenomenon:

Seen with is oflurane

- NEUR   OLEPT ANALGESIA:

  Tranquilizar ↓ + opiod ↓ → thus, patient remains conscious but pain free

  {doperidol} ↓ {fentanyl} ↓

- NEUROLEPT ANESTHESIA:

  Neurolept analgesia + (65% N2O + 35 % O_2)

- The action of long acting muscle relaxants used during GA may be terminated by NEOSTIGMINE (cholinergic drug)
- Laryngospasm during GA is relieved by Sch (succinylcholine)
- The action of long acting muscle relaxant used during GA is terminated by neostigmine (cholinergic drug)

LAST 5-YEAR QUESTIONS FROM THIS TOPIC

1. **Highest percentage of clinical failures are seen with which nerve block?** *(KCET 11)*

Ans. IAN block (Ref: Malamed's LA 5/e p47)

2. **Mucous membrane on the buccal aspect of the upper alveolar process is innervated by buccal nerve and** *(COMEDK 11)*

Ans. Superior alveolar nerve/PSA (Ref: Malamed LA 5/e p179)

3. **Among the following pain theories, the most accepted theory is** *(COMEDK 11)*

Ans. Gate control theory (Ref: Pain control by norman trigger 2/e p13)

4. **All of the following nerves are encountered during submandibular gland resection except:** *(COMEDK 11)*
   a. Lingual nerve
   b. Hypoglossal nerve
   c. Accessory nerve
   d. Marginal mandibular nerve

Ans. c. Accessory nerve

5. **Non-myelinated axons differ from myelinated onesIn that they:** *(COMEDK 11)*

Ans. Lack nodes of ranvier (Ref: Monheim's LA and pain controlIn dental practice 7/e p64)

6. **the use of vasoconstrictors adrenaline/Non adrenaline with LA is contraindicatedIn patients on:** *(COMEDK 11)*

Ans. TCA (Ref: Malamed's LA 5/e p53)

7. **Which of the following LA is active topically:** *(KCET 10)*

Ans. Lidocaine and Benzocaine

8. **Openings of the posterior alveolar canals are seen on:** *(COMEDK 11)*

Ans. Posterior maxillary surface (Ref: Balaji's textbook of oral and Maxillofacial surgeryIst edition)

9. **High tuberosity technique is used to anesthetize:** *(COMEDK 10)*

Ans. Maxillary nerve

10. **During mandibular nerve block which nerve also gets damaged:** *(AIIMS Nov. 12)*

Ans. Facial (Ref: Balaji is ted. p642)

11. **Gate control theory was Ist proposed by:** *(AIIMS Nov. 12)*

Ans. Melzack and wall (Ref: Moheem's 7/e p5)

12. **Last option for dental anaesthesia is** *(AIIMS May 12, AIPG Q)*

Ans. Intrapulpal (Ref: Malamed's LA 5/e p255, 266)

13. **Regarding OPD general anaesthesiaIn dental chair absolute contraindication is all except:** *(AIIMS Nov. 12)*
   a. Children
   d. Serious medial disease

c. Edema of floor of mouth
d. Trismus

Ans. a. Children (Ref: McDonold p298)

14. Transient bell's palsy during mandibular nerve block afterInjection of LA occurs due to needle piercingInto: *(AIPG-12)*

Ans. Paroted gland (Ref: Malamed 5/e p234)

15. Most common route for premedicationIn children is: *(AIPG 09)*

Ans. Oral (Ref: Millers anaesthesia 6/e p2381)

16. N2O acts by: *(AIPG 09)*

Ans. Non specific CNS depression (Ref: Ajay yadav 2/e p55, 59)

17. In a case of trismus,IfIAN, mylohyoid nerve, lingual nerve and long buccal nerve all need to be simultaneously blocked, which technique will be most suitable: *(AIPG-10)*

Ans. Vazirani Akinosi (Ref: Malamed LA p228/5/e p)

18. Route not used for sedationIn child is: *(AIPG 09)*

Ans. Subdermal (Ref: Mcdonalds 7/e p305-313)

19. Paravertebral block can extendInto all except: *(AIIMS Nov. 09)*

Ans. The subarachnoid space (Ref: Finucaine complication of regional anesthesia 2/e p108)

20. Gate control theory of pain is modulated by: *(AIPG-12)*

Ans. Substantia gelatinosa (NBDE Q)

21. All of the following are true regarding the use of articaineIn a child except: *(AIPG-12)*

a. It is amine based and is metabolizedIn the liver
b. Half life is 90 minutes
c. Infiltration produces adequate anesthesiaIn 1° molar so need for block anesthesia is eliminated
d. Increased breakdown is responsible for less toxicity

Ans. b. Half life is 90 minutes

22. SlowI.v.Infusion of methylene blue 1% (1-2 mg/kg) body weight is used for Rx of: *(AIPG-12)*

Ans. Methemoglobinemia

23. The anaesthetic drugInjected for paravertebral block is bast likely to diffuse to: *(AIIMS May 11)*

Ans. Subarachnoid space (Ref: Finucane complication of regional anesthesia 2/e p108)

24. Which of the following is Not a sign of successful stellate ganglion block? *(AIIMS May11)*

a. Nasal stiffness
b. Guttman sign
c. Horner's Syndrome
d. Bradycardia

Ans. d. Bradycardia (Ref: Yadav 2/e p113)

25. Which of the followingInhalation anaesthetic agent has analgesic property? *(AIIMS Nov. 10)*

Ans. Nitrous oxide

26. Ist LA to be used clinically was: *(AIIMS Nov. 10)*

Ans. Cocaine (Ref: Katzung 10/e p412)

27. Which nerve fiber has the largest diameter and fastest conduction velocity? *(AIIMS Nov. 10)*

Ans. A-α (Ref: Malamed 4/e p5)

28. ParaesthesiaInInferior alveolar nerve block occurs mainly due to: *(AIIMS May 10)*

Ans. Contact of needle to nerve trunk (Ref: NBDE)

29. The sudden appearance of dumb-bell shaped surlling during posterior superior alveolar nerve block is mainly due to: *(AIIMS May 10)*

Ans. InjectionIn pterygoid plexus (Ref: Kruger 6/e p244)

30. Sodium bicarbonate is given as an adjunct to LA because: *(AIIMS Nov. 09)*
Ans. Sed onset of action and duration
31. Which combination forms day care anaesthesia? *(AIIMS Nov. 09)*
Ans. Fentanyl, propofol, is oflurane
32. Which anesthetic agent is contraindicated forIntrathecal use? *(AIPG-11)*
Ans. Remifantanly (Ref: Fundamentals of anesthesia by colin pinnock, lin, smith 2/e p627)
33. WhichI.v. anesthetic is a potent bronchodilator/choice of agentIn asthmatic patient: *(AIPG-11)*
Ans. Ketamine (Ref: Goodman-gillman 10/e p347)
34. All are true about propofol, except: *(AIPG-11)*
a. Cause vomiting
b. Hase rapid recovery rate
c. Used forInduction and maintenance of anesthesia
d. Cause sedation
Ans. a. Cause vomiting
35. Administration of which of the following anesthetic agints is associated with reducedIncidence of light headedness and rapid recovery: *(AIPG-11)*
Ans. Propofol
36. On the administration of LAIn the area ofInfection, most of the LA is presentIn the form of: *(AIPG-11)*
Ans. IncreasesIn cationic form
37. Eutectic mixture of 2.5% lidocaine and 2.5% prilocaine is primarily usedIn: *(AIPG-11)*
Ans. Topical skin application (Ref: Malamed 5/e p77)
38. Infra orbital nerve block will anesthetize: *(PGI June 11)*
Ans. Anterior and middle superior nerve (Ref: Handbook of LA 5/e p198)
39. Which of the following is not anesthesized with mental nerve block? *(PGI June 11)*
a. Ist M
b. Permanent molars
c. Canines
d. Incisors
Ans. b. Permanent molars (Ref: Malamed 5/e p246)
40. The Ist sensation to be lost following administration of LA is: *(PGI Dec. 10)*
Ans. Pain (Ref: Monheim's 7/e p133)
41. Most common anesthetic complication within Ist 24 hrs. after surgery unde GA is. *(PGI Dec. 10)*
Ans. Atelectasis (NBDE Q)
42. Topical anesthesia used are effective upto the depth of: *(PGI Dec. 10)*
Ans. 2-3 mm (Ref: malamed 6/e p75)
43. AmmoniumInhalation used during synocope acts by producing? *(PGI Dec. 11)*
Ans. Respiratory stimulation (Ref: Vinod kapoor 2/e p606)
44. LA blocks nerve conduction by: *(COMEDK 12)*
Ans. Decreasing the membrane permeability to Na+Ions there by stabilizing nerve membrane
45. Na metab isulfite is used In LA asIt acts as: *(COMEDK 12)*
Ans. Anti-oxidant for vasoconstrictor
46. DuringInferior alveolar nerve block needle is insertedInto: *(PGI Dec. 09)*
Ans. Pterygomandibular space (Ref: Monheims 7/e p105)
47. Computerize controlled LA delivery system is known as: *(PGI Dec. 09)*
Ans. WAND (Ref: Malamed 5/e p92)
48. Surface anesthetic alone is not much usefullIn: *(KCET 12)*
Ans. Incision and excision

EMERGENCY AND IT'S MANAGEMENT

- Altered Conciousness:

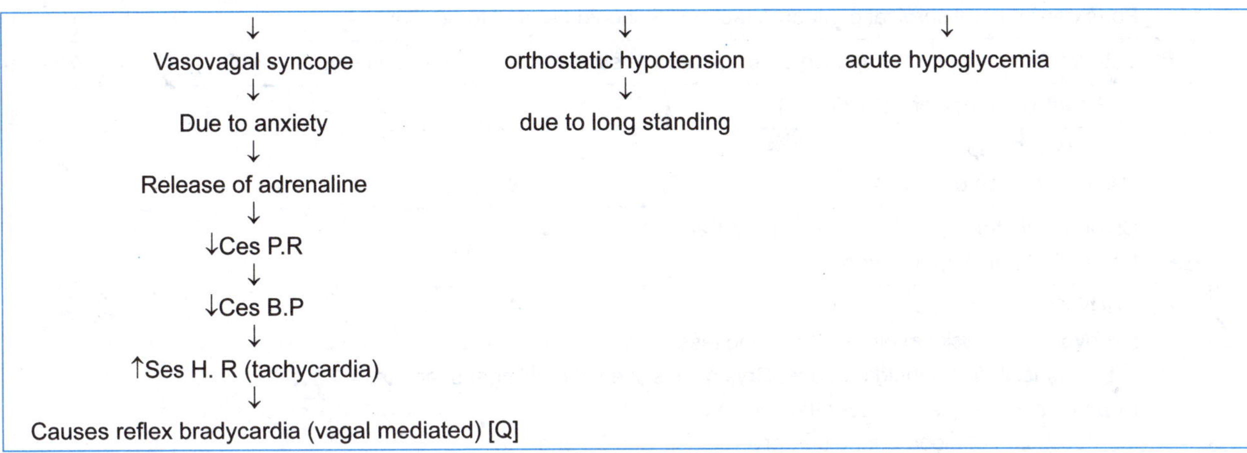

- HyperventillationIn Anxious Patients:

↑SeIn pco_2 – Respiratory alkalosis.
Water – 65% of body wt.

- 1st SIGN:

• Of syncope = PALLOR [Q]
• Of shock = TACHYCARDIA [Q]
• Of O_2 want = TACHYCARDIA [Q]

- Syncope:

Most common emergency (53 % of total)
Most common emergency adverse reaction of LA/dental surgery
Cerebral blood flow to maintain consciousness is 30 ml of blood/100 g of Brain tissue/minute.
Normal – 50–55 ml of blood/100 g of Brain tissue/minute
Anxiety ↓ Adrenalive release ↓ ↑sed PR ↓ ↑sed B.P. ↓ ↓ced HR ↓ Reflex Bradycardia (Vagal mediated)

- Hemorrhage and Shock:

- **Banked blood:**
  - Poor Source of platelets
  - Absent factor – 5, 8
    (Fresh blood – calledIf administered within 2hrs of donation)

• 1 unit platelet rich plasma – ↑ses platelet count by 7000 –10,000
• 1 unit Fresh Blood – 1 gm% Hb sed, 3% Hematocrit *(AIPG 2012)*
• For extensive oral surgical procedure factor VIII should be sed to 50–75%
• Both fresh frozen plasma and Cryoprecitpitate are stored at – 30°c Blood is stored at 4°C *(PGI 2012)*
• FFP contains – Factor VIII (200 ug)
• FactorIX (200 ug) • Use is t/t of Hemophillia B
• CryoprecipitateIn t/t – F VIII (100 ug) No FactorIX • UseIn the t/t of Hemophillia A
• **SHOCK:** Hypovolumic shock develops after blood less of 40% Initial resuccitation should be done, Crystalloids like saline/Ringer's lactate. Dopamine is the vasopressor oflst choice (i.v.) If Pt looses 1 l of blood during surgery–replace with 3 l of blood. Septic shock – is mostly by gram(-)ve bacteria. Septic shock – Persistent hypotension because of low PR due to substance produced byInfections agent. Cardiogenic shock – because of anIntrinsic problemIn myocardium or valve (related to long standing MI) Hypovolemic shock developes after loss of 40 % blood *(KCET 2012 Q)*
• **Rx for shock:** • Initial resuccitation should be done with crystalloid like SALINE/RINGER LACTATE • Dopamine is the vasopressor of 1st choice [Q] • If patient looses 1 liter blood during surgery replace with 3 liter (3 times) fluid

- Hypertension:

DBP > 110 mmHg
SBP > 150 mmHg
Guanathidine + Bretyllium – Inhibits release of NA so usedIn severe HTN

- vWBD is also called pseudo haemophillia
- Adrenalinein anaphylax is given = 0.5 Mgin 1: 1000i. M
- Patient Position:

Condition	Position of The Patient
MostImportant patient positions during recovery from SYNCOPE	Semireclined and trendeleburg positions [Q]
During CPR patient should be keptIn	Supine position
A patient with suspected cervical fracture should be keptIn	BODY and neck extended (NBDE Q)
A patient with maxillofacial trauma	Lateral [Q]
Preferable positionIn recovery room after ambulatory GA	Lateral [Q]
Pregnant patientsIn syncope should be keptIn	Left lateral position [Q]
Patient affected with orthostatic hypertension	Reclined/supine position

Pregnancy patient during surgery	Upright position/with her trunk slightly to one side
Congestive failure patients	Upright position [Q] so that blood flows towards gravity and reduces load on heart. supine position should be avoided

- CPR:

RATE OF COMPRESSION = 80 to 100/min (if Q is askedIn NEET/AIIMS and 60/min is givenIn option thenIt means thatIt's a direct pick from NBDE Q bank. so, go forIt)
Depth of compression – 1.5 to 2Inch
Compression should not be delayed for more than 10 sec
Rate of rescue breadtingIn child = 20 times/min
Rate of rescue breadthingIn adults = 12 times/min
Compression: rescue breadth {In 1 rescuer = 30: 1 In 2 rescuer = 15: 1}

- ASA(American Society of Anesthesiologists) physical status classification:

Used to assess fitness of patients before surgery: • Normal healthy patient • Patient with mild systemic disease • Patient with severe systemic disease • Patient with severe systemic disease that is a constant threat to life • Moribund patient who is not expected to survive without operation • Patient declared brain dead and whose organs are being removed for donor purposes

- Rx Status Epilepticus:

Diazepam 10 mgI.v/thiopentone Na/phenytoin (NOT carbamazepine)

- Average daily adult fluidIntake – 1800ml. (Remember: plaque – 80% H2O, Dentrifrice –20-30% H2O)
- In hemophilllics – Both field block and nerve Block are contraindicated.

LAST 5-YEAR QUESTIONS FROM THIS TOPIC

1. **O_2 as an emergency drug is contraindicatedIn:** *(KCET 11)*

Ans. Hyperventilation

2. **In Glasgow coma scale, rataing is given to patient on the basis of his level of consciousness. The minimum score that can be given is:** *(AIPG-12)*

Ans. 3.

3. **A morbid patient unlikely to survive 24 hrs with/without surgery is classified as:** *(KCET 11)*

Ans. ASA V (Ref: Malamed's LA 5/e p14)

4. **The head tilt procedure while dealing with an unconscious patientIn dental chair is done to ensure:** *(COMEDK 09)*

Ans. Patient airway

5. **In an emergency which of the following blood group can be transfused with cross matching:** *(KCET 09)*

Ans. O - ve

6. Commonest cause of postoperative shock is: *(KCET 09)*

Ans. Hypovelemia (hypocalcemia)

7. Most common sign of airway obstruction: *(AIPG-12)*

Ans. Strenous breadthing

8. On applying pressure on angle of jaw while maintaining patent airway which nerve is likely to be damaged: *(AIIMS Nov. 12)*

Ans. 7th CN (Ref: BDC 3/e p249)

9. In a patient with oral and maxillofacial trauma cervicalInjury is not ruled out,Intubation of preference will be: *(AIIMS Nov. 12)*

Ans. FiberopticIntubation (Ref: Fonseca 3/e. Vol. 1 p151, 153)

Airway is

10. In oral surgery best way to secure airway is: *(AIIMS Nov. 12)*

Ans. Nasal RAE

11. The recommended position to keep a person who faints during extraction? *(PGI Dec. 11, 10)*

Ans. Trendelenberg position (Ref: Monheims 7/e p238-240)

12. A ladyIn 2nd trimester of pregnancy develops syncope while extraction of the 2nd maxillary molar. She should be placedIn: *(AIPG 12)*

Ans. Left lateral position

13. The head tilt procedure while dealing with and unconscious patientIn dental chair is done to ensure: *(COMEDK 12)*

Ans. Patient airway

14. Tracheostomy is done throught: *(PGI June 09)*

Ans. 2th to 4th tracheal ring

15. Sequence is CPR is: *(KCET 12)*

Ans. Airway, Breadthing, circulation

16. A patient is in shock with gross comminuted #Immediate treatment is to give: *(KCET 10)*

Ans. Ringer's lactate solutionI.v.

17. Endotoxic shock is intiated by: *(AIPG 12)*

Ans. Injury to endothelial cells

18. A patient with trauma suffers form 15% blood loss. What should be done: *(AIPG 09)*

Ans. No treatment

TRAUMA AND IT'S MANAGEMENT (Favorite Q of AIIMS and NEET)

- Airway Managementin Severe Maxillofacial Trauma: (Imp. for AIIMS)

IDEAL management - cricothyrotomy Next best optionIf "cricothyrotomy "not mentioned – orotrachealIntubation preffered over nasotrachealIntubation. *(AIIMS Nov 2010 MED. Q)*
TRACHEOSTOMY – is time taking. so, does not have much roleIn emergency Airway management
Laryngotomy/cricotomy/tracheotomy are always preffered over TRACHEOSTOMY to maintain airway

laryngotomy/cricotomy/tracheotomy are done through CRICOTHYROID membrane. *(NBDE Q)*
SubmentalIntubation – useful alternative to tracheostomy with minimal complicationIn case of panfacial fracture [Q]
LMV used where endotrachealIntubation is C/I
In maxillofacial trauma patient: lateral position + head tilt – chin tilt done (donot confuse NOT head tilt chin lift followedIn CPR).

- GLASGOW coma scale: (trick = VME)

Verbal Motor Eye opening
Minimum value = 3 (comma patient)
Maximum value = 15 (fully concious patient)

- Trauma deaths:

• 1ST peak –Immediate death due to Brain and spinalInjuries and major CVS damage
• 2nd peak – early death (after few hours) due to hemorrhage/hematoma (epidural/subdural hematoma) + airway compromise
3rd peak – death days/weeks afterInjury. multiorgan failure +Infection (sepsis) is the cause

- DIRECTIMPACT on bone will produce comminuted #
- BUCKET HANDLE # seenIn edentulous patient
- mandibular #:

The most common anatomic site of # = angle (NBDE Q. So,If Q is askedIn NEET/AIIMS then go for this answer as they DIRECTLY PICK from NBDE)
BUT most commonly seen # = body > angle > condyle

Otorrhoe, Battle's sign, Racoon's eye seenIn CRANIAL base #. Also Rhinorrhoea is seen.

- Masticatory forces produce TENSIONAL forces at alveolar border and COMPRESSION forces at lower border of mandible
- ANGLE #:

It is compound #
More chances ofInfection. so, difficult to treat.
It is the weakest point of mandible where # occurs

- Swelling BEHIND the ear suggest CONDYLAR # (Donot confuse with ZMC #)
- lateral pterygoid effectIn condylar # anteromedial pull [Q]
- Medial pterygoid effect seenIn angle # # segments moveIn medial, Lingual and superior direction
- RADIOGRAPHIC sign of #:

• Abnormal linear density – Bright signIn ANTRAL #
• Trapdoor signIn orbital ROOF #
• Rail road/parallel line signIn lateral orbital wall #

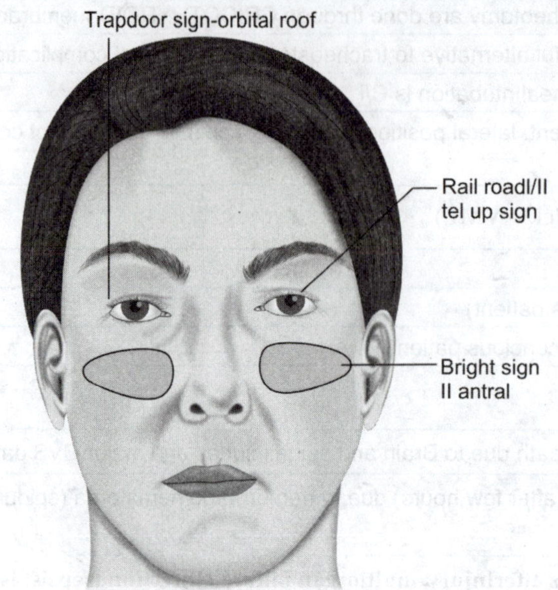

Fig. 10.3: Radiographic sign of #

- If occlusion is normal with any #,NO need of T/t. EvenIMF not needed [Q]
- Rx of mandible #In children:

Treated best by acrylic cap splint with circumferential wiring

- Period of Immobilisation:

CONDYLAR #	OTHER MANDIBULAR #
Children = 10 to 14 days [Q]	Children = 3 weeks
Adults = 2 to 3 weeks	Adults = 5 weeks
	Old/infected = 6 – 7 weeks

- If Q is just about # of mandible then answer should be 6 weeks (BOUCHER's MCQ)
- Complication of condylar #In children:

Most common complication is ANKYLOSIS. so, to avoid this early mobilization/active treatment is given

- Deviation towards same side as defect:Trick–HAS

H–Hypoplasia of condyle
A–Ankylosis
S–Sub condylar #

- CHAMPY'S plates/miniplates:

Semirigid monocorticated plates [Q].

Advantages:
- Minor degree of movement is not considered as disadvantage.
- Miniplates provide quick fixation
- They reduce risk of malocclusion
- Better bone healing seen
- Stable result over compression plates

- BONE plating for mandibular #

• Mandibular body #: 1 plate with monocortical self tapping screw at the base of the alveolar processI.e middle of body (AIPG 2012 Q). It is theIdeal osteosynthes is line corresponding to the line of tension at the alveolar base.
• # behind the mental foramen: 1 plate can be appliedImmediately below the dental roots and above theInferior alveolar canal
• # at angle of the jaw: 1 plate at the broad surface of EXTERNAL oblique ridge as high as possible [Q]
• Anterior b/w mental foramina: 2 plates, one cervical plate + one near lower border of the mandible [Q] • A gap of 4.5 mm should exist b/w the 2 plates This is done to neutralize torsional forces [Q]
• ATROPHIC mandible #: give reconstruction plates/2.4 universal # plates

- RISDON WIRING used for symphyseal #
- optimum length of screw for fixationIn mandible – 4mm
  Length of LAG screw – 20mm
- Splint:

Edentulous	Dentulous
Gunning splint	Cap splint

- Concept:

Rx of # of mandible NOTInvolving dental arch is by open reduction as absenceInInvolvement of teeth resultsIn absence of guidance for closed reduction

- Intraoral approach to reduce zygomatic arch is called "KEEN'S Technique "
  It is through buccal sulcus
- Eburnation:

Rounding off and sclerosis of bone ends seenIn NON – UNION
In edentulous mandibleIt is called as "Elephant foot deformity "
Non union can be caused due toINFECTION [Q]

- Anisocorea – DifferenceIn pubillary size
- Electrolytes requiredIn maxilla facial trauma:

Na^+ - 100 mmol
K^+ - 60 mmol
1g protein

- For Nasal fracture:

• Water's/OM projection • Lateral view of nasal bone **NB:** Water's view is best for – maxillary sinus and coronoid process.
– Diplopia after Fracture vesults from entrapment ofIR (Inferior rectus) >>IO (Inferior Oblique) muscles *(COMEDK)*

- Enopthalmus: is not seenIn leforII #
- Epiphora:

Excessive secretion of water from eye due to obstruction of lacrimal duct.
SeenIn lefortII, III and NOE compex #

- Compression osteosynthesis – earlier was used for fibrous/Non union.

- Hess chart: use to measure degree of diplopia. *(AIIMS 2012)*
- In children – LeforIII/craniofacial dysjuction rarely seen. Because of poorly developed ethmoidal and sphenoidal sinus. So Bone is thicker than Adult bone.
- CSF Rhinorrohea:

Tramline/Hallo on pillow effect seen.

- In children:

↑ sed vascularity ↓ ↑ sed haemarthrosis ↓ ↑ sed chances of ankylosis

- Blow-out Fracture:

Most commonInvolved site is posteromedial aspect of orbital floor.
Most difficult area to repair is posteromedial
Overlapping sign = Double density/cortical duplication sign

- CSF otorrhoea:

7th and 8th CN palsies
seenIn condition associated with CSF otorrhoea (b'coz 7th and 8th CN lies togetherInInternal acoustic meatus)

- Flial chest: rib cage is separated from rest of chest wall, due to severe blunt trauma.

LAST 5-YEAR QUESTIONS FROM THIS TOPIC

1. **The weakest part and most vulnerable part for fractureIn the mandibile is:** *(KCET 11)*

Ans. Condylar neck (Ref: Neelima mailk is ted. p619)

2. **The "Hanging drop" sign,If visualizedIn the waters projection of the traumatized faceIndicates:** *(KCET 11)*

Ans. Orbital floor # (Ref: Kelly and K 5/e p47)

3. **Case report:** *(COMEDK 11)*

A 35 year old man with a Le fortIII # complains of blood tinged watery discharge from nose 2 days after trauma. CT scan confirms NOE # as well.

a. **What clinical features surggest that the discharge is CSF leak.**

Ans. Appearance of tramline/halo rings

b. **WhatInvestigation is most confirmatory for detecting CSF leak**

Ans. Presence of B-tansferrin

c. **The most common complication of CSF rhinorrhea is**

Ans. Ascending meningitis

4. **Miniplate fixation is effective at:** *(COMEDK 10)*

Ans. Zone of tension

5. **Bird face appearance is seen in:** *(COMEDK 10)*

Ans. Zygomatic bone #

6. **Flattening of the check is seenIn:** *(COMEDK 10)*

Ans. Zygomatic bone #

7. **Transosseous wiring is an e.g of:** *(KCET 11)*

Ans. IMF with Osteosynthesis (Ref: Williams HaxilloficialInjury 2/e p341)

8. **Craniofacial dysjunction seen in:** *(COMEDK 11)*

Ans. LefortIII # (Ref: Killey's textbook)

9. **A fractured coronid process of mandible displace upwards by the action of following muscle:** *(COMEDK 11, 09) (COMEDK 11)*

Ans. Temporalis (Ref: Killey's fracture of mandible 3/e p11)

10. **The most common anatomic site of # of mandible is the:** *(KCET 10)*

Ans. Angle (Mark this answer for KCET only)

11. **LefortI is characterized by:** *(KCET 10)*

Ans. BleedingInto antrum

12. **Restricted mouth openingIn zygomatic arch # is due toImpingement of:** *(COMEDK 10, AIPG-2000)*

Ans. Coronoid process

13. **Gillies approach done through:** *(COMEDK 09)*

Ans. Temporal region

14. **Rowe's disimpaction forceps usedIn treating:** *(COMEDK 09)*

Ans. Maxillary #

15. **Paresthesia over nasal and upper lip following # zygoma is because ofInvolvement of:** *(KCET 09)*

Ans. Infraorbital nerve

16. **Use of acrylated arch bars for closed reduction of mandible # was described by:** *(KCET 09)*

Ans. Schuchardt (1956)

17. **"Moon face" appearance ss seen in:** *(KCET 09)*

Ans. LefortII andIII #

18. **After Le-FortI osteotomy the blood supply of maxilla is maintained by:** *(AIIMS Nov. 11)*

Ans. Ascending palatine branch of facial artery (Ref: Plast Reconstr. Surg 1997 Sep, 100 (4): 843-51, Blood supply of the Le fortI maxillary segment: an anatomic study)

Note: Also supplied by anterior branch of ascending pharyngeal artery.

19. **The joint which histologically and Morphologically best stimulate the TMJ is:** *(AIIMS Nov. 11, 12)*

Ans. Sternoclavicular joint

20. **Maximum complication of angle # while treating with:** *(AIIMS Nov. 11)*

Ans. IMF

21. **High velocity gunshotInjury with periosteal denudation and Comminuted # is best treated as:** *(AIIMS Nov. 11)*

Ans. Initially debridement is done then load bearing reconstruction plates, and graftingIn secondary procedure (Ref: Neelima malik p298)

22. **In children # line of mandible is:** *(AIIMS Nov. 11, AIPG-12)*

Ans. Zig Zag due to permanent tooth buds

23. **Open reduction of # is stronglyIndicatedIn:** *(AIIMS Nov. 11)*

Ans. Lateral displacement of condyle (Ref: Balaji p589)

24. **CSF leakage is diagnosed by all except:** *(AIIMS Nov. 11, 12)*

a. Tramline
b. β-2 transferrin level
c. IncreaseIn glucose
d. IncreaseIn proteins

Ans. d. IncreaseIn proteins (Ref: Fonseca 3/e p222)

25. **Most common site of # of Zygomatico-temporal suture:** *(AIIMS Nov. 11, 12)*

Ans. Posterior to zygomatico temporal suture (Ref: Stone's plastic surgery facts and figures by Tor wo chiu p 62)

26. Check pointIn zygomatic reductionIn case of maxillary arch fractures is: *(AIPG-12)*

Ans. click sound (Ref: Neelima Malik p363)

27. Sorting a patient of trauma of headInjury on basis of need of care and availability of resources: *(AIIMS Nov. 12)*

Ans. Triages (Ref: Taber's cyclopedic medical dictionary 19/e p2141)

28. An adult patient with panfacial trauma Rx should start from: *(AIIMS Nov. 12)*

Ans. Mandible

29. Which of the following is used to diagnose diplopiaIn maxillofacial trauma: *(AIIMS Nov. 12)*

Ans. Hess chart (Ref: Neelima mallik 2/e p361)

30. Excessive bleeding during oral surgery can be decreasedIn which position: *(AIIMS Nov. 12)*

Ans. Head Up (Ref: basics of blood management by petra seeber, aryeh shander p192)

31. B/L circumorbital ecchymosis is commonly seenIn which # ? *(AIPG 12)*

Ans. LefortIII (Ref: Fonceca vol 3/e p254)

32. In Gille's approach for reduction of zygomatic arch fractures, the rowe's forcep is Inserted between: *(AIPG 12)*

Ans. Temporalis fascia and temporalis muscle

33. Most common site of CSF rhinorrhea is: *(AIPG 12)*

Ans. cribriform plate (Ref: Fonseca vol. 3 p187)

34. In U/L condylar #, the mandible deviates to which side on opening: *(AIPG 12)*

Ans. Same (Ref: Fonseca 3/e p536)

35. Paresthesia of lower lip is most commonIn fracture of: *(AIPG 12)*

Ans. Body (Ref: Fonseca p491)

36. The most complicated # of the mandible is: *(AIIMS May 11)*

Ans. Angle (Ref: malik p352)

37. A patient is admitted with headInjury GCS < 8, severe midface fractures, frequent aponea and low oxygenation, airway management is best done by: *(AIPG 09)*

Ans. Orotracheal airway (Ref: fonseca 3/e p140.

38. In mass casuality, patient treatedIst are: *(AIPG 09)*

Ans. Patient with maximum chances of survival with minimum available resources

39. Champy plate is: *(AIPG 09)*

Ans. Monocortical non compressive (Ref: Head, face and neck trauma comprehensive management by Michael G. Stewart p95)

40. When a case is transferred toICU, mandibular fracture is evaluated in:

Ans. 1° Survey

41. A/C rule of tension and compressional forces acting along the condylar border, best way to stabilize a condylar # against these forces would require: *(AIPG 09)*

Ans. One plate at anterior border, one at posterior border (Ref: Peterward booth p291-292.

42. Based on champy's principle of tension and compression, angle # is best treated with: *(AIPG 09)*

Ans. Fixation of segments with bone plate according to AO principles (Ref: Peterson 2nd vol. 1 p371-381)

43. Mandible would require use of: *(AIPG 09)*

Ans. Reconstruction plates with centric screws

44. Type of healing seen after compression plating is: *(AIPG 09)*

Ans. 1° (Ref: Peterson 2nd vol. p371-381)

45. Following a B/L # of the mandibleIn the canine region, the anterior fragment of the mandible is displaced posteriorly by the action of the: *(AIIMS Nov. 10)*

Ans. Anterior belly of diagastric muscles, geniohyoid and genioglossus muscles (NBDE oral surgery july 1978, Q-25.

46. A patient with LefortII,III and NOE # treated withIntermaxillary fixation is bestIntubated by: *(AIIMS May 10)*

Ans. SubmentalIntubation (Ref: Paetkau etal. Submental orotrachealIntubaleun for maxillofacial surgery, Anesthesiology, mar 2000, Vol. 92, Issue 3, p912)

47. A 40 year male has got a blow on the angle region of mandible and he is asymptomatic. The X-ray of that region shows a radiopaque line with very sharp undercutIn the lower border of the mandible, which may be due to: *(AIIMS May 10)*

Ans. Overlapping sign (Ref: Petu ward booth 1/e. Vol. 1 p273)

48. MaximumInjury to the protective layer is seen with: *(AIIMS Nov. 09)*

Ans. Intrusion (Ref: Trope clinical management of the avulsed tooth (Roots summit monterry mexico 2005)

49. Open reduction and fixation of # of mandibular condyle is indicated when: *(AIIMS Nov. 09)*

Ans. Shortening of ramal height is more than 5mm

50. TheIncision used for treatment of traumatic telecanthus is: *(AIIMS Nov. 09)*

Ans. BicoronalIncision (Ref: balaji 2007 p632)

51. A patient with an accident is presented in a casuality, what will be the least Glasgow coma index to measure his responsiveness: *(AIPG 11)*

Ans. 3

52. The Ist and most important step in management of a case of trauma is: *(AIPG-11)*

Ans. Clearing the airway

53. Objective method of pain assessment: *(AIPG 10)*

Ans. Facial pain scale

54. In which mandibular # the tongue fall backwards? *(PGI June 11, 10)*

Ans. B/L Parasymphysis # (Ref: BDC 4/e p252)

55. Keen's Approach is for? *(PGI June 11)*

Ans. Intraoral reduction of zygoma # (Ref: Neelima malik 2/e p370)

56. Which of the following is not cause of exopthalmos? *(PGI June 11)*

a. BlowIn #
b. Hyperthroidism
c. Blow out #
d. Throtoxicosis

Ans. c. Blow out # (Ref: Neelima malik 2/e p340)

57. Blow out #Involves which part of the orbit? *(PGI June 11)*

Ans. floor and medial wall (Ref: Neelima malik 2/e p361)

58. Which of the following is the best method for # stabilization? *(PGI June 11)*

Ans. Arch bar with wiring (Ref: Peterson 2/e p538)

59. A child aged 5yrs suffers U/L # occlusion is normal, there is only pain on movement what is the recommended treatment? *(PGI June 11)*

Ans. active movement (Ref: killey's mandibular # 4/e p100)

60. Fracture of theInfraorbital margin will lead to: *(PGI Dec. 10)*

Ans. Anesthesia of upper lip (Ref: Killey's # of the middle 3rd of facial skeleton 5/e p37)

61. LefortI # is characterized by: *(PGI Dec. 10)*

Ans. Bleeding from the antrum (Ref: Vinod kapoor 2/e p289)

62. Floating maxilla is typically found in: *(PGI June 10)*

Ans. LefortI/Geurin # (Ref: Killey's midfacial # 3rd volume 5/e)

63. Battle sign is seen with (PGI June-10)

Ans. # of middle cranial fossa (Ref: Killey's Mandibular fracture 4/e p61)

64. Most serious complications of open #is: *(PGI Dec. 09)*

Ans. Infections (Ref: Neelima malik 2/e p400)

65. According to champy's principal for extened condylar # how many plates are given: *(PGI Dec. 12)*

Ans. 2

66. Racoon eye is not seen in: *(PGI Dec. 12)*

Ans. LefortI

67. The 'Search lines' to detect fracture line on occipitomental radiographic view of mid-facial skeleton # was described by: *(KCET 12)*

Ans. Mcgrigor and Campbell

68. In which of the following conditions doesInternal derangement cause mandibular diviation to same side? *(KCET 12)*

Ans. U/L disk displacement anteriorly without reduction

69. Which technique of facial # treatmentInvolved purely closed reduction: *(KCET 12)*

Ans. Maxillo – mandibular fixation

70. In patient with fresh blow out of the orbit "best" management is: *(AIIMS Nov. 09)*

Ans. Titanium mesh

Note: If Immediate management is asked,It should be wait and watch

71. In case of # biomechanics seen at the alveolar border are: *(AIPG 11)*

Ans. Tension

72. A Patient with a history of fall after hypoglycaemic episode presents with painIn b/L preauricular region and deviation of the mandible to right side on mouth opening. The probable diagnosis will be: *(AIIMS Nov. 09)*

Ans. Fracture of the right condyle (Ref: Ghom, oral radiology, 2008/e p591)

73. Mandibular fracture managed by adapting mini-plates: *(AIIMS Nov. 09)*

Ans. Load sharing osteosyntheseo (Ref: kerawala and newlands, oral and maxillofacial surgery 2010, p36)

74. The cause of death during 2nd peakIn a patient with severeInjuries is: *(AIIMS Nov. 09)*

Ans. Subdural/Subarachnoid hematoma (Ref: CMDT 13/e p176)

75. The common site for CSF rhinorrhoea is:

Ans. Ethmoid sinus (Ref: Fonseca, OMFS trauma Vol. 2, 3/e p676 vol. 1 p117)

76. Mandibular fracture with bone loss shouldIdeally be treated with: *(AIIMS May 09)*

Ans. Bone grafting with load bearing (Ref: Fonsica, OMFS trauma Vol-2, 3/e p1146)

77. GCS does notInclude which of the following? *PGI June 11)*

a. Sensory response
b. Motor response
c. Verbal response
d. Eye movement

Ans. a. Sensory response (Ref: Bailey's and love 23/e p277)

78. Which survey has the purpose of examining the fracture of the condylar neck of mandible? *(AIIMS May 09)*

Ans. Reverse towne's view (Ref: Fonseca OMFS trauma Vol 1, 3/e p422)

79. A patient had a fall resulting in midsymphyseal guardsman # while reducing the # lingual splaying of the segments was noted. This will causeIncrease in: *(AIPG 09)*

Ans. Interangular distance

80. A case of subcondylar # with fragment overlap of > 5mm and deviation of > 37° would required: *(AIPG 09)*

Ans. ORIF (Ref: Peter ward booth p282)

81. **In fracture through mental foramenIn mandible through mental foramenIn mandible with less than 10 mm of bone loss, treatment would be:** *(AIIMS May 09)*

Ans. Reconstruction plates (Ref: Fonseca OMFS trauma vol. 2 3/e p1146)

EXODONTIA

- Rubber band extraction – Method of extractionIn Bleeding disorder
- Ash Forceps – For extraction of lowerIncisors.
- Cowhorn Forceps – 16, 23 – Mandibular 3rd molar
- (For Grossly decayed molar) 88 – Maxillary 3rd molar
- Remember: Patients on long term antiplatelet and corticosteroid do't need to alter their dose.
- Extraction can be safely done.
- **Absolute C/I to Extraction:**

Central hermangioma and A-V fistula.

- During extraction all teeth moved buccally/labially except mandibular posterior (lingually) and Maxillary LI (Palatally)
- Maxillary centralIncisors – Rotatory movements are used for extraction
- **AcuteInfection and Extraction:**

Most rapid resolution ofInfection is obtained whenInfected tooth is removed as early as possible. ie, AcuteInfection should not be a C/I to extractionIf proper LA and antibiotic coverage given.
Maxillary lateralIncisors are palatallyInclined cause palatal abscess.

- Inhaled foreign body enters Right bronclus [Q]
- Maximum difficultyIn extraction – Mandibular Ist molar.
- Maximum chances of fracture of root – Maxillary Ist PM.
- Most easiest tooth for extraction – Mandibular Ist PM
- Odontectomy – Transalveolar extraction.
- Postage stamp method- is a method of bone removalIn transalvealar extraction.
- Open window Technique: use to extractionof Maxillary PM where buccal cortical plate should beIntact as for orthodontic purpose.
- Stobies Tech.: use of elevator by usingInterdental bone as fulcrum for extraction of adjacent multiple teeh.
- Position of operator while extraction.

• For all mandibular and maxillary teeth, position is in "FRONT"
• For mandibular posterior – Both front and Behind position can be used.

- After multiple extraction Black – blue marks over neck after several days is "ecchymosis"
- Teeth removed by rotation – Maxillary CI and Mandibular Ist PM
- Swelling over extraction Wound with crackles on palpation – Emphysema.
- Non surgical extraction Site heals by 2°Intention.
- Impaction:

Winter's line: W – White line (Below occlussal plane) A – Amber line Amount of Bone covering tooth R – Red line (Red-means Difficulty) – Depth of toothIn bone

WHARFE assessment: DifficultyIndex for removal ofImpacted 3rd molars.

Classification	DifficultyIndex valve
Angulation (Winter's classification)	
• Mesioangular	1
• Horizontal	2
• Vertical	3
• Distonangular	4
Depth	
Level A	1
Level B	2
Level C	3
Ramus Relationship/Space available (Pell and Gregory classification)	
ClassI	1
ClassII	2
ClassIII	3
Very Difficult	7 – 10
Moderately	5 – 10
Minimally	3 to 4

W – Winter's classification
H – Height of mandible
A – Angulation of 3rd molar
R – Root shape
F – Follicle
E – Path of Exit of tooth during removal.

Lingual split bone technique/kelsy fry TECHQ:

- For removal of linguallyImpacted mandibular 3rd molar
- Only chisells used *(PGI 2011)*

Lateral trephination:

- For removal ofImpacted mandibular 3rd molarIn age group of 9-16 yrs.
- 'S' ShapedIncision is given.

Bulls eye is seenIn – lingullay placed 3rd molar.

Line of withdrawl of tooth is determined by root pattern

Maxillary 3rd molarImpaction:
Most common – vertical
Most easiest to remove – Distoangular
Most Difficult to remove – mesio angular (Just opposite of lower 3rd molarImpaction)
Position of tooth B-L ly determines difficulty of removal.

WhenIAN canal crosses 3rd molar root apex, there is reductionInIts diameter. This narrowing/converging of canal is called HOUR GLASS appearance.

- After multiple extraction sutures are placed on –Intendental septum
- Dry Socket:

Is delayed healing but is not associated withInfection.
No usual sign and symptoms ofInfection like fever, swelling and crythema.
Moderate to severe dull aching pain.
Commonest complication after Molar extraction – Dry socket
Dry socket commonly caused by T. denticoli.

- Most common complication of extraction of maxillary 3rd molar is – Fracture of Tuberosity (Do Not confuse – M.C. complication of any tooth extraction is root fracture)
- Commonest complication mandibular Distoangular Impaction is # of Ramus.

LAST 5-YEAR QUESTIONS FROM THIS TOPIC

1. **Antibiotic coverage for extractionIn a prosthetic mitral valve patient is:** *(AIIMS Nov. 11)*

Ans. 2 mg amoxicillin 1 hr. before surgery. (Ref: Neelima malik I/e p106)

2. **In war lines, red lineIndicates:** *(COMEDK 09, AIIMS Nov. 12)*

Ans. Depth ofImpacted tooth

3. **Radiograph of mandibular 3rd molar shows fading of the trabeculations and narrowing of canalIn apical region of tooth. What will be the diagnosis?** *(AIIMS Nov. 11, AIPG 11)*

Ans. Deep grooving of root and loss of dense costical wall of the canal (Ref: Neelima malik, is ted. P119)

4. **A patient who underwent extraction of 3rd molar reports with painIn socket after 3 days. On examination the socket is tender and extremely sensitive with No fever. What is the treatment:** *(AIPG 12)*

Ans. Irrigate the socket and place a sedative dressing.

5. **Which of the following is least likely to be damaged during extraction of lower 3rd molar:** *(AIPG 11)*

Ans. Lingual artery

6. **For maxillary 3rd molar extraction position which is wrong?** *(PGI June 09)*

Ans. 12 O'clock

7. **Last tooth to be extractedIn whole mouth extraction case:** *(PGI Dec. 10)*

Ans. Canine (Ref: Vinod kapoor 2/e p51)

8. **In lingual split osteotomy technique which of the following is used to cut the bone?** *(PGI June 11)*

Ans. Chisel (Ref: Neelima malik, 2/e p132)

9. **Which of the following method can be used for controlling blood from extraction socket?** *(PGI Dec. 09)*

Ans. Bone wax (Ref: Vinod kapoor 2/e p353)

10. **Which of the following is easiest tooth for extraction?** *(KCET 12)*

Ans. Mandibular Ist PM

11. **Howe and payton (1960. developed a criteria to diagnose the:** *(KCET 12)*

Ans. Relationship of the root apices ofImpacted 3rd M to theInferior alveolar canal

12. **A patient is on regimen of steroid therapy and need for extraction of chronicallyInfected teeth require premedication with:** *(AIIMS Nov. 12, Nov. 10)*

Ans. Antibiotics (Ref: NBDE oral surgery and pain control july 1978, Q-23 p40)

13. **Cardiac dysarrythmia during extraction is caused by:** *(AIIMS Nov. 12)*

Ans. Trigeminal nerve (Ref: Dental hypothesis Vol. 1 No. 1, 2010, Arakeri's reflex: an alternative pathway for dentocardiac reflex mediated syncope).

INFECTION

- **Fascia –** Greatest barrier toInfection.
- **Deep Fascia –** Absent over face except massetesic fascia [Q]
- **Trismus:**

Most common cause is infection of muscle of mastication.

- **Oro Antral Communication and Fistula:** (QAC and OAF)

OAC (Oro-Antral Communicaton) Small opening < 2 mm Rx – Surgical Closure is not necessary. Blood Clot is organized and retained.
<u>T/t of small cases:</u> No treatment allow clot to form.

T/t of Early cases: Cases where OAC is srecent and formation of fistula is not established. t/t: • Immediate surgical repair to achieve 1° Closure. • Simultaneous Antibiotic prophylayis to prevent sinusInfection.
T/t of Delayed cases: Approximately after 3 weeks until gingival edges shows sound healing.
FlapsIn the treatment of OAC/OAF: • Buccal advancement flap of rehman's • Berger's flap– modified rehrman buccal advancement flap. Adv: double closure [Q] • Ashley's palatal pedicle rotational advancement flap: – Follow the cause of Greater palatine artery – The Abundant blosed supplyIn palatal tissue promotes satisfactory healing. – Kruger's Modification: A 'V' Shaped excision to the lessel curvature of the flap to minimize folding.
– Non resorbable suture should be removedIn 7-10days when placed over OAC/OAF
Intranasal Antrostomy: Performed throughInferior meatus *(AIPG)* To close an oro-antral fistula To remove a tooth or a root from sinus PackIs removal on 4th day
Caldwell Luc procedure: SemilunarIncision extending from canine to 2nd molar.. Method of gaining entryInto the maxillary sinus via canine fossa with nasal antrostomy • For closure of Oro-Antral fistula and Chronic maxillary sinusitis. • For removal of foreign body/root from the max. sinus A semilunarIncision is plannedIn the buccal vestibule from carrure to 2nd molar area just above the gingival attachment
Denker's operation: Modification of Caldwell luc. Maximum chances of damage of ASA

- Osteomyelitis of Jaw (OM):

Streptococci (most common)+organism causing dentalInfection.
Other than Jaw – Staphylococcous aureus.
Rx – Clindamycin, Penicillin and Fluoroquinolones. (Good Bone penetration)
Decortication and Saucerization: Both done to gain access to the medullary cavity.

- Consending osteitis/Focal scterosing OM:

Remember: Associated with Both vital and non vital tooth

- Garre's Osteomylitis:

Most commonIn children and young adult.
No lymphadenopathy, fever and leukocytosis
T/t: No need of seqestrectory/De cortication, Removal ofInfected tooth/RCT. Surgical recontouing.

- OM:

Condesing Osteitis – T/t: For tooth – Extract/Extripate
Sclerotic lesion – does't require any surgical removal until Asympomatic

- 1° Spaces:

Mandible	Maxilla
SpacesIn volvedIn ludwing's angina+ Buccal space	**TRICK:** CBI Canine BuccalInfratemporal

- HBO Therapy:

Indication: OM, ORN (Osteo radionecrosis) of jawIn patients refractory to usual surgical and Medical treatment. These patients are associated with marked pain and trismus
Out come: HBO treatment account for marked se is pain, trismus and fistula closer and complete radiological and clinical healing.

- Marx protocol:

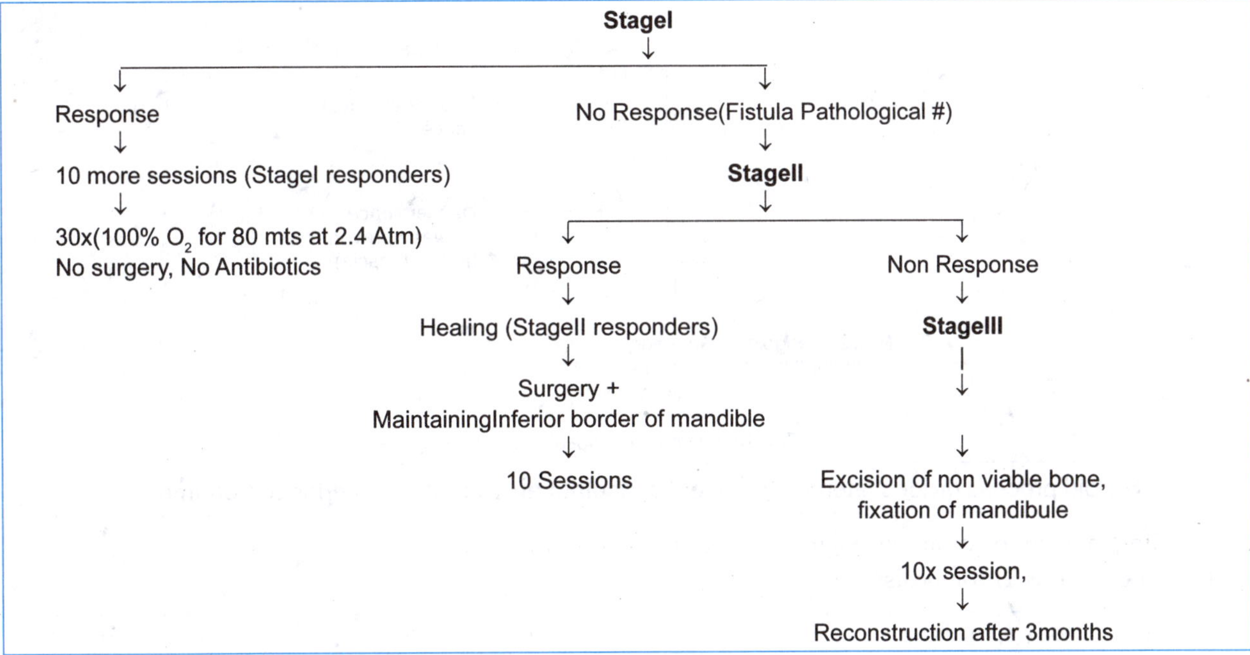

- Spread of infection:

Teeth Involved	Space Infection
Mandibular anteriors	Submental space
Mandibular PMs and Ist molar	Sublingual space
Mandibular 2nd Molar and 3rd Molar	Submandibular space
Maxillary laterals and Palatal Roots of maxillyar posteriors	Palatal abscess
PericoronalInfection from 3rd molar spaceInfection	Lateral pharyngeal, pterygomandibular submasseteric
Buccal roots of max. 2nd and 3rd Molar	Infratemporal space
Maxillary and mandibular Posterior teeth	Buccal space (Mostly from maxillary teeth)
Infection throughIANB	Pterygomandibular space
Infection through PSA	Infratemporal space.

- Lateral pharyngeal space:

– Lies b/w medial pterygoid and superior constrictor
– Most common causes ofInfectionIn this space is odontogenicInfection
–Infection from this space is life threatening because ofItsIntimate relation with CAROTID SHEATH *(AIIMS 2011)*
HOT potato voice seanIn: Lateral pharyngeal space *(COMEDK 2011)*, Retropharyngeal space, Ludwig's Angina, Peritonsillar abscess.

- Retropharyngeal and danger space:

These spaces lies b/w pharyngeal constrictor and preventebral fascia.
IfInfectionInvolves danger space-high risk of mediastinities. *(PGI 2006)*

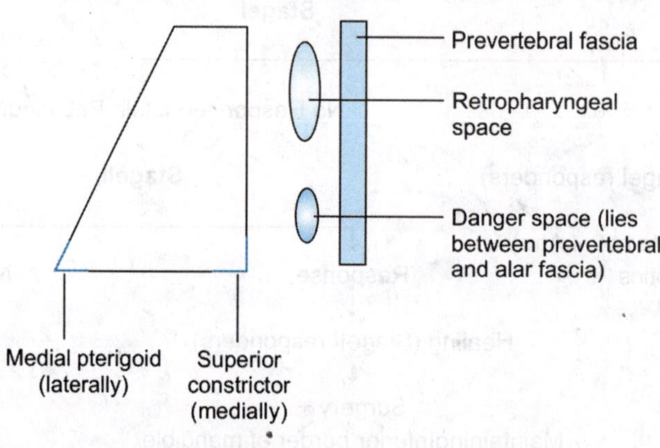

Fig. 10.4: Retropharyngeal and danger space

- Styloid process divides lateral pharyngeal spaceInto anterior and posterior compartment.

- Swelling may not be prominent sign of masticator spaceInfection.
- Cavernous sinus Thrombosis:

Most commonly spreads by Opthalmic vein (From lip and Face) and Pterygoid plexus (From DentalInfection). *(PGI 07)*
The Dangerous area of the face are – VALVELESS-so, retrogradeInfectionIn the form of cavernous sinus thrombosis.
Eagelton criteria for diagnosis of cavernous sinus thrombosis *(PGI 2012)* • Known site ofInfections • Paralysis of 3,4, 6 nerves. • Propoptosis of eyes due to sed venous pressureIn superior andInferior veins of orbit.
Rx of cavernous sinus thrombous: Rapid early aggressive heparinizaion.

- Submental, Submandibular and Buccal space are most commonlyInvolved while canine space is rarelyInvolved.
- Pterygomandibular space:

Remember: Long Buccal nerve and Auriculotemporal nerve are not presentIn pterygomandibular space
Site of 2°Infection from pterygomandibular space- • Infratemporal space and Retropharymgeal space • Buccal and submandibular space (Uncommon)

- **Ludwig's angin:** All 3 spaces submandibular, sublingual and submental areInvolved. Also called PHLEGMON
- **Masticator spaceInfection:**

The Masticator space-Masseteric, Pterygoid and Temporal are well differentiated but communicate with each other and with buccal, submandibular and parapharyngeal spaces.
• **Infection:** Mosts Commonly fromInfection of 3rd molar, can also result from contaminated mandibular block anestheticInjections. Infection may also result from direct trauma.
• The Hallmark of masticator spaceInfection-"TRISMUS"
• Swelling may not be a prominent sign of masticator spaceInfection.

- Pericoronitis:

SpaceInvolved:
- Masticator space
- Lateral pharyngeal space

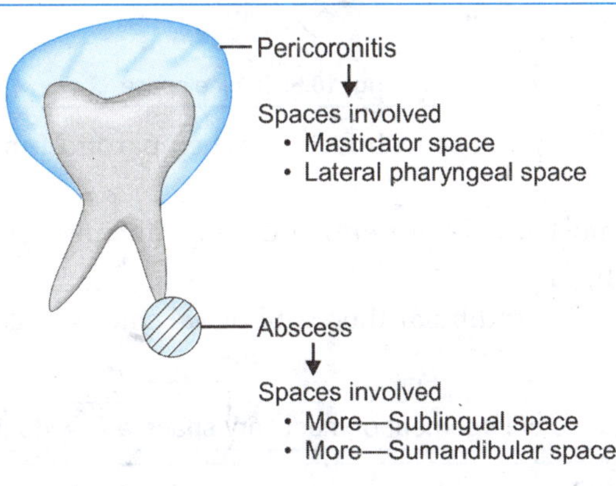

Fig. 10.5: Pericoronitis

- SpacesInvolvedIn:

Ist molar-sublingual space
2nd and 3rd molar-submandibular space

- Boundaries of Pterygomandibular space:

Anteriorly	• Pterygomandibular raphae.
Posteriorly	• Parotid gland
Inferiorly	• Pterygomasseteric slign *(PGI 2012)*

- Canine Space:

Levatolabi superioris Levator anguli oris (Caninus) Orbicularis oris

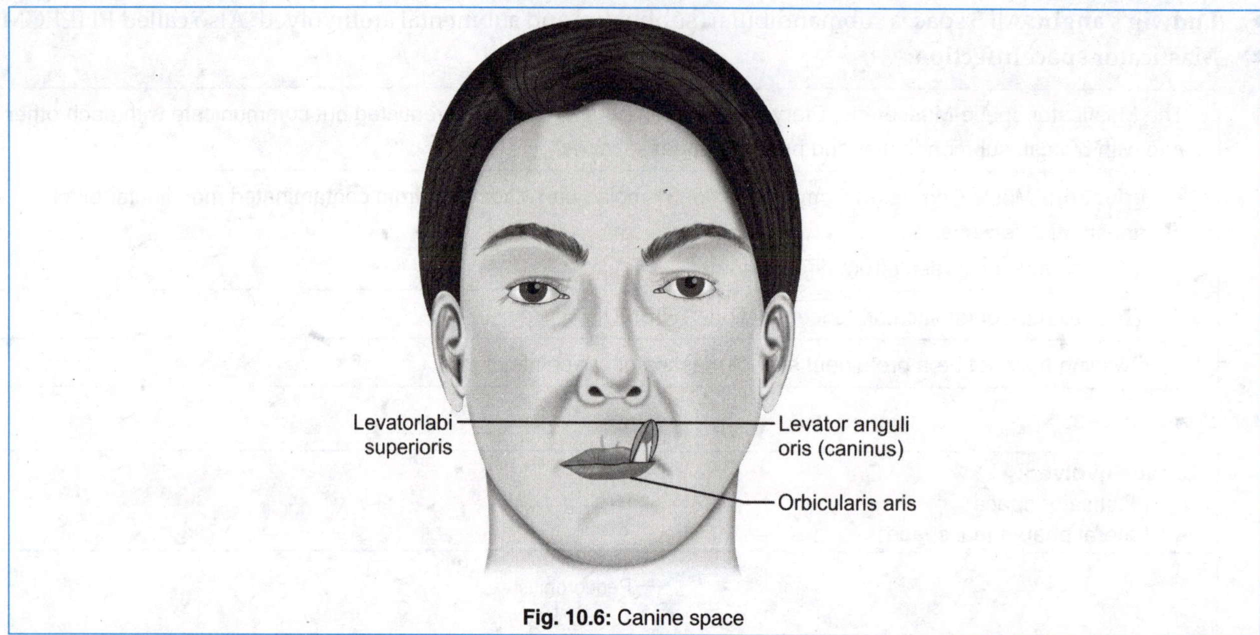

Fig. 10.6: Canine space

- Dumb-bell shaped swelling – Temporal spaceInfection+when parotid tumor extendsInto paraphrygeal space.
- OdontogenicInfection:
  - Anaerobic bacteria are almost always presentIn odontogenicInfection
  - Drug of choice – penicillin
- **Ludwing's Angina:** BeginsIn submandibular then sublingual chief source ofInfection – Mandibular molars.
- Osteomylitis (OM):

"Moth eatnn appearance" is due to enlargement of medullary space and widening of volkman's canal.

Cellulitis	Abscess
Firm	Soft, Fluctuant
Diffuse swelling	
No pus (Inflammatory Exudate)	Localized collection of pus
T/t – Antibiotic (High dose penicillin/Ciprofloxacin) Heat and Fluid	T/t –Incision and drainage

- BacteriaInfection vs ViralInfection:

Neutrophillia (Except typhoid)	Neutropenia Lymphocytosis

- Rheumatoid Arthritis – ESR is ↑sedIn all pateint.

LAST 5-YEAR QUESTIONS FROM THIS TOPIC

1. **Case Report: COMEDK 12**

   A 58 year-old healthy man was evaluated for a toothache of 2 days duration. He was treated with oral penicillin and an opiate analgesic and advised to have the affected teeth pulled. He returned less than 24 hrs later reporting sever swellingIn the neck, sore throat, chills and chest pain. On examination the floor of his oral cavity wasIndurated and woody, and he had marked tendernessand adenopathy through out his neck. He had erythema spreading from his neck down over his anterior chest wall where his chest pain was localized

a. The patient is suffering from:

Ans. ludwing's angina

b. This condition is an emergency asIt can lead to:

Ans. Airway obstruction

c. TheInfection spreads to the

Ans. Submental, sublingual and submandibular space.

d. The treatment of choicIn such acute condition is:

Ans. Surgical drainage, antibiotic andIntensive care:

2. Lundwig's angina is caused due to pus collection in: *(COMEDK 12)*

Ans. Submandibular space

3. A male patient had a pin point Oroantral communication. The treatment is: *(COMEDK 11)*

Ans. Nothing needs to be done (Ref: Textbook of maxillary antrrum by Kelly 3/e)

4. Ludwig's angina is usually caused by: *(KCET 10)*

Ans. Streptococci and various mixed anerobes

5. AnInhaled foreign body, most likely to: *(KCET 10)*

Ans. Enter right bronchus

6. The most serious complication which can occur following surgeryIn maxillaryIncisor region is: *(KCET 10)*

Ans. Cavernous sinus thrombosis

7. Which is not seenIn cavernous sinus thrombosis? *(PGI June 09)*

a. Increases venous pressureIn orbit
b. MeningealIrritation
c. Septicemia
d. NoInfection site is present

Ans. d. NoInfection site is present

8. Radiographically sequestrum appears as? *(PGI Dec. 11)*

Ans. More radiopaque than normal bone (Ref: Neelima malik 2/e p642)

9. The recommended time gap b/w the radiation exposure and surgery to avoid osteoradionecrosis is: *(PGI Dec. 09)*

Ans. 4-6 weeks (Ref: 4-6 weeks, Ref. Peterson 3/e p110)

10. Head shaking test is done to diagnose: *(COMEDK 10)*

Ans. Position of rootIn relation of maxillary antrum

11. Berger flap procedure is used forL: *(COMEDK 09)*

Ans. Oroantral communication

12. Acute osteomyelitis is commonly caused by: *(KCET 09)*

Ans. S. aureus

13. Protein concentration of cystic fluid is: *(KCET 09)*

Ans. 5–11 g/dl

14. Hyperbaric oxygen is contraindicatedIn all except: *(AIIMS Nov. 11)*

Ans. Glaucoma (Ref: Ash high Roda Tokskol 1993 Sep., 44(3), 239-47)

15. In oral and maxillofacial surgery danger space is known as: *(AIIMS Nov. 11)*

Ans. Space between Alar and prevertebral fascia (Ref: Textbook of oral and maxillofacial surgery by neelima malik is ted. p564)

16. Cavernous sinus thrombosis takes place whenInfection traverses through: *(AIIMS Nov. 11)*

Ans. Pterygoid plexus of veins (Ref: Neelima malik p590)

17. **There is a swellingIn a patient with respect to maxillary LI, since last 48 hrs, the swelling is hot and Palpable, rebound on pressure, the treatment of choice is:** *(AIIMS Nov. 11, 10)*

Ans. Incision and drainage (Ref: Neelima malik, p554)

18. **In ludwig's angina, Ist step when patient report to emergency room:** *(AIIMS Nov. 12)*

Ans. Tracheostomy under L.A. (ref.: Serious soft tissueInfections of the head and neck by Robert D. Herr. American family physician sep. 1991, Vol. 44, No. 3, 878-888)

19. **Most common 3rd molarImpaction is:** *(AIPG 09)*

Ans. Mesioangular

20. **After calwell luc operation nasal antrostomy is performed through:** *(AIPG 12, PGI Dec. 11)*

Ans. Inferior meatus (Ref: Laskin's/21)

21. **Ludwig's Angina is characterized by:** *(AIIMS May 12)*

Ans. Raised tongue (Ref: Neelima malik 2/e p624-626)

22. **Masticator spaceInfection is due toInfection from:** *(AIIMS Nov. 09)*

Ans. The mandibular molar

23. **Osteomyelitis beginsIn?** *(PGI Dec. 11)*

Ans. Medullary bone (ref.: neelima malik 2nd ed p636)

24. **Trismus can results from theInfection of which space?** *(PGI Dec. 10)*

Ans. Submasseteric space (ref.: Neelima malik p194)

25. **Following splenectomyIn children, which one of the following is recommended?** *(COMEDK 12)*

Ans. pneumococcal vaccination

26. **Entery of Caldwell procedure is made through:** *(COMEDK 12)*

Ans. Canine fossa

27. **'Hot potato ' voice is characteristically seen in:** *(COMEDK 12)*

Ans. Lateral phaygeal spaceInfection

28. **Tooth which isInvolvedIn the most common cause of oroantral communication is:** *(COMEDK 09)*

Ans. Ist molar

CYST AND TUMOR

- Protein concentration of:

cystic fluid – 5–11 gm/dl
< 4 gm/dl is highly suggestive of OKC [Q]

- Salivary Gland Tumors:

Benign	Malignant
No associated nerve sign	May cause cranial nerve palsies. (Facial nerve palsy, lingual and Hypoglossal nerveInvolvement)
Ex-pleomorphic Adenoma (PA)	Ex- malignant PA, Mucoepidermoid CA, Adenoid Cystic CA

- Erythematous granular mucosal lesionIn high risk area like soft palate, floor of mouth, ventral surface of tongue that persist for 7–12 days without apparent etiology should be suspected as sign of asymptomatic squarmous CA.
- Sublingual Dermoid cyst – presentIn floor of mouth butIn midline.
- Mucocle vs Salivary duct cyst:

Mucocle	Salivary duct cyst
Other names: Mucus extravasatin cyst (Ranula)	Mucus duct cyst/sialocyst/mucus retention cyst.
No Epithelial lining	Epithelial lining present
Not A true cyst	True cyst.

- Epidermoid cyst = Sebaceous cyst
- Cock's Peculiar tumor – Ulcerated Sebaceous cyst.
- Dermoid cyst – Bony defect present.
- Lymphangioma = cystic hygroma of neck
- Lymphangioma and Ranula + Hydrocele + Meningocele have H2O content so, fluctuant and Brilliantly transilluminate.
- Branchial cyst:

2nd Branchial arch [Q]
Under the cover of upper anterior 1/3rd Sternocleido mastoid muscle

- Branchial fistula:

From 2nd Bronchial cleft [Q]
Ist cleft persist as External Auditary meatus. While 2nd, 3rd and 4th dissappeard.

- Thyroglossal cyst and Thyroid swelling Both move with Deglutition.
- But with protrusion of tongue only thyroglossal cyst moves.
- T/t of Thyroglossal Cyst – "Sistrunk operation"
- Biopsy:

Indications for Biopsy: • Any lesion that persist for more than 2 weeks with no apparent etiologic basis. • AnyInflammatory lesion that does't respond to local treatment after 10-14 days (ie, after removing localIrritant) • Persistent hyperkeratotic changesIn surface tissue • An lesion that has the characteristics of malignancy.
Excisional biopsy: < 1 cmIn diameter
Excisional Biopsy – wire guided biopsy a special type of biopsy for breast.
Stereotactic needle biopsy – New technique for breast lesion

- Biopsy segment:

Better to take Deep narrow biopsy rather than wide shallow as even connective tissue changes can be visualizedIn deep narrow biopsy.

- "Biopsy" from floor of mouth:

Suturing is C/I after taking biopsy from floor of mouth b'coz during biopsy there are chances of damage of wharton's duct and sleepage of salivaInto sub mandibular spaceIf place suture.

- Rx for tumor:

• Tumor notInvolving the lower border of mandible–Enbloc resection to preserve continuity.
• TumorInvolving lower border: segmental resection/Hemimandibulectomy.
• Benign, Non Aggressive tumors: • ex-odontoma, Ameloblastic febroma, Pindberg tumor, AOT, ABC, COC – Enucleation and/or curettage
• Benign Aggressive tumor: • Ameloblastoma, pindborg tumor myxoma, SOT– Enbloc Resection (Marginal or partial resection) • Unicystic Ameloblastoma – Enucleation *(AIPG 2012)*
• Malignant tumor – Complete resection

- Maxillary tumors have poorest prognosis as they remain asymptomatic for a long time (as they canInvadeInto Maxillary sinus/nasopharymx)
- In anIrridiation field – Optimal time for surgery = 4-6 weeks.
- Most frequentlyIndicated treatment for odentogenic cyst – Enucleation.
- Aspiration of airInto needleIndicates traumatic bone cyst or, entryInto maxillary sinus.
- Marsupilization = Decompression = PartschI.
- Marsupilization + Enucleation = Waldron operation = PartschII
- Treatment of Dentigerous cyst:

Children – Marsuplization and allow tooth erupt + prevent damage to developing tooth bud.
Adult – Enucleation.

- Enucleation with curettage:

• In OKC (with High recurrence rate)
• In any cyst which recurs after what was expected to be completely removed.
• Traumatic Bone cyst: Open the cavity andInduce bleeding is the treatment.

- Perepheral gaint cell granuloma: T/t – surgical excision
- Central G.C.G.:

– Curettage/surgical excision
– X-ray contraIndicated.

- Irritational fibroma – T/t – simple excision.
- Enucleation of Cyst:

If small cyst – enucleation via socket after tooth removal
If cyst is large – enucleation by making a mucoperiosteal flap and removing the cyst through an opening madeIn alveolar bone (osseous window)

- Carnoy's Solution:

3 mins application of carnoy's solution.
Use: In OCK [Q]
Treatment of pathological lesions with carnoy's solution may lead to nerveInjury.

- Neck Disection:

• Classical Radical neck dissection: Cervical lymphnodes +Internal jugular vein+ accessory nerve + submandibular gland + sternomastoid musle (All resected)
• Modified Radical Neck dissection/Functional neck dissection: Accessory nerve + Sternomasloid +Internal jugular preserved
• Selective neck dissection: One/more major lymph nodes+ Sternomastoid + acussory nerve +Internal jugular vein preserved.

- Commando operation:

RND+Hemimandibulectomy + Radical glossectomy

LAST 5-YEAR QUESTIONS FROM THIS TOPIC

1. Treatment of choice for BCC of skin is: *(KCET 11)*

Ans. Surgical excision (Ref: Bailey and love's short practice of surgery 23/e p181)

2. **Pleomorphic adenomas arising from the minor salivary glands can be treatment with:** *(KCET 11)*

Ans. Local excision with 5mm margin (Ref: Bailey surgical textbook 23/e p660)

3. **Aspirate which is creamy white viscoid with the value of total protein less than 5.0 g/100 ml is suggestive of?** *(COMEDK 11, 09)*

Ans. OKC (Ref: Neelima malik 2/e p424)

4. **A patient with fibrous dysplasia can be treated by:** *(KCET 10)*

Ans. Conserative surgery

5. **A patient with ameloblastoma of the jaw can be treated by:** *(KCET 10)*

Ans. Surgical removal followed by cauterization

6. **A tumor arising of a burns scar is likely to be:** *(COMEDK 10, PGI Dec. 11)*

Ans. Marjolins ulcer (NEXT best option is SCC)

7. **Chemical cauterization of OKC is done by:** *(KCET 07, COMEDK 10, AIPG 12)*

Ans. Carnoy's Solution (Ref: Peterson 2/e p245)

8. **Case Report:** *(COMEDK 12)*

A 15 year old boy report with a rapidly growing swelling of the mandible with Intermittent pain. Patient gives history that the swelling occurred after an episode of trauma radiographs reveal formation of layers of new subperiosteal bone producing onion skin appearance the patient also has lip paraesthesia and elevated WBC

a. Based on clinical and radiographic picture one of the following condition could be considered in provisional diagnosis:

Ans. Ewing's sarcoma

b. One the following conditions produces onion skin appearance of the jaws on radiography

Ans. Osteomyelitis with proliferative periostitis

c. There is considerable clinical and H/P overlap of Ewing's sarcoma with

Ans. PNET

d. True statement for Ewing's sarcoma

Ans. An episode of trauma often precedes development of Ewing's sarcoma

9. **Throid carcinoma with pulsating vascular skeletal metastasis is:** *(COMEDK 09)*

Ans. Follicular metastasis

10. **Which of the following statements is true regarding thyroglobulin:** *(COMEDK 09)*

Ans. Elevation after complete therapy suggests recurrence In well – differentiated thyroid malignancies (Ref: Davidson 17/e p699)

11. **The following lesions are premalignant except:** *(KCET 09)*

    a. Bowen's disease
    b. Solar keratosis
    c. Radio keratosis
    d. Epidermoid

Ans. d

12. **In functional neck dissection, the following structures are preserved:** *(KCET 09)*

Ans. Sternomastoid muscle, spinal accessory nerve and IJV

13. **Rx of choice In cold nodule of thyroid:** *(KCET 09)*

Ans. Hemithyroidectomy

14. **Commonest site of Ca of tongue:** *(KCET 09)*

Ans. Lateral magin

15. **In case of nodal metastasis, which is not seen on CT scan:** *(AIIMS Nov. 11)*

    a. Spiculated node

b. Size more than 6mm

c. Necrotic node

d. Rounded node

Ans. a (Ref: The otolaryngologic clinics of north America vol. 31, No. 4 Aarg 1998 p646 and 647)

16. StageIII lymphomaIn ann Arbor classification of lymphoma is: *(AIPG 11)*

Ans. Involvement of lymph node regions/lymphoid structures on both sides of the diaphragm

17. Excisional biopsy is done by: *(AIPG 09)*

Ans. Removal of entire lesion with a margin of uninvolved normal border tissue.

18. Ameloblastoma's pathologicallyInvade and spread by: *(AIIMS Nov. 11)*

Ans. MMP's (Ref: Annals of maxillofacial surgery year 2011, Volume: 1, issue: 2, p145-149)

19. There is < 2 cms painful sweling responsive to salicylates, this is: *(AIIMS Nov. 11, 12)*

Ans. Osteoid osteoma (Ref: White and Pharoah 5/e p443, 452, 550)

20. In 35 year old man there is recently developing classIII malocclusion, there is a bony mass seen protruding towards lateral ptergoid on panorex, condition is: *(AIIMS Nov. 11, 12)*

Ans. Osteochondroma (Ref: White and Pharoh 5/e p550, 443, 44 4.

21. Standard treatment of unilocular amloblastoma is: *(AIPG 12, 11)*

Ans. Enucleatoin

22. Most common primary malignant tumor of long bones is: *(AIPG 10)*

Ans. Osteosarcoma

23. The type of UV radiation known toInduce skin cancer: *(COMEDK 12)*

Ans. UV-B

24. A negativeIncisional biopsy report of a highly suspicious oral lesion suggests that: *(AIIMS May 09)*

Ans. Repeat biopsy (Ref: Person OMFS 3/e p521)

25. Type of carcinoma developedIn Marjolin ulcer is: *(PGI Dec. 11)*

Ans. SCC (Ref: Manipal manual of surgery p91)

26. Which of the following radiopaque mass surrounded by radiolucent line? *(PGI Dec. 11)*

Ans. Compound odontoma (Ref: Shafer's 5/e p404)

27. Reed Sternberg cells are seen in: *(PGI June 11)*

Ans. Hodgkin's disease (Ref: Robbins 7/e p268)

28. The most important factor associated with causation of head and neck Ca is: *(COMEDK 12)*

Ans. Tobacco use

29. TNM staging does notInclude: *(PGI June 11)*

a. Tumour size

b. Tumour site

c. NodalInvolvement

d. Metastasis

Ans. b. Tumour site (Ref: Bailey's and Love 23/e p154-155)

30. Which lesion arises from sunlight? *(COMEDK 12)*

Ans. BCC

31. In a 3 year old child which of the following is the most common cyst locatedIn midline of neck: *(PGI Dec. 10)*

Ans. Thyroglossal cyst (Ref: Baily and love 23/e p777)

32. TheInc isional biopsyIndicatedIn all conditions, except: *(KCET 12)*

Ans. When lesion < 1 cmIn diameter

33. Ameloblastoma of the mandible is definitively treated by: *(KCET 12)*

Ans. Wide local excision

34. Prophylactic throidectomyIndicated in: *(KCET 12)*

Ans. Medullary carcinoma

35. Treatment of choice for pleomorphic adenoma of the parotid is:

Ans. Superificial parotidectomy

36. Nasolabial cysts arises from: *(AIIMS Nov. 11)*

Ans. Remant Embryonic part of nasolacrimal duct (Ref: Shafer's 5/e p92)

TMJ

- **TMJ:** Diarthroidal and Ginglimoidal joint [Q]
- **NOTE:** Joint between C1 and C2 – synovial joint *(KCET 2010)*
- Ankylosis:

Condylectomy – Fibrous Ankylosis
Gap arthroplasty – Minimum gap of 1-1.5 cm to prevent reankylosis

- Frequent dislocation:

Dye to spasm or excessive contraction of muscle mastication. (Lateral pterygoid)

- Repeated Dislocation of condyle:

<u>T/t:</u> Dautry's Zygomatic arch procedure Mayer's grafting techqnique on eminence. Removal of obstacles – condylectomy, Eminectomy.

- Condyle: Growth persists until age of 20 yrs and even more
- Bilateral ankylossis – Bird face

LAST 5-YEAR QUESTIONS FROM THIS TOPIC

1. The most common dislocation of TMJ is: *(COMEDK 09)*

Ans. Anterior

2. Mandibular subluxation is associated with: *(AIIMS Nov. 11)*

Ans. Prochlorperazine (Ref: KDT 4/e p180)

3. Not a treatment for ankylosis: *(PGI Dec.12)*

Ans. High condylar shaving

4. Which is not a theory of TMJ ankylosis? *(AIIMS Nov. 11)*

a. Fractured segments moves backward and fuse with zygomataic arch
b. Synovial fluid leakage attracts Ca2+
c. Calcification of soft tissues
d. Condyle burst

Ans. b. Synovial fluid leakage attracts Ca2+

5. Which is initial clicking of TMJ while opening is due to: *(AIIMS Nov. 11)*

Ans. Retruded condyleIn respect to articular disc (Ref: Neelima malik p226)

6. **For detection ofImpacted maxillary right canine the most clinically valid view is:** *(PGI June 10)*

Ans. IOPA X-ray with tube shift technique (Ref: Ghom p185)

7. **A 8 year old child suffered trauma to TMJ at the age of 5 years causing ankylosis. The Rx of choice would be:** *(AIPG 12, 10, PGI Dec. 11)*

Ans. Gap arthroplasty withInterpositional graft. (Ref: Balajhi)

8. **Medial dislocation of condylar segmentIn cases with condylar # occurs due to action of:** *(AIPG 12, AIIMS May 10)*

Ans. Lateral pterygoid (Ref: Moore 5/e p213)

9. **A patient attempt protrusion, then mandible deviates to the right side, the muscle unable to contract is:** *(AIIMS May 12)*

Ans. Righ lateral pterygoid (Ref: BDC head and Neck p117)

10. **Obstructive sleep apnoea caused by following:** *(AIIMS Nov. 12)*

Ans. B/L TMJ ankylosis (Ref: Surgery of TMJ under LA.Indian J plastic serg july December 2008 Vol. 4, issue 2)

11. **Ankylosis of TMJ is most commonly caused by:** *(AIIMS Nov. 12, May 12, AIPG 11, 10)*

Ans. Trauma (Ref: Shafer's 5/e p1012)

12. **BestIncision for TMJ for surgery:** *(PGI June 10)*

Ans. Alkayat bramlyIncision (Ref: Neelima malik 2/e p222)

MISCELLANEOUS

- Factor VIII andIX: (AIIMSQ)

• The minimal level needed for adequated hemostasis is 25% - to lead Normal life.
• The majorities of haemophillics patients have factor VIII less than 5%
• For extensive oral surgical procedure – Factor VIII Level raised to 50-70%
• Minimal acceptable value for hematocrit for electlve oral surgery-30% [Q]

- Hemophillia A vs Hemophillia B:

Hemophillia A	Hemophillia B
Rx– cryoprecipitate	Rx–Fresh frozen plasma/factorIX concentrate.

- Promethazine–Antihistaminics
- Phenothiazine–Typical Antipsychotic
- Synthetic Opioids: Ex-Mepiridine (pethidine), Methadone, Fentalyl
- Jorgensen tech.

i.V. administration of opioids like pethidine, mepisi dine, pentobarbital, scapalamine (Hyoscine)– ForI.V. sedation.

- Ketorolac:

Weak Anti-inflammatory but potent analgesic+ Anti pyretic
It has equal efficacy of morphine but does notInteract with opioid receptors.
Can be given orally/I.m
Not recommended for use for > 5 days.

- Site of Action of BZD and Barbiturates:

BZD – limbic system + RAS (Ascending reticular formation)
Barbiturates – RAS

- ACEInhibitors – Causes Swelling of tongue
- Cocaine causes Palatal and Nasal septal perforation
- **Phenytoin:** What % age of persons taking phenytoin will develops gingival hyperplasia – 50-60%
- Best oral sedative for dentistry – BZD (Diazepam)
- Phlebitis after diazepamInjection is due to propylene glycal [Q]
- Dose of TT (tetanus toxoid) = 0.5 ml (both 1° and booster)
- Opioid:

Tramadol – opioid analgesic
Pentazocin – complex agonist – Antagonist opioid Main action agonist so not givenIn morphine addicts.

- Opiods (Ex-Morphine, Codeine) – Actions on respiration

Respiratory center	Bronchial smooth muscle
Depressant	Broncho Construction (AsIt release Histamine)

- **NOTE:** So, Both Morphine and CodeineIe. Opioid is C/IIn Asthmatics
- Atropine – is a parasympatholytic
- Aspirin – Should be avoidedIn G-6PD deficiency as causes hemolysis
- Penicillin:

Major problem with penicillin is Allergy.
Mostly with procaine penicillin G.
• As D.O.C. for – OdontogenicInfection, syphilis, pregnancy [Q]
• Does't cause – SLE, lichenoid Reaction

- Antibiotic prophylaxis forI.E.:

Continued for 2 days post operatively
HBV can transmit through saliva (Do't confuse with HIV)
RecomemdedIn: valvular heart diseaseIncluding prosthetic heart valve+congenital heart disease + Haemodialysis+ Previous history ofI.E. (Infective andocarditis)+ Those who have a total joint replacement.

- Antibiotic Prophylaxi and Dental procedures:

RecommendedIn	Not recommendedIn
• Extraction	• Restorative procedures
• Periodontal procedures	• Routine LA
• Implant placement	• Intracanal endodontic therapy
• Apical endodontics	• Suture removal
• Orthodontic bracket placement	• Removable appliance placement
• Intraligamentary L.A.	• Impression making
• Oral prophylaxis	

- Savlon Concentration: 1.5% CHX (V/V) + 3% (W/V) cetrimide
- AMG's are effective against – G (-)ve bacteria.
- Sketetal muscle relaxant:

Depolarizing Blocker – ex-sch. Decamethorium

Sch. Combines Nm (Neuomurscular)
↓
Depolarization
↓
Transient twitching of muscle (Initially)
↓
Don't dissociate rapidly from the receptors
↓
Continued depolarization
↓
Flaccid paralysis (As Na^+ channelInactivated)
("TypeI block" due to continuous depolarization) [Q] Reversed restored muscle activity
↓
Prolonged and High dose of sch
↓
Desensitization of Ach. Receptors
↓
Flaccid paralysis
(TypeII Block)

- Dermatome–used for harvesting skin graft.
- **Thickness of Grafts:**

Free Gingival graft –1-1.5 mm *(KCET 2011)*
Skin graft – Full thickness – > 1 mm
Split thickness – 0.3 to 0.5 mm [Q] – Most commonly usedIn oral surgery.

- **Abbey**–Estlandar flap– is used for reconstruction of lip.
- **Elevators:** Works on all the three principles but lever is most common.

Elevator	Principle
Stright elevator	– Lever and wedge
Cryer elevator	– Lever
Apex elevator	– Lever and wedge
Cross bar elevator	– wheel and axle
Elevators fitting well b/w thumbs and finger is warwick-James elevator.It is used to displace deciduous roots not grasped by forceps.	

- Mechanical advantage of

  - Wheel and Axle – 4.6
  - Wedge – 2.5
  - Lever+wedge – 3

- Blades forIntra Oral use:

Blade	Use
11, 12	– Gingivectomy
15	– Oral surgery
11	– For stabIncision (Incising an abscess)
10	– For skinIncisions
12	– ForIncising PDL abscess

- **Bibevelled chisel:** Called Osteotome used primarily for splitting of bone.
- Chisel – (1) Cutting the bone (2) Splitting the toothIn difficult extraction
- Sterilization:

Dry heat – Protein Denaturation + Oxidative damage. The main disadvantage of dry heat method – Time consuming.
Autoclave – Protein Denaturation + Protein coagulation.

- Suture materials:

Absorbable	Non Absorbable
Natural • Catgut-resorbsIn 70 days • Chromic catgut-ResorbIn 90 days **Synthetic** • Polyglycolic acid (VICRYL) • Polyglactin • Prolene-minimal tissue adhesion *(ACPG 2012)*	Silk-most commonIntraoral suture. Nylon-popular skin suture vitallium

- Non resorbable suture – causes gall stone/Renal stone.
- Suture material:

Catgut/chromic gut – monofilament
Silk – Braided.

- **Suture material:**

SILK: hasIncreased risk ofInfection. Silk rarely units Braided suture (SILK) is most PLIABLE Catgut/silk – undergo proteolysis/enzymatic (Natural suture) digestion
Polyglycolic acid (VICRYL) has highest knot strength
Polypropyline and nylon are high memory sutures (have high tendency to unite)
Synthetic absorbable – undergo hydrolysis suture
Packing of Gut suture:In isopropyl alcohol, Na Benzoate, Diethyl ethanolamine

- Suturing technique:

• Interrupted suture – M.C used.
• Figure of 8 suture – used for extraction socket closure.
• Horizontal mattress suture – needle is passed from one edge to another and again from latter to 1st edge and Knot is fitted HZ mattress suture is often used forInterproximal area of diastema or, wideInterdental space to adaptInterproximal papilla against bone.
• Vertical mattress suture: Similar to HZ mattress suture except when needle is brought back from 2nd to first, the depth of penetration is more superfiscial. So, that with contracture during healing this will become flat and produces desired cosmetic result that is vertical M. suture is used for wound closure to evert wound margin.
Note: Skin suture also given to evert wound margin so that with contracture during healing this will become flat with a desired cosmetic result. [Q]
Suturing provides little or no benefitIn protection of clot.
In sub cutaneous tissue absorbable suture is uses (Catgut)

- Incisions:

• **SkinIncision:** ***SubmandibularIncision***: Placed 2 cm below theInferior border of mandible to avoid cutting the marginal mandibular branch of facial nerve. ***Risdon'sIncision:*** Slightly curvedIncision placed 2 cm below the lower border of mandible. Both are used for the surgery of angle and ramus area. ***Pre-auricularIncision:*** Provide acces to TMJ. It is made anterior to ear. The upper margine is curved anteriorlyIn order to save "Auriculotemporal nerve" TheIncision should neve be extend downward beyond pinna to avoidInjury to facial nerve. ***Alkayat-BramleyIncision:*** Modification of the pre-auricularIncision where the upper part of theIncision is extendedIn a question mark fashion over the temporal area. ***GillesIncision:*** ItIs made within the hair line at an angle of 45° to the zygomatic arch for the reduction of fractured zygoma.
• **IntraoralIncision:** Used for elevating murcoperiosteal flaps.It isImportant to maintain theIntegrity of papilla. **Wards'Incision:** 'L' shapedIncison for raising L-shaped soft tissue flap for the removal ofImpacted 3rd molar

- Malocclusion and Surgical treatment:

Malocclusion	Surgical treatment
• ClassII with skeletal Open bite	• lefort–I osteotomy with maxillaryImpaction to correct open bite. • Sagittal split osteotomy for mandibular advancement. **Note:** lefort-1 osteotomy: gives stable resultIn open bite even when primarily deformity • In mandible.
• Skeletal classI with mandibular Retrognathism	• Sagittal split osteotomy with mandibular advancement.
• ClassII due to maxillary protrusion	• Maxillary segmental (Anterior) set back.
• ClassIII due to mandibular prognathism	• Sagittal split osteotomy with mandibular set back.
• ClassIII due to maxillary retrusion	• LefortI with maxillary advancement
• Bimaxillary protrusion	• Maxillary and Mandibular Segmental osteotomy with set back of anterior maxilla and Mandible.
• Long face due to maxillary excess	• LefortI with maxillaryImpaction.

- Implant:

Recommnded osteointegration time: Maxilla – 4-6 Months Mandible – 2-3 Months (As denser boneIn mandible)
minimum thickness of keratinized tissue around anImplant is – 1.5 mm
Survival rate – 5–10 yrs.

- Apicoectomy – Amount of root respected – 3 mm (Remember: Post and Core – 4 mm of GP left)
- **Cryosurgery:**

Temprature Varies b/w – 20° C to 180°C
Below – 20°C cryogenic necrosis occurs due to dehydration and desaturation of LIPID molecules [Q]
Used – For superfiscial hemangioma + Papillary hyperplasia.

- Distraction Osteogenesis:

NewImmature formed bone is called – Regenerate [Q]
Rate: 1 mm/dayIn adult 1.5 mm/dayIn children.
Rhythum – 1-2 times/day
Latency phase: 5-7 daysIn adult 0-2 daysIn children.
Consodilation phase – 8-12 weeks.

- Trismus:

Breakage of needleInto muscle causes trismus after some weeks (4 weeks) while spaceInfection or, other causes trismus –Immediately

- Normal CD4 count – 400-1600/mm3 (800–1200 (AIIMS)
- **Hematoma:** Painless swelling relieved by application of cold and pressure – COLD compression.
- Ecchymosis – No treatment required.
- Ridge Augmentation:

• Onlay Grafting–Height maintained but widthInadequate.
• Visor osteotomy
• Modified visor osteotomy.

- Sinus lift procedure: used along with the placement ofImplant [Q]
- Moore or, weber fergusoonIncision:

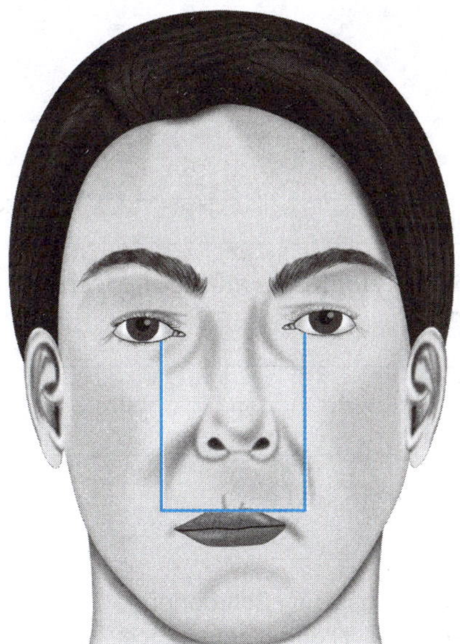

Fig. 10.7: Single stroke incision used in hemimaxillectomy (KCET 2013)

- If fracture of tuberosity with murcoperiosteumIntact – Repositioned and Splinted for 4 weeks
- Antiseptic technique –Introduced by J. lister.

- Ankylosis + myositis ossificans:

Trauma is the most common cause *(PGI 2012)*
Adeno ameloblastoma = AOT
Admantinoma = Ameloblastoma.

- Surgical T/t For Madibular Deformity:

• BSSO – use for both prognathic + Retrognathic mandible "OBWEGESER" [Q] – Transverse movement Not possible (AIPG 12)
• Sub condylar osteotomy – SET back – for mandibular prognathism Robinsoin and Hinds *(COMEDK 07)*
• Vertical Ramus osteotomy – set back for mandibular prognathism – Caldwell and letterman Modifications –Inverted L/C Ostiotomy – main [Q] use for retronathism but can be used for both.

- Hemostasis:

1° – by platelet plug formation. Occurs within seconds ofInjury. Most commonly used test for 1° hemostais – B.T. [Q]
2° – Activation of clotting process. Strengthens 1° hemostatic plug. CompletedIn several mins. And is ImportantIn bleeding from large vessels.
vWF is associated with both 1° and 2° hemostasis.

- % age of WBC:

Neutrophile – 40–70% Lymphocyte – 25–40% Eosinophile – 1–6 % Bassphile – 0–1%

- Ideal Rx for Maxillary tori:

Section with bur and remove with chisel.

- Z-plasty is used for the treatment for ankyloglossia and labial frenum
- **Minor salivary Gland:**

Retromolar – Carmalt's gland
Tonsillar – Weber's gland

- Rhytidectomy – Removal of skin wrinkles (KCET)
- Implant:

Ossedintegration are called functional ankylossis by Schroeder Successful cases have been between 30–95% ofImplant surface.

- Sialolith:

Parotid stones unlike submandibular stone are radioluscent and can not be detected on radiographys.

- Ohngren's line:

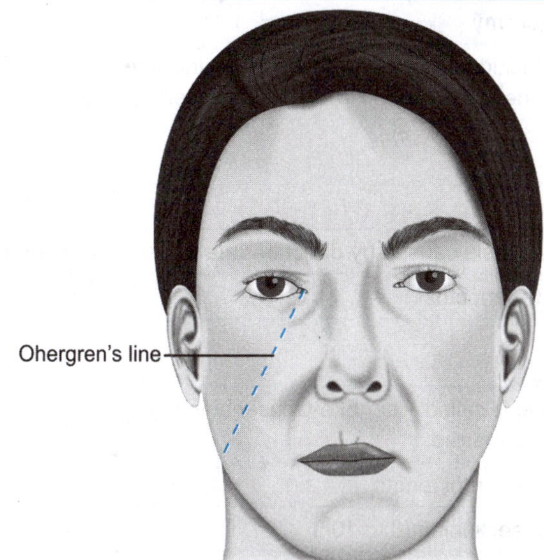

Fig. 10.8: Ohngren's line

Tumors above this line hase poorer prognosis compared to thoseInferior to this line due to the proximity to the orbit and carnial cavity.

- Absorption of Absorbable suture material:

Natural (Catgut)	Synthetic (Polyglocolic/vicryl, Polylactic)
Enzymatic digestion/ Proteolysis	Hydrolysis

- **Nasolacrimal duct** – OpeningIntoInferior meatus is guarded by "HASNER's valve". This valve doesn't permit entery of airInto duct.
- Enlargement of salivary Gland:

• Sialos is/Sialdenosis: NonInflammatory, Non neoplastic painless enlargement of salivary gland. Female > Male Parotid gland gland is commonlyInvolved.
• Sialadenitis:Inflammatory enlargement of gland
• Sialodochitis – is related to "DUCT"

- FREY's Syndrome:

Parasympathetic Cholinergic reinervation *(AIIMS 2012)*
Parasympathetic nerve fibres of auriculotemporal nerve reinervate Sweat gland (Sympathetic cholinergic supply normally)

- Nerve Damage and Surgical Procedure:

Surgical procedure	Anatomical sturtureInjured
Excision of Ranula	Submandibular duct
Excision of submandibular gland	lingual nerve (most common) Hypoglossal nerve
Parotidectomy	Marginal mandibular nerve (branch of facial nerve) Facial nerve
Excision of brachial cyst	hypoglossal nerve accessory nerve

- **Frenectomy vs Frenetomy**

Frenectomy	Frenotomy
Complete removal of frenumIncludingIts attachments to underlying bone.	Incision of frenum. Generally suffices for PDL purpose

- NerveInjury:

Paresis –Incomplete paralysis
Paresthesia – Persistent anesthesia caused by direct trauma to nerve by tip of needle.
Note:Injured nerve repairsIn 3-6 months

- **Apicoectomy:**

Submarginal envelop flap used is called – Lenbke-Ochsenbein flap. But full mucoperiosteal flap is preferred.
Sectioning of root <1/3rd of entire root length
No Bevel angle advocated for sectioning (0 to 10°)

- FNAC – 22-25 Gauze needle use.
  (Note: 27 Gauze is used for canalIrrigation) (PGI)
- **Sialography:**

Can't be performedIn acuteInfection like viral parotitis + Pts allergic tolodine + During thyroid function test.

- Best Graft:

For oral region – posteriorIlliac crest.
For TMJ – Costochndral (Obtained throughInframammary approach through 7th rib)
The graft which resembles TMJ Morphologically is – Sternocavicular *(AIIMS 2012)*
Codman's tumor = Chondrosarcoma

- Most common Rythm disturbance post operatively is – Tachycardia
- CBCT (Cone Beam CT):

• Compact, safe and faster version of regular CT.
• Radiation doses and Time needed for scanning are dramatically used.
• Developed for Angiography.
Indications: • Implant site Assessment • Position ofImpacted and Supernumerary tooth and their relation to adjacent structures *(AIIMS Nov 2011)* • Localisation ofInferior alveolar canal • TMJ • Assessment of many conditions of jaw such as periapical disease, fractured tooth, PDL disease

- Teeth Pigmentation:

Chloradontia – Tooth discaloratoin due to bilirubin *(AIPG12)*
Ochronosis – Blue – Black discoloration seenIn Alkaptonuria

- *Thrombocytosis: Causes: Tricks – Make – Maps*

M – MPD (Myeloproliferative disorders) ex-CML A – Acute hemorrhage K – Kawasaki E – Essential thrombocytosis (a from of MPD) M – Malignancy A – Acute/ChronicInflammation P – Post operative S – Splenectomy

- **Thyroid Gland**:

Grave's disease	Papillary and Follicular	Meullary CA of Thyroid
	CA. of thyroid (Well Differentiated)	
T/t: Over 45 yrs – Radiotherapy Under 45 yrs Rx: Surgery + Anti Thyroid drug Surgery – Sub total [Q]	Near Total thyroidectomy [Q]	Total Thyroidectormy [Q]

- All Solitary Nodules – Treatment is "Hemithyroidectomy"
- Best Diagnositc Modality for Parotid Swelling – FNAC
- Ca, P, ALP levels:

Serum	Ca	P	ALP
Oteoporosis	N	N	N (N= Normal)
Osteomalacia		OR	

NOTE: Osteomalocia – sed osteoid maturation time (mean mineralizaton log time more than 100 days) as law Ca.

- **Ulcers:**

• Arterial ulcer – seen is atherosclerosis + Burger's disease + Raynaud's disease very painfull punched out
• Venous ulcer – Post-phlebitic patients/Varicosal painless (Commonest ulcer)
• Infective ulcer – Pyogenic ulcer
• Tropical ulcer – Malnutrition, anemia, avitaminosis Rhumatoid arthritis Underminded edge
• Cryopathic ulcer – due to coldInjury, fraostbite
• Martorell's ulcer – Hypertensive patient Deep punched out *(KCET 12)*

Ulcer	Edge
TB ulcer	undermined (COMEDK -13)
Gumma + Arterial + Deep trophic+ Martorells	Punched out
Traumatic/venous	Sloping (healing ulcer)
Rodent ulcer (BCC)	Raised, Pearly white beaded
SCC/ulcerated [Q] adinocarcinoma	Rolled out/everted [Q]

Neurogenic ulcer –called perforating ulcer e.g. Trophic ulcer (Bed sole), diabetic neuropathy, leprosy
BRAZIN's ulcer: exclusively seenIn young women
Soft Chancer/Chancroid – caused by H. ducreyi
Black mass at base of Ulcer – Malignant melanoma
Traumatic ulcer – footballer's ulcer seen on SHIN (Injected with staphylococcus)

LAST 5-YEAR QUESTIONS FROM THIS TOPIC

1. **No surgical procedure should be performedIn patients with thrombocytopenia untill the platelet count is:** *(KCET 12, 11)*

Ans. > 80,000 (Ref: Neelima malik is ted. P676)

2. **The orthognathic surgery that is commonly carried out for correction of mandibular prognathism is:** *(KCET 11)*

Ans. Sagittal split osteotomy (Ref: Neelima malik is ted. p27)

3. **Carmalt' glands are:** *(KCET 11)*

Ans. Minor salivary gland (retromolar area) (Ref: Peterson p435-436)

4. **Dilation of the salivary duct 2° to epithelial atrophy as a result of repeatedInflammatory/infections process is:** *(KCET 11)*

Ans. Sialodochitis (Ref: Peterson p440)

5. **Rhytidectomy is:** *(KCET 11)*

Ans. Removal of skin wrinkles (Ref: Peterson's 2/e p1365)

6. **According to the "rule of nine"In burns, what is the percentage of burnsIf both the upper limbs and lower limbs areInvolved:** *(KCET 11)*

Ans. 54% (Ref: A concise textbook of surgery by S.Das 4/e p52)

Note: "Rule of 9"

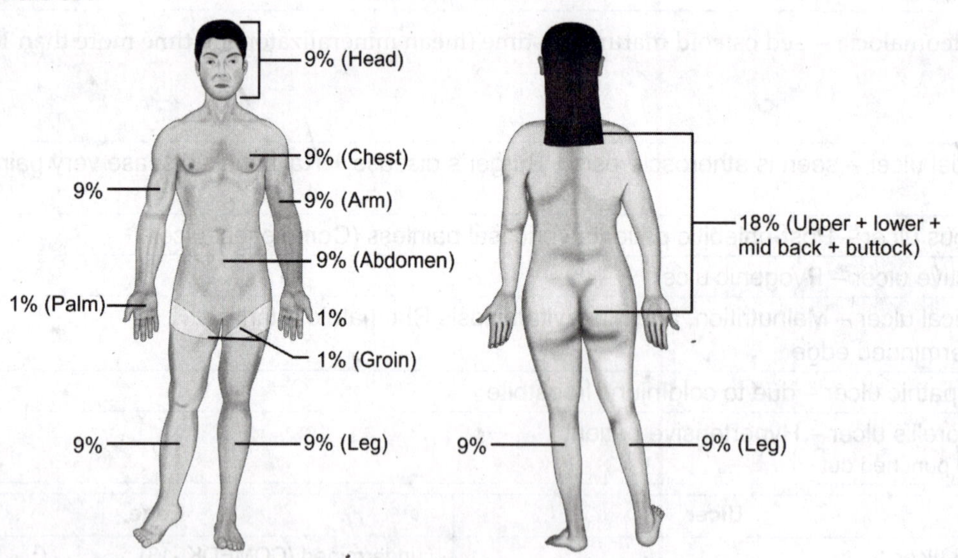

Fig. 10.9: Rule of 9

7. **Commonest location of a thyroglossal cyst is:** *(KCET 09,11)*

Ans. Subhyoid (Ref: Concise textbook of surgery by S. Das 4/e p427)

8. **Rule of nine is usedIn burns for estimation of:** *(KCET 10)*

Ans. extent of burn

9. Commonest thyroid carcinoma is: *(KCET 10)*

Ans. Papillary

10. Hilton's method deals with: *(KCET 10, COMEDK 10)*

Ans. drainage of abscess

11. A direct connection between living bone and load bearing endosseous implant at the light microscopic level: *(KCET 11)*

Ans. Osseointegration (Ref: Carranza 9/e p885)

12. In blood bank, platelets are stored at: *(COMEDK 12)*

Ans. 20 to 24°C for 3 to 5 days

13. Primary antomic structure of concernIn posterior mandible periradicular surgery: *(KCET 10)*

Ans. Neurovasuclar bundle coursing through mandibular canal

14. The suture material most commonly usedIntraoral wound closure is: *(KCET 10)*

Ans. Silk

15. Which of the following suture material will lead to maximum tissue response? *(PGI Dec. 09)*

Ans. Catgut (Ref: Laskin is ted. p265)

16. Which of the following will cause postoperative haemorrhage? *(KCET 10)*

Ans. Salicylates + Liver cirrhosis + prolonged antibiotic administration

17. During submandibular gland excisions which of the following nerve getsInjured: *(PGI Dec. 10)*

Ans. Hypoglossal nerve (Ref: Bailey and Love 23red p663)

18. 2° haemorrhage occurs: *(KCET 10)*

Ans. 7 to 14 days after surgery

19. Treatment of calculus within submandibular salivary gland is: *(KCET 10)*

Ans. Removal of gland

20. During surgery on the submandibular gland: *(COMEDK 10)*

Ans. The submandibular gland is seen to wrap around the posterior border of mylohyoid

21. Tinel's test is:

Ans. Percussion produces tingling sensation

22. Which one of the following medical conditions DOES not mimic acid acute abdomen? *(COMEDK 10)*

Ans. Hypokalemia

23. A complicationIn the Ist 48 hrs of total parenteral nutrition is: *(COMEDK 10)*

Ans. Hyperglycemia (Ref: Sepastin surgery 2/e p130)

24. Which of the following has greater bone density: *(COMEDK 09)*

Ans. Anterior mandible

25. Z-plasty is performedIn cases of: *(COMEDK 09)*

Ans. High frenal attachment (Ref: Carranza 10/e p1023)

26. Cystic hygroma is: *(KCET 09)*

Ans. Lymphangioma

27. Wound healing is: *(KCET 09)*

Ans. More rapidIn young than in old

28. Echymosis and hematoma is treated by: *(KCET 09)*

Ans. IntermittentIce pack

29. distraction is performed by activating the screw at the rate of: *(COMEDK 09)*

Ans. 1 mm/ day

30. Epulis fissuratum is: *(KCET 09)*

Ans. Inflanmmatory fibrous hyperplasia

31. NeurotransmitterIn frey's syndrome is: *(AIIMS Nov. 11)*

Ans. Acetylcholine (Ref: the Dalhousie medical journal may 1999 issue)

32. Orphan annie eyed nuclei is the characteristic histologic appearance seen in: *(KCET 12)*

Ans. Papillary carcinoma thyroid

33. The combination of rest pain, colour changes, oedema and hyperaesthesia with/without is chaemic ulceration, is frequently reffered to as: *(KCET 12)*

Ans. Pre-gangrene

34. Genioplasty refers to: *(KCET 12)*

Ans. Surgical procedures which after the shape, size/position of the chinIn all 3D of space.

35. A majorIndication for orthognathic surgery before puberty is: *(KCET 12)*

Ans: Ankylosis of mandible

36. Surgical approaches for open thymectomyInclude all except: *(COMEDK 12)*

a. Transcervical thymectomy

b. Median sternotomy

c. Thoraco abdominalIncision

d. Partial midian sternotomy

Ans. c. Thoraco abdominalIncision

37. Latent period of distraction osteogenes is in a 8 month old child is: *(AIIMS Nov. 11)*

Ans. 0-2 days (Ref: Maxillofacial distraction Osteogenes is by dr. Hatem W. AL Rashdan/ Craniofacial distraction Osteogenesis by Mikhail L. Samchukov p216)

38. Distraction osteogenesis is doneIn pediatric patient which of the following is considered: *(AIIMS Nov. 11, AIPG 12)*

Ans. Increased rate (Ref: Maxillofacial distraction osteogenesis by Dr. Hatim W.AL Rashdan/Craniofacial Distraction Osteogenesis by Mikhail L. Samchukov p216.

39. Tuft cells are receptor for: *(AIIMS Nov. 11)*

Ans. Salivary duct epithelium (Ref: Anat sciInt. 2007 Dec. 82. (4.187-99)

40. When Soft palate is paralysed, which is not seen: *(AIIMS Nov. 11)*

a. Clefting of palate

b. Nasal regurgitation

c. Nasal twang

d. Flat palate

Ans. a. Clefting of palate (Ref: BDC 3rd ed. Vol. 111 p181)

41. Compression osteosynthesis wasInitially used for: *(AIIMS Nov. 11)*

Ans. To prevent callus formation (Ref: Fonseca 3rd ed. P1140 vol.II)

42. After surgery of cleft palate most common finding is: *(AIIMS Nov. 11)*

Ans. Anterior cross bite (Ref: Profit 4th ed. P323-24)

43. A patient with haemophilia B is posted for surgery, he will requires: *(AIIMS Nov. 11)*

Ans. 80-100 units factor 9/24 hourly

44. CBCT is most usefulIn diagnosis and treatment planning of which malocclusion? *(AIIMS Nov. 11)*

Ans. B/LImpacted canine

45. Clamshell technique refers to: *(AIIMS Nov. 11)*

Ans. Illiaco cancellous bone grafting (Ref: Reconstructive andImplant surgery by fonseca, P367)

46. Latency period of distraction osteogenesis is: *(AIIMS Nov. 12, AIPG 12)*

Ans. 4-7 days

47. Best way to monitor perfusion of flap: *(AIIMS Nov. 12, AIPG 12)*

Ans. Prick test (Ref: Stell and Marror's head and neck surgery 4th ed. P137)

48. Cleft lip is treated by all of the following methods except: *(AIIMS Nov. 12)*

a. Von langenback
b. Millard's method
c. Tannison rindall method
d. Le-mesurier

Ans. a. Von langenback (Ref: Neelima malik 2/e p558)

49. Thyroid storm can be treated by all the following drugs except: *(COMEDK 12)*

a. Propylthiouracil
b. Dexamethasone
c. Propranolol
d. Aspirin

Ans. d. Aspirin

50. Bell's Palsy is: *(AIIMS Nov. 11, PGI Nov 13)*

Ans. LMN disorder (Ref: Neelima malik is ted. P667)

51. Most common clefts of lip and palateIn population are: *(AIIMS May 12, AIPG-12)*

Ans. Unilateral cleft lip and palate (Ref: Neelima malik 2/e p546)

52. Type of movement not possible with BSSO is: *(AIPG 12)*

Ans. Transverse (Ref: Revision surgeryIn otolaryngology by edelstin 2008, p47)

53. During 3rd molar surgery, lingual flap elevation is done by using: *(AIPG 12)*

Ans. Broad surface retractor (Ref: Fonseca Vol 1, p268)

54. A 16 year old boy needs reconstruction of cleft palate with an autogenous bone graft. TheIdeal material would be: *(AIPG 12)*

Ans. posteriorIliac crest

55. AnteriorInferior cerebellar arteryInfract is associated with lesion of: *(AIIMS Nov. 09)*

Ans. The vestibular nucleus

56. Which is more dangerous after a thyroidectomy resultingIn acute respiratory distress? *(COMEDK 12)*

Ans. B/L partial section of recurrent laryngeal nerve

57. Suture with least adhesion to tissues and high plasticity is: *(AIPG 12)*

Ans. Prolene (Ref: Balaji 2007 p107)

58. A 2½ year old child with horizontal bone loss but cementum appears normal. What is the disease? *(PGI June 11)*

Ans. Hypophosphatasia (Ref: Harrison 17th ed. P2408.

59. Necrotizing fascitisInvolve: *(PGI June 11)*

Ans. Fascia + skin + underlying muscle (Ref: Bailey and love 23rd ed p171)

60. Matted cervical lymphademopathy is seen in: *(PGI June 11)*

Ans. TB (Ref: Bailey and Love's 23rd ed p704)

61. In a post-operative patient, 21 years old with 70 kg weight, 1 unit of packed RBC will raise the hematocrit by: *(AIPG 12)*

Ans. 3-5% (Ref: Essentials of general surgery by Lawrence, Bell, Dayton, 2006 p99)

62. Better levels of factor VIII are achieved byInfusion of: *(AIPG 12)*

Ans. Cryprecipitate (ref.; Blood: physiology and circulation by Rogers, Britannica Educational publishing 2010 p220)

63. Buerger's disease is caused by: *(AIPG 12)*

Ans. Cigarette smoking

64. Inverted L-shaped osteotmy is done for: *(PGI Dec. 09)*

Ans. Used for treating mandibular retrognathism (Ref: Vinod kapoor 2/e p535)

65. In hemophilia, drug administration before a surgical procedure is: *(AIPG 09)*

Ans. E-Amino coproic acid (Ref: Schwartz 8th ed. P67)

Note: 15-30% blood loss – CrystaloidInfusion

30-40% blood loss – Always require blood transfusion

66. Chronic burrowing ulcer is caused by: *(AIPG 09)*

Ans. Microaerophilic streptococci

67. Goldenhar syndromeIncludes: *(PGI June 11)*

Ans. Epibulbar dermoid

auditory appendices

vertebralInvolvement (Ref: Shafer's 5th ed. P4)

68. Submucous palatal defect is: *(PGI June 09)*

Ans. mucosaIntact and underlying bone bear notching at posterior margin of palate+appear as blue discolorationIn the region of mid palatal suture (Ref: vinod kapoor 2nd eg. P584)

69. A patient is giving symptom of sweating while having his food most probably he has undergone a surgery of: *(PGI June 09)*

Ans. Parotid gland (Ref: White and pharoach 5th ed. P375)

70. Side effect of methaemoglobinemia is seen with which drug? *(PGI June 09)*

Ans. Phenacetin

71. OSMF, True is? *(PGI June 09)*

Ans. Vesicle, petechiae, melanosis, Xerostomia + stomatopyrosis + blotchy marble like pallor and progressive stiffness of subepethelia

72. Most common cause of mysoitis ossificans: *(PGI June 09)*

Ans. Trauma

73. Oral submucous fibrosis is caused by: *(PGI June 12)*

Ans. Chewing areca nut

74. Catabolic phase after surgery: *(PGI June 12)*

Ans. 2-5 days

75. Most commonly used sutureIn oral cavity is: *(KCET 12)*

Ans. Silk

76. The earliest operative procedure undertakenIn the management of a complete U/L cleft lip with alveolus and palate is: *(KCET 12)*

Ans. Chilorrhaphy

77. Prophylaxis against bacterial endocarditis is directed primarily against: *(KCET 12)*

Ans. hemolytic streptococci

78. Which statement with respect to mucoceles is false? *(KCET 12)*

a. Psudocysts contain viscous saliva but lack a true epithelial lining

b. Patients relate a history of filling, rupture and refilling

c. Preventing recurrence requires removal of associated major salivary gland.

d. Preventing recurrence requires removal of associated minor salivary gland.

Ans. c. Preventing recurrence requires removal of associated major salivary gland.

CHAPTER

11 Anatomy

Topic

- Nerves
- Muscle
- Blood Vessels
- Miscellaneous
- Questions

NERVES

- Sensory nerve supply of scalp:

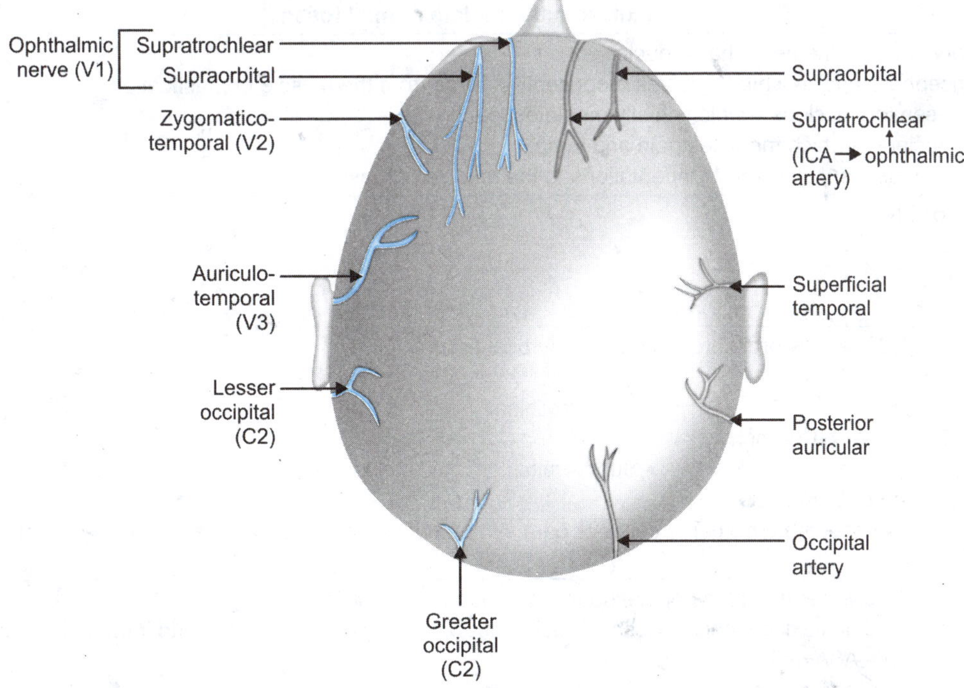

Fig. 11.1: Sensory nerve supply of scalp

- Motor nerve supply of SCALP:

In front of auricle – temporal branch of facial nerve.
Behind auricle – post. Auricular branch of facial nerve.

- Cranial nerves:

3, 4, 6, 12 – MOTOR
1, 2, 8 - SENSORY
REST – MIXED.

- Olfactory and Optic nerve – NO CN nuclei in brainstem
- CILIARY ganglion - located at the apex of orbit b/w OPTIC NERVE and Lateral rectus.[Q]
- Trochlear nerve:

Only CN whose all fibres cross to contra lateral side.[Q]
Only CN arising from dorsal side of brain stem.[Q]
Has longest intradural course.[Q]
Smallest CN in terms of axon it contains.

- ABDUCENT CN:

Follows extradural course so abducent nerve palsy develops in meningitis and subarachnoid hemorrhage.

- CN 3, 4,6 and ophthalmic division of Trigeminal nerve passes through superior orbital fissure. [Q]
- CN 3 and 6 passes through common tendinous ring of extraoccular muscle.
- Trigeminal nerve:

Exit from the middle cranial fossa.
The sensory nerve of the head, has 4 nuclei: • Mesencephalic nuclei- which receives propriceptive fibres from the muscle of mastication. • Pontine sensory nucleus – which chiefly mediates touch. • Spinal nucleus – which mediates pain and temp. • Motor nucleus – supplies motor innervations to the muscle of mastication.
3 divisions of T.N: OPTHALMIC MAXILLARY MANDIBULAR
1. OPTHALMIC – enters orbit through superior Orbital fissure. BRANCHES – Frontal – LARGEST branch → Supratrochlear; → Supraorbital. Lacrimal nerve- SMALLEST **NOTE:** the branch of ophthalmic nerve conveys para sympathetic from facial nerve along the zygomatic nerve to the lacrimal gland.[Q]
2. MAXILLARY div. – enters pterygopalatine fossa through foramen rotundum [Q]. THE branches of maxillary nerve passes through infraorbital fissure Zygomatic and infraorbital nerve [Q]. Infraorbital n.= ASA+PSA MSA(middle superior alveolar)= seen in 28% people.

3. MANDIBULAR div. – passes through foramen ovale. Branch from Main trunk – meningeal branch + nerve to medial pterygoid. Posterior div. – auriculotemporal,lingual,IAN. Auriculotemporal – supplies pinna, TMJ Masseteric nerve- supplies TMJ Mylohyoid nerve – branches from IAN just before mandibular foramen. Mylohyoid nerve supplies – mylo hyoid + anterior Belly of diagastric nerve to medial pterygoid – supplies tensor villi palatine+ tensor tympani. buccal nerve only sensory branch. Tip of nose is supplied by – ophthalmic nerve Side and ala of nose by – maxillary nerve.

- Root value of phrenic nerve is - c3 c4 c5.
- Facial nerve:

NTS (NUCLEUS OF TRACTUS SOLITARIUS): caries afferent signals from visceral organ through 7, 9, 10 CN. [Q]

- Superior salivatory nucleus gives Parasympathetic fiber to the submandibular and sublingual gland through 7th CN. [Q]
- Inferior salivatory nucleus to parotid gland through 9th CN.[Q]
- Nerve Of Pterygoid Canal = greater petrosal branch of facial nerve + deep petrosal nerve.
  - Nerves intermedius [see AIIMS May 2012 question and write]
- Glossopharyngeal nerve:

Leaves cranial cavity through jugular foramen (also 10th and 11th).
• **Branches:** – Pharyngeal branch- innervates constrictor muscle of the pharynx(pharyngeal branch join with the vagus nerve to form pharyngeal plexus) – Branch to STYLOPHARNGEUS [Q] – Tonsillar branches – main nerve supply to tonsil.
• **Function:** – Parasympathetic presynaptic fibres are sent to the OTIC ganglion through tympanic and lesser petrosal nerve and post synaptic fibres are distributed to PAROTID, Buccal and labial gland. [Q]
Gag reflex can be lost due to paralysis of 9 th CN.

- Vagus nerve:

Has most extensive distribution of all CNs.
Vagus nerve branches in the neck: • Pharyngeal branches • Sup. laryngeal nerve • Right recurrent laryngeal nerve • Left recurrent laryngeal nerve • Cervical cardiac branches.

- All laryngeal muscles are supplied by recurrent laryngeal nerve except CRICOTHYROID MUSCLE which is supplied by EXTERNAL LARYNGEAL NERVE which is a branch of superior laryngeal nerve. [Q]
- Internal laryngeal nerve (branch of sup. Laryngeal nerve) is sensory branch supplying throhyoid membrane and tongue.
- Damage of nerve of larynx:

Unilateral destruction of the recurrent laryngeal nerve leads to hoarseness of voice and bilateral destruction leads to respiratory distress(dyspnea).
Internal laryngeal nerve – anesthesia of larynx.
External laryngeal nerve – loss of timber of voice.

- Accessory nerve:
  - Cranial root of the accessory nerve is now considered as a part of the vagus nerve. The cranial fibres distributed via the vagus nerve while the spinal root fibres continue as spinal accessory nerve.
  - Innervates Trapezius and SCM.
  - Effects of nerve injury:
    - Trapezius paralysis –Drooping of shoulder on affected side and diificulty raising arm above H-Z plane.
    - Sternocleidomastoid paralysis: torticolis (WRY NECK) ie, difficulty in turning head.
    - Uvula moves to the opposite side if accessory nerve is damaged.
- Hypoglossal nerve:
  - Supplies all muscles of tongue (except palatoglossus) +thyrohyoid + geniohyoid.
  - Hypoglossal nerve lesion – tongue deviates AWAY from the lesion.
- SOMATIC EFFERENT – 3, 4, 6, 12 CN(motor CN) – supply muscles like tongue and eye ball muscles. [Q]
- VISCERAL EFFERENT – 3, 7, 9, 10 CN – Supply smooth muscle and gland. [Q]

MUSCLE

- Tongue:
- Genioglossus is the main muscle of the tongue.
- The Safety muscle of the tongue.
- All infrahyoid muscles are supplied by ansa cervicalis except thyrohyoid which is supplied by C1 through hypoglossal nerve as of geniohyoid. [Q]
- all muscles of soft palate are supplied by cranial root of accessory nerve except tensor villi palate which is supplied by mandibular nerve (nerve to medial pterygoid). [Q]
- Summary:
  - Tensor villi palati + tensor tympani – supplied by nerve to medial pterygoid (mandibular nerve).
  - Geniohyoid + thyrohyoid – c1 through hypoglossal nerve.
  - Muscles of ear osscicles –
  - Tensor tympanii – supplied by mandibular nerve.
  - Stapedius - facial nerve
    - Protect the internal ear.
    - Palatoglossus – is common to both soft palate and tongue but its nerve supply is similar to soft palate i.e., c1 through spinal accessory nerve.
- Muscles of pharynx:

Musles	Origin
• Superior constrictor - attached to mandible [PGI]	Pterygoid hamulus Pterygomandibular raphae
• Middle constrictor	Hyoid bone (lesser + greter cornua) Stylohyoid ligament. [Q]
• Inferior constrictor	Thyropharyngeal part – thyroid Crico – cricoid

- At the posterior wall thyropharyngeal part is called KILLIANS dehiscence as it is not overlapped by superior And middle constrictor.
- Palatine aponeurosis – is tendon of tensor villi palatine. [Q]
- Muscle of mastication:
  - Medial and lateral pterygoid – both protrudes the mandible.
  - Temporalis retracts the protruded mandible.

- Masseter:
  - Dual action in CD
  - Powerful bcoz of MULTIPINNATE arrangement. [Q]
  - Most commonly affected in MYOSITIS OSSIFICANS. [PGI]
- Fan shaped muscle – temporalis and genioglossus.[Q]
- Buccinator – is a C shaped muscle.muscle of facial expression is supplied by buccal branch of facial nerve NOT by mandibular nerve.
- MPDS – most commonly affected muscle is lateral pterygoid.
- Superficial neck muscles:
  - Platysma – muscle of facial expression
    - Insertion -mandible
    - Innervations by cervical branch of facial nerve [PGI].
  - Trapezius – motor nerve:accessory nerve
    - Pain and proprioception: cervical plexus (c2, c3).
  - Sternocleidomastoid – same nerve supply of trapezius.
    - Insertion – mastoid process, occipital bone (sup. Nuchal line).
- Suprahyoid muscles:
  Diagastric muscle:
  Ant. belly – supplied by mylohyoid nerve (v3)
  Post. Belly – supplied by facial nerve [Q]
- Traingles:
  - Anterior triangle is divided by diagastric muscle and superior belly of omohyoid into different.
  - Post. Triangle is divided by inferior belly of omohyoid into large upper occipital and small lower supraclavicular triangle.
- Post belly of diagastric divides diagastric triangle from carotid triangle.
- Floor of mouth/oral diaphragm is formed by mylohyoid.
- Buccinator prevents accumulation of food in buccal vestibule.
- Passavant's muscle is formed by palatopharyngeus fibres.
- No deep fascia on face except except parotid fascia (masseteric) and over buccinators. [PGI]
- Levator palpebrae is an extraoccular muscle. [do not confuse]
- TMJ:
  - Articular disc – weeping lubricant
    AVASCULAR fibrous connective tissue.[Q]
  - Superior head of the lateral pterygoid attached to the articular disc.
    And inferior head to the neck of condyle.
    Nerve supply – Auriculotemporal
    Masseteric.
    Blood supply – Superficial temporal artery
    – Maxillary artery (deep auricular branch)
  - Dislocation of TMJ – dislocation may occur if the head of the mandible slides past the articular tubercle.
- Lateral pterygoid: only among the muscle of mastication which has attachment to the CONDYLE.
- Structure b/w two heads of lateral pterigoid – maxillary Artery and buccal nerve. *(PGI 06)*

BLOOD VESSELS

- ARCH OF AORTA – Brachiocephalic trunk
  Left common carotid
  Left subclavian artery
- Subclavian artery is principle artery of upper limb.
- Internal carotid artery (ICA)
  - The ICA arises from the bifurcation of the common carotid artery at
  - The level of upper border of thyroid cartilage.[Q].
  - Curvature of ICA – forms S- shaped figure called CAROTID SIPHON OF ANGIOGRAM.
  - Branches: [Q]
    - Cervical part – no branches
    - Petrous part – corticotympanic artery, pterygoid artery.
    - Cavernous part – cavernous branches, meningeal branches,
    - Cerebral part – ophthalmic [Q], Ant. and Middle cerebral, posterior
    - Communicating, anterior Choroidal, superior Hypophyseal artery.
- Carotid bifurcation – at the level of upper border of thyroid cartilage. [AIPG]
- Branches of ext. Carotid artery (eca):

  Anterior branch
  - Superior thyroid artery - glandular branch to thyroid gland, superior laryngeal artery, SCM branch
  - Lingual artery – to base of tongue, sublinlual artery (to sub lingual gland, tongue, oral floor)
  - Facial artery – ascending palatine a.(to pharyngeal wall, soft palate,pharyngotympanic tube), tonsillar branch(to palatine tonsils, MAIN SUPPLY TO THE TONSIL), submental a.(to oral floor, submandibular gland), labial a., angular a(to nasal root)
- Chances of damage of facial artery during circum

  Mandibular wiring [q].

  Medial branch:
  - Ascending pharyngeal artery

  Posterior branch
  - Occipital branch – to posterior neck muscle
  - Posterior auricular a.

  Terminal branches:
  - Superficial temporal artery – supply Ext. Auditory canal.

    Transverse facial artery – is a branch of sup. Temporal artery supplies to soft tissue below the zygomatic arch.
  - Maxillary artery – artery of 1st pharyngeal arch [q]

    Origin – near neck of condyle.
- Branches of maxilllary artery:
  - Lateral pterygoid divides maxillary artery into 3 parts[Q].

    1ST PART/Mandibular part – trick – DAM I AM

    D – Deep auricular(to TMJ, ext. Auditory canal)

    A – Anterior tympanic

    M – middle meningeal artery – COMMONEST area of extradural hematoma[Q]

    I – Inferior alveolar artery

    AM – Accessory meningeal

2nd part/pterygoid part / muscular branch- supplies muscle of mastication.

- Masseteric artery (Origin – near SIGMOID NOTCH), deep temporal artery, pterygoid branches, buccal a.

3Rd part / pterygopalatine part – trick – pig pas

P – PSA, I – infraorbital, G – greater palatine, P – pharyngeal branch

A – artery of pterygoid canal, S – Sphenopalatine artery

- Sphenopalatine artery – Supplies the wall of nasal cavity. excessive nasopharyngeal bleeding from the branches of the sphenopalatine artery may necessitate ligation of maxillary artery in the pterygopalatine fossa.
- Veins of the head and neck:
  - The veins of the head and neck drains into the BRACHIOCEPHALIC vein.[Q]
  - IJV – drained interior of skull including brain.
    Is a direct continuation of sigmoidal sinus. [Q]
- Connection of facial vein:
  - To superior ophthalmic and supraorbital vein
  - And deep facial vein
    The facial vein through these connections communicate with cavernous sinus – DANGEROUS AREA
  - FACIAL VEIN lies INFERIOR to submandibular gland *(PGI 2011)*
- Venous sinuses:
  - Unpaired sinuses – Superior and inferior sagital sinuses, straight sinus, occipital sinus and ant. and post intercavernous sinus.
- Cavernous sinus:
  - Superior and inferior petrosal sinus connects cav. Sinus to the sigmoidal sinus.
  - Relations of cavernous sinus:

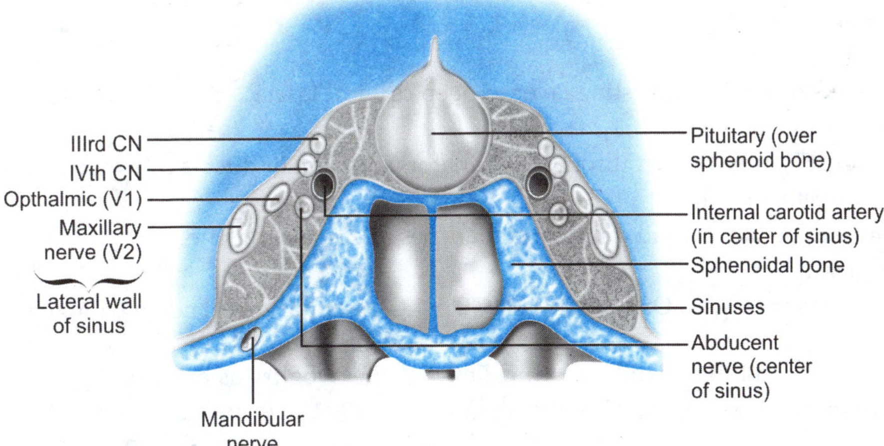

Fig. 11. 2: Cavernous sinus

MISCELLANEOUS

- Parotid – purely serous. Facial nerve divides parotid gland into superficial and deep part.
- Sublingual – predominantly mucus.(Mixed)
- Submandibular – predominantly serous (Mixed)

- SCALP :Layers

S – Superficial skin
C – Connective tissue (superficial fascia)
A – Aponeurosis (has occipitofrontalis)
L – Loose areolar tissue (dangerous area of scalp because has emissary vein draining directly into sinuses.)
P – Pericranium

- Tracheostomy – Done in retrothyroid region after retracting isthmus.
  - Done b/w T2 – T4.
  - Both trachea and oesophagus begins at the level of lower border of cricoid cartilage.
  - Trachea bifurcates at the sternal angle which is at T4.
  - Arterial supply of trachea – inferior thyroid artery.
- Sex determination of mandible:
  In males – the angle of mandible is everted(projected outward)
  In females – the angle of mandible is everted.
- Palatine aponeurosis – is formed by Tensor villi palatine. Levator villi palatine is inserted into it. [DO NOT CONFUSE]
- Lacrimal gland:
  - Levator palpebrae superioris divides lacrimal gland into ORBITAL AND PALPEBRAL part.
  - VALVE OF HASNER – an imperfect valve at the lower end of nasolacrimal gland.
  - The upper eyelid shows a characteristic S- CURVE during acute inflammation.
- Eye lid:
  - Levator palpebrae superioris – an extraoccular muscle which elevates the eyelid.
    Supplied by 3rd C.N.
- Orbitalis occuli – muscle of facial expression, supplied by facial nerve.
  It closes the eyelid.
- Parotid gland: Purely serous.
  - Parotid capsule – formed by investing layer of deep cervical fascia.
  - Parotid duct – 5cm long.
  - Bcoz of OBLIQUE course of duct through buccinators,inflation of duct is prevented during blowing.
  - Development – ectodermal.
  - Blood supply – ECA (ext. carotid artery)and branches arising near gland.
- Submandibular gland:
  - 3 structures are below HYOGLOSSUS: TRICK- GLaS 1.Glossopharyngeal nerve 2. Lingual artery 3. Stylohyoid ligament.
  - Deep part of submandibular gland with duct lies over the hyoglossus muscle.
  - Hyoglossus – inserted into the SIDE of the tongue.
- Tongue:
  - Muscles – 1. EXTRINSIC –have bony attachment and move tongue as a WHOLE.
  - GENIOGLOSSUS – control PROTRUSION of the tongue.
- **INTRISIC** – have no bony attachment. Alter shape of tongue.
  Superior And inferior Longitudinal, transverse and vertical.
- Pharynx and Soft palate:
  - Palatoglossus – closes the oropharyngeal isthmus.
  - Passavants ridge – fibres of palatopharyngeus form passavants muscle deep to sup. Constrictor contol opening of isthmus b/w naso and oropharynx.

- Pharyngeal/lateral recess/fossa of Rossenmuller – present behind the tubal elevation in nasopharynx.
- Pyriform recess – in laryngopharynx.
  - Blood supply of soft palate:
    1. Greater palatine branch of maxillary artery
    2. Ascending palatine branch of facial artery
    3. Ascending pharyngeal branch of ECA.
  - NERVE SUPPLY of pharynx:
    1. nasopharyx – pharyngeal branch of pterygopalatine ganglion suspended by maxillary branch of TN.
    2. Oro and laryngopharynx and constrictor – by 9th and 10th CN (BY pharyngeal plexus)
- Inferior constrictor Receives additional supply from external Laryngeal nerve.
- Stylopharyngeus – by glossophayngeal only. [Q].

- Tonsils:
  - Main nerve supply – 9th cn
  - Main blood supply – facial artery (tonsillar branch)

  Development –from ventral part of 2nd pharyngeal pouch.
- Waldayer's ring: Formed by pharyngeal, tubal, lingual,lateral band along salphingopharyngeal fold and palatine tonsil.
- Auditary tube/pharyngotympanic tube: 36mm length.
  - Blood supply:
    - Ascending pharyngeal [AIPG, AIIMS 12]
    - Middle meningeal
    - Artery of pterygoid canal

  NOT by superficial temporal artery(it supplies TMJ).
  - Nerve supply -1. Same as nasopharynx – for ostium
    - Nervus spinosus branch of mandibular nerve-cartilaginous part
    - Tympanic plexus formed by glossopharyngeal nerve- bony part
  - Infection from throat to middle ear in children is more frequent due to shorter and straight tube.
- **Lymphatics:** The bodies chief lymph vessel ie, thoraxic duct and right Lymphatic duct both drains to junction of left and right IJV and SUBCLAVIAN vein respectively.
- LARYNX:
  - The larynx consists of 5 laryngeal cartilages – epiglotic,thyroid,cricoid and paired arytenoids and corniculate cartilage.

    They are connected to each other, the trachea and the hyoid bone by ELASTIC ligaments.
  - Arytenoid cartilage is PYRAMIDAL shape.
  - Hyoid bone – is the only bone which is not attached to any other bone. [Q]
  - Action of laryngeal muscles:

    Cricothyroid and vocalis – tightens the vocal folds.

    Thyroarytenoid, transeverse arytenoid and lateral cricoarytenoid – adducts the vocal folds(closes glottis).

    Posterior cricoarytenoid – abducts the vocal folds(open glottis)

    – Only abductor. [Q]
- **In simple**:
  - These arytenoids cartilage control the opening b/w two the two vocal folds and this opening is called GLOTTIS.
  - ONLY those muscles which are attached to the arytenoids cartilage controls the opening and closing of glottis.
  - Post. Cricoarytenoid is the only abductor.

- **Blood supply:**
  - Upto the level of vocal fold – Superior laryngeal artery (branch of sup. Thyroid artery).
  - BELOW – By inferior laryngeal artery (a branch of inf. Thyroid artery)
  - Nerve supply: vagus nerve.
  - Sensory -
  - Upto the level of vocal fold – the internal laryngeal nerve.
  - Below – recurrent laryngeal nerve.
- Motor:
  - All laryngeal muscle – inferior laryngeal nerve except cricothyroid which is by external Laryngeal nerve.
- Thyroid:

  Development -

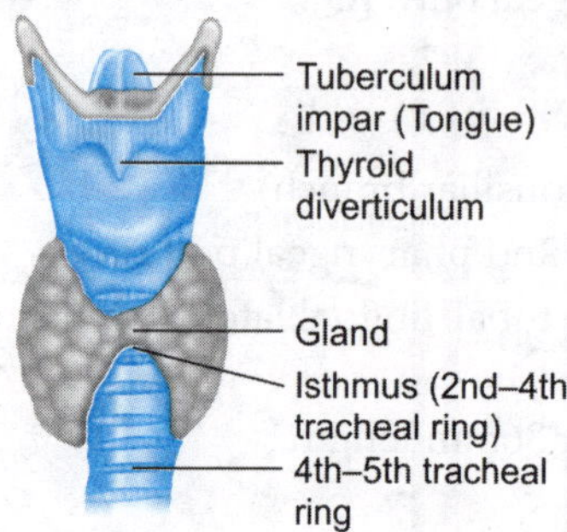

Fig. 11.3: Thyroid

- From THYROID DIVERTICULUM – lower part of thyroid diverticulum gives thyroid gland and the remaining portion gives THYROGLOSSAL DUCT which soon disappears.
- The persistence of thyroglossal duct gives rise to – THYROGLOSSAL CYST / FISTULA. [Q]
- Location of thyroid gland –against c5,c6,c7,T1. (C3-C6 For larynx).
- ISTHMUS- 2nd- 4th tracheal ring.
- Gland is larger in female and further increases during menstruation and pregnancy.
- Capsule:

True – By condensation of connective tissue of gland itself.

False - Pretracheal layer of deep cervical fascia [Q]

- Forms suspensory ligament of berry which attaches gland to cricoids cartilage.
- Arterial supply:
  - Superior thyroid artery – the 1st branch of ECA.

    During surgery ligate it as close as possible. [Q]
  - Inferior thyroid artery – a branch from THYROCERVICAL TRUNCK.[Q]
- Ligate as far as possible.

  Veins – superior, middle and inferior thyroid vein.

  A fourth thyroid vein of kocher may emerge b/w middle and inferior thyroid vein and drains into ijv.

  Nerve supply – Superior, middle and inferior cervical ganglion.
  - Blood supply of PARATHYROID GLAND – same as thyroid gland BUT mainly from inferior thyroid artery.
  - NASAL CAVITY and NASAL SEPTUM:
- Nasal septum – formed by vomer + perpendicular plate of ethmoidal bone. [Q]
- Arteris and nerves of the nasal cavity:

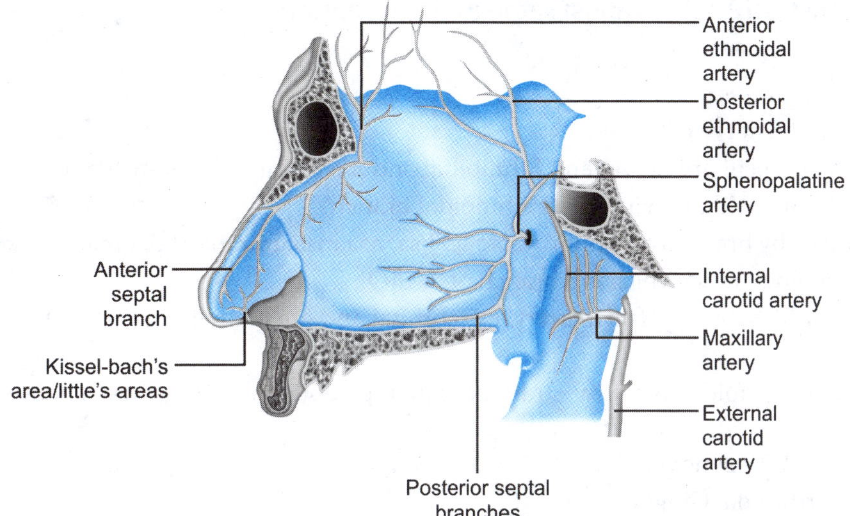

Fig. 11.4: Arteries

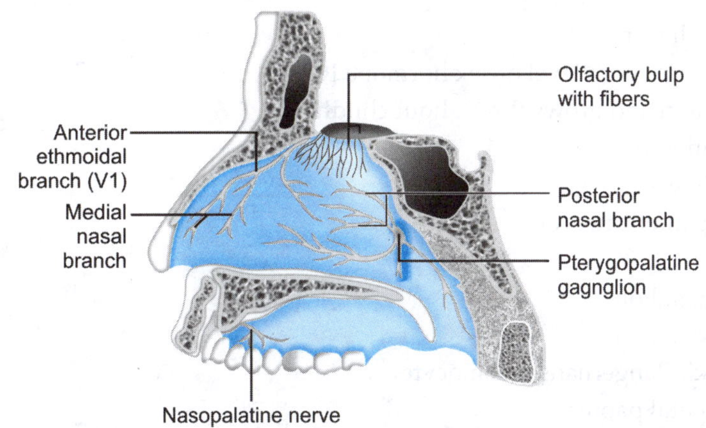

Fig. 11. 5: Nerves

- CLINICAL – vascular supply to the nasal cavity arises from both the internal and external carotid arteries. The anterior part of nasal septum contains a very vascularized region referred to as KIESSELBACH'S AREA. this area is the most common site of significant nose bleed.

- Lateral Wall of Nose:

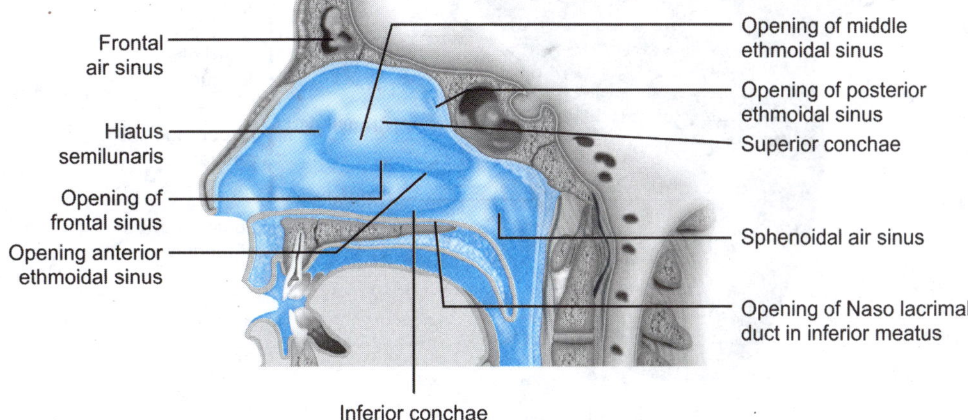

Fig. 11.6: Lateral wall of nose

NERVE AND ARTERIAL SUPPLY – Almost same as nasal septum.

- Paranasal sinuses:
  Innervation of nasal sinuses:
  - Frontal – by frontal nerve (v1)
  - Ethmoidal – by nasocilliary nerve (ant. Ethmoidal and post ethmoidal branch of nasociliary nerve)
  - Sphenoidal – by nasocilliary nerve(post ethmoidal branch)
  - Maxillary sinus – by branch of v2 (max nerve ie. Psa, asa,msa, infraorbital, greater palatine)

  NOT by ant. Ethmoidal nerve which is a branch of V1.[Q].
  - Blood Supply of Max. Sinus – facial artery, infraorbital and greater palatine artery.
- Embryology:
  - Epiglottis and vocal fold – lined by stratified squamus epithelium [Q]. Rest lined by ciliated columnar epithelium.
  - Joint b/w C1 and C2 = synovial [Q]
  - TMJ joint – Diarthroidal Ginglimoidal [Q]
  - Amphiarthrosis – Slightly Movable Joint [Q]
  - Thymus – Bilobed assymetrical [Q]

  Location – Superior mediastinum.
  Regresses at puberty due to high level of sex hormone [Q]
  Well developed in children and grows throughout childhood.
- Neural crest cell derivatives:
  - Muscle of head andneck
  - Post ganglion sympathetic neuron
  - Schwan cell. *(KCET 07)*
  - Dorsal nerve root ganglion
  - Adrenal medulla
  - Dendritic cells of skin(langerhans.melanocyte)
  - Odontoblast and dental papilla
- Tongue:

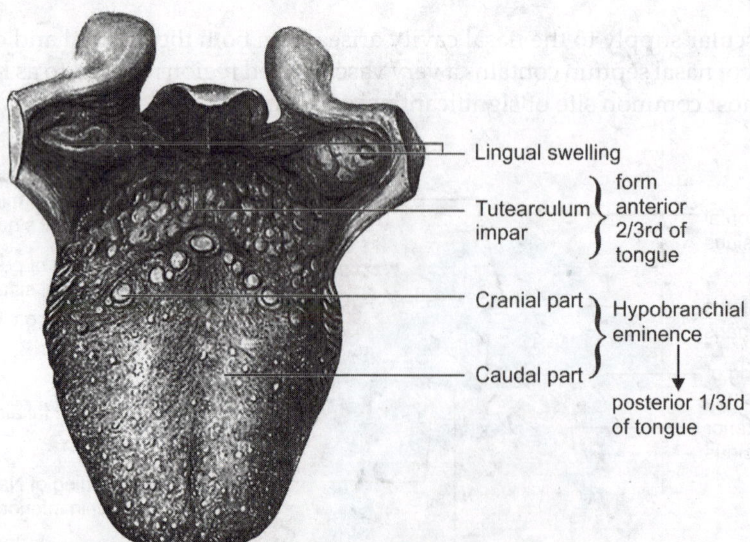

Fig. 11.7: Development of tongue

1ST arch gives rise to 3 swellings – 2lingualand 1 tuberculum impar which forms ant. 2/3rd of tongue and 3rd and 4th arch forms median swelling called hypobranchial eminence which forms post. 1/3rd of tongue.

So tongue develops from 1st, 3rd and 4th arch.

- Occipital somites- gives rise to muscle of tongue.[Q]
- Nerve supply of tongue [Very Imp.]

Sensory: ANT. 2/3rd by lingual, POST1/3rd by glossopharyngeal,posterior most part by internal laryngeal branch of vagus.

TASTE –ant2/3rd by chorda tympanii except vallate papilla, post1/3rd by glossopharyngeal including vallate papilla, posterior most part by internal laryngeal branch of vagus.

MOTOR: all the intrinsic and extrinsic muscles except the palatoglossus, are supplied by HYPOGLOSSAL nerve. the palatoglossus is supplied by the cranial root of the accessory nerve through the pharyngeal plexus.

- Lymphatic drainage:
  - Of tongue – jugulo omohyoid L.N
  - OF tonsils – jugulo diagastric L.N
- Muscles of tongues –
  - Genioglossus causes protrusion of tongue and retraction of tip of tongue.[Q]
  - - Styloglossus retracts the post. 1/3rd of tongue(upward and backward).
  - Styloglossus is attached to the side of tongue.
  - - Both genioglossus and hyoglossus depresses the tongue.
- Glands:
- Apocrine: ex- mammary gland, holocrine –sebaceous gland
- Others most of them are merocrine gland only.
- Merocrine gland discharge their content by exocytosis only.

OSTEOLOGY

- Cervical vertebra:
  - 1, 2, 7 – Atypical cervical vertebra.
  - Rest 3 to 6 are typical.
  - C1 atlas – no body and no spinous process.[Q]
  - C7 is called the vertebra prominens for its long, palpable spinous process.[Q]
  - C6 – anterior tubercle of c6 is large called carotid tubercle.
  - Dens/odontoid process – tooth like process.
  - The most common injuries of the cervical spine are fracture of dens of the axis,traumatic spondylolisthesis and atlas fracture.
  - Transverse foramen – Vertebral artery and veins and inferior cervical ganglion.
    - Tori – Commonly present above mylohyoid line.
- Skull:
  - Metopic suture – separates two halves of frontal bone. Rare/or present in 3-6% of people.

- Skull suture:

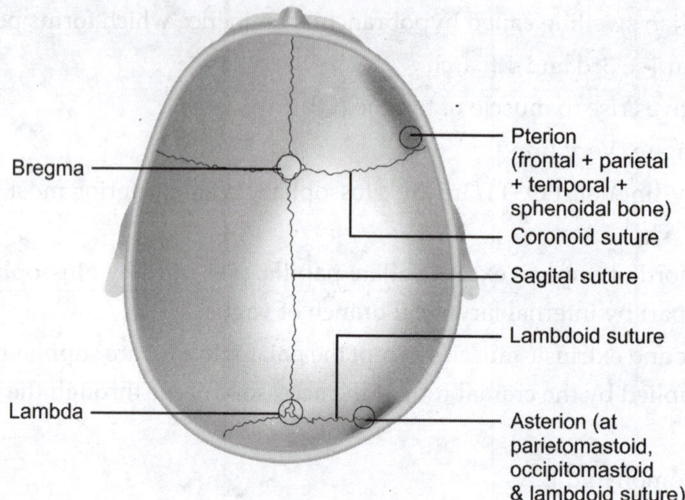

Fig. 11.8: Skull sutures

- Mandible is 2nd bone next to clavicle to ossify in body. [Q].
- Foramen present in GREATER wing of sphenoid – trick = ROSE [Q]
  R – rotundum, O – ovale , S – spinosum ,E – emissary vein
  LESSER wing has OPTIC CANAL.

• Foramens/canals/fissures and structures passing through:
  - Foramen magnum: 11th cn, lower medulla oblangata, vertebral arteries. [Q]
  - Foramen ovale – trick – male [Q]
    M – Mandibular nerve
    A – Accessory meningeal artery
    L – Lesser petrosal nerve
    E – Emissary vein
  - Foramen spinosum – trick – all meningeal branch.
    Middle meningeal artery(branch of max artery)

• Meningeal branch from mandibular nerve.
  - Anterior condylar canal / hypoglossal canal
    Hypoglossal nerve
  - Jugular foramen:
    Middle part – 9, 10, 11 cn [Q]
  - Stylomastoid foramen – facial nerve
  - Optic canal – optic nerve and ophthalmic artery.
  - Foramen rotundum- maxillary nerve [Q]
  - Carotid canal – internal carotid artery
  - Internal acoustic meatus-
    - Motor and sensory root of facial nerve
    - Vestibule cochlear nerve
    - Labyrinthine branch of basilar artery.
  - Superior orbital fissure: [Q]
    Trick- live free to see absolutely no insult.
    L – lacrimal nerve

F – Frontal nerve
T – Trochlear nerve
S –
A – Abducent nerve
N – Nasociliary nerve
I – Inferior opthalmic nerve.

- Inferior orbital fissure: [Q]
  Infraorbital and zygomatic nerve.
- Mental foramen – mental nerve and vessels.
- Mandibular foramen – inferior alveolar nerve and vessels.

• **Misclaneus:**

- Hassal corpuscle – seen in thymus. *(KCET 12)*
- Cortex of lymph node – lymphatic nodule.
- Cords of billroth – red pulp of spleen
- Umbilical cord – 2 umbilical arteries and 1 umbilical vein.
- Sweat gland → Eccrine (general body) – sympathetic cholinergic
  → Apocrine (pubis, axilla. Mammary gland) – sympathetic adrenergic.
- Ann Arbor staging – for LYMPHOMA.

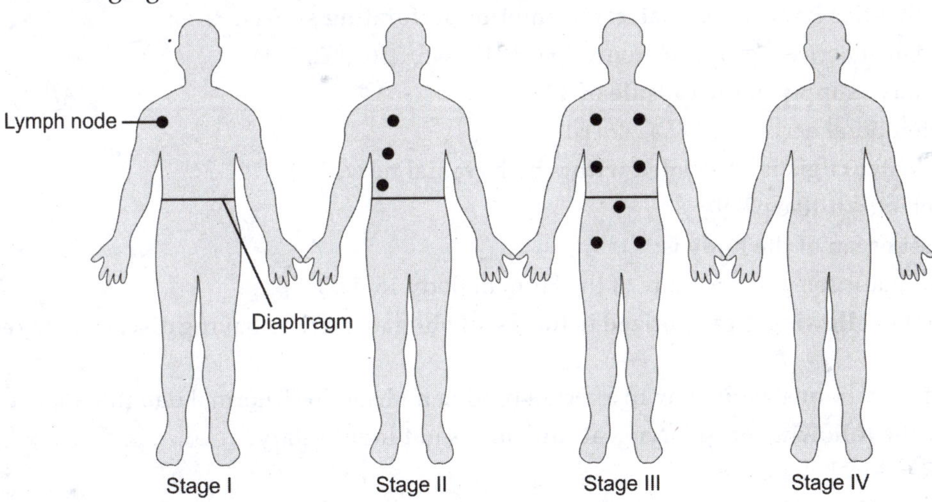

Fig. 11.9: Ann Arbor staging

Stage 1 – Single ipsilateral l.N
Stage 2 – Multiple ipsilateral l.N
Stage 3 – Multiple l.N on both sides and both above and below the diaphragm. *(AIIMS Nov 2012)*
Stage 4 – Diffuse.

- *Level of lymph nodes:*
  Level 1 – Submental + submandibular
  Level 2 – Upper jugular
  Level 3 – Middle jugular
  Level 4 – Lower jugular
  Level 5 – Post. Triangle cervical
  Level 6 – Ant. Compartment
  Level 7 – Upper mediastinal

- In 8% individuals thyroid is supplied by thyroidema artery.

- **Gag Reflex:**
  - Gagging can be triggered by stimulation of soft palate, post. Part of tongue and the fauces.
  - Mostly due to overextended maxillary denture.[Q]
  - Also due to extended distolingual (DL) mandibular denture, inc V.D and unstable denture.
  - Old denture wearer adapt to it, if persist it may be due to GIT and respiratory disorder.
- Deglutition/Swallowing:
  - Centre – medulla oblongata.
    Afferent by 5th(oral region), 9thand10th (pharyngeal region) C.N.
    Efferent by 9th, 10th and 12th (oral region).
    Phases:
    - Oral – voluntary
    - Pharyngeal –involuntary

  Tongue moves upward and touches palate to prevent food back to the oral cavity. Soft palate – backward and upward to prevent food entry into nasopharynx.
  - Oesophageal
- Pterygopalatine/sphenopalatine/hay ganglion – largest ganglion.

LAST 5-YEAR QUESTIONS FROM THIS TOPIC

1. **The area that lies immediately lateral to anterior perforating substance is:** *(AIIMS May 11)*

Ans. The limen insulae. (Ref: gray's anatomy 40/e p317, 346, 356, 383, 391)

2. **Sensory nerve supply to the capsule of TMJ is:** *(AIIMS Nov 10, May 11)*

Ans. Auriculotemporal nerve (Ref: BDC 4/e p151)

3. **Geniculate neuralgia is associated with which cranial nerve?** *(AIIMS Nov 10)*

Ans. Facial (Ref: burkit 10/e p329)

4. **The largest organ of the body is:** *(AIIMS Nov 10)*

Ans. Liver (Ref: pattinson. the Anatomy of the Human Body 18/e p385)

5. **Which of the following is categorized in the list of obligate carriers having disease with recessive trait?** *(AIIMS Nov 10)*

Ans. Phenotypically normal woman with affected brother and son BUT normal daughter.

6. **Which of the following oropharyngeal function is not involuntary?** *(AIIMS May 10)*

Ans. Speech (Ref: McNiell p252 – 254)

7. **Fibroblast in the pulp produce collagen of:** *(AIIMS Nov 09)*

Ans. Type 1 and 3 (Ref: orbans 13/e p124)

8. **All of the characteristic to differentiate a typical cervical vertebra from a thoracic vertebra EXCEPT that:** *(AIIMS May 09)*
   a. It has a triangular vertebral canal
   b. It has a foramen transversarium
   c. Superior articular facet is directed backwards and upwards
   d. It has a large vertebral body

Ans. d. (Ref: BDC 4/e vol 3 p40)

9. **All of the following are true regarding heart muscle, EXCEPT:** *(AIIMS May 09)*
   a. That it acts in a syncitium
   b. That it has multiple nuclei
   c. That it has gap junctions

d. That it has branching

Ans. b. (Ref: singh. etxbook of human histology p13)

10. Infraorbital nerve exits through the: *(AIIMS May 09)*

Ans. Inferior orbital fissure (Ref: BDC 4/e vol. 3 p25 – 26)

11. Proprioreception is carried from head and neck by all EXCEPT: *(AIIMS May 09)*

a. Trigeminal
b. Facial
c. Glossopharyngeal
d. Spinal accessory

Ans. d. (Ref: tripathi. concise textbook of physiology for dental students p430)

12. The only sensory branch of anterior division of mandibular nerve is: *(AIPG 10)*

Ans. Long buccal nerve (Ref: BDC 3rd ed vol 3 p123)

13. Anterior ethmoidal nerve supplies all EXCEPT: *(AIPG 11)*

a. Maxillary sinus
b. Interior of nasal cavity
c. Dural sheath of anterior cranial fossa
d. Ethmoidal air cells

Ans. a. (Ref: BDC 4/e vol 3 p234)

14. the sensory supply of the palate is through all of the following, EXCEPT: *(AIPG 11)*

a. The facial nerve
b. The vagus nerve
c. The glossopharyngeal nerve
d. The trigeminal nerve

Ans. b. (Ref: BDC 4/e vol 3 p212)

15. Slightly movable articulations in which the contiguous bony surfaces are either connected by broad, flattened disk of fibrocartilage / united by intraosseous ligament are known as: *(AIPG 10)*

Ans. Amphiarthrosis (Ref: BDC p51)

16. Which of the following is NOT neuroectodermal derivative? *(AIPG 10)*

a. Paneth cells
b. Neurons
c. Schwann cells
d. Odontoblasts

Ans. a. (Ref: Inderbir singh 5 /e p41 – 43, 50 – 51)

17. Insertion of hyoglossus is at: *(AIPG 10)*

Ans. Side of tongue (Ref: BDC 4/e p252 – 253)

18. The deepest layer of cervical fascia is: *(AIPG 10)*

Ans. Prevertebral fascia (Ref: BDC 4/e p67)

19. Which cells are not present in cerebral cortex: *(AIPG 10)*

Ans. Purkinje cells (Ref: Demeyer 3rd ed p300 – 302)

20. Infection spreading via lymphatics from the lower lip, 1st enters the blood stream at the: *(AIPG 10, 12, AIIMS Nov 11)*

Ans. Brachiocephalic vein (Ref: BDC 3rd ed vol 3 p180)

21. All of the following are derived from connective tissue EXCEPT: *(AIPG 10)*

Ans. Clara cells (Ref: grays anatomy 38/e p1666 - 1667

22. **Action of styloglossus muscle:** *(AIPG 10)*

Ans. Upward and backward pull of tongue (Ref: BDC 4/e p252 – 253)

23. **Lacrimal gland secretion is affected by injury of:** *(AIPG 10, 12)*

Ans. Greater petrosal nerve (BDC 4/e vol 3 p103)

24. **The middle pharyngeal constrictor is attached to the:**

Ans. Body of hyoid bone (Ref: BDC 4/e vol 3 p221, 223)

25. **A person showing 2 cell lines derived from a single zygote is called as:** *(AIPG 10)*

Ans. Mosaicism (Ref: moore, embryology 7/e p145)

26. **Which nerve originates from the dorsal surface of the brain?** *(AIPG 10)*

Ans. Trochlear (Ref: BDC 4/e vol 3 p25 – 26, 108, 115)

27. **Routine technique for karyotyping using light microscopy is:** *(AIPG 10)*

Ans. G – banding (Ref: robbins 6/e p165)

28. **lining of the blood vessels in the blood - brain barrier IS FORMED OF:** *(AIPG 10)*

Ans. Endothelial cells (Ref: guyton 7/e p377)

29. **Which of th e following is NOT derived from viscerocranium?** *(AIPG 10)*
   a. Sphenoid
   b. Lacrimal
   c. Vomer
   d. Zygomatic

Ans. a. (Ref: guyton 7/e p377)

30. **Common carotid artery bifurcates:** *(AIPG 10)*

Ans. At the upper border of thyroid cartilage (Ref: grays anatomy 39/e p543 – 545)

31. **Which are the composite muscles?** *(AIPG 09)*
   a. Pectineus
   b. Biceps femoris
   c. Adductor magnus
   d. All

Ans. d. (Ref: Gray's anatomy 38/e p873 – 875)

32. **Which of the following is NOT a tributary of cavernous sinus?** *(AIPG 09)*
   a. Superficial middle cerebral vein
   b. Deep cerebral vein
   c. Inferior petrosal sinus
   d. Superior petrosal sinus

Ans. b. (Ref: Hasan. general anatomy and osteology of the head and neck p102)

33. **What type of joint is between the ossicles of ear?** *(AIPG 09)*

Ans. Synovial joint (Ref: BDC 4/e vol 3 p262)

34. **Sensory branch of mandibular nerve are all EXCEPT:** *(AIPG 09)*
   a. Mylohyoid
   b. Lingual
   c. Temporal
   d. Buccal nerve

Ans. a. (Ref: Last's Anatomy 11/e p517 – 518)

35. **Motor supply of tongue is by:** *(AIPG 09)*

Ans. Hypoglossal

36. Which is NOT a branch of the cavernous part of INTERNAL carotid artery: *(AIPG 09)*

a. Cavernous branch
b. Inferior hypophyseal
c. Meningeal artery
d. Ophthalmic artery

Ans. d. (Ref: BDC 4/e vol 3 p177 – 179)

37. Which of the following supplies the capsule of TMJ?

Ans. Auriculotemporal nerve (Ref: BDC 4th p151)

38. Infection spreading via lymphatics from the lower lip 1st enters the blood stream at the: *(AIMS Nov. 11)*

Ans. Brachiocephalic vein (Ref: BDC 3rd ed vol 3 p180)

39. All the following muscles are attached to the oblique line of thyroid cartilage EXCEPT: *(AIIMS Nov. 11)*

a. Superior constrictor
b. Inferior constrictor
c. Thyrohyoid
d. Sternothyroid

Ans. a. (Ref: BDC 3rd ed vol. 3 p221)

40. Muscle spared by complete transaction of cranial part of accessory nerve: *(AIIMS Nov. 12, AIPG 12)*

Ans. Stylopharyngeus (Ref: Gray's anatomy 40/e p571)

41. In case of progressive bulbar palsy where nucleus ambiguous in the brain stem is involved, function of which of the structure listed below will NOT be affected: *(AIIMS Nov. 12)*

a. Muscle of pharynx
b. Cardiac ganglia
c. Intrinsic laryngeal muscle
d. Parotid gland

Ans. d.

42. Facial nerve lies: *(AIIMS Nov. 12)*

Ans. Below SMAS and below parotidomassetric fascia (Ref: maxillofacial surgery ; vol. 2 2nd ed by peterward booth p1309)

43. Tensor palate is supplied by: *(AIIMS Nov. 12)*

Ans. Trigeminal nerve (Ref: BDC 4/e vol.3 p155)

44. Parotid fascia extends anteriorly as: *(AIIMS Nov. 12)*

Ans. Massetric fascia (Ref: Topazian oral and maxillofacial infection 4/e p189)

45. Sublingual space is divided from submandibular space by: *(AIIMS Nov. 12)*

Ans. Fibres of mylohyoid (Ref: neelima malik 2nd ed p614)

46. Nerve for motor function of buccinators muscle: *(AIIMS May 12)*

Ans. Facial nerve (Ref: BDC 4/e vol 3 p153, 155, 151)

47. Derivative of 2nd branchial arch is: *(AIIMS May 12)*

Ans. Muscle of facial expression (Ref: inderbir singh 7/e p115)

48. Pharyngotympanic tube is supplied by all EXCEPT: *(AIIMS May 12, AIPG 12)*

a. Ascending pharyngeal
b. Ascending palatine
c. Middle meningeal artery
d. Artery of pterygoid canal

Ans. b. (Ref: BDC 4/e vol. 3 p225)

49. Taste sensation is carried by all EXCEPT: *(AIPG 12)*

a. Facial nerve

b. Glossopharyngeal nerve

c. Vagus nerve

d. Trigeminal nerve

Ans. d. (Ref: BDC 4/e vol. 3 p253)

50. Pain in ethmoid sinusitis is carried by: *(AIPG 12)*

Ans. Nasocilliary nerve (Ref: BDC 4/e vol. 3 p118, 229)

51. All are branches of occulomotor nerve EXCEPT: *(AIPG 12)*

a. Medial rectus

b. Superior rectus

c. Twig of ciliary ganglion

d. Lacrimal nerve

Ans. d. (Ref: BDC 4/e vol. 3 p118, 229)

52. Cavernous sinus thrombosis caused when infection spreads through: *(AIPG 12)*

Ans. Pterygoid venous plexus (Ref: vinod kapoor 2nd ed p167, 168)

53. Why a child is able to breathe and suckle at the same time: *(AIPG 12)*

Ans. Highly placed pharynx (Ref: gray's anatomy 40/e p584)

54. Which of the following attains adult size before birth: *(AIPG 12)*

Ans. Ear ossicles (Ref: gray's anatomy 40/e p623)

55. Pneumatic bone is all EXCEPT: *(AIPG 12)*

a. Mastoid

b. Mandible

c. Maxilla

d. Ethmoid

Ans. b. (Ref: cunningham's textbook of Anatomy 12th ed)

56. Common carotid is palpated at: *(AIPG 12)*

Ans. Upper border of thyroid cartilage (Ref: BDC 4/e p103, 177)

57. Facial nerve injury occurs just above the branches of chorda tympani nerve, which is NOT seen: *(AIPG 12)*

a. Decreased salivation

b. Paralysis of facial muscle

c. Loss of taste

d. Hyperacusis

Ans. d. (Ref: Burket's 9/e p335)

58. All are supplied by anterior division of the mandibular nerve EXCEPT: *(AIPG 12)*

a. Kedial pterygoid

b. Lateral pterygoid

c. Masseter

d. Temporalis

Ans. a. (Ref: BDC 4/e vol. 3 p151)

59. Artery supply to floor of mouth and suprahyoid muscle is: *(AIPG 12)*

Ans. Lingual artery (Ref: BDC 4/e vol.3 p252)

60. Spaces in healthy individual are filled by: *(AIPG 12)*

Ans. Loose connective tissue (Ref: neelima malik 1/e p563)

61. Lacrimation is lost in lesion of? *(AIPG 12)*

Ans. Greater petrosal nerve (Ref: BDC 5/e p65)

62. The following arteries provide a rich blood supply to the face, EXCEPT: *(KCET 09)*

a. Buccal artery
b. Mental artery
c. Posterior auricular artery
d. infraorbital artery

Ans. c

63. Bell's palsy results in the inflammation of one of the following nerve: *(KCET 09)*

Ans. Facial nerve

64. Secretomotor fibres for the parotid gland are relayed in one of the following ganglion: *(KCET 09)*

Ans. Otic ganglion

65. Median cleft of the upper lip occurs as a result of defective formation of the: *(KCET 09)*

Ans. Frontonasal prominence

66. Injury to one of the following arteries results in extradural hematoma: *(KCET 09)*

Ans. Middle meningeal artery

67. Lymphocytes are located in each of the following tissues / organs EXCEPT: *(KCET 09)*

Ans. Brain

68. Umbilical cord contains: *(COMEDK 09)*

Ans. 2 arteries and 1 vien (Ref: Langman embryology 9/e p137)

69. CSF is directly returned to venous system by: *(COMEDK 09)*

Ans. Subarachnoid villi (Ref: BDC vol.3, 4/e p305)

70. The abductors of the vocal cords are: *(COMEDK 09)*

Ans. Posterior cricoarytenoid

71. Nerve supply to vocal cords is by: *(COMEDK 10)*

Ans. Internal and recurrent laryngeal nerves

72. Which of the following venous sinuses is more likely to be affected with thrombosis in chronic otitis media and mastoiditis? *(COMEDK 10)*

Ans. Sigmoid

73. Meiotic division of male germ cells commence: *(COMEDK 10)*

Ans. By around 16 years

74. The lingual surface of epiglottis is lined by: *(COMEDK 10)*

Ans. Stratified squamous epithelium

75. The 1st evidence of cartilage getting converted to bone in craniofacial skeleton occurs during: *(COMEDK 10)*

Ans. 8 prenatal week

76. The type of suture represented by sagittal suture of the cranial vault is: *(COMEDK 10)*

Ans. Serrate

77. The maxillary sinus drains into: *(KCET 10)*

Ans. Middle meatus

78. The meckle's cartilage is derived from: *(KCET 10)*

Ans. 1st branchial arch

79. The joint between atlas and axis is all EXCEPT: *(KCET 10)*

a. Synovial

b. Closely related to 1st cranial nerve

c. Allow rotation of the head

d. Supported by alar ligaments

Ans. b

80. All the cranial nerves provide innervations for the structures in head and neck EXCEPT one, that additionally supplies the thorax and abdomen: *(KCET 10)*

Ans. Vagus

81. Which part of the body is underdeveloped at birth: *(KCET 10)*

Ans. Face

82. Hypoglossal nerve is: *(KCET 10)*

Ans. Purely motor

83. Infection from the dangerous area of face spreads via one of the following veins: *(COMEDK 11)*

Ans. Ophthalmic veins

84. All of the following canals open on the posterior wall of the pterygopalatine fossa EXCEPT: *(COMEDK 11)*

a. Greater palatine canal

b. Foramen rotundum

c. Pterygoid canal

d. Palatovaginal canal

Ans. a

85. Hypoglossal nerve supplies all the muscles EXCEPT: *(COMEDK 11)*

Ans. Palatoglossus

86. Motor nerve for occipital belly of occipitofrontalis: *(COMEDK 11)*

Ans. Posterior auricular

87. Which of the following muscle is attached to posterior part of pterygomandibular raphe? *(KCET 11, 12)*

Ans. Superior constrictor

88. Injury to which nerve causes non – closure of eyelids, sagging of mouth and dribbling of saliva: *(COMEDK 12)*

Ans. Facial nerve

89. Failure of descent of thyroid analage can be seen in the tongue: *(COMEDK 12)*

Ans. Near the base of the tongue close to foramen caecum

90. Lymph from the teeth drains into all of the following nodes EXCEPT: *(COMEDK 12)*

a. Submandibular nodes

b. Deep cervical nodes

c. Retropharyngeal nodes

d. Sub mental nodes

Ans. c

91. Posterior ethmoidal air sinus opens into: *(COMEDK 12)*

Ans. Superior meatus

92. Facial vien communicates with cavernous sinus through: *(COMEDK 12)*

Ans. Deep facial vien

93. Mandibular fossa is a part of: *(COMEDK 12)*

Ans. Temporal bone

94. Cortical plates are thickest in the: *(COMEDK 12)*

Ans. Premolar and molar region of the mandible on the buccal side

95. Which of the following organ has most permeable capillaries? *(COMEDK 12)*

Ans. Liver

96. Right anterior quadrant of the scalp is supplied by the following arteries EXEPT: *(COMEDK 12)*

a. Right supraorbital artery
b. Right supratrochlear artery
c. Right superficial temporal artery
d. Right maxillary artery

Ans. d

97. Which of the following is a fourable prognostic indicator in Bell's palsy? *(KCET 12)*

Ans. Persistence of stapedial reflex

98. Cardiac Pain may be transmitted to the jaw due to overlapping of: *(KCET 12)*

Ans. 5th cranial nerve, 3rd cervical nerve and 1st thoracic nerve

99. What is the type of joint formed between the tooth and alveolar socket? *(KCET 12)*

Ans. Gomphosis

100. Philtrum of upper lip developes from: *(KCET 12)*

Ans. Frontonasal process

101. The cortex of lymph node contains: *(KCET 12)*

Ans. Lymphatic nodules

102. Hyaline cartilage is: *(PGI June 12)*

Ans. Mesodermal

103. The submandibular ganglion is associated anatomically with: *(PGI June 12)*

Ans. Lingual nerve

104. Maxillary antrum dips in the region of? *(PGI Dec 11)*

Ans. Between 2nd premolar and 1st molar (Ref: orbans 12/e p314)

105. Tongue on protrusion is deviated to left, the nerve injured is? *(PGI Dec 11)*

Ans. Left hypoglossal (BDC 4th p253)

106. Anterior ethmoidal sinus drains into? *(PGI Dec 11)*

Ans. Hiatus semilunaris (BDC 4/e p231)

107. Which of the following structures passes through foramen rotundum? *(PGI June 11)*

Ans. Maxillary nerve (Ref: BDC 4/e vol 3 p236)

108. Keisselbach's plexus is present? *(PGI June 11)*

Ans. Anterioinferior surface of nasal septum (Ref: BDC 4/e VOL 3 p229)

109. In which of the following aspects growth is completed soon after birth and shows no further growth with age and remains same in size throughout? *(PGI June 11)*

Ans. Width of oropharynx

110. which muscle helps in protrusion of tongue? *(PGI June 11)*

Ans. Genioglossus (Ref: BDC 4/e p252)

111. Which of the following lies in the posterior cranial fossa of a 5 year old child? *(PGI June 11)*

Ans. Jugular foramen (Ref: BDC 4/e p23)

112. Which of the following does NOT lie mesial to submandibular gland? *(PGI June 11)*

a. Facial vein
b. Mylohyoid muscle
c. Hyoglossus
d. Styloglossus

Ans. a (Ref: BDC 4/e p23)

113. An area having multipotent cell can give rise to cell of: *(PGI Dec 10)*

Ans. 1 germ layer only, ectoderm, mesoderm and endoderm

114. The nerve that emerges from the 2 superfacial heads of lateral pterygoid muscle is: *(PGI Dec 10)*

Ans. Buccal branch of mandibular nerve (Ref: BDC 4/e p147)

115. Epithelium of nasal, tracheal and nasopharyngeal mucosa: *(PGI Dec 10)*

Ans. Resemble pseudostratified epitheliu histologically (Ref: Inderbir singh)

116. Infection in danger area of face most commonly leads to: *(PGI June 10)*

Ans. Cavernous sinus thrombosis (Ref: BDC 4/e p59)

117. Trauma to nerve resulting in paraesthesia is termed as: *(PGI Dec 09)*

Ans. Neuropraxia (Ref: Neelima malik 1/e p650)

118. Which type of nerve cells are present in trigeminal ganglion: *(PGI Dec 09)*

Ans. Pseudounipolar (Ref: BDC 3/e p100)

119. Cartilages differs from bone in that: *(PGI Dec 09)*

Ans. Interstitial growth pattern (Ref: Profit 4/e p40)

120. The types of collagen fibers found in lamina lucida of basement membrane: *(PGI June 09)*

Ans. Type 4 (Ref: Tencates 6/e p66)

121. Which is a type of non – fibrillar collagen? *(PGI June 09)*

Ans. Type 9 (Ref: Tencates 16/e p66)

CHAPTER

12 Biochemistry

Topic

- Carbohydrate
- Lipid
- Amino Acid and Protein
- Nucleic Acid
- Vitamins
- Enzymes
- Miscellaneous

CARBOHYDRATE

- Number of ATP generation from different cycle:

Glycolysis Anaerobic glycolysis – 2 molecules of ATP for each molecule of glucose. Aerobic glycolysis – 8 molecules of ATP for each molecule of glucose.
TCA cycle – 12 molecules of ATP per molecule of Acetyl Co A
Fatty acid oxidation: Oxidation of 1 molecule of palmitate yield 129 ATP.

- Glycogenolysis:

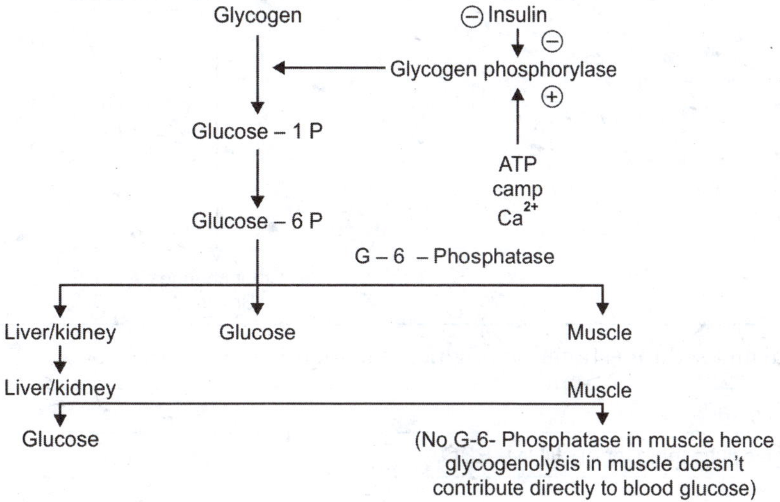

Fig. 12.1: Glycogenolysis

- Phosphorylase:

Phosphorylase a (active form)	Phosphorylase b (inactive form)
Factors maintain phosphprylase In active form – CAMP, ATP, Ca IN Muscle – only ATP	Factors maintaining phosphorylase in inactive form is INSULIN

- Glucose Transporters:

Insulin sensitive glucose transporters – GLUT 4 Essentially Found in Muscles (skeletal + cardiac) & Adipose tissue. [Q] Glucose transporters in muscles and adipose tissue are dependent on insulin so these transporters (GLUT 4) are reduced in FASTING when insulin levels are low.
Insulin insensitive glucose transporter – GLUT 1, GLUT 2, GLUT 3, GLUT 5 FOUND in rest of the tissues like BRAIN, RBC, HEPATOCYTES etc.

- LAC OPERON:

STRUCTURAL gene	REGULATOR gene
Z – β GALACTOSIDASE ↓ lactose→Glucose+ galactose	Positive regulator ex-CAP
Y –PERMEASE	NEGATIVE – Repressor gene e.g – LAC I

- Bacteria use only glucose for energy production.

LAC operon operates when glucose is NOT available for bacteria ↓ Lac operon is ON – CAP regulator gene initiates transcription of Structural gene.
when glucose is present - REPRESSOR (LAC I) binds to operator region and LAC operon turns off.

- Glucose estimation test:

Use enzyme OXIDASE and PEROXIDASE [Q].

Reaction:

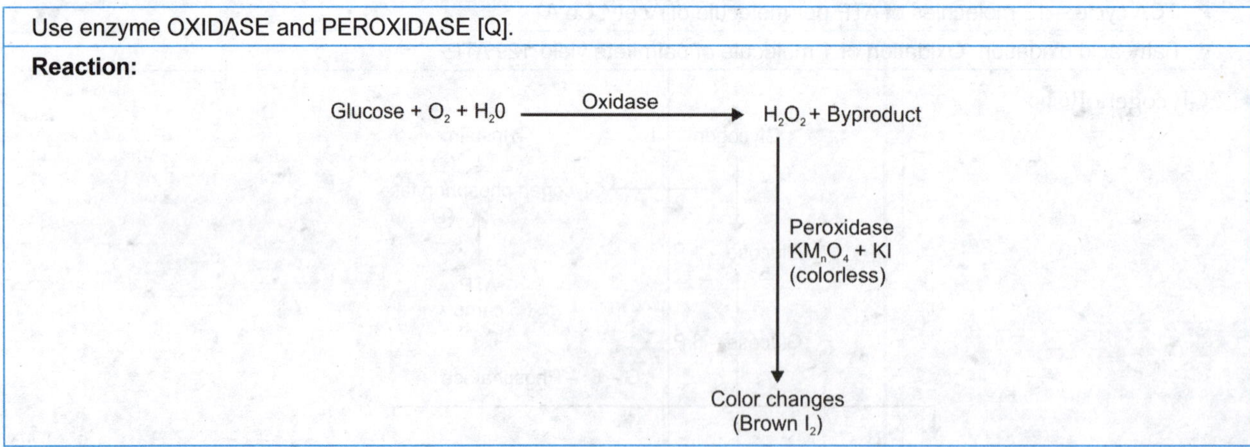

- Standard anticoagulant used for estimation of glucose in blood:

Potassium oxalate + NaF.
NaF – used as a glycolytic inhibitor of still live RBC.
Citrate is preservative.

LAST 5-YEAR QUESTIONS FROM THIS TOPIC

1. **The total number of ATP molecules that are generated per molecule of glucose under aerobic conditions are:** *(KCET 10)*

Ans. 38

2. **Von Gierke's disease, a type of glycogen storage disease, is caused due to deficiency of the enzyme:** *(KCET 10)*

Ans. Glucose – 6 phosphatase in liver

3. **Which of the following enzymes provides a link between glycolysis & citric acid cycle?** *(COMEDK 10)*

Ans. Pyruvate Dehydrogenase

4. **Insulin increases the activity of:** *(COMEDK 10)*

Ans. HMG – CoA reductase

5. **Maltose which is produced as a breakdown of starch is:** *(AIPG 12)*

Ans. Disachharide (Ref: Satyanarayana 3/e p18)

6. **Carbohydrate when taken in excessive form is stored in which form:** *(AIPG 12)*

Ans. Glycogen (Ref: Satyanarayana 3/e p263)

LIPID

- On electrophoresis CHYLOMICRONS do not move.
- Acetyl-CoA:

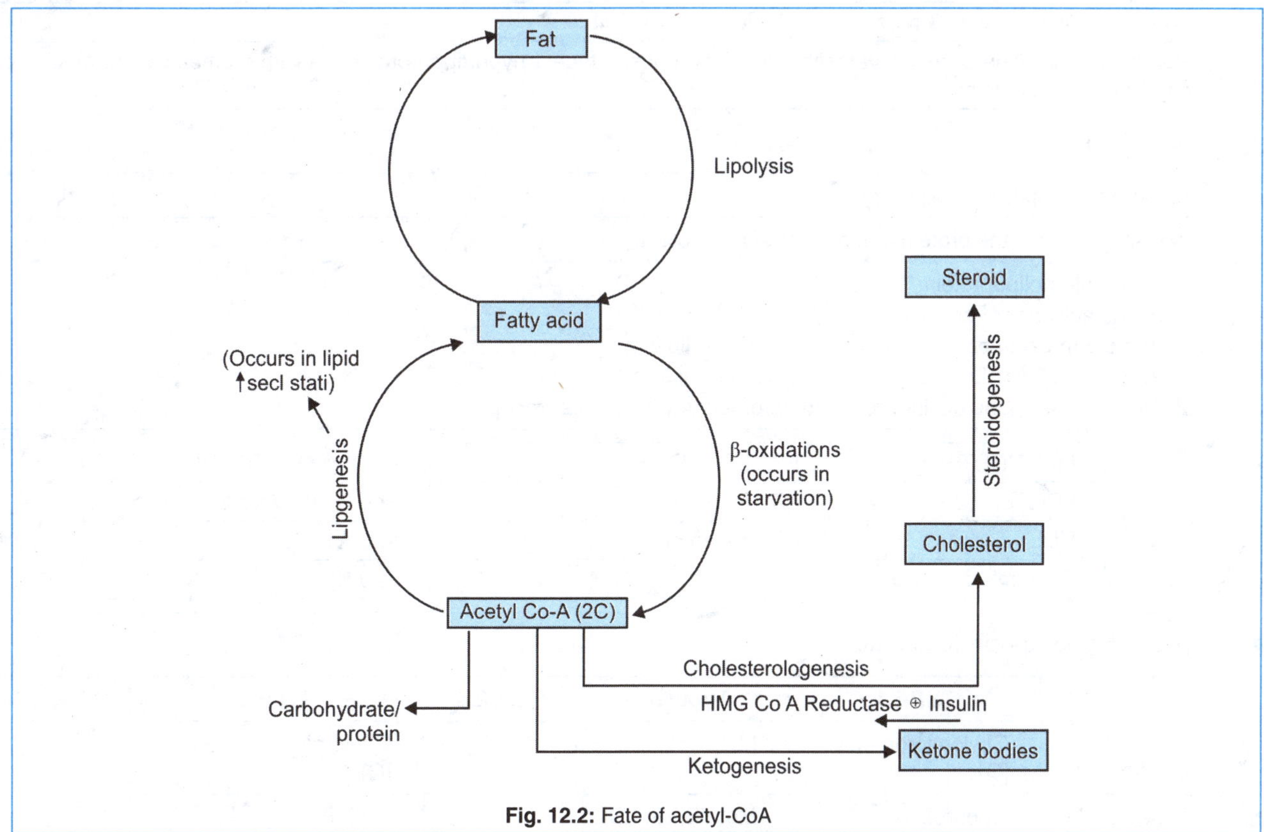

Fig. 12.2: Fate of acetyl-CoA

Fatty acid, cholesterol, and ketone bodies all can be synthesized from Acetyl- coA.

Maximum Content of TG (triglycerides) – chylomicrons.
Maximum content of exogenous TG - chylomicrons
Maximum content of endogenous TG - VLDL.
Maximum content of cholesterol - LDL

- Synthesis of TRIACYL GLYCEROL:

Synthesis of triacyl glycerol requires Glycerol – 3 phosphate which is synthesized from glycerol in the presence of GLYCEROL KINASE.
Glycerol kinase ↓ Glycerol → Glycerol -3 phosphate→Triacyl glycerol
Glycerol kinase is not expressed in ADIPOSE tissue so, glycerol kinase can not performed any function in ADIPOSE TISSUE.

- Role of Insulin in Lipogenesis:

Insulin promotes lipogenesis by increasing activity of ACETYL CO A CARBOXYLASE ACTIVITY, the principal enzyme of lipogenesis.
Insulin also activates PYRUVATE DEHYDROGENASE which catalyzes pyruvate into Acetyl co A, the building blocks of fatty acids.

- Lipoprotein Lipase:

Found in adipose tissue & muscles. NOT found in liver. [Q]
Requires apoprotein C_2 as activator.its deficiency leads to type 1 hyperlipoproteinemia with dramatic accumulation of chylomicrons in plasma .

- Lipoprotein:

Lipoprotein = lipid + apolipoprotein
So, apoprotein is the protein component of lipoprotein.
Function of apolipoprotein: 1. act as activator of enzymes – Apo c 2 (most important), apo c1 – lipoprotein lipase Apo A 1 – LCAT (Lecithine cholesterol acyl transferase) 2. functions as ligand on lipoprotein for interaction with cellular receptor.

LIPOPROTEIN	RECEPTOR	APOLIPOPROTEIN
LDL	LDL receptor	Apo B 100, Apo E
HDL	HDL receptor	Apo A1
Chylomicron, VLDL		Apo E

- Types of Hyperlipoproteinemia:

	TYPE 1	**Type 2a**	**Type 2 b**	**Type 3**	**Type 4**
Lipoprotein elevated	Chylomicron only [Q]	LDL		Chylomicron + VLDL [Q]	VLDL
Molecular defects	Lipoprotein lipase,APO C 2	Mutation in LDL receptor[Q]		APO E	

- Hmp/Pentose Phosphate Pathway:

Synthesis of NADPH→reducing equivalent for synthesis of Fatty acid, reduced glutathione.
Pentose – nucleic acid.
Site – liver, RBC, testes[Q], adiposites. [Q]

- Lipid Accumulating Disease:

Disease	Enzyme deficiency	Lipid accumulating
Gaucher's disease	B- galactosidase	glucosylceramide
Niemann-Pick disease	Sphingomylinase [Q]	sphingomylin
Tay-Sachs disease	Hexosaminidase A	GM2 ganglioside

MUSCLE	ADIPOSE TISSUE
Glucose – 6 phosphatase absent. So glycogenolysis in MUSCLE does not contribute DIRECTLY to blood glucose .	Glycerol kinase absent .

LAST 5-YEAR QUESTIONS FROM THIS TOPIC

1. **The main pathway for " de – novo" synthesis of fatty acids occur in:** *(KCET 10)*

Ans. Cytosol

2. **In Nieman – Pick disease, which of the following substance accumulates in CNS in excess?** *(AIPG 11)*

Ans. Sphingomyelins (Ref: Satyanarayan 3/e p307)

3. **The highest percentage of PUFAs are present in:** *(AIPG 10)*

Ans. Margarine

4. **Which of the following fatty acids cannot be synthesized in humans?** *(KCET 09)*

Ans. Linoleic acid

5. **The most lipogenic carbohydrate is:** *(AIPG 10)*

Ans. Fructose (Ref: Satyanarayan biochemistry 1/e p287)

6. **The most important source of reducing equivalents for fatty acid synthesis in the liver is:** *(AIPG 10)*

Ans. HMP pathway (Ref: Harper 25/e p230)

7. **Calorific value of fat is near to:** *(AIPG 12)*

Ans. 9 (Ref: Satyanarayana 3/e p503)

8. **Under metabolic conditions associated with a high rate of fatty acid oxidation, the liver produces:** *(COMEDK 10)*

Ans. Acetoacetate

AMINO ACID AND PROTIEN

- Branched chain a.a (amino acids):

Leucine, Isoleucine, Valine.

- Marple Syrup urine disease:

Defect in decarboxylation of branched chain ketoacids.
Due to inherited defect in branched chain ketoacid dehydrogenase enzyme.

- Essential a.a:

Trick – Today The PM Very ILL
Tryptophan, **t**hreonine, **p**henylalaline, **v**aline, **i**soleucine, **l**eucine, **l**ysine.

- Semiessential a.a:

Arginine, Histidine.

- Acidic a.a:

Aspartic and Glutamic Acid

- Basic a.a:

Arginine, Histidine, Lysine

- HARTNUP disease: defect in transport of neutral a.a.
- a.a that forms succinyl Co A:

TRICK – MTV+ Isoleucine (Methionine, Threonine, Valine)

- a.a that forms α- ketoglutarate:

TRICK – GPA + Histidine (Glycine, Proline, Alaline)

- Classification of a.a based on the nature of metabolic end product:

KETOGENIC	GLYCOGENIC+KETOGENIC	GLUCOGENIC
Leucine, **L**ysine [TRICK – **L**] [Q]	**TRICK** – PITT [Q] P – phenylalaline I – Isoleucine T – tryptophan T – tyrosine	Rest are GLYCOGENIC

- Glycine – is required for the synthesis of HEME [Q]
- 3 a.a are required for the biosynthesis of CRETININE:

Glycine, arginine and methionine.

- a.a with ALIPHATIC side chain:

Seen in Isoleucine, alaline & valine
So Homologous substitution can occur between them.

- Amino acid migrating FASTEST on chromatography:

NEUTRAL a.a
Valine > glycine [Q], as valine is more non polar.

- Aromatic a.a:

All aromatic a.a absorb UV rays.
E.g.- tryptophan, tyrosine at 280 nm.

- G- protein:

Gα has inherent GTPase activity.

- Ribozyme:

Peptidal transferase is the only enzymatic activity of r-RNA.
It is specific to 23S r-RNA found in 60S subunit. So it is called RIBOZYME.

- Differential RNA processing:

Leads to various forms of Ig.
E.g. – membrane & secretary form.

- Translation:

Poly A translates into POLYLYSINE. [Q] .

- Nitric Acid Synthesis:

NO synthase ↓ Arginine→citruline ↓ NO (by product)

- Carrier of NH_3 to liver (from peripheral tissue for its conversion to urea)

From most tissue – by GLUTAMINE.
From MUSCLES – by ALALINE. [Q]

- Function of protein depends on:

As long as protein ligand interaction are conserved, function of protein will essentially be CONSERVED. ↓ Most important factor to be conserved in protein for its function is LIGAND BINDING RESIDUE. [Q]
FIBROUS protein – maintain structure, shape & strength of cell. Ex- collagen, keratin, myosin.

- Structure of protein:

Primary – the linear SEQUENCE OF a.a forms the backbone.
Secondary – Helix, loops & bends
Tertiary – three dimensional structure. – most important for function & most conserved. [Q]
Quatenary – DIMER/TRIMER [Q]

- Proteoglyc:

Glycosaminoglycan + protein
They are polyanions so attract Na ion and thus hold large amount of water [Q].
All have sulphate at the end sulphated.
Ex – chondratin sulphate, keratin sulphate, heparin, heparin sulphate.
Note: hyaluronic acid is glycosoaminoglycan but NOT proteoglycan as NOT SULPHATED.

- Distribution of various GAG (GLYCOSAMINOGLYCANS):

Hyaluronic acid – synovial fluid, vitreous humor.[Q]
Chondroitin sulphates – cartilage, bone, cornea.
Heparan sulphate – aortic wall, skin fibroblasts.
Heparin – mast cell.

PROTEOMICS	GLYCOMICS
Study of structure & function of protein in disease process	Structure & function of chains of sugars.

- CHAPERONS – Enable proper folding of other proteins without themselves.
- Pathway of protein degradation: (of misfolded)

In Lysosome	Ubiquitine-proteosome pathway
ATP independent	ATP dependent.

- Proteosomes are organelles involved in → degradation of misfolded protein.
- Ammonium sulphate precipitation:

Is a method of protein purification by alteration of protein SOLUBILITY.
Method is known as SALTING OUT.

- Alkaptonuria:

Caused due to deficiency of HOMOGENTISIC ACID OXIDASE.
AR disorder of TYROSINE metabolism.
TRIAD of: homogentisic acid urea, black pigmentation, arthritis(calcification of intervertebral disc)

LAST 5-YEAR QUESTIONS FROM THIS TOPIC

1. In the body, metabolism of 10g of protein would produce approximately: *(COMEDK 12)*

Ans. 41 kcal

2. Mannose – 6 – phosphate containing freshly synthesized proteins are directed to: *(COMEDK 12)*

Ans. Lysosomes

3. The nitrogen content in 50 g of a typical dietary protein is most likely to be: *(COMEDK 11)*

Ans. 8 g

4. Phenylketonuria is a disease due to: *(AIPG 12)*

Ans. Improper metabolism of amino acids (Ref: Robbin's pathology 7/e p488)

5. False about denaturation of protein is all, EXCEPT: *(AIPG 09)*

A. Unfolding occurs
B. Disruption of secondary structure
C. Sequence of amino acid remains the same
D. Biological activity is retained

Ans. b (Ref: Stoker. General, Organic & Biological Chemistry pg 684)

NUCLEIC ACID

- Dna Hybridisation:

Study variation in gene sequence/expression.	
Single gene sequence	Multiple gene/ entire genome
DNA – sothern blot	MICROARRAY microarray is the BEST technique for detection of variation in DNA sequence and gene expression.
RNA – northern blot	

- Detection of Aneuploidy:

FISH & PCR are used.
NOTE: Microarray are currently not used for detection of aneuploidy
(Western blot – for protein synthesis, South Western blot – protein DNA interaction)

- DNA primase – provides RNA primer .
- Codons:

Genetic codes are Degenerate: 1 a.a coded by more than 1 codon. Exception methionine and tryptophan which is coded by 1 codon.
Unambiguous/ specificity - one codon code only one a.a.
Stop codon: UAA (ochre), UAG (opal), UGA (Amber)

- Enzymes involved in DNA Replication:

Helicase – unwind the DNA to provide single stranded DNA.
Topoisomerase – relieve torsional strain that results from helicase induced unwinding.
DNA primase – initiates synthesis RNA primer.(do not confuse)
DNA Polymerase – polymerises DNA Polymerase 1 – Gap filling & synthesis of LAGGING strand. Polymerase 2 – DNA proof reading & repair . Polymerase 3 – LEADING strand synthesis (5' – 3' direction)
DNA ligase – seals the nick between okazaki fragments on lagging strand.

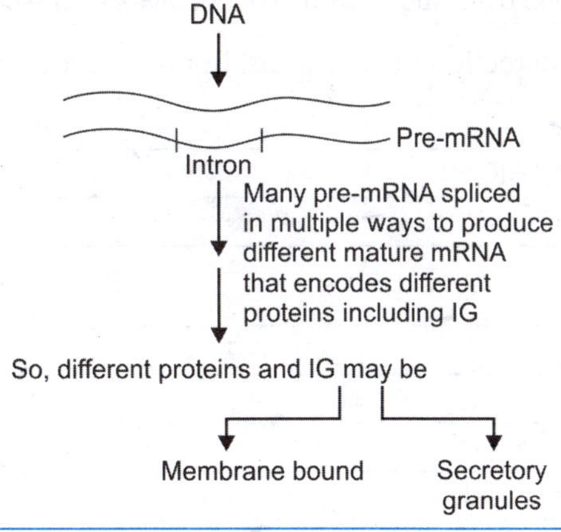

- Micro RNA:

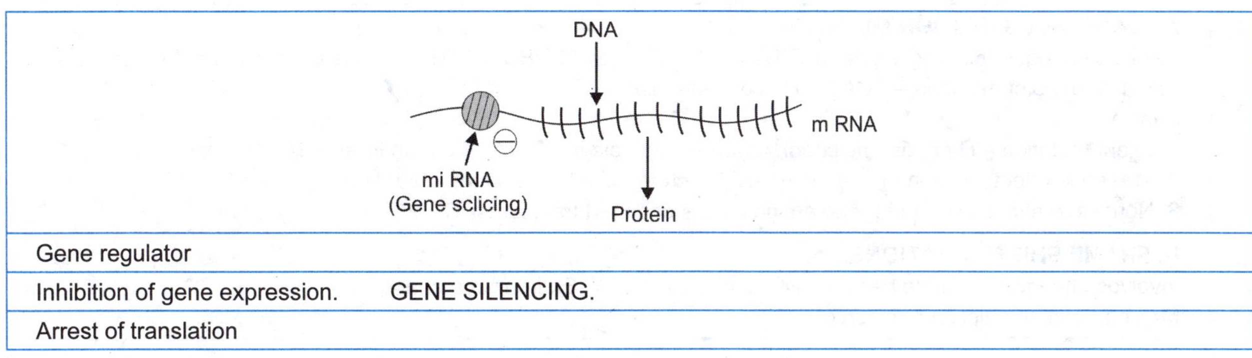

Gene regulator	
Inhibition of gene expression.	GENE SILENCING.
Arrest of translation	

SnRNA→ Splicing → Occur to Remove Introns.

Structure of Nuclear Receptor (androgen)

AF-1	DBD	LBD
N –terminal	Central domain Highly conserved	C- terminal
AF-1 = activating transcription	DBD – DNA binding domain.	LBD - Ligand binding domain [Q]

- Prokaryotic RNA polymerase:

Sigma sub unit recognises PROMOTER region on DNA.

- t - RNA has %age of modified bases.
- Mitochondrial DNA:

Only non- chromosomal DNA in human cells.
Always inherited MATERNALLY.
Has NO INTRONS.

- PCR:

Ion required are – Magnesium, Mn. [Q]
Requires: • Primer • Taq polymerase(heat stable) • dNTP • Mg and Mn • SYBER GREEN DYE (Cyanide dye. Nuceic acid stained, gives fluorescent signal.)

- Blue White Screening – Use for detection of successful ligation & identify desired DNA into plasmid vector.
- Chrosomal structure:

X chromosome – SUBMETACENTRIC
Y chromosome – ACROCENTRIC.

- LESCH NYHAN syndrome:

Defective PURINE metabolism.
X- linked
male affected
mental retardation + increased uric acid .

- Different types of Mutations:

A. BASE SUBSTITUTION MUTATION: Involves changes to a single base (POINT MUTATION) and SUBSTITUTION of the base with another base. Example of point mutation – SCA (sickle cell anaemia). Effects: 1. Silent mutation – changes one codon for an amino acid into another codon for the SAME amino acid. 2. Missense effect – codon of one amino acid is changed into codon for ANOTHER amino acid. 3. Nonsense effect – codon for one amino acid is changed translation TERMINATION CODON.
B. FRAME SHIFT MUTATIONS: Involves change to a single base but NO SUBSTITUTION .Entire frame changes. May be seen as deletion or insertion.

- Lysosomal storage disorder (LSD):

Molecular changes in LSD - mutation of gene encoding lysosomal hydrolase . [Q]

- **LAST 5-YEAR QUESTIONS FROM THIS TOPIC**

1. **Hybridisation of 2 homologous BUT not identitical DNA strands can be increased by:** *(AIIMS May 11)*

Ans. Increasing salt concentration/polyethylene glycol (Ref: Kendrew & Lawrence the encyclopedia of molecular biology p504)

2. **Denaturation of DNA meAns.** *(AIPG 10)*

Ans. Reversible separation of DNA (Ref: Satyanarayan 2/e p80)

3. **DNA recombination technique is possible due to:** *(AIPG 10)*

Ans. Restriction endonuclease (Ref: Harper 25/e p489)

4. **DNA estimation can be done by:** *(AIPG 12)*

Ans. Spectrophotometer

5. **In RNA interference all are involved EXCEPT:** *(AIPG 12)*
   a. Dorsha
   b. Pasha
   c. m RNA
   d. mi RNA

Ans. d

VITAMINS

- Visual Cycle:

Rhodopsin (visual purple) (11-cis retinal + opsin) ↓ PHOTOISOMERISATION GENERATION OF visual IMPULSE All trans retinal + opsin
Visual impulse is initiated as a result of photochemical isomerisation [Q] reaction when RHODOPSIN is exposed to light.

- Vitamin A intoxication:

Excess of vit A can cause lysosomal membrane rupture. [Q]
Acute toxicity – ADULT – 150mg, CHILDREN – 100mg
Chronic toxicity – ADULT – 15mg/day for several months, children – 6mg/day.

- All Dehydrogenase (Except LDH) depend on Vit B_1, B_2, B_3
- Thiamine:

For Transketolase reaction (in HMP pathway), pyruvate dehydrogenase & α- keto gluterate dehydrogenase complex.
Central role in energy yielding metabolism especially of carbohydrate.
TPP (thiamine pyrophosphate) is the active form .
Thiamine deficiency: Wet beriberi – cvs symptoms Dry beriberi – cns symptoms Wernicke's encephalopathy.
The laboratory diagnosis of thiamine deficiency is usually made by enzymatic assay of TRANSKETOLASE ACTIVITY.[Q]

- LDH only require Vit. B_3
- Transamination/ Deamination require Vit. B6
- All Carboxylase Depend on Biotin.
- VIT B_{12} dependent:

• Homocysteine methyl transferase
• Isomerisation of methyl malonyl Co A To succinyl co A

- Vit. C – larger dose of Vit. C used in acidifying urine & treatment for UTI.
- Vitamin K:

Is required for synthesis of Ca binding protein (osteocalcin, BMP).
So, WARFARIN if used in pregnant mother decreases vit K level in foetus leading to bone defects.
Vit k is a necessary cofactor in OXIDATIVE PHOSPHORYLATION.

LAST 5-YEAR QUESTIONS FROM THIS TOPIC

1. Which of the following factors are associated with vit. K? *(AIIMS May 10)*

Ans. 2, 7, 9, 10 (Ref: ganong 22/e p544)

2. NOT true about vitamin D: *(PGI June 10)*

a. UV light helps in formation of it
b. Increased parathyroid hormone secretion is seen in renal failure
c. Hydroxylation of 25 – hydroxycholecalcitrol occurs in kidney
d. 25 – hydroxycholecalciferol is used in treatment of renal failure

Ans. d

3. Pernicious anaemia occurs due to deficiency of: *(AIIMS May 10)*

Ans. Cobalamine (Ref: Shafer 5/ed p1043)

4. Pellagra is seen in deficiency of: *(KCET 11)*

Ans. Niacin

5. Biotin is required for the activity of: *(KCET 09)*

Ans. Pyruvate carboxylase

6. Vitamin D *(KCET 09)*

Ans. Along with PTH, increases Ca2+ resorption from bone

7. Burning feet syndrome occurs due to deficiency of: *(COMEDK 09)*

Ans. Pantothenic acid

8. Wernicke – korsakoff psychosis is due to: *(AIPG 10)*

Ans. Thiamine (Ref: Satyanarayan 2nd ed pg 186)

9. Which of the vitamin deficiency leads to lactic acidosis? *(AIPG 12)*

Ans. Thiamine (Ref: Harper' biochemistry 28/e p473)

10. Vitamin B6 is also known as: *(AIPG 12)*

Ans. Pyridoxine (Ref: Harper's biochemistry 26th ed pf 488, 489)

11. Thiamine deficiency causes decreased energy production because: *(AIPG 09)*

Ans. It is a coenzyme for transketolase in pentose phosphate pathway (Ref: Harper's 26/e p488 – 489)

ENZYMES

- Functional and Non Functional Enzymes:

Functional enzyme	Non functional enzymes
Normally present in higher concentration in plasma and their substrate is always present in plasma.	Enzymes present at low concentration in plasma and higher concentration in tissue and their substrate are absent from plasma.
E.g – LPL (lipoprotein lipase) [Q]	Most of the enzyme.

- Ca dependent enzyme /CALMADULIN – " Cyclase "

Adenyl cyclase, guanyl cyclase, glycogen synthase [Q]

- Mg dependent – 'KINASE"

Hexokinase, pyruvate kinase
ENOLASE.

- Zn dependent:

MMPase, alcohol dehydrogenase, ALP

- Liver Enzymes: Tells about hepatocellular damage.

Cytosolic	Mitochondrial	Membrane bound
SGPT, SGOT, LDH	SGOT(AST), GDH	GGT, ALP, 5- NUCLEOTIDASE ↓ tells about cholestasis

- PROTEASE:

The laboratory diagnosis of thiamine deficiency is usually made by enzymatic assay of TRANSKETOLASE ACTIVITY. [Q]	
ENDOPEPTIDASE	**EXOPEPTIDASE**
E.g. Pepsin, trypsin,Chymotrypsin, elastase So, chymotripsinogen is a zymogen. [Q]	Carboxypeptidase, aminopeptidase

- Competitive & non competitive inhibition of enzyme:

COMPETITIVE	NON COMPETITIVE INHIBITION
K_m is increased but V_{max} is constant.	K_m constant, V_{max} decreased.

- Note: V_{max} never increases in inhibition it either remains constant or decreases.
- Enzyme creatinine assay – estimate blood creatinine level most accurately.

LAST 5-YEAR QUESTIONS FROM THIS TOPIC

1. **Which of the following liver enzymes is predominantly mitochondrion?** *(AIIMS Nov. 10)*

Ans. SGOT/AST

NOTE: SGPT is only cytosolic

2. **Enzymes which play an important role in calcification are:** *(PGI dec 11)*

Ans. Alkaline phosphatase & pyrophosphatase (Ref: Satyanarayan 2/e p125)

3. **LDH has following number of isoenzymes:** *(KCET 11)*

Ans. 5

MISCELLANEOUS

- Test for Haemoglobin estimation: [Q]

Used method – Sahli's, Specrophotometry (most accurate), Drabkins, oxyhaemoglobin method.

- Prenatal Diagnosis of Haemophillia:

Direct mutational analysis	Indirect linkage analysis
Based on PCR technique	
Method of choice.	

- Sickle cell disease:

Due to substitution of valine for glutamate – STICKY PATCH/HYDROPHOBIC PATCH generated at Hb ↓ Leads to REDUCED SOLUBILITY [Q] ↓ Causes SICKLING of RBC

- Some Important Biochemical Tests:

SUGARS (reducing sugars)	PROTEIN	Bile pigments	BLOOD	KETONE BODIES
Benedict's test Fehling's test	Heat coagulation test Nitric acid test.	Fouchet's test Bile salts - Hay's test Urobilinogen- Ehrlich's test.	Benzidene test	Rothera's test. [Q] Gerhardt's test.

- BOTH simple and facilated diffusion are BIDIRECTIONAL & active transport is UNIDIRECTIONAL .
- Neutral molecules are transported by SIMPLE diffusion (favoured by hydrophobicity)
- Golgi body – functions:

Glycosylation.
Sorting of protein for their correct destination.[Q]

- Endosome:

Ligand receptor uncoupling occurs in endosomes due to low PH.

- Urea synthesis and gluconeogenesis occurs in both cytosol & mitochondria.
- 2, 4 Dinitrophenol:

Causes uncoupling of oxidation & phosphorylation within respiratory chain.

- Eukaryotic plasma membrane:

Made of Carbohydrate, Lecithin, Cholesterol NOT TAG (triacylglycerol). [Q]

- Fire flies produce light due to ATP.
- Refsum disease:

Due to deficiency of phytanic α- oxidase. [Q]

- MMP requires Zn ion.

- Prebiotics:

Undigestable agents in upper GIT like inulin used to deliver prebiotic agents (lactobacilli, bifidobacter). [Q]
Resist digestion due to β- configuration anomeric C2. [Q]

- Lytic & lysogenic phase of bacteriophase:

In Lysogenic pathway – the lambda DNA integrates into the host genome and remains dormant until activated.
In Lytic phase – the lambda DNA integrates into the host genome & starts replicating until it has made several copies of the complete virus after which the virus particles are released by lysis.
Note – lytic & lysogenic phase cannot occur together .[Q]

- Resting energy expenditure (REE) & BMR:

REE = BMR + energy used in digestion of food → BMR is energy expanded in resting & fasting state.
Both BMR & REE are related to LEAN BODY MASS [Q]
Adipose tissue is inert in REE & BMR (not contribute).

- lignin is the only plant product not fermented by GIT bacteria.
- Copper metabolism:

Copper is excreted from body by liver into bile. So any disease which hampers biliary excretion will lead to accumulation of copper in liver and increased urinary excretion of copper.
E.g- primary biliary cirrhosis, primary sclerosing cholangitis, Wilson disease.
MENKE'S DISEASE–X–linked disorder of Cu metabolism (kinky hair syndrome)

- The 40 nm gap between tropocollagen in collagen serve as a site of bone formation, occupied by Ca ion. [Q]
- Cyanide inhibits complex 4 of ETC (electron transport chain).

LAST 5-YEAR QUESTIONS FROM THIS TOPIC

1. **The half life of plasma albumin is approximately:** *(COMEDK 12)*

Ans. 20 days

2. **In prolonged starvation the main source of energy to brain is:** *(KCET 11)*

Ans. Ketone bodies

3. **Plasma ceruloplasmin is a:** *(COMEDK 11)*

Ans. Alpha – 2 globulin

4. **Ehrlic test is done to detect:** *(COMEDK 11)*

Ans. urobilinogen

5. **The fluid mosaic model of membrane structure was proposed by:** *(KCET 10)*

Ans. Singer & Nicolson

6. **Free radicals are chemical species which have:** *(COMEDK 09)*

Ans. Single unpaired electron in an outer orbit

7. **Serum creatine kinase – 3 (CK-3) is elevated in:** *(COMEDK 09)*

Ans. Muscular dystrophy

8. **Bilirubin is formed from:** *(KCET 09)*

Ans. heme

9. **Rothera' s test is used for the detection of:** *(AIPG 11)*

Ans. Ketones (Ref: Satyanarayan 3/ep295)

10. **The type of collagen present in hyaline cartilage is:** *(AIPG 11)*

Ans. Type 2 (Ref: harpers illustrated biochemistry, 26/e p551 – 552)

11. **What is the function of serum albumin?** *(AIPG 11)*

Ans. Oncotic pressure maintenance (Ref: Puri Textbook of medical biochemistry 3/e p87)

12. **Sickle cell anemia substitution of valine in place of glutamic acid is by:** *(AIPG 10)*

Ans. Missense mutation (Ref: Satyanarayan 2/e p445)

13. **Oxygen dependent killing is done through:** *(AIPG 10)*

Ans. NADPH oxidase (Ref: Robbins 7/e p60)

14. **All of the following have receptors which are transcription factor EXCEPT:** *(AIPG 10)*
    a. Insulin
    b. Oestrogen
    c. Glucocorticoids
    d. Vit. D

Ans. a (Ref: KDT 5/e p145, 214)

15. **Eicosapentaenoic acid is present in:** *(AIPG 10)*

Ans. Fish oil (Ref: Park 20/e p482)

16. **ATP is the store house of:** *(AIPG 10)*

Ans. energy (Ref: Guyton 7/e p809)

17. **True regarding Ehler – Danlos syndrome (EDS) is all EXCEPT:** *(AIPG 09)*

Ans. X – linked dominant (Ref: Harper's illustrated Biochemistry 26/e p538)

18. **Actual measurement of energy of cells is done by:** *(AIPG 12)*

Ans. ATP (Ref: Guyton 11/e p881)

19. **Color of bile is due to:** *(AIPG 12)*

Ans. Bile pigments

20. **Iron absorption is least affected by:** *(AIPG 12)*

Ans. Sodium chloride (Ref: Guyton 11/e p425)

21. **Bile acid pool is recycled how many times:** *(AIPG 12)*

Ans. 8 times/day (Ref: Lippincott's 4/e p224 – 227)

CHAPTER

13

General Pathology

Topic

- General Pathology and Histopathology
- Systemic Pathology

GENERAL PATHOLOGY AND HISTOPATHOLOGY

- Reversible and Irreversible cell injury: Irreversible cell injury → Membrane damage → Amorphous density in mitochondria[Q]
- Apoptosis:

The most characteristic feature is nuclear pyknosis[Q]
Other • Cellular shrinkage • Chromatin clumping • Intact cell membrane • Cytoplasmic eosinophillia
Apoptosis is phagocytosis without release of inflammatory mediators → Inflammation is virtually absent.
Inter nucleosomal cleavage of DNA seen in apoptosis (AIIMS 05)

- Necrosis:

1. Tissue Architecture is preserved only in Coagulative necrosis.
2. Caseous Necrosis is a Distinctive form of Coagulative necrosis. Affected tissue – Cheesy white appearance. Characteristically seen in TB[Q]
a. Coagulative Necrosis – Characteristically associated with sudden severe Ischemia resulting in hypoxic cell death. Characteristic site – Heart (MI), Kidney b. Liquefaction Necrosis – Resulting from dissolution of dead cells by hydrolytic enzymes Characteristic Site → Brain c. FAT Necrosis → results from damage of adipocytes. Characteristically seen in Acute pancreatic and breast
Note: In liquefactive necrosis enzymatic digestion is a predominant feature

- Apoptosis vs Necrosis:

Apoptosis	Necrosis
Cellular shrinkage	Cellular swelling
Nuclear compaction (Most characteristic)	Karyolysis
Plasma membrane intact	Plasma membrane disrupted

- In Karyolysis there is complete disappearance of nuclear chromatin *(AIIMS 07)*
- Karyohexis there is just nuclear fragmentation
- Neutrophilic leucocytes completely engulf bacteria *(AIIMS 06)*
- Paraganglioma → Characterized by the presence of dense neuroendocrine granules.
- Usual interstitial pneumonia: (UIP)

H/P – Presence of Heterogeneous, Patchy fibrosis with Several fibroblasts is characteristic[Q]

- Acute inflammation:

• Hall mark of Acute inflammation vascular permeability factor.

- Thrombin → Main link between clotting system and acute inflammation
- Patterns of altered permeability:

• Increased permeability in acute inflammation may occur in 3 patterns: • Immediate transient leakage – Endothelial cell Contraction • Delayed sustained leakage– Endothelial cell Retraction[Q] – Direct effect of injurious agent

- Scavengers of free Radicals – Superoxide Dismutase, Catalase, Glutathione.
- Most effective bactericidal system – Hydrogen peroxide – MPO – Halide system [Q]
- Types of Hypersensitivity Reaction:

1. Type I → (IgE) Local → Eczema , Hay fever, Asthma (ATOPY) (Atopy → A genetic predisposition towards development of immediate hypersensitivity reaction Ex–Allergic Rhinitis, ASTHAMA)
2. Type II → (IgG and IgM) – Cytotoxic, complement mediated lysis Grave's disease, Myasthenia Gravis Blood disease – Agranulocytosis, ITP, Hemolytic Anemia
3. Type III → Immune Complex (IgG and IgM) Local – Arthus reaction Systemic – Serum sickness Ex– SLE, PAN, EM, Steven Johnson, Pencillamine Toxicity → Drugs Related
4. Type IV Delayed hypersensitivity reaction (Cellular immunity) Includes – Tuberculline test, Lepromin test, Contact dermatitis, Graft Rejection NB: Hypersensitivity Pneumonitis – is associated with Both Type III and IV Hyersensitivity[Q] Type III > Type IV

- Thyroid Gland:

• Papillary CA of Thyroid is characterized by the presence of Psammoma bodies and Orphan Annie Eye Nuclei [Q] • Psammoma bodies never found in follicular and Medullary CA
• Hashimoto's Thyroiditis → Hurthle cell seen

- Different Marker's:

Melanoma – HMB 45, S–100
GIST – CD117 **Note:** CD–117 marker– for GIST, (Myeloid series)[Q] Granulocytic sarcoma (Chloroma)[Q]
• Hodgkin's Lymphoma – CD15, CD30
• Burkeit lymphoma – t (8,14)[Q] (Most common), t (2, 8)[Q], CD 15, 30
• Synovial Sarcoma- t (x, 18)
• Mantle cell lymphoma – (+)ve for CD5, 20, 43 and (–) ve for CD 23[Q]
• Langerhan's Histocytosis – CDIa, S-100, HLA-DR , Langerin[Q]
• Granulocytic Sarcoma is (–)ve for CD45 RO[Q]
• Myeloid series – CD4, 11, 13, 15, 33, 117
B– cell – 10, 19, 20, 21, 22, 23, 79 ↓ Present in immature B cell so absent in mature B-cell ex-Burkett lymphoma (Lymphoma of mature B cell)
• Ewing sarcoma – MIC-2/CD 99[Q]
• Anexin V – Early marker of Apoptosis

- Immuno histochemical markers:

• Cytokeratin → Carcinoma
• Vimentin → Sarcoma, Lymphoma, Melanoma, Tumor derived from uterus and ovary[Q]
• Cadherin → Breast cancer
• Desmin → Tumors muscular origin

- Proapoptic factor vs Anti apoptic factor

Proapoptic factor	Anti apoptic factor
BaK, Bas, Bim[Q] P53, Cyt C, Caspase, TNF	Inhibit Apoptosis → Tumorogenesis Bcl–2 , Bcl-X[Q])

- Tumor suppressor genes → NF-1, PTEN, APC, P53, WT-1, RB gene[Q] *(AIIMS 08)*
- RAS gene is associated with tumor development.
- **Oncognes:**

• PDGF (Platelet derived growth factors) → Sis Oncogene
• Nuclear Regulatory protein – myc, foc, jun
• Cell cycle control → Bcl, mdm-2 (p53 Antagonist) CDK 4

- CD7 + Pro T-cells are earliest identifiable cells of T-cell lineage during maturation[Q]
- CD4 helper T cells:

• Native and memory T cells display characteristic surface markers that can be used to distinguish them: Native T cell → CD45 (CD 45 RA) → High Molecular Wt. Memory T cell → CD45 (CD 45 RD) → Low Molecular Wt.
• CD4 T helper cell help the cytotoxic T cells 1° response develops independently → Helper independent. however restimulation of memory cytotoxic T cell requires CD4 helps.

• Interaction between helper T-cell and B-cells required for → B cell memory → Long lived plasma cells production Production of Ab producing Plasma cells and Memory B cell ↙ Extra follicular pathway → No interaction → • Production of short lived plasma cells and low Affinity Ab • No memory B cells[Q] ↘ Follicular pathway → Interaction between T helper cell and B cell → Long lived plasma cells and Memory B cells
• CD4 helper cells also required for opsonization: ↓sed production of C3b and IgG.

- HLA complex (MHC complex):

Class I (MHC I)	Class II (MHC II)	Class III (MHC III)
Found on surface of all nucleated cells and platelets So Not on RBC (AIIMS 05)	Found only on the cells of immune system (APC → B cells, Macro phases, dendritic cells)	Involve in Autoimmune disorders.
• MHC I present Ag to Cytotoxic CD-8 T cells	• MHC II is associated with • APC → have groove for Ag [Q] • MHC II present Ag to CD4– T cells [Q]	
Responsible for: • Graft rejection • Cell mediated cytolysis (Virus, cancer cells)	• Responsible for GVHR (graft versus host response)	

NB: NK-cells kill those cells which fail to express MHC I (AIIMS Nov. 2012)

- **Complement pathway:**

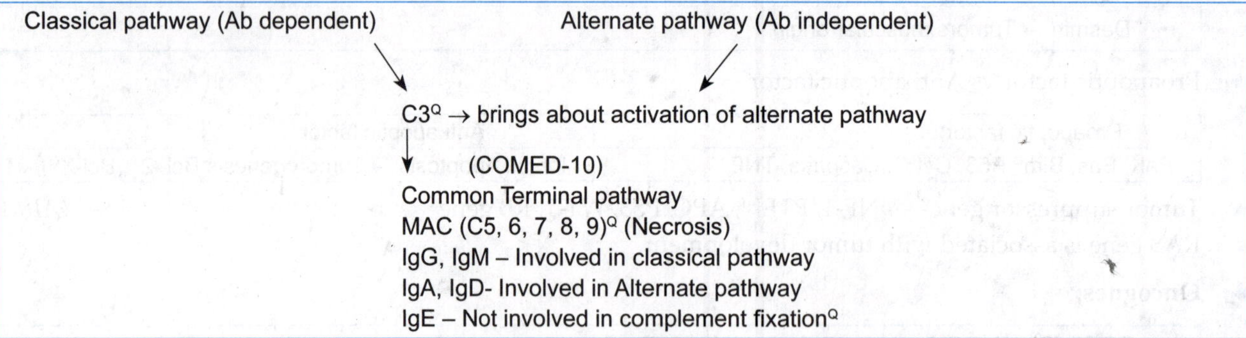

- **Tissue injury:**

Ist initial 24 hrs → Neutrophilia [Q]
24-48 hrs → Monocytosis / Macrophases

- Trans differentiation vs De Differentiation

Trans differentiation	De Differentiation
Change of cells from one Differentiated stage to → Another differentiated state and perform function of New lineage[Q]	Cells → Differentiated cells De-Differentiation (Lower life)

- Genomic Imprinting:

• Prader willi Syndrome → Deletion of Paternally derived chromosome
• Angelman syndrome → Deletion of Maternally derived chromosome
• Genomic imprinting – is Differential expression of same gene depending on parent of origin[Q]

- Composition of BM (Basement membrane):

• Laminin, fibronection, Entaction (Nidogen), Tenascin, heparin sulfate, proteoglycan, type IV collagen
• Type IV collagen → chicken wire appearance[Q]

- Rey's syndrome: Mitochondrial dysfunction HHP– Glycogen depletion[Q]
- Michaelis gutmann bodies → Melakoplakia[Q]
- Metalloproteinase – Degradation of Basement membrane *(ALPORT Syndrome)*
- Microscopic changes in MI patients:

• 3-5 days – Large PMN's at border of Coagulative Necrosis.
• 6-7 days – Marked Granulation tissue
• 10 days – Collagenous tissue

- Staining:

• For lipids → Unconjugated → Oil Red O, sudan, fillipin
• conjugated lipid (glycolipid) → PAS → Glycogen+fungal cell wall
• For fungus → PAS, Methamine silver, mucicarmine
• KOH wet mount → Rapid method for fungal hyphae *(KCET 2012)*

- In kleinefelter's Syndrome XXY seen, i.e. 47, XXY or 46, XY *(AIIMS 08, AIPG 12, 11)*
- **Transduate vs Exudate:**

Transduate	Exudate
• Associated without changes in endothelial permeability	Associated with increased vascular permeability
• Non-inflammatory edema	Inflammatory edema
• Glucose → same as blood	Glucose → low
• Specific gravity → < 1.012 *(KCET 12)*	Specific gravity > 1.012
• LDH → Low	LDH → High
• e.g. → Heart, Liver, Kidney→ Failure	Infections like TB malignancy

- Haptoglobin:

– Carier free Hb in plasma
so ↓sed haptoglobin when ↑sed consumption ex-hemolytic disease
↑sed Haptoglobine when ↓sed consumption ex-Billiary obstruction[Q]

- Transfer of Ig from mother to child across placenta is an example of natural passive immunity.
- Haptenes:

• They are partial antigen.
• Itself does not stimulate antibody production But can stimulate antibody production when combined with carrier protein

- Proteins are most antigenic

- CD Markers for B-cell lineage:

CD 10, 19, 20., 21, 22, 23, 24, 79
↓
Stem cell (CD 34+ve)
↓
Immature B-cell – CD 10 and CD 34 Lost
↓
Mature B-cell (Ex-Burkeit lymphoma
↓
Acquire CD 10 again during activation so only CD 34 (–)ve[Q]
↓
Mature B-cell activation Plasma cells (CD 38+ve)
↓
Memory B-cell (CD 38+ve)

- So Mature B cell markers are – 10, 19, 20, 21, 22, 23, 79, sIgM, sIgG, Bcl-6
- Burkeit lymphoma is a mature B-cell lymphoma so CD–37–ve and surface Ig → IgM +ve + BCL–6
- NB: Burkeit lymphoma never expresses anti apoptic Bcl-2

- Inflammatory Mediators:

• Vasodilation → Prostaglandins, histamine, Bradykinin, Histaminia
• ↑sed Vascular Permeability → Bradykinin[Q], Histamine, No, Leukotrienes
• Chemotaxis → C5a
• Phagocytosis → C3b, IgG
• Anaphylotoxins → C3a, C5a
• Necrosis → C5b, 6, 7, 89 – MAC (Membrane attack complex) → Common terminal pathway
• Pain → Prostaglandins, Bradykinins
• Fever → IL–1, TNF, Prostaglandins
• Tissue damage → Neutrophills, Macrophages, Oxygen metabolites No.

- Peripheral nerve regenerate at rate of 1 mm/day
- Super antigens do not bind to the cleft or the antigen[Q] binding groove in the MHC II molecule. They bind at a site which is distinct from the cleft and located on the lateral side of the cleft
  Ex- Toxic shock syndrome, Kawasaki syndrome
- Follicular dendritic cells/ Mature dendritic cells are the most patient stimulator of nerve T-cells *(AIPG 07)*
- Rheumatoid Factor (Rheumatoid factor) in Rheumatoid Arthritis → IgM class, Directed against Fc Fragment of IgG[Q]
- **Bone Formation Marker vs Bone resorption Marker:**

Bone Formation Marker	Bone resorption Marker
Tetracycline Osteocalcin Alizarin Von Korsa, ALP Procollagen	TRAP Deoxyphyridino lene (PYD) cross linked N-Telepeptide

- Markers for rate of newly synthesized osteoid mineralization if → Tetracycline[Q]
- Lipofuschin:

• Also called lipochromic / wear or tear / aging pigment
• Tells about free radical injury / oxidative stress

- Tumor suppressor gene p53 induce cell cycle arrest at late G1/G1-S phase *(AIIMS 05)*

• Myeloperoxidase is Not a mediation of Inflammation *(AIPG 12, AIIMS 05)*
• IL-1, MMP, TNF, Prostaglandin are mediators of inflammation.

- P53 is called guardian of genome *(AIIMS 05)*
- Most of the cells like macrophages, NK cells, complements are part of innate immunity. T-cells and B-cells are part of acquired immunity[Q]
- Oncogene → Inhibits apoptosis → Cancer develops
- Tumor suppressor gene:

Promote Apoptosis → Prevent cancer development
Ex- p53 RB → Retinoblastoma WT-1→Wilm's tumor BRCA → Breast Cancer

- Staining:

DNA and RNA → Acridine orange
DNA → Best method fuelgen
RNA → Methyl green

- Neointimal hyperplasia in vascular graft failure:

Vascular injury
↓
Smooth muscle cell activated and proliferate [Q]
↓
Migrate into internal layer
↓
Sets activation response
↓
Vascular injury (Occlussive neointimal disease)

- APC (Antigen presenting cell):

• Most common APC → Immature dendritic cell
• Most potent stimulator of native T. cell → Mature dendritic cell
• APCs are – Dendritic cells, Langerhan's cells, B-cell, NOT T-cell

• HLA – chromosome 6 (short arm)
• BRCA – 1 – Chromosome 17 (Breast cancer)
• Folate carrier protein – Chr. 21

- PAP smear:

• Based on neoplastic cells are Non-cohesive.
• It's a type of exfoliative cytology (Used for mass screening of cervical CA)

LAST 5-YEAR QUESTIONS FROM THIS TOPIC

1. **Which of the following statements is not true regarding its association with increased aging?** *(AIIMS May 11)*
   a. Damage of the tissues due to free radical injury
   b. Increased superoxide dismutase
   c. Increased accumulation of the free radicals.
   d. Increased cross-linkages in collagen

Ans. b (Ref: Robbins 7/e p42-44)

2. **Best marker for dyslipidemia:** *(AIIMS)*

Ans. APO-1 level

3. **Hyponatraemia with increased Na+ concentration in the body is seen with:** *(AIIMS Nov.10)*

Ans. Nephrotic syndrome (Ref: Fauci, Harrison Manual of medicine p4-6)
Note: Other answers can be CCF, liver cirrhosis

4. **Which of the following is categorized in the list of obligate carriers having disease with recessive trait?** *(AIIMS Nov.10)*

Ans. Phenotypically normal woman with affected brother and son but normal daughter

5. **Fading of nuclear chromatin of a necrotic cell is called:** *(AIIMS May 10, AIPG 07)*

Ans. Karyolysis (Ref. Robbins 7/e p21-22)

6. **When malignant cells resemble more primitive undifferentiated cells than those from which they arose, they are said to be:** *(AIIMS May 10)*

Ans. Anaplastic (Ref: Robbins 7/e p272-273)

7. **Cells that secrete maximum amount of antibodies are:** *(AIIMS May 10)*

Ans. Plasma cells (Ref: Robbins 7/e p81-82)

8. **Which hormone has greatest effect on granulation tissue in wound healing?** *(AIIMS May 10, AIPG 07)*

Ans. Cortisol (Ref: Robbins 7/e p114, 207)

9. **A mother donated her kidney to her daughter what type of graft is it?** *(AIPG 11)*

Ans. Allograft (Ref: Lindhe 4/e p662)

10. **Down syndrome is characterized by translocation of:** *(AIPG 11)*

Ans: 46 xy, t (14, 21)

11. **Acute infection causes:** *(AIPG 11, 09)*

Ans. Leukocytosis (Ref: Robbin;s 7/e p664)

12. **Excisional biopsy is done by:** *(AIPG 11)*

Ans. Removal of entire lesion with a margin of uninvolved normal border tissue

13. **Fibrin degradation products help in detection of:** *(AIPG 11, 10)*

Ans. DIC

14. **Which of the following tests is not used for detection for species aneuploidy?** *(AIPG 11)*
   a. Fish
   b. QF–PCR
   c. Microarray
   d. RT–PCR

Ans. c (Ref. Harrison's 17/e p406)

15. **Defect in DNA repair mechanism is associated with:** *(AIPG 11)*

Ans. Xeroderma pigmentosum (Ref: Medical genetics by Jorde–Carry 3/e p39)

16. **ORF stands for:** *(AIPG 10)*

Ans. Open reading frame (Ref:Biomacromolecules: introduction to structure, function and informatics by stan Tsai, 2007, p563)

17. Which of the following disorder involves a defect in primary hemostasis: *(AIPG 10)*
Ans. Platelet disorder (Ref: Robbin's and Cotran 7/e p124, 125, 653)
18. Sequence of cellular events in a ischemic brain infract is all except: *(AIPG 12)*
a. Intense neuronal eosinophilia
b. Influx of PMNs
c. Proliferation of astrocytes
d. Ingress of macrophages and apoptosis
Ans. d
19. Components of innate immunity that are active against viral cells includes: *(AIPG 10, 09)*
Ans. NK cells (Ref: Robbin's and Cotran 7/e p198-201)
20. Prostate specific antigen is: *(AIPG 10)*
Ans. Tumor marker (Ref: Robbin's 7/e p339)
21. Earliest transient change following tissue injury will be: *(AIPG 09, 08)*
Ans. Neutrophilia (Ref: Robbins 7/e p56)
22. Differential leucocyte count is used for diagnosis of: *(AIPG 09)*
Ans. Eosinophilia *(NBD Q)*
23. An infant with cleft lip, cleft palate, polydactyly, microcephaly with holoprocephaly and ectodermal scalp defects is suffering from: *(AIPG 09)*
Ans. Trisomy 13 (Ref: Syndromes rapid recognition and perioperative implications by bissonette B Ist 800-802)
24. CAT eye syndrome is: *(AIPG 09)*
Ans. Partial trisomy 22 (Ref: Dorland 28/e p1626)
25. Which of the following does not present antigens:
a. NK cells
b. Dendritic cells
c. Langerhans cells
d. Macrophages
Ans. a (Ref: Robbins 8/e p113)
26. Xeroderma pigmentosum is characterized by: *(COMEDK 12)*
Ans. Inability to repair sunlight induced damage to DNA
27. Anti-D (Rh) immunoglobulin is used for the prevention of: *(COMEDK 12)*
Ans. Haemolytic disease of newborn
28. Non-Caseating granulomas are characteristic of:
Ans. Sarcoidosis
29. The predominant cell in an established lesion is:
Ans. Plasma cell *(COMEDK 12)*
30. HLA-B27 is seen in: *(COMEDK 12)*
Ans. Ankylosing spondilitis
31. The activation of caspases is likely to lead to:
Ans. Apoptotic cell death *(COMEDK 12)*
32. The dominant histologic feature infarction is: *(KCET 09)*
Ans. Coagulative necrosis
33. Mutation of oxidative enzymes (Peroxisomes) could lead to: *(COMEDK 12)*
Ans. Zellweger's syndrome
34. Examples of preventive antioxidant is: *(COMEDK 12)*
Ans. Catalase
35. In the body, metabolism of 10g of protein would produce approximately: *(COMEDK 12)*
Ans. 41 Kcal

36. Coating of bacteria particles with host proteins to facilitate phagocytosis is known: *(COMEDK 12, 08)*
Ans. Opsonization

37. Free radicals can be inactivated by following enzymes excepts: *(KCET 09)*
a. Glutathione peroxidase
b. Catalase
c. Superoxide dismutase
d. Myeloperoxidase
Ans. d (Ref: Harper's biochemistry 26/e p622)

38. The necrotic tissue and deposits of immune complexes complement and plasma protein produce a smudgy eosinophilic deposit is termed as: *(KCET 10)*
Ans. Fibrinoid necrosis

39. The major enzyme responsible for oxidative killing mechanism in neutrophil is: *(KCET 10)*
Ans. Hypochlorous acid

40. Which of the following cytokines cause bone resorption: *(KCET 10)*
Ans. IL-1

41. In Troisier's sign the lymph node involved is: *(COMEDK 11)*
Ans. Left supraclavicular nodes (Ref: General and systematic pathology by James cressee 5/e p974)
Note: troisier's sign seen in Gastric adeno-Carcinoma. Associated with virchow's node

42. Carcinoembryonic antigen (CEA) is associated with: *(KCET 11)*
Ans. Carcinoma of colon (Ref: Robbins 7/e p208, 585)
Note: also associated with Ca. of pancreas, lung, stomach, Heart

43. TIGERED effect of heart is seen in: *(KCET)*
Ans. Fatty change (Ref: Robbins 7/e p208, 585)

44. Somatic mutation of PTEN is seen in: *(KCET 11)*
Ans. Endometrial carcinoma (Ref: Robbins 7/e p693)

45. Which of the following is not a constituent of Virchow's triad? *(KCET 11)*
a. Damage to endothelium due to injury / inflammation
b. Diminished rate of blood flow
c. Increased coagulability of blood
d. Increased venous blood pressure
Ans. d (Ref: Robbins 7/e p90)

46. IL-1 and TNF are secreted by: *(PGI Dec. 11, Dec. 10, 09)*
Ans. Activated macrophages (Ref: Robbins 7/e p63)

47. Receptors for which of the following are present on Osteoclasts / Osteoblast and plays an important role in bone remodeling? *(PGI June 11)*
Ans. PTH (Ref: white and pharaoh 6/e p454-456)

48. Icterus is checked in sclera because? *(PGI June 11)*
Ans. has higher content of elastin (Ref: Harrison 17/e p261)

49. Hypokalaemia is not present in: *(PGI June 10)*
a. Vomiting
b. Diarrhea
c. Patient on diuretics
d. Chronic renal failure
Ans. d (Ref: Davidson 20/e p483)

50. Endotoxins are by nature: *(PGI 09)*
Ans. Lipopoly saccharides (Ref: Carranza 10/e p317)

51. Immunity present in a group of individuals in a community is: *(PGI June-12)*

Ans. Herd Immunity

52. In humans preterm birth refers to birth of a baby of less than: *(PGI June 12)*

Ans. 37 weeks gestational age

53. A patient with male androgenic characters and a genetic make up with 2x and more than I Y chromosome would have: *(AIPG 12)*

Ans. Klinefelter syndrome

54. Apoptosis is: *(AIPG 12)*

Ans. Programmed cell death

55. Which of the following is Not a mediator of inflammation: *(AIPG 12)*

a. TNF
b. Interferon
c. Prostaglandin
d. Myeloperoxidase

Ans. d (Ref: Immunopathology, Immunology and immunity by sell, max. 2001 p78)

SYSTEMIC PATHOLOGY

- Endocarditis:

• Most friable vegetation is present in IE (Infection endocarditis). so, highest risk of embolisaton
• Libman sacks endocarditis seen in SLE

- Carcinoid Heart disease:

• Fibrous thickening of right ventricle, Tricuspid value, pulmonary valve
• It's a paraneoplastic syndrome

- **Transmural infarct (All layers of ventricular wall) vs Subendocardial infarct:**

Transmural infarct	Subendocardial infarct
• Due to coronary artery atherosclerosis with super imposed thrombosis of a coronary artery	• Usually multifocal as it most often results from reduction in perfusion
• Usually associated with single coronary so unifocal	• Usually don't cause Ventricular Aneurysm[Q]
• Cause ventricular Aneurysm	

- Berry's Aneurysm / Saccular Aneurysm / Brain Aneurysm → Rupture is common
- Infarcts → Not commonly seen in lung and liver due to dual blood supply
- Appearance of Infract:

• Red/ Hemorrhagic → Lung, intestine
• Both Red + White → Brain

- % age of emboli progressing to MI = 5-15%[Q]
- Benign HTN vs Malignant HTN

Benign HTN	Malignant HTN
• Microscopic finding	Necrotizing/Fibrinoid arteriosclerosis
• Hyaline Arteriosclerosis	

- In PNH:

Associated with deficiency of GPI anchored protein including DAF and MIRL on hematopoietic cells.

- Nephrotic syndrome:

• Loss of Antithrombin III and Protein C and S → hypercoagulable state.
• Loss of Transferrin → Microcytic Hyprochromic anemia.
• Loss of Thyroxin binding globulin → Hypothyroidism

- Renal system:

• Nephrin – A mutation in Nephrine gene → Heriditary form of Congerital nephritic syndrome (Finnish type)[Q]
• Podocin – Mutation in podocine gene (NPHS2) Leads to focal segmental glomerulonephritis[Q]

- MC paraneoplastic Syndrome in RCC – Polycythemia, Hypercalcemia, HTN
- RCC (Renal cell carcinoma), Hodgkin's Lymphoma
- Liver and kidney:

NB: Amyloidosis of kidney is most common in patients on long term hemodialysis for renal failure develop Amyloidosis due to deposition of B2- Micro globulin[Q]
• B-pleated structure of Amyloidosis seen on X-ray crystallography *(AIPG 07)*

- Plasmacytoid lymphoma associated with IgM:

• B cell lymphoma
• Old individual

- Vasculitis:

• Large vessel vasculitis Ex-Giant cell Arteritis • Takaysu Arteritis
• Medium vessel vasculitis PAN (Poly arteritis nodose, Kawasski disease, Buerger's disease)
• Small vessel vasculitis- Wegner's vasculitis

- Giant cell Arteritis is also called temporal Arteritis:
- Systemic vasculitis:

Granulomas	Necrotizing
Giant cell Arteritis	PAN[Q]
Takaysu	Churg straurs syndrome
Wegner's	Microscopic polyangitis

- Granulomatos Vs Non Granulomatous or Necrotizing Vasculitis:

Granulomatos Vasculitis	Non Granulomatous Vasculitis
• Ex–Gaint cell vasculitis	Ex–PAN
• Wegner's	
• Takaysu	
• Churg Straus	

- Hodgkins lymphoma:

EBV is associated with mixed cellularity and lymphocytic depleted Hodgkin's lymphoma
Types
• Nodular Sclerosing → lacunar cells

• Mixed Sclerosing → Classical RS cells (Reid Steinberg cells)
• Lymphocytic Depleted → Reticular variant of RS
• Lymphocytic predominant → Popcorn cells

- Leukemia:

AML: Subtypes
• M3 → PML (Promelocytic Leukemia) → DIC is associated[Q]
• M4, M5 → Gum hypertrophy
• M4 is called Acute Monocytic Leukemia *(AIIMS 2011)*
• Non Specific esterase is Not a feature of M0, M1, M2, M6[Q] of AML
• ALL → L36 subtypes are termed as tumors of Mature B cells
• Ex- Burkett lymphoma

- Acute leukemia:

• Increased frequency seen in – Down syndrome, Bloom Syndrome, Kleinefilter, Wiskott Aldrich

- ANCA (Anti neutrophil cytoplasmic antibody):

C– ANCA	P-ANCA
• Cytoplasmic protenase 3 is the target antigen[Q] *(AIPG-07)*	• Perinuclear myeloperoxidase[Q] is the major target antigen.
Ex- Wegner's Granulomatosis[Q]	• Ex-PAN
	• Churg Straurs syndrome
	• Good Pasteur's syndrome

- Amyloidosis:

The most important amyloid proteins and their clinical scenarios include:
1. AL (Amyloid light chain) → This is derived from plasma cell and contains immunoglobulin light chain
• Associated c 1° Amyloidosis
• Multiple myeloma[Q]
• Heart and Skeletal muscles
2. AA (Amyloid associated protein) → Synthesized from Reticuloendothelial cells of liver associated with 2° Amyloidosis.

- Diagnosis of Amyloidosis:[Q]

• Rectal biopsy / Gingival – 80%
• Abdominal FAT aspirate – 70-80%
• Bone marrow biopsy – 50%

- Appearance of Amyloid:

• On congo Red → Yellow green bifringes
• On EM → Non Branching fibrils of indefinite length[Q]
• On X-ray crystallography → B-sheet conformation[Q]

- Chronic Inflammatory conditions:

• TB (COMEDK 10, 12) – Osteomyelitis
• Bronchietasis

- Connective tissue disorders:

• RA (Most common),
• Ankylosing Spondylitis
• 1° Billiary cirrhosis

- Multiple myeloma Vs plasmacytoma: (BOTH are Associated Plasma cell)

Multiple myeloma	Plasmacytoma
• Older	Younger Variant of Multiple myeloma
• Plasmacytoid lymphoma	
• B-Cell neoplasia	
• Associated with IgM	

- Different bodies associated with disease:

• Ferruginous bodies – Asbestosis
• Russel's bodies – Multiple myeloma
• Psammoma bodies – Papillary CA of thyroid
• Negri bodies – Rabies
• Paschan and Gunari bodies – Small pox
• Pick's Bodies– Picks disease
• Civette bodies – Rheumatic carditis
• Cowdry type A – Herpes virus yellow fever (virus)
• Cowdry Type B – Adenovirus (Basophilic)
• Both nuclear and cytoplasmic inclusions can be seen in measles.

- Proteins defective in Hereditary spherocytosis:

Ankyrin > Protein 3 (Anion transport protein) > Spectrin > Palladin[Q]

- Risk factors for gastric Carcinoma:

• Loss of gastric acidity – Atropic gastritis, Partial gastrectomy (Peptic ulcer surgery), Pernicious anemia
• Infection with H pylori
• Intestinal Metaplasia → Most significant risk factor[Q]
• Gastric ulcer and Polyps (No association has been found between duodenal ulcer and gastric ulcer)
• Blood group A
• Long term ingestion of high concentration of nitrate in dried smoke and salted foods.
NB: Pernicious anemia associated Gastric CA is seen in Fundus[Q] Part of stoma.

- DNA repair defects: (Genomic instability)

Mismatch repair	Nucleotide excision repair	Recombination repair AR disorder
• Heriditary colon Cancer Syndrome	• Xeroderma pigmentosum	• Ataxia Telangectasia
• Bloom's syndrome		

- NARP:

• Neurogenic Weakness
• Ataxia
• Retinopathy
• Pigmentation (Mitochondrial disease)

- Neutrophil disorder:

• Neutrophil Agranulocytosis → Aggressive periodontitis
• Chediak Higashi syndrome → sed neutrophil chemotaxis and secretion. Neutrophil fuse to form MEGA bodies. Chr. I defective[Q] AR[Q] Mutation seen in LYST gene line. Aggressive periodontitis + oral ulceration. Lysosomes are unable to fuse with phagosomes to form phagolysosomes[Q]
• Papillon Lefever syndrome – Myeloperoxidase deficiency. Defective chemotaxis and Phagocytosis[Q] Chromosome 11 defective. Aggressive periodontitis
• LAD 1 → Chr. 21 mutation → CD 18/ integrin 32 defect
• LAD 2 → Chr. 11 mutation → CD 15 defective

- Organs affected commonly in GVHD (graft versus host disease) → Skin, liver GIT[Q] Infection with CMV is very common
- Chronic Granulomation disorder:

• Is a disorder of phagocytes.
• Lack fully functional NADPH Oxidase[Q]
• Nitro blue tetrazoline Test → Test for phagocytosis[Q]

- LE body/ Haematoxyline body → Feature of SLE
- Retinoblastoma: (RB)

• Is a tumor associated with loss of heterozygosity (means both allele becomes mutant)
• No normal tumor suppressor gene.
• Almost certainly results in tumor genesis Ex-Familial RB

- CNS involvement in AIDs:

• Very common after lymphoid
H/P
• Perivascular infiltration of giant cell.
• Microglial nodule
• No inclusion bodies seen[Q]
• Vacuolar degeneration
Vasculitis is characteristically absent in CNS involvement of AIDS

- Councilman's bodies:

Acute viral hepatitis

- Pancytopenia with cellular BM:

PNH
Megaloblastic anemia
Mylodysplastic syndrome

- Heavy metals and sites of renal damage:

• Hg → PCT damage
• Pb → Entire tubule

- Cerebral malaria:

• Duck's Gramuloma – Pathognomic
• H/P: Kuffer cell hyperplasia

- BNP and ANP:

• Both degraded by neutral endopeptidase
• BNP → Reduces preload on heart → Nesiritide

- Carcinogens and associated cancer:

• Aromatic amines (Aniline dyes) → Bladder cancer
• Androgen → Prostrate cancer
• Alkylating agent → AML
• H. pylori → Gastric cancer
• HIV → Non-Hodgkin's Lymphoma, Kaposi Sarcoma, SCC, HPV
• EBV → Burkeit lymphoma
• Arsenic → Lung cancer, skin
• Asbestos → Lung
• HTLV-1 → Leukemia / lymphoma
• Nitrogen mustard gas – lung, Head and Neck
• vinyl chloride → Liver cancer

- Acid phosphatase:

• Highest levels are found in monocytes (Macrophages)
• Nearly all of the acid phosphatase in normal individual comes from platelets and erythrocytes

- PTLD (Post transplant lymphoproliferataive disorder) are majority of B-cell origin and contain EBV
- GVHD → Associated with CMV
- **EBV vs HPV**

EBV	HPV
• Burkeit lymphoma, naso- Pharyngeal CA, OHL, Cervical cancer	• Squamous papilloma (HPV 6, 11) Cervical cancer (MC cause) Heck's disease (HPV 13, 32)

- Basophillia > 10% is characteristically seen in PS (Peripheral Smear) CML
- IL–1 → Leukocyte activating factor ↓ses bone resorption with TNF
- Lepra cells → Foamy macrophages
- Marker's of MI:

• CPK → Earliest
• SGOT → 2-3 days
• LDH → After 3 days (late marker)

- HOX gene – patterning of limb vertebra polysyndactyly
- SSh gene – Regulate organogenesis

- PSA (Prostrate Specific Antigen) → Tumor marker used in early diagnosis of CA of prostrate
- PATAU vs Edward syndrome

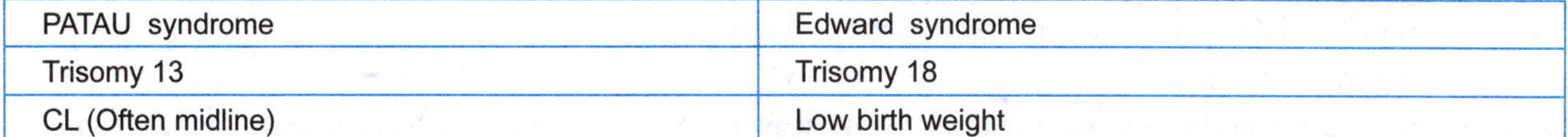

PATAU syndrome	Edward syndrome
Trisomy 13	Trisomy 18
CL (Often midline)	Low birth weight

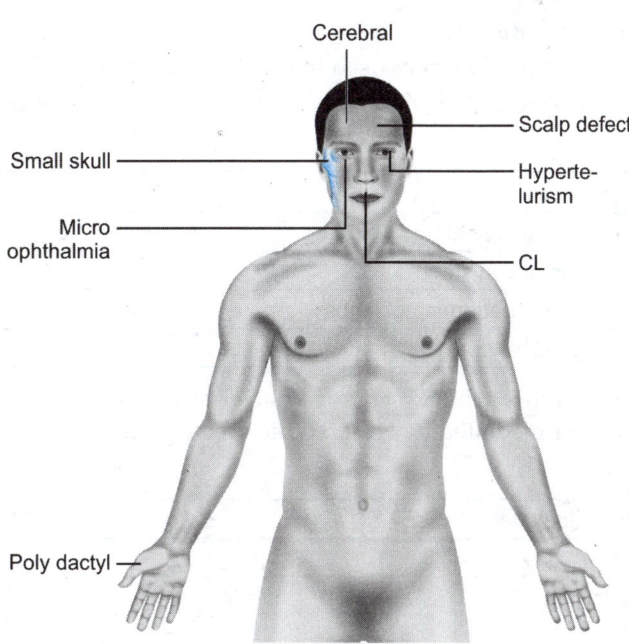

Fig. 13.1: Patau syndrome

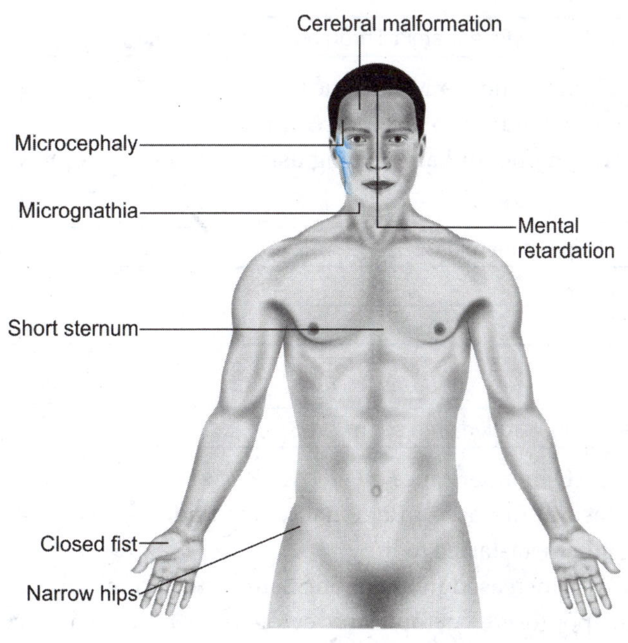

Fig. 13.2: Rocker bottom feet

- Silicosis: (Associated with TB)

• Most prevalent chronic occupational disease world wide
• Seen in sand blasting, quarrying, mining, stone cutting
• Quality most toxic
• Silicolic nodules in upper zone of lungs. Honey comb pattern+ egg shell calcification of lymph nodes seen

- PT is increased in warfarin therapy *(AIIMS 08)*
- Hard tick is the vector in lyme's disease *(AIIMS 08)*
- Myogenin → Immunohistochemical marker used in rhabdomyosarcoma *(AIIMS 08)*
- Addison's disease is associated with: *(AIIMS 08)* Hypoglycemia, Hypotension, Hyponatraemia, Hypercalcemia
- Genes and their functions:

• SRY gene determines sex	*(AIIMS 08)*
• MSX → regulates tooth development	
• Defective → tooth arrested in bud stage	
• HOX gene → associated with patterning of limbs	
• Shh → Regulates oncogenesis	

- NK cells have Toll like receptors which recognize bacterial products and stimulates immune response by transcription of nuclear factor mediated by NF-kB which recruits cytokines *(AIIMS 08)*
- Raynaud's phenomenon:

Rashes on Face + Fever + Joint pain → SLE[Q]	
X– thalassemia → Hb H	
Hb Bart → Have high affinity for O_2 ↓ Does Not release O_2 to fetal tissues	*(AIIMS 08)*

- Thalassemia is associated with: *(AIIMS 08)*

↑sed erythrocyte fragility
Haemolysis Hypochromic, Microcytic anaemia Thrombocytopenia

- Most common malignant bone tumor → Metastatic Ca
- Most common bone tumor in children → Osteosarcoma *(AIIMS 06)*
- G-banding is the routine technique for karyotyping using light microscopy *(AIIMS 06)*
- Papillary Ca thyroid:

Most common histological type of thyroid Ca	*(AIIMS 06)*
Psammoma bodies seen	
orphan eye cells seen[Q]	

- In osteomalacia:

↑sed osteoid mineralization/ maturation time seen	*(AIIMS 06)*

- Familial retinoblastoma is AD in inheritance *(AIIMS 05)*
- Most common site of metastatic disease → Regional lymph node → Liver is 2nd most common.
- Jaw tumors most commonly metastasize to lung
- Urinary excretion of VMA is increased in melanotic neuroectoclermal tumor of infancy *(AIPG 08)*
- Caspases are involved in apoptosis[Q] + cytoplasmic cytochrome c also plays same role

- Hypoproteinemia occurs in:

Liver cirrhosis, nephritic syndrome, chronic malnutrition

- In iron deficiency anemia TIBC ↑ses, ↓sed ferritin *(AIPG-07)*
- Casts:

• Hyaline cast → seen in fbrile illness after strenuous exercise
• RBC casts → Acute glomerulonephritis[Q]
• WBC casts → pyelonephritis, interstitial nephritis
• Red tubular cell casts → Acute tubular necrosis interstitial nephritis

- Extrahepaitc cholestasis shows:

↑sed Bilirubin in urine + Increased billirubin in Serum[Q]

- Clay colored stool+dark urine characteristic of obstructive Jaundice[Q]
- Immediate transient ↑sed permeability in Acute inflammation is caused by endothelial gaps by histamine *(AIPG-08)*
- Direct injury and Necrosis caused delayed increased permeability
- **Fanconi anemia:**

• There is mutation in DNA repair gene *(COMEDK 11)*
• Inherited form of aplastic anemia (AR)
• Increased risk of malignancy of AML, SCC of head and neck congenital anomaly of all system seen.

- TB shows caseation necrosis *(COMEDK -07, 08)*
- Saddle embolus blocks pulmonary arteries to cause sudden
- Phagocytes kill bacteria through both oxidative and non-oxidative mechanism *(COMEDK 08)*
- If liver disease is present for a minimum of 6 months then only chronic hepatitis is diagnosed *(COMED K -07)*
- Tongue is the most common site of tuberculous lesion in oral cavity *(COMEDK -06)*
- Left ventricular Sub Endocardial region is most prone to infarction *(COMEDK -06)*
- white infarcts occur in heart[Q]
- CVC lung shows heart failure cells[Q]
- SAGO spleen is the term used to describe the gross appearance of spleen in Amyloidosis
- Hg is toxic because it binds to sulfahydryl group
- Lepra cells in leprosy are vacuolated histocystis Virchow cells are compact globular masses / cigarettes in a pack are seen leprosy.
- Elie methnikoff discovered process of phagocytosis
- **Other names of lipofuscin:**

• Lipochrome
• wear and tear pigment
• Aging pigment

- Renal papillary necrosis is seen in sickle cell anemia.
- Nutmeg liver is seen in CVC liver
- "Chicken wire" appearance of enlarged bone marrow space is seen in B-thalassemia major[Q]
- Hepatomegaly → 3 causes → 3 C's

C → Cirrhosis
C → Carcinoma
C → Cardiac failure

- G-6PD deficiency:

  - Due to this deficiency → Failed to develop adequate level of Reduced Glutathione in their red cell, which protects RBC against oxidation
  ↓
  - Oxidation and precipitation of Hb within RBC forming "Heinz bodies"

LAST 5-YEAR QUESTIONS FROM THIS TOPIC

1. CVS complications of HIV infection includes all of the following, except: *(NEET 13, AIIMS May 11)*
   a. Pericardial effusion
   b. Cardiac tamponade
   c. Congestive cardiac failure
   d. Aortic aneurysm

Ans. d (Ref: Harrison 17/e p1172)

2. Which gene is responsible for hereditary Non-polyposis colon carcinoma? *(AIIMS May 11)*

Ans. MLHI (Ref: Fisher, Tumor suppressor Genes in Human cancer p219)
Note: APC gene is associated with Hereditary polyposis

3. A patient presents following parameters: pH = 7.5 PCO_2= 30 mm Hg, PO_2 = 102 mm Hg and HCO_3=16 meq/L which of the following correctly describes the compensatory mechanism? *(AIIMS Nov. 10)*

Ans. Metabolic acidosis (Ref: Longmore, etal oxford handbook of clinical medicine 5/e p684)

4. All of the following statements about S.aureus are true, except: *(AIIMS Nov. 10)*
   a. Most common, source of infection is cross infection from infected people
   b. About 30% of population is healthy nasal carriers.
   c. Epidermolysis and TSS toxins are superantigens
   d. Methicillin resistance is chromosomally mediated

Ans. a. (Ref: Harrison-17/e p873-9)

5. Which stage of P. vivax is infective to mosquito?

Ans. Gametocyte

6. About pseudomonas, all are true, except: *(AIIMS Nov.)*
   a. Strict aerobe
   b. Can grow
   c. Infection is mostly due to endogenous source
   d. Most common organism in burn patient

Ans. c (Ref: Ananthanarayan 7/e p315)

7. All are true about Widal test, except: *(AIIMS Nov. 10)*
   a. base line differs depending on the endemicity of disease.
   b. O antibodies last longer and hence are not an indicator of recent infection
   c. H antigen cannot differentiate between subtypes
   d. High titre value in a single widal test not confirmative.

Ans. b (Ref: Ananthanarayan 7/e p299)

8. Most common cause of pulmonary embolism is:

Ans. Thrombophlebitis (Ref: NBDE Dec. 1996 set, micropatho) *(AIIMS Nov.10, AIPG 09)*

9. CO has limited diffusion because: *(AIIMS Nov. 10, AIPG 12)*

Ans. It has high affinity for Haemoglobin (Ref: Rhoads,and Bell Medical physiology-Principles for Clinical medicine p350)

10. Infections mononucleosis is caused by: *(AIIMS Nov. 10)*

Ans. EBV (Safer 6/e p774)

11. A patient presents following parameters: pH = 7.45, PCO_2 = 30mm Hg and PO_2 = 102 mmHg. Which condition describes Pre compensated stage/mechanism? *(AIIMS Nov. 10, AIPG 12)*

Ans. Respiratory alkalosis

12. Which is true about Haemophillia A? *(AIIMS May 10, PGI)*

a. Increased BT
b. Increased PT
c. Increased PTT
d. Increased platelet count

Ans. Increased PTT (Ref: Harrisson 15/e p359)

13. Which of the following is the Ist sign that appeared in hemorrhagic shock? *(AIIMS May 10, 08)*

Ans. Tachycardia (Ref: Robbins 7/e p141)

Note: also O_2 want is the Ist sign

14. Cooley's Anemia is commonly known as: *(AIIMS Nov. 09, PGI)*

Ans. b. Thalassaemia major (Ref: The gale encyclopedia of genetic Disorders: A-L p156)

15. Dengu hemorrhagic fever is caused by: *(AIPG 11)*

Ans. Virus

16. Interferon act against virus during: *(AIPG 11)*

Ans. Protein synthesis phase

17. Bence Jones proteinuria may been seen in: *(AIPG 11, PGI Dec 09)*

Ans. U-heavy chain disease (Ref: Harrison 17/e p707)

18. Haemophilia A is due to defective gene for which one of the following factors? *(AIIMS May 09, AIPG 11)*

Ans. Factor VIII

19. Protein that precipitates on heating at 46°C and redissolves on boiling is: *(AIIMS May 09, AIPG 12)*

Ans. Bence Jones proteins

20. Fibrous dysplasia is associated with: *(AIIMS May 09)*

Ans. Ground glass density

21. After obtaining incisional biopsy a negative report in face of a clinically suspicious lesion means: *(AIPG 11)*

Ans. Second biopsy should be taken:

22. All of the following are STD except: *(AIPG 11)*

a. Herpes
b. Scabies
c. Candida
d. Leprosy

Ans. d

23. Most common malignancy seen in AIDs: *(AIPG 11, COMEDK 12)*

Ans. Kaposi sarcoma

24. Disorder characterized by craniosynostosis, craniofacial anomalies, symmetrical clinodactyly of hands and feet along with preaxial polysnydactylyly and variable soft tissue syndactyly is: *(AIPG 11, 07)*

Ans. Carpenter syndrome (Harrison's 17/e p466, 412)

25. All are secondary causes of polycythemia except: *(AIPG 11)*

a. High attitude
b. Hemangioblastoma
c. Myeloproliferative disorder
d. Pheochromocytoma

Ans. c (Robbins 7/e p649/696, 697)

26. Decreased BMR is seen in: *(AIPG 11)*

Ans. Obesity (Ref: Ganong 23/e p462)

27. Which of the following causes of orofacial pain is not associated with vascular origin: *(AIPG 11)*

a. Cluster headache
b. Giant cell Arteritis
c. Anesthesia dolorosa
d. Chronic paroxysmal hemicraria

Ans. c

28. Mutation seen in heterozygous sickle cell anemia provides protection against: *(AIPG 11)*

Ans. Malaria (Ref: Robbin's 8/e p387)

29. Hepatolenticular degeneration is seen in: *(AIPG 10)*

Ans. Copper poisoning (Ref: Davidson's medicine 20/e p975)

30. Pigmentation occurs in all of the following disease, except: *(AIPG 10)*

a. Addison disease
b. Cushing syndrome
c. Albright syndrome
d. Peutz jeghers syndrome

Ans. Cushing syndrome (Ref: Shafer's p972)

31. In Bacterial meningitis, CSF changes includes: *(AIPG 10)*

Ans. High protein (Robbins 7/e p1370)

32. Ist clinical Sign of Vit. A deficiency is: *(AIPG 10, KCET 08)*

Ans. Night blindness/Nyetalopia

33. Which is a T-cell derived tumor: *(AIPG 10)*

Ans. Mycosis fungoids

34. In a 70 kg adult, the fasting blood sugar level is 180 mg/ 100 ml, this is indicative of: *(AIPG 12)*

Ans. Hyperglycemia (Ref: Diagnosis and classification of diabetes mellitus: American Diabetes Association)

35. In a Lung with complete blockage of blood flow, which of the following would be seen: *(AIPG 12)*

Ans. Ventilation perfusion ratio approaches infinity

36. Infraction occurs due to: *(AIPG 12)*

Ans. Arterial occlusion (Ref: Pathology by Holliman / p17)

37. Edema in nephritic syndrome occurs due to: *(AIPG 12)*

Ans. Hypoalbunemia

38. Aschoff's nodules are seen in: *(AIPG 12)*

Ans. Rheumatic endocarditis

39. Reed Sternberg cells are seen in: *(AIPG 12)*

Ans. Hodgkin's disease

40. Wilm's tumor is a tumor of: *(AIPG 12)*

Ans. Kidney (Ref: Devita, Hellman and rosenderg's Cancer: Principles and practice of Oncology 8th ed. Vol. p. 2050)

41. Which of the following conditions predisposes to colonic carcinoma: *(AIPG 12)*

Ans. Ulcerative colitis (Ref: Gastro entistinal oncology by Abbruzzese, 2004, p22)

42. Biochemical change seen in wilson's disease is: *(AIPG 10)*

Ans. Urine copper increased + serum ceruloplasmin decreased

43. In HIV infection, which of the following cells are affected the most: *(AIPG 10)*

Ans. CD-4 (Ref: Robbins 7/e p248)

44. A malignant tumor arising from voluntary muscle is a: *(AIPG 09)*

Ans. Rhabdomyosarcoma

45. Bone lytic lesions along with increase in B-cells derived from hyperplastic bone marrow are seen in: *(AIPG 09)*

Ans. Multiple myeloma

46. Absolute increase in RBC count and haemoglobin with increase in blood volume is seen in: *(AIPG 09)*

Ans. Osler's disease (Ref: Shafers 4/e p731)

47. Disorder characterized by craniosynostosis polysyndactyly of feet, scalp defects and syndactyly of soft tissue is: *(AIPG 09)*

Ans. Carpenter syndrome

(Ref: Syndrome rapid recognition and perioperative implication by B issonetttet al 1/e p9)

48. 'Aur rods' are seen in: *(COMEDK 10)*

Ans. Myeloblast (Ref: Robbins 8/e p462)

Note: These are seen in case of AML

49. What is seen in acromegaly: *(AIPG 09)*

Ans. Large tongue (Ref: Neville 2/e p719)

50. Type I diabetes mellitus is associated with: *(COMEDK 10)*

Ans. Islet cell autoantibody (Ref: Robbins 8/e p777)

51. Hemorrhagic infract is invariably seen in: *(COMEDK 10)*

Ans. Lung (Ref. Robbins 8th ed., Pg-100)

52. Venous emboli are most often lodged in: *(COMEDK 09)*

Ans. Lungs (Ref: Harsh mohan 3/e p212)

53. Ghon complex of the lung usually: *(COMEDK 12)*

Ans. Undergoes calcification

54. Parathormone in normal parathyroid gland is secreted by: *(COMEDK 10)*

Ans. Chief cells (Ref: Robbins 8/e p772)

55. In lobar pneumonia, the presence of fibrino suppurative exudates with disintegration of red cells is seen in the stage of: *(COMEDK 10)*

Ans. Grey hepatization (Ref: Robbins 8/e p511)

56. Codman's triangle is one of the radiographic features observed in: *(COMEDK 11)*

Ans. Ewings sarcoma (Ref: Robbins 8/e p812, 816)

57. Hypoparathyraoidism is seen in all of the following except: *(COMEDK 12)*

a. Digeorge syndrome
b. Chronic renal failure
c. Wilsons disease
d. Haemochromatosis

Ans. b

58. The type of UV that is known to induce skin cancer is: *(COMEDK 12)*

Ans. UV-B

59. Hpokalemia is likely to be seen in: *(COMEDK 12)*

Ans. Insulin therapy

60. Otomycosis is caused by: *(COMEDK 12)*

Ans. Aspergillus niger

61. DiGeorg's Syndrome is due to: *(COMEDK 12)*

Ans. Congenital thymic aplasia

62. The type of AML associated with a high incidence of disseminated intravascular coagulation is: *(NEET 13, KCET 09)*

Ans. Acute promyelocytic leukemoid

63. Abnormal function of epithelial chloride channel protein is cause of: *(KCET 09)*

Ans. Cystic fibrosis (Ref: Robins pathology 6/e p477)

64. Abnormality in clotting of blood is seen in all of the following, except: *(AIPG 12)*

a. Patient taking ibuprofen
b. Thalassaemia
c. Christmas disease
d. Von willebrand disease

Ans. b

65. The most common site of origin for venous thrombi leading to pulmonary embolism to:

Ans. Deep leg veins *(KCET 09)*

66. Giant cell tumor of bone is otherwise called as: *(KCET 10)*

Ans. Osteoclastoma

Note: Epiphysis → Osteoclastoma *(NEET 13)*
Metaphysis → Osteomyelity, Osteosarioma *(COMEDK 13)*
Diaphysis → Ewings sarcoma

67. Collar stud abscess occurs is: *(KCET 10)*

Ans. Cervical TB lymphadenitis

68. Increased levels of Haemoglobin A2 is characteristic of: *(COMEDK 11)*

Ans. Thalassemia minor

69. Squamous metaplasia in the respiratory epithelium is induced by deficiency of: *(COMEDK 11)*

Ans. Vit. A (Ref: Robbins 5/e p48)

70. Malignant ulcer is differentiated from Benign by: *(COMEDK 11)*

Ans. Heaping up of margins (Ref: Robins 7/e p818)

71. Which of the following true of thyroglobulin: *(COMEDK)*

Ans. Elevation after complete therapy suggests recurrence in well differentiated thyroid malignancy: (Ref: Robbins 7/e p1182-1183)

72. Diamond Blackfan anemia is characterized by: *(PGI June 11)*

Ans. Erythroidaplasia (Ref: Diamond LK, Black fan KD (1938) "Hypoplastic anemia" Am.J. Dis. Child 56: 464-467

73. PTT is prolonged in case of: *(PGI June 10)*

Ans. Heaemophilia – A (Ref: Davidson 20/e p1063)

74. Which of the following is a feature of Iron deficiency anemia? *(PGI June 10)*

Ans. Decrease MCV (Ref: Harshmohan 3/e p446)

75. Type of carcinoma developed in Marjolin ulcer is: *(PGI 09)*

Ans. SSC (Ref: S.Das surgery 3/e p108)

76. Gas gangrene is most commonly caused by: *(PGI 09)*

Ans. Clostridium perfringens

77. General lack of bone marrow activity is seen in which type of anemia? *(PGI June 12)*

Ans. Aplastic anemia

CHAPTER

14

Microbiology

Topic

- General Microbiology
- Bacteriology
- Virology
- Parasitology and Miscellaneous

GENERAL MICROBIOLOGY

- Disinfectants:

– Phenol, HOCl, formaldehyde, Glutaraldehyde → All four are viricidal
– Sporicidal → Formaldehyde, Glutaraldehyde
– Organic compounds are not inactivated by organic matter so, only HOCl will be inactivated by organic matter.

- Prion → is most resistant to antiseptic. 2nd is spore
- 100% Alcohol is never used as disinfectant [Q]
- Glutaraldehyde:

2% called → Cidex		
Used for sterilizing endoscope as gentle on lens/cements of instrument.		
Critical items	Semi critical items	Non-critical items
Needs sterilization	High level disinfection	Intermediate/ low level disinfection
E.g. of High level disinfection	e.g. of intermediate level disinfectant	
Eg. 2% Glutaraldehyde 8% formaldehyde 1% Sodium hypochlorite Pasteurization [Q] Ethylene oxide gas	e.g. → Phenols Iodophores Quaternary Amnonium compounds 0.1% sodium hypochlorite	

- Dry heat damage:

– Denaturation, oxidative damage

- Moist heat damage:

– Denaturation of protein, coagulation
Vaccine sterilized by moist heat < 100°C

- Pasteurization:

Holder method → 63°C for 30 mins.
Flash method → 72°C for 15-20 sec.
Pasteurization kills all bacteria except thermoduric

- Indicators of sterilization:

Hot air → Clostridium tetani spores
Moist heat method → spore of Bacillus sterarothermophillus.
Riedel walker/phenol coefficient → Salmonell typhii bacilli

- Allograft → Sterilized by γ-radiation/e⁻ beam radiation
- Ig (Immunoglobulin) structure:

• Isotopic variation (class of antibodies) is due to variation in amino acid sequence in Heavy chain [Q] Not due to variation of both heavy and light chain.
• The Antigenic specificity of an Ig is associated. C variable region of Both heavy and light chain [Q]

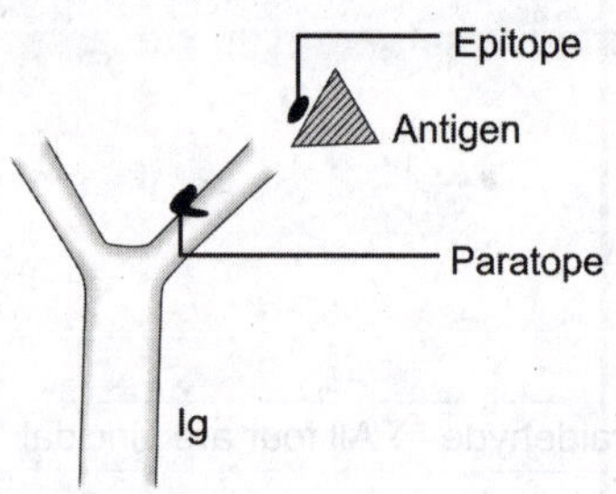

Fig. 14.1: Ig (Immunoglobulin) structure

- Haptens:

Is a partial Ag.
Unable to stimulate antibody production but induces hypersensitivity.

- Constant region heavy chain determines class of Ig.
- Hybridoma:

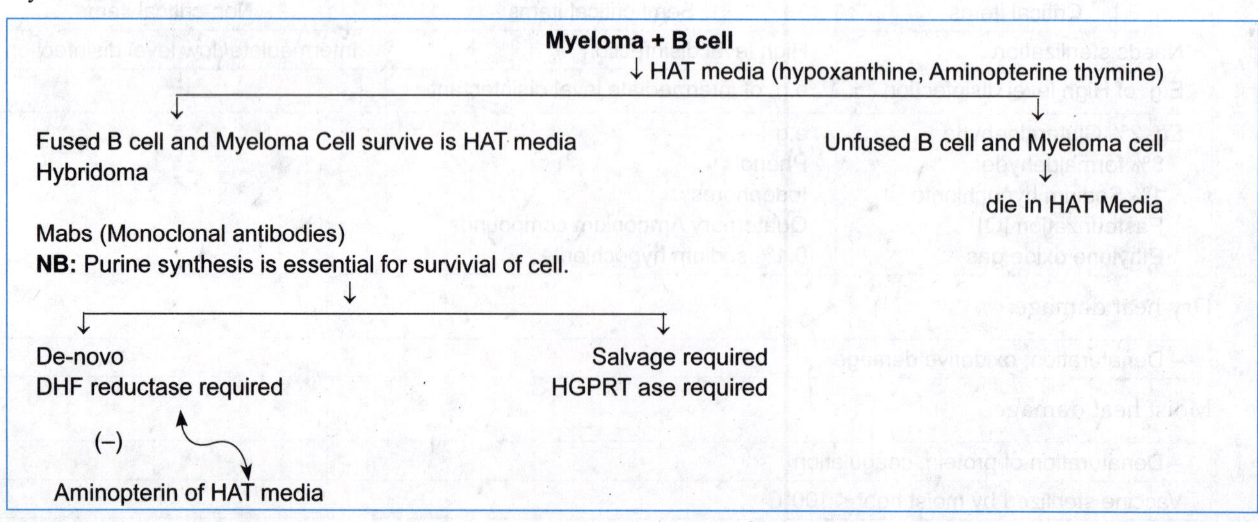

- IgG:

IgG1–65% > IgG2 (25%) IgG3 > IgG4 [Q]

- IgG:

Fc	Fab
Insoluble	(Antigenic binding site)
Complement binding site	Determines by Variable regions of Both heavy and light chain [Q]
On - CH2 domain	
Constant region of heavy chain determines Ig class (Isotypic variation of Ig)	

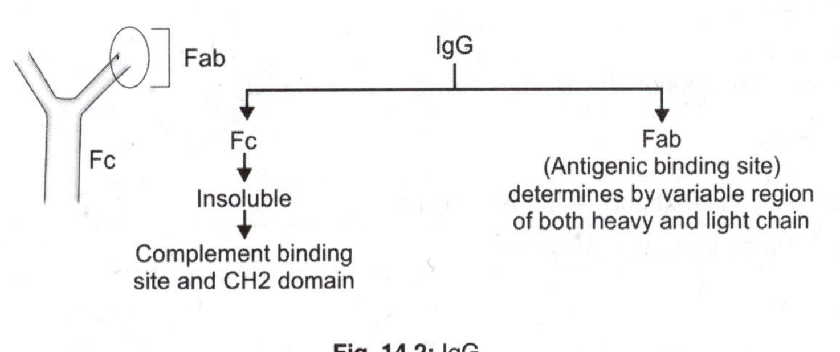

Fig. 14.2: IgG

- In 1° immune deficiency, γ-globulin is ↓ ced
- IgG shows maximum amount of immunoglobulin after 2° humoral immune response.
- IgA is used to prepare caries vaccine
- IgM → produced during 1° immune response
- IgE → Does not fix complement
- FTA – ABS is most specific for diagnosis of syphilis
- Negative phase is seen in active immunity [Q]
- Peptide binding site on MHC (for processed Ag)

MHC I → b/w distal domain of α– subunit [Q]
MHC II → b/w distal domain of α and β subunit

- NK cells and INF: Provide innate immunity which doesn't require any prior exposure to any antigen and Do not have any memory
- Interleukins:

IL-1 → LAF (Leukocyte activating factor) + Bone resorption promoter C TNF
IL-8 → Chemotactic cytokine

- Leukotriene e.g. → Lipoxins
- T-cell has infection of lymphokine production and delayed hypersensitivity.
- Culture media:

• **Simple medium/Basal medium:** There are basal medium, provides essential substance required for growth of micro-organism Ex- Nutrient broth [Q], Nutrient Agar [Q]

• Enriched medium: Blood, serum or egg are added to a basal medium Ex- Blood agar, chocolate agar [Q]
• **Selective medium (Solid media):** Particular substances are added to a solid media that inhibit or poison the growth of few organism. This facilitates the isolation of particular species from a mixed inoculum. Ex-L.J. Medium (for M. Tuberculae) [Q], Wilson and Blair media – S. Typhii [Q] Deoxycholate citrate media
• **Enrichment media:** Addition of selective substance to a liquid medium that have stimulating effect on the bacteria to be grown or an inhibitory effect on its competitors produces enrichment media. Ex- Selenite F broth → Salmonella, Shigella Tetrathionate broth → Typhoid – Parathyphoid bacilli
NB: Agar: Agar is a substance used to solidify culture media. It is not a culture media by itself Obtained from sea weeds. It has No nutritive value and is not affected by growth of bacteria [Q]

- 2 most important media:

BCYE (Buffer charcoal yeast extract) → For legioniella
TCBS (Thiosulfate citrate bile salt) → V. cholera

- Mode of Transmission:

Pasturella multocida → Animal bites and Scratches
Tetanus is transmitted by spores and dust (Not by droplet)
Listeria – Refrigerated food
Legionella – aerosol of A.C.
Leptospirosis – Rat urine (Direct man to man transmission Rare) • (Vetenary doctor, Slaughter house) • Ingestion, inhalation or direct contact contact c infected tissue • No person to person [Q]
A typical mycobacterium/Non TB mycobacterium – M. avium M. Kangassi → Environmental source No man to man
Anthrax – By contact with infected animal/product (usually occupational) → Vetenary doctor, farmer, clinical feature → painless ulcer chylamydia prittacosis → Bird Droping (Poultry)
Histoplasmosis → By inhalation of spores (No Man to man)

- Disease Transmitted by Vectors: Arthropods

• **Mosquito:** All 3 can cause filaria Anopheles → Malaria Culex → Japanese encephalitis, West nile fever, Bancrofitian filariasis. Aedes → Yellow fever, Dengu, Dengu hemorrhagic fever,Chickengunya fever, Rift valley fever
• Sand fly – Kala Azar Oriental store [Q]
• Tse-Tse fly – African sleeping sickness → by T. Gambieus
• Reduived bug – American sleeping sickness → causative organism is traypansoma cruzi.

• Louse born → Epidemic types (R. Prowazaki), Epidemic Relapsing fever (B. recurrentis), Trench fever *Trick:* Louse born is always associated with Epidemic
• Rat Flea → Bubonic plague, Endemic plague, Leptospirosis, Brucella. Endemic typhus (R. typhii)
• Ticks → Soft tick → Q fever, Relapsing fever [Q] Hard tick → Tick typhus, KFO, Tularamia NB.: Q-Fever→ has No human vector (Transmitted by aerosol in man) [Q]
• Thromboculid mite → Scrub typhus (Orientia Tsutsu gamushi)

- Nosocomial infection:

Ist most common – UTI (Urinary catherisation)
2nd Most common – Pneumonia
3rd Most common – elective surgery.

- Hospital acquired infections:

• M.C. hospital acquired pneumonea → caused by Psuedomonas
• M.C. nosocomial infection in ICU → Enterococci
• M.C. mode of transmission → by hands of hospital personnel.
• M.C. and mode serious causes of infection in Burns → Psuedomonas.

- Infection associated with i.v. catheter:

• Most common – Coagulase (–)ve staphylococcus. Amongst pseudomonas most common is P. aeruginosa

- Biosafety level:

I – Low risk (Lactobacilus, E. coli)	
II – Bacteria (all cocci+All bacilli except anthrax)	Virus Herpes, Influenza virus
III – Bacteria Anthrax Brucella Coxiella burnetti Mycobacterium	Virus
IV - Ebola, Lasa	

- Drug resistance:

• Can be transferred by both conjugation and Transduction. But conjugation → Most common and most important mode of transfer of Antibiotic transfer in bacteria [Q]
• May involve chromosomal or extra chromosomal (Plasmid) DNA transfer.
• Gene carrying resistance factor transferred only in presence of RTF (Resistance transfer factor)

- Test for mutagenesis done on mammalian cells → Styles tests [Q]
- If the test done on bacterial cell (S. typhimurium) → Ame's test
- Lepromin Test:

• Used to assess prognosis not treatment plan [Q]
• Used to assess immune station [Q]

LAST 5-YEAR QUESTIONS FROM THIS TOPIC

1. **Sunlight has sterilizing effect because:** *(AIPG 12)*

Ans. it has short wavelength

2. **Which of the following investigations should be done immediately to best confirm a non matched blood transfusion reaction?** *(AIIMS Nov. 10)*

Ans. Direct coombs test (Ref: Harrison 17/e p710)

3. **Which of the following is not a part of koch's postulate?** *(AIIMS Nov. 10, 08)*
   a. Bacteria may/may not cause disease in experimental animals.
   b. Bacteria should be isolated from the diseased animals
   c. Bacteria should be cultivable outside the animal
   d. Bacteria should be able to cause the same disease/condition when inoculated in another animal.

Ans. a (Ref: Ananthanarayan Textbook of microbiology 8/e p5)

4. **A rabbit is injected with horse serum. Two weeks later it is again injected with the same serum in the skin. The type of necrotizing skin reaction observed at the site of 2nd infection is:** *(AIIMS Nov. 10, 08)*

Ans. Arthus reaction (Ananthanarayan 8/e p166)

5. **Which of the following is not used as disinfectant?** *(AIIMS nov. 10, 09)*

Ans. 100% Alcohol (Ref: Ananthnarayan 7/e p30)

6. **Expression of receptor in malignant epithelial cells is mediated by:** *(AIIMS Nov. 10)*

Ans. Laminin

7. **Which of the following is true about endemic typhus?** *(AIIMS may 10)*
   a. man is the only reservoir of infection
   b. Flea is a victor of the disease
   c. a rash developing into an eschar is characteristic of the disease.
   d. Culture is the diagnostic modality

Ans. b (Ref: Ananthanarayan 7/e p415)

8. **phase contrast microscopy is based on:** *(AIIMS Nov. 09)*

Ans. Difference in refractive index

9. **NK cells are effective against viral infected cells only if the cell with infection:**

Ans. Unable to express MHC class I proteins (Ref: Robbins 8/e p186)

10. **Which of the following microbial cell is most resistant to antiseptics and disinfectants:** *(AIIMS Nov. 12)*

Ans. Prions (Ref: centre of disease control and prevention Guideline for disinfection and sterilization in health care facilities, 2008

11. **Vector for sleeping sickness is:** *(AIPG 10)*

Ans. Reduvid bug (only given is option. Like this actual answer should be Tse-Tse fly)

12. **The term epitope refers to:** *(COMEDK 09)*

Ans. Smallest antigen determinant

13. **Tissue graft rejection can be prevented by suppression of:** *(KCET 09)*

Ans. T-cell

14. **Immunoglobin class which crosses the placenta is:** COMEDK 09, 10)

Ans. IgG

15. **Cold sterilization refers to the process of sterilization by use of:** *(COMEDK 09)*

Ans. X-rays (Ref: ananthanarayan microbiology 7/e p30)

16. **Which one of the following does not present antigens?** *(COMEDK 10)*
   a. NK cells　　b. Dendritic cells
   c. Langerhan's cells　　d. Macrophages

Ans. a

17. Ability of a material to elicit an appropriate biological response in a given application in the body is called: *(KCET 10)*

Ans. Biocompatibility

18. Negative phase is seen in: *(KCET 10)*

Ans. Active immunity

19. out of the following hypersensitivity reactions, in which type a single dose of the antigen can act as both the sensitizing and shocking dose: *(KCET 11)*

Ans. Serum sickness (Ref: Ananthanarayan 7/e p165)

20. Most antigenic is: *(PGI Dec. 11, 10, June 07, 06)*

Ans. protein (Ref: Ananthanarayan 7/e p80, 81)

21. Which is the ideal method to sterilize snap-a-ray film holder? *(KCET 12)*

Ans. Autoclave

22. CD4 cells recognize the antigens in association with: *(KCET 12)*

Ans. MHC-II

23. The function of Langerhan's cells is: *(KCET 12)*

Ans. Antigen presentation to lymphocytes

24. Most cell secretion during an immediate hypersensitivity reaction is stimulated when antigens combine with: *(KCET 12)*

Ans. IgE antibodies

BACTERIOLOGY

- Psychrophilic → grow in temperature < 20°c
- Mesophilic → grow in temperature 25°C – 40°C [Q]
- Flagella types:

Flagella types
Peritrichous e.g. typhoid bacilli
Monotrichous Cholera vibrios
Lophotrichous Spirilla
Amphitrichous

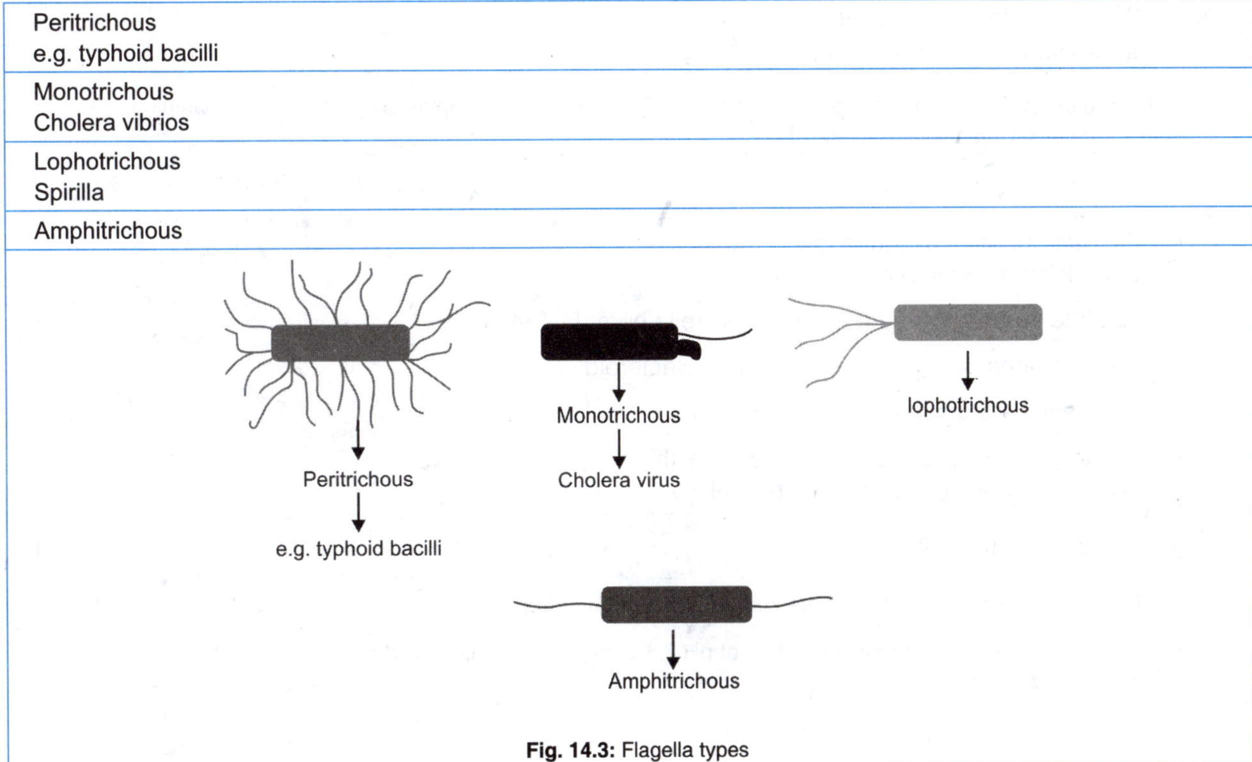

Fig. 14.3: Flagella types

- Virulence factor:

Polysaccharide capsule → Mostly in all bacteria including H. influenza.
Polypeptide capsule → Anthrax.

- Bacterial fimbriae → are antigenic, demonstrated by haemoglutination.
- Pilli are present only in Gram (–ve) bacteria except diphtheria
- Bacterial Toxin:

Exotoxin	Endotoxin
Gram +ve	Gram –ve
Protein in nature	LPS (PGI)
Highly Antigenic [Q] (PGI)	Low antigenicity
NB: Teichoic Acid Is present on the cell Wall of gram +ve Organism.	LPS has three regions Region I → Antigenic Specificity Region II → Activities (KCET) Region III → Responsible for endotoxic

- Mechanism of resistance in penicillin (very imp):

Production of lactamase	Altered PBP	Impaired penetration
M.C. in both G+ve and G(–)ve	Primarily in G+ve	Only in G–ve

- NB: PBP = Penicillin binding protein
- Pencillin resistant organisms: (IMP)

BCR + Enterococi + Logionella + most strains of N. Gonorrhoea + Mycoplasma (as has no cell wall) BCR = Brucells, Chlamydia, Ricketessia

- Oxygen Requirement of Bacteria:

• Microaerophillic – (Require low O_2 tension) Campylobacter, Borrelia burg, H. Pylori
• Obligate aerobes – Pseudomonas, Borrelia burg, H. Pylori
• Obligate anaerobes – Closteridium and Bacteroid
• Facultative anaerobes – E.coli, Klieshiella
• Capnopillic – Require. extra CO_2 for growth Ex- Brucella, Pneumococci, gonococci.

- Growth Requirement of Bacteria:

• All Medically important bacteria are Heterotrophs not autotrophs.
• Most medically important bacteria grow at pH 7.4 except lactobacilli – Acidic V. Cholerae – Alkaline

- Bacterial growth Curve:

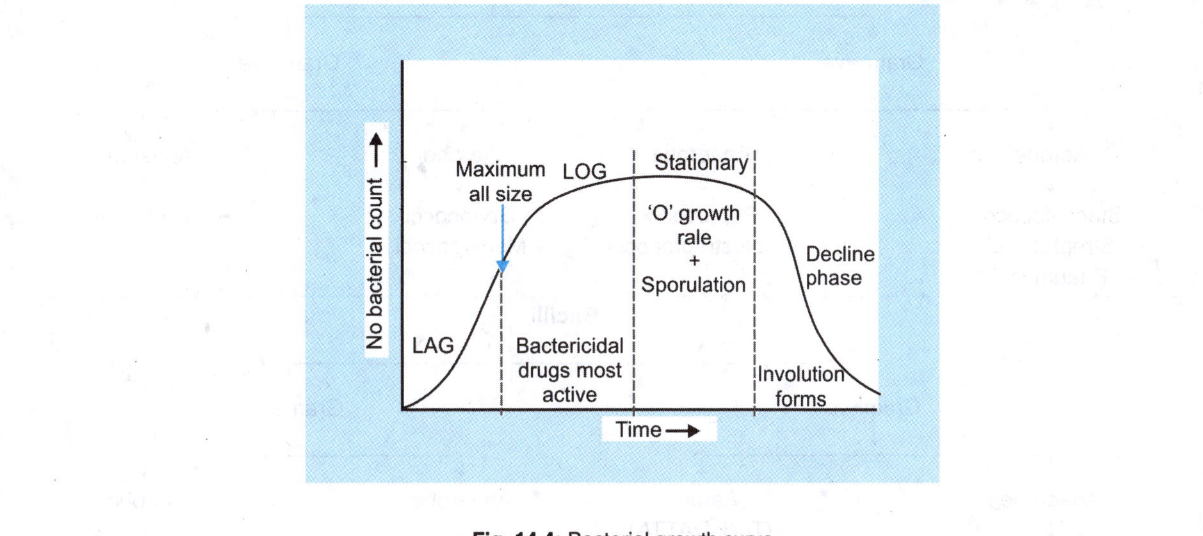

Fig. 14.4: Bacterial growth curve

- Staining:

• Albert stain – C. diptherae
• Zeil nelson stain – M. tuberculosis (KCET 09, 11), Nocardia, Leprae
• Mc Fayden Reaction – B. Anthracis (Meduse head appearance)
• Wayson stain/Giemsa stain – Y. pestis.
• Trichome methylene Blue – Anthrax
• Nagler Reaction – Clostridium perfringes (For toxin detection)
• For Rapid detection of TB– Auramine and Rhodamine
• Spirochetes and Bacterial flagella – Fontana's Staining
(Trichome methylene blue staining of Anthrax → MC Fayden Rn)

- GRAM staining:

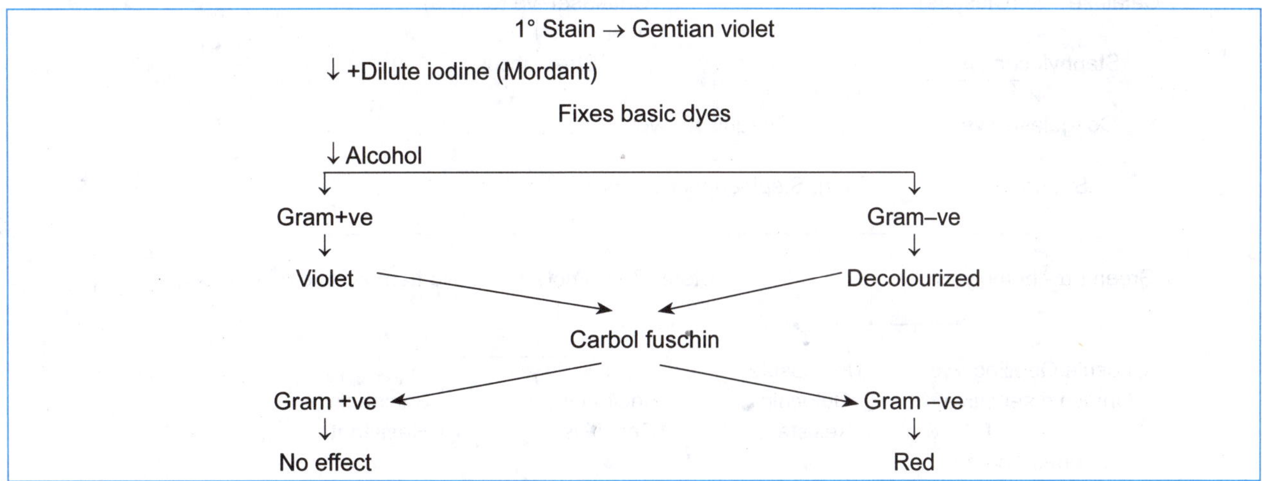

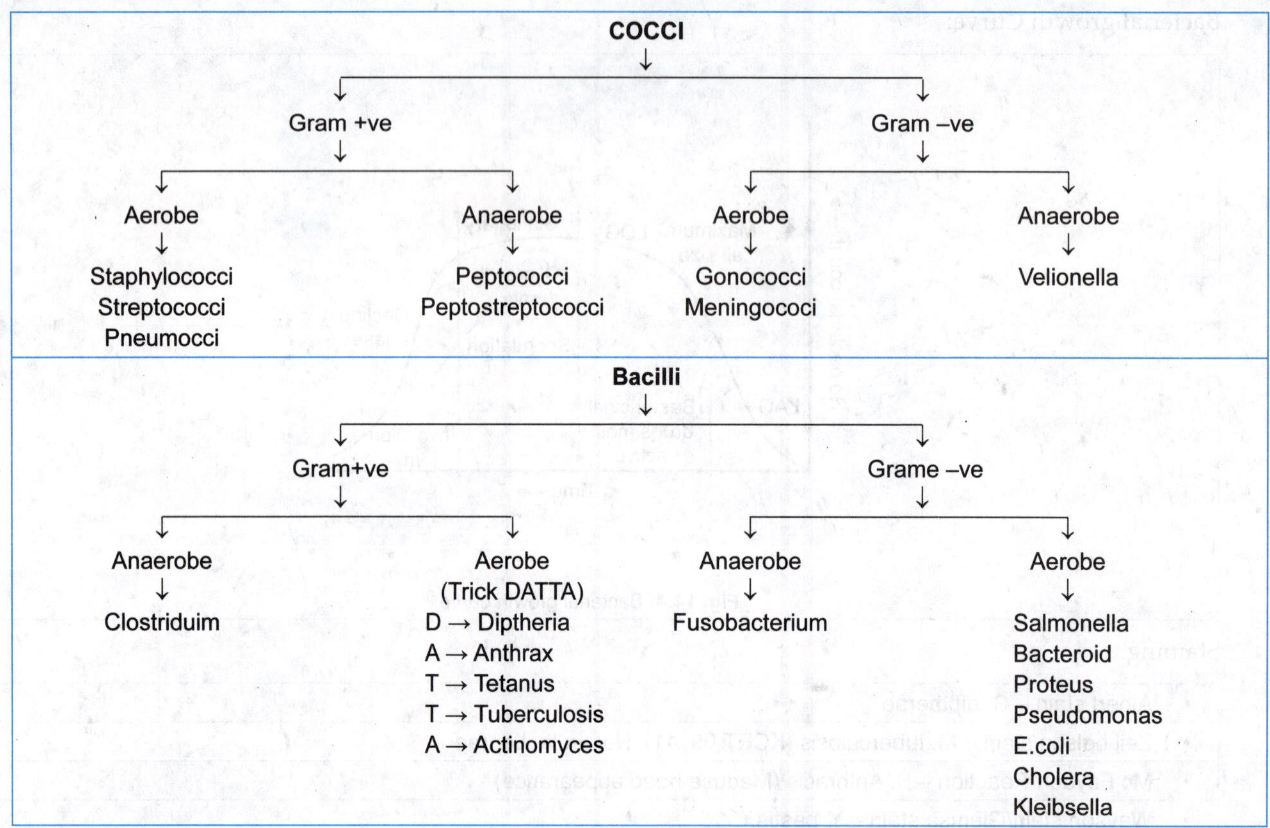

- Gram stain (V.imp):

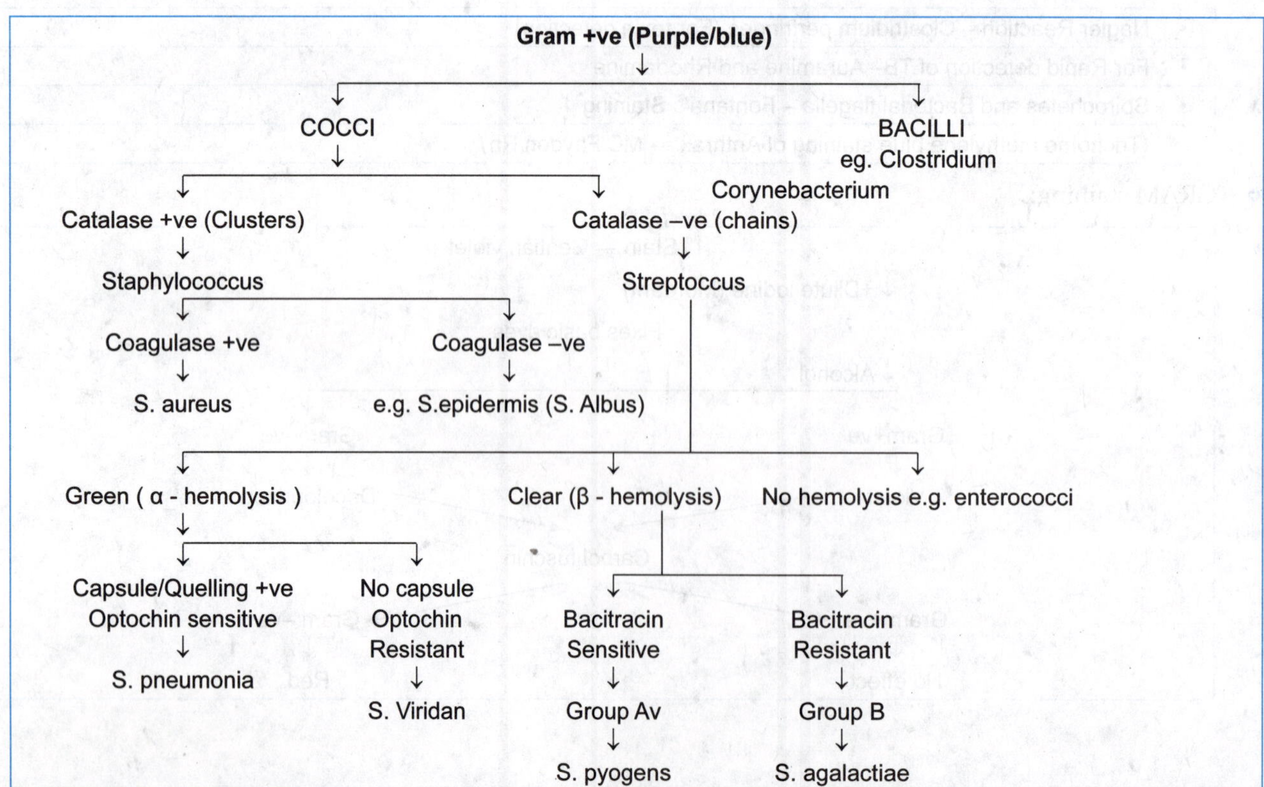

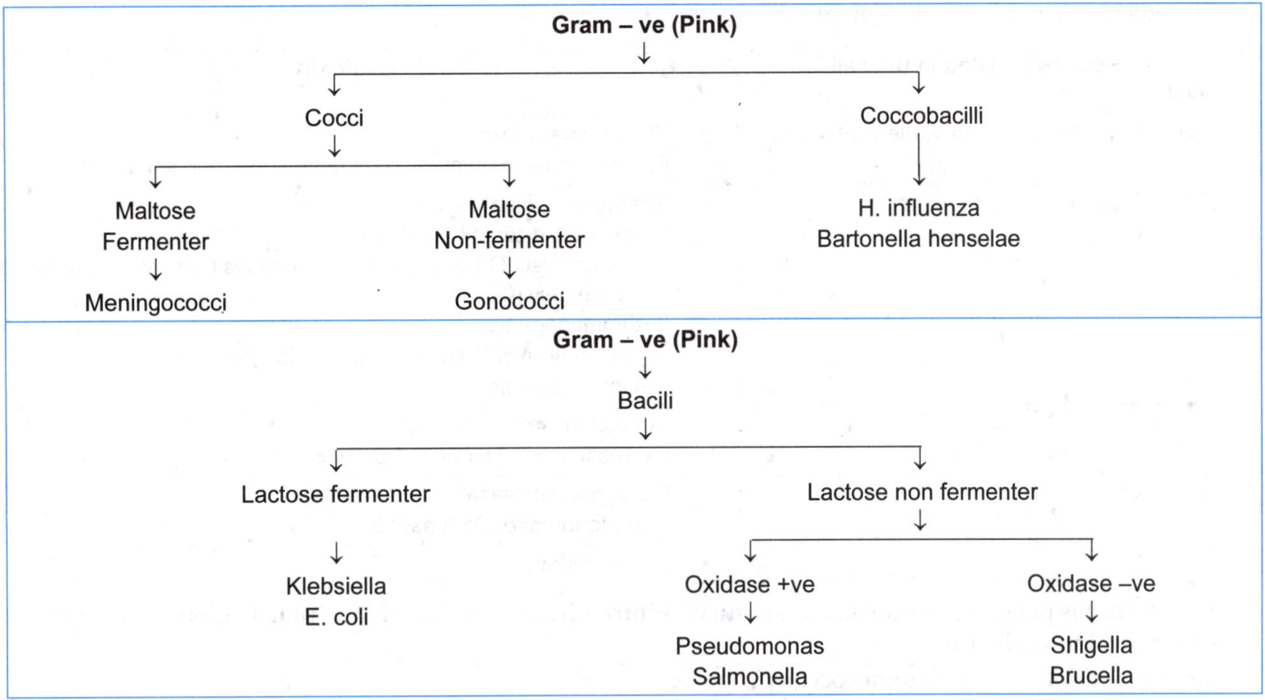

- Streptococcus: Hemolysis (Very Imp.)

α **Haemolysis**	β **Hemolysis**	**Gamma-haemolysis (No haemolysis)**
Optochin sensitive Bile Solubility ↓ Yes → S. phenumonae No → S.viridans	Bacitracin sensitive ↓ Yes → S. Pyogens No → CAMP test CAMP test Yes → S. Agalacitae CAMP test No → Other hemolytic streptococci	Grow on 6.5% Nacl ↓ Yes → Enterococci no → Other Gr D streptococci

Species	**Lancefield group → based on cardohydrate (Antigen) (AIIMS 08)**
S. Pyogens –	A [Q]
S. Agalacitae –	B
Enterococcus	C

- Staphylococcus:

2 toxins seen → TSST, Epidermolysin toxin (causing staphylococcus scaled skin syndrome)

- Streptococci:Virulence factor for streptococcus

Factors situated in the cell wall	Exotoxin
• "M protein" →Major virulence factor	• Pyrogenic exotoxin Bacteriophase mediated. They have super antigen activity.
• Capsule	• Streptolysin (Hemolysin) Produces 2 distinct hemolysin – Hemolysin O (Oxygen labile) – causes hemolysis in reduced state only [Q] • It is immunogenic. – Hemolysin S (Serum soluble) – Oxygen stable • Not immunogenic
	• Streptokinase or, Fibrolysin Expressed on all strains of S. Pyrogens
	• Deoxyribo nuclease (Streptodornase, DNA as) [Q]
	• Hyaluronidase

- Streptococcus pyogens → is not known to survive intracellularly. Neisseria, S. typhii, Legionella are well known to survive intra cellularly.
- Group A streptococci → Streptococcus pyogens:

• Acute Rheumatic fever and Acute GN are 2 imp. Non-suppurative sequel of S. pyogens infection.
• Skin → Erysipeals and Impetigo [Q]
• Scarlet fever (Pastia lines)

- TSS (Toxic shock syndrome) – is due to pyrogenic exotoxin type C and Extotoxin type E
- Common inhabitant of tonsil and throat → S. viridians (hemolytic)
- Selective medium commonly used for S. mutans is MSA (AIIMS Q)
- Most common organism causing:

SABE → S. Viridans [Q] (AIPG-11)
Bacterial endocarditis in healthy i.v. drug user affects tricuspid valve caused by S. valve bacterial
endocarditis in prosthetic heart valve patient → S. albus

- Viridans streptococci (e.g. mitis, salivarius, sangeus) ⊚ Produces greenish colony on blood agar *(AIPE 08)*
- Grp. A streptococci causes Erysipelas
- S. mutans can be distinguished from other streptococci by producing hemolysis on blood agar *(AIPG 08)*
- Staphylococcus saprophyticus: Normally non pathogenic may cause UTI in female
- Staph. Aureus:

Is associated with i.V drug user endocarditis [Q]
Tricuspid valve is most commonly involved [Q]
S. Aureus food poisoning after consumption of dairy products (2-6 hrs after consumption)
NB: Carbuncle → Staph aureus [Q]

- Cholera:

• Cholera enterotoxin has no effects on any other tissue except intestinal epithelium [Q]
• Human is the only reservoir

• All vibrios are halophillic except V. Cholerae [Q]	
• Sorbitol Mc conkey media is screening media for EHEC 0157:11 7 (E.Coli) [Q]	
• V. Cholerae 01 → Produces 01 LPS	
• 0139 (Chennai, Bengal) → Doesn't produce	
• Cholera Enterotoxin (+ Pertusis toxin):	
A subunit	**B Subunit**
Active subunit	(Binding subunit)
Acts by sing cAMP	Binds to GM1 ganglionic receptor of jejunum epitheliam Cell
ADP ribosylation of G-protein → Activate G-protein → Activate A denylate cyclase	
• In infections with V. Cholera → Rice water stool is seen	

- Salmonella:

Typhoid associated salmonella	Non typhoid asso. Salmonella
Humans are only reservoir	Humans are not only reservoir
	Multiple animal reservoir

- Babesiosis:

Presence of Maltese cross (Characteristic tetrad configuration in RBC)
Maltese cross – Also seen in C. neoformans

- Leptospirosis: Weil's syndrome → Ictero-Haemorrhagic fever

Diagnosis – Serology and Darkfield microscopy
Diagnostic medium – Korthoff medium
Antibody detected in 2nd week [Q]

- Brucella → Oxidase +ve gram - ve Bacilli_ similar as Pseudomonas.
- Pneumococci:

Flame shaped → Capsule → gives quelling reaction

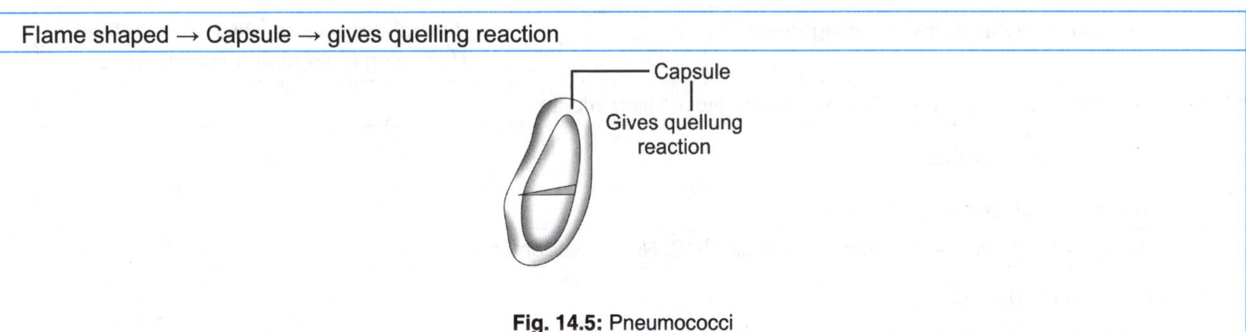

Fig. 14.5: Pneumococci

- Capsultaed – capsule can be demonstrated as clean walls in india ink [Q]

- Enterococci:

Are part of normal enteric flora.
Present in intestine, genital tract and saliva.
• M.C. cause of Nosocomial infection particularly in ICU [Q]
• The most common mode of transmission of enterococci is on the hands of hospital personnel [Q]

- Bacteroid Fragilis:

The LPS (Endotoxin) of B. Fragilis are less potent than other bacteria → This biological inactivity leads to lower frequency of DIC and purpose [Q] So LPS of B. fragilis is different from conventional endotoxin

- Mycobacterium:

– M. tuberculosis + M. Bovis → Equally pathogenic for man	
– M. Kansasi → Produces infections disease indistinguishable from TB [Q]	
Mycobacterium TB Complex ↓ – M. Tuberculosis - M. Bovis - M. Africanum	Non TB mycobacteria (atypical mycobacteria) – Environmental source of infection [Q] – No person to person infection ↓ – Ex– Mycobacterium Avium - Mycobacterium kansassi

- Plague (Yersenia pestis) Characterized by:

Axillary and Inguinal lymphadenopathy
Stalactite growth
Specific stain → Wayson stain
Bubonic plague → No person to person transmission
Pneumonic plague → person to person transmission

- Clostridium perfringes = Clostridium Welchi
- Clostridium perfringes:

Gas gangrene	Food poisoning
Toxin phospholipase (Most imp. Toxin, demonstrated by Nagler reaction)	– By ingestion of heat resistant spores.
Other toxin – Hyaluroridase, Collagenase	– Only those strains which causes food Poisoning have heat resistant spores
caused by – C. perfringes (80%) Septicum, Novi, Histolyticum	

- Psuedomembrane colitis:

Organism → Clostridium difficile
Antibodies associated – Tetracycline (AIIMs 2012, Nov.) Clindamycin

- Clostridium Difficile:

Causes Psuedomembrane colitis
Toxin → Type A → Enteropathic → Responsible for diarrhea
Type B → Cytopathic
H/P: Early lesion → type I summit lesion
Type II Glandular lesion → Diagnostic of Psuedomembrane colitis
Diagnosis – Demonstration of toxin in stool

- Anthrax:

• Cutaneus Anthrax is the most common form of Human Anthrax
• Acquired by contact with infected animal or their products (Usually occupational – Veterinaries, Farmers are commonly affected) • In abattoir/slaughter house people working are at special risk.
• Cutaneus anthrax (Malignant pustule) – Occurs on exposed surface of arms and hands (popular stage → vesicular → ulcerative stage)
• G+ve aerobic bacilli – polypeptide capsule ("Bamboo stick" appearance)
• Special appearances on Culture → Frosted glass appearance, medusa head appearance, and Inverted fir tree appearance.

- Botulinum toxins:

• Botulinum toxin affects the PNS. The CNS is not involved it blocks the release of acetylcholine.
• Characteristically produces symmetric ascending paralysis.
• Botulinum toxin is heat labile but spores are heat resistant

- Calymmatobacterium Granulomatis:

Calymmatous penile ulcer + organism within macrophages

- Neisseria Gonorhoea: "Obligate pathogen"

Female → Most common site of infection – Endocervix, urethra mostly asymptomatic [Q]
Male → M.C. site urethra urethra discharge is the M.C. symptom. Mostly symptomatic [Q]
Gonrrhoea is Neonates – B/L conjunctivitis (Opthalamia neonatarum) infection is acquired from mother during delivery.
Treatment → Neisseria G. has become resistant to numerous antibiotics including penicillin.
Treatment of choice → Ceftraxmic

- Lyme disease:

• Borrelia Burg
• Infection progresses even after good humoral immunity.
• Lyme meningitis: CSF shows (1) Lymphocytosis (Not PMN Leukocytosis) (2) Presence IgM, IgA Intrathically confirms the diagnosis.

- Hemophilus influenza:

Means blood loving → Requires blood containing media for their growth → usually chocolate blood agar.
• Requires 2 Erythrocyte factors for growth Factor X, Factor V
• Pathogenesis: Polysaccharide capsule is known to be major factor in virulence [Q]
• M.C. invasive infection caused by H. Influenzae → Meningitis

- Widal test:

• Tube agglutination test
• Typhii – 'H' and 'O' antigen, Paratyphii – H antigen
• H antigen lasts longer

• H-antigen differentiate typhii and paratyphii
• Single tests is Not confirmatory instead 4 fold rise in antibody titre b/w 2 successive test is considered more diagnostic.
• Timing of Test → 2nd, 3rd and 4th week
• To differentiate various strains of S. typhii → Vi Antigen is used. So, H–antigen can't differentiate different strain/ types of S. typhii (Only differentiate S. typhii from para typhii)

- Campylobacter:

is Microaerophillic.
Causes GB syndrome and Reiter's syndrome

- Nocardia:

• AFB (Acid Fast bacilli)
• Stain used → AF stain + mucin stain (mucicarmine + Alcian blue
• No kiram stain used [Q]
• Rx – Sulphonamides

- Brucella:

• Brucellosis/Malta fever/Medittarian fever/undulant fever.
• Castenda method of blood culture.

- HACEK group:

Refers to a group of fastidious slow growing bacteria normally resident in the mouth which can cause severe infection particularly endocarditis
H → Haemophillus A → A.a C → Cardio bacterium E → Eikenella K → Kingella

- Diptheria:

The organism does not penetrate deeply into the tissue. The systemic features are due to the production of toxins.
Elek test → The toxigenicity of bacteria is demonstrated by Elek test shick test → Susceptibility test.
Diptheria toxin acts by inhibiting protein synthesis

- Diphtheria is when infected with B-phase
- E. Coli when infected with $\lambda - K_{12}$
- In Gut – Anaerobes to Aerobes ratio= 1000: 1
- Furospirochaetosis/ANUG:

Caused by → Borrelia vincenti/Treponemia vincenti

- Causative organism for CAT scratch disease is → Bartonella
- Syphillis:

Phospholipid used to investigate syphilis by regain test is → Cardiolipin

- Typhoid carriers organism present in Gall bladder.

- Human is the only reservoir in following cases:

Cholera
E. Histolytica
Typhoid associated salmonella

- Pneumocystis jerovici:

Infection can occur in either healthy or immune compromised individuals but disease ie, pneumocystis pneumonia occurs only in immunocompromised individual
Usually diagnosed by sputum examination.

- Spores of Non toxic strains of clostridium tetani is used for determining sterilization efficiency
- Yeresina lipopolysaccharide:

forms endotoxin as it is gram –ve
It has bipolar appearance grows at 25°C
Transmitted by bite of fleas.

- Both E.coli + Lactobacillus Leishmanni is used for microbiological assay of Vit. B_{12}
- Donavan bodies are seen in bone marrow and splenic aspiration smears in infection with ◉ Leishmania donovani [Q]

LAST 5-YEAR QUESTIONS FROM THIS TOPIC

1. **Black pigmented anaerobes include all of the following except:** *(KCET 12)*
   a. Tannerella
   b. Porphyromonas
   c. Bacteroides
   d. Prevotella

Ans. c

2. **Kolmer test is a screening test done for:** *(KCET 12)*

Ans. Syphilis

3. **The property of splitting sugars by bacteria is called:** *(AIPG 12)*

Ans. Sacchrolysis (Ref: www.answers.com)

4. **some bacteria get encapsulated to:** *(AIPG 12)*

Ans. to achieve protection from phagocytosis
Note: It also increases virulence

5. **Gas gangrene is caused by all except:** *(AIIMS May 11)*
   a. C. histolyticum
   b. C. novyi
   c. C. septicum
   d. C. sporogenes

Ans. d (Ref: Horrison 17/*e p*903)

6. **Culture media of Leptospirosis is:** *(AIIMS May 11)*

Ans. Korthof (Ref: Ananthanarayan 7/*e p*392)

7. **Which of the following is microaerophilic?** *(AIIMS May 11)*

Ans. Campylobacter (Ref: Harrison 17/*e p*965)
Note: Other e.g. are H. pylori + Bonrelia burgdorferi

8. **All of the following statements about S.aureus are true, Except:** *(AIIMS Nov 10)*
   a. Most common source of infection is cross infection from injected people.

b. About 30% of population is realthy nasal carriers
c. Epidermolysis and TSS toxins are super antigens
d. Methicillin resistance is chromosomally mediated

Ans. a (Ref: Harrison 17/*e* *p*873-9)

9. About pseudomonas aeruginosa, all are true, except: *(AIIMS Nov. 10, 09)*

a. Strict aerobe
b. Can grow in disinfectant in hospital
c. Infection is mostly due to endogenous source
d. Most common organism in burn patient

Ans. c (Ref: Ananthanarayan 7/*e* p315)

10. All about Neisseria gonorrhoeae , are true Except: *(AIIMS Nov. 10, 09)*

a. Most common cause of urethritis in males
b. All strains are susceptible to penicillin G
c. Some strains are found in disseminated form
d. Found exclusively in human beings

Ans. b (Ref: Ananthanarayan 7/*e* *p*225-227)

11. All are true about widal test, except: *(AIIMS Nov. 10, 09)*

a. Baseline differs depending on the endemicity of disease.
b. O antibodies last longer and hence are not an indicator of recent infection
c. H-antigen cannot differentiate between subtypes
d. High titre value is a single widal test is not confirmative.

Ans. b (Ref: Ananthnarayan 7/*e* *p*299)

12. Average number of bacteria present in saliva is? *(AIIMS Nov. 10)*

Ans. 750 millions/ml

13. Regarding staphylococcus lugdunensis, all are true, except: *(AIIMS Nov. 10)*

a. Causes skin infection
b. Does not show coagulase activity
c. Is susceptible to many antibodies
d. Causes native valve endocarditis

Ans. c.

14. A farmer with pustules, which shows gram positive cocci on smear culture. The organisms show B-hoemolysis and are catalase negative. To show that the identified organism is Grp. A streptococci, which of the following test should be done: *(AIIMS May 10)*

Ans. Bacitracin sensitivity (Ref: Ananthanarayan 7/*e* *p*203-205)

15. Brucella is transmitted by all, Except: *(AIIMS May 10)*

a. Through the placenta of animal
b. Aerosol
c. Person to person
d. Eating uncooked food

Ans. c (Ref: Park 19/*e* *p*242)

16. Which of the following organism produces a toxin that acts by adenylate cyclase? *(AIIMS May 10)*

Ans. V. Cholerae (Ref: Ananthanaryan 7/*e* *p*310)

17. Which of the following is Not true about bacteroids? *(AIIMS Nov. 09)*

a. Bile resistant anaerobe
b. Most total form is bacteroids fragilis
c. Most common in mixed infection

d. Highly susceptible to broad spectrum of antibioties

Ans. d (Ref: Clinical laboratory sciences, university of missisippi accessed 7/e October 2011)

18. DPT vaccine is NOT contraindicated in: *(AIIMS May 09)*

a. Immunocompromised patient
b. Progressive neurological disease
c. Severe reaction to Ist dose/subsequent dose
d. Uncontrolled convulsions.

Ans. a

19. Which of the following is true? *(AIIMS May 09)*

a. Agar has nutrient properties
b. Chocolate medium is a selective medium
c. Addition of selective substances in a solid medium is called enrichment medium
d. Nutrient broth is a basal medium

Ans. d (Ref: Anathanarayan and panikar 8/*e p*39, 40)

20. Culture was done on a child with infective skin lesions of the leg, which showed gram true cocci in chains and haemolytic colonies, which test best identifies the organism? *(AIIMS May 09)*

Ans. Bacitracin sensitivity test

21. Which of the following is not true of vibrio cholera?

a. It is halophibic
b. It grows on simple media
c. Man Is the only natural host
d. It can servive outside human intestine

Ans. a (Ref: Murray and baron manual of clinical microbiology 8/e)

22. An elderly male patient is presented with fever, chest pain and dry cough. Spectum culture showed growth of charcoal yeast extract medium. The organism is of charcoal yeast extract medium. The Organism is: *(AIIMS May 09)*

Ans. Legionella (Ref: Ananthanarayan and paniker 8/*e p*400)

23. After splenectomy patient becomes more prone to: *(AIIMS Nov. 09)*

Ans. Encapsulated bacteria (Ref: Harrison's principle of internal medicine 16/e Vol 1 p348)

24. With referenc to bacteroide fragilis the following statement are true except: *(AIIMS Nov. 12)*

a. B. fragilis is the most frequent anaerobe isolated from clinical samples.
b. B. fragilis is not uniformly sensitive to metronidazole
c. The lipopolysaccharide formed by B. fragilis is structurally and functionally different from conventional endotoxin.
d. Shock and D/C are common in bacteriods bacteremia.

Ans. d (Ref: Harrison 8/*e p*1079)

25. All are true about Legionella pneumopehila except: *(AIIMS May 12)*

a. Aquatic bodies are main habitat
b. It can replicate in amoeba
c. Urine test is a reliable method
d. Person to person transmission

Ans. d (Ref: ananthanarayan 8/*e p*400)

26. All are true regarding B pertussis except: *(AIPG 11)*

a. Nasopharyngeal swab is taken as a simple for diagnosis
b. Antibody immunoassay is diagnostic
c. children and adults who are vaccinated can have disease later in life
d. Causes whooping cough.

Ans. d (Ref: Parija p346, 347)

27. All are true relation to scrub typhus, Except? *(AIPG 11)*

a. Mites act as reservoir
b. Tetracyline is the drug of choice
c. Transmitted when adult mites feed on host
d. Caused by O. Tsutsugamushi

Ans. c (Ref: Microbiology by Walker pg. 228-229)

28. All are true regarding donavanosis Except: *(AIPG 11)*

a. The causative organism is calymmatobacter granulomates
b. Causes painful ulcerative genital lesions
c. Endemic in tropical areas
d. Syphilis can occur con comitant with it.

Ans. b

29. All are true about leptospirosis, Except: *(AIPG 10)*

a. Pen G is drug of choice
b. Urine and faces are main mode of transmission
c. IgM is formed in 5 days
d. Latent period is 10 days

Ans. c

30. True about mycobacterium other than tubercular bacilli: *(AIPG 09)*

a. Causes disseminated infection
b. Diagnosis is by demonstration of trophozoite is CSF
c. Feco-oral transmission occurs
d. More common in tropical climate

Ans. d (Ref: Harrison 17/*e p*1279, 2632)

31. The ability of different species of plaque micro organisms to adhere to one another is: *(KCET 09)*

Ans. Coaggregation

32. Pathogenesis of diphtheria is attributed to: *(COMEDK 09)*

Ans. Exotoxin (Ref: Robbins pathology 6/*e p*273-274)

33. ASO test is used for the diagnosis of: *(COMEDK 10)*

Ans. Rheumatic fever

34. Lyme disease is: *(COMEDK 10)*

Ans. Diagnosed by demonstration of specific IgM antibody+ the etiological agent can be grown in modified kelley's medium

35. Pseudomonas aeuroginosa: *(COMEDK 11)*

Ans. Causes shanghai fever (Ref: Textbook of microbiology by Ananthanarayan 6/*e p*295)

36. Injection abscesses due to use of contaminated vaccines occurs in infections caused by: *(COMEDK 11)*

Ans. M. Chelonae (Ref: Textbok of microbiology by Ananthanarayan 7/*e p*367)

37. The most frequent non-sporing anaerobic bacilli isolated from clinical specimens is: *(COMEDK 11)*

Ans. Bacteroids fragilis (Ref: Textbook of microbiology by ananthanarayan 7/*e p*268-69)

38. A full course of immunization against tetanus with 3 doses of tetanus toxoid, confers immunity for how many years: *(COMEDK 11)*

Ans. 10 years (Ref: Park's Textbook of social and preventive medicine)

39. Which of the following organisms does Not react with gram's stain? *(KCET 11)*

a. Actinomyces israelli
b. Candida albicans
c. M. Tuberculosis

d. S. mutans

Ans. c (Ref: Ananthanarayan 7/*e p*351)

40. In which phase of the bacterial growth curve involution forms of the bacteria can be observed?

Ans. phase of decline (Ref: Ananthanarayan 7/*e p*21) *(KCET 11)*

Note: In stationary phase sporulation is seen

41. General paresis in neurosyphilis is a feature of: *(KCET 12)*

Ans. 3° Stage of syphilis

42. Actinomycosis is an: *(KCET 12)*

Ans. Anaerobic bacterial disease

43. Prophylaxis against bacterial endocarditis is directed primarily against: *(KCET 12)*

Ans. hemolytic streptococci

44. The lactoperoxidose thiocynate system present in saliva is against: *(KCET 12)*

Ans. Streptoccus

VIROLOGY

- Viruses are very heat labile
- In viral infection there is production of interferon which is not seen in bacterial infection
- DNA virus Vs RNA virus:

HBV, varicella Zoster, EBV, HSV, simian 40, Parvo virus B19	ds RNA → Rheovirus, Rotavirus Colorado tick fever virus
HPV – ss DNA	
ss DNA virus – Parvovirus B19, HPV	

- HIV:

<table>
<tr><td>P24 Antigen– Major core antigen that can be detected in early stage of HIV infection before appearance of IgM antibodies (Appears in 4-6 wks) followed by IgG.
If viral load is small (needle stick injury) process is delayed</td></tr>
<tr><td>Window period 2-6 months.
Antibodies appear after window period so, Elisa and Western blot are negative during window period.</td></tr>
<tr><td>Small non-particulate protein leading to entranced replication of HBV and HIV is HBx Ag</td></tr>
<tr><td>HIV tests:<table><tr><th>Screening</th><th>Supplemental</th></tr><tr><td>Elisa, rapid test</td><td>Western blot, RIPA, indirect immunoflorescent assay</td></tr></table></td></tr>
<tr><td>HIV binds to CD4 and CCR5 molecules on macrophages</td></tr>
<tr><td>Salivary leukocyte proteinase inhibitor is the salivary protein which prevents transmission of HIV via saliva.</td></tr>
<tr><td>Most common oral lesion – Candida</td></tr>
<tr><td>Most common genital lesion – HSV</td></tr>
<tr><td>“HIV” Associated diarrhea:<table><tr><td>• Isospora and Cryptosporidium → Acid fast → parasites associated</td></tr><tr><td>• Microsporidea</td></tr><tr><td>NB: Cyclospora – Acid fast organism, Causing Chronic diarrhea But Not associated with HIV.</td></tr></table></td></tr>
</table>

- Hepatitis:

• Chronic HCV and Alcohlic liver disease → M.C. cause for liver transplant
• HCV and HBV cause Hepatocellular carcinoma (HCC)
• HBV → only DNA virus
• HCV causes co-infection c HBV→ ses risk for HCC
• Only hepatitis virus that can be cultured → HAV
• **HBV antigen:**

• HBsAg → Live virus (Acute/chronic/carrier)
• Anti HBsAg → Patient protected + immune cure (good prognosis) [Q]
• Anti HBcAg → Not protective used to predict how long the infection has been going IgM [Q] predicts New infection IgG [Q]
• HBeAg → High infectivity + active disease
• Anti HBeAg → Low infectivity

- Parvovirus B19:

(ssDNA)
Smallest virus
• Crosses placental > 30% cases → Hydrops foetalis
• Causes aplastic crisis and severe Anemia (Congenital hemolytic)
• The most common manifestation of P. B19 is Erytherma infectiosum/fifth disease.

- Enterovirus:

Ex- coxsaki, herpangina, hand foot and mouth disease, polio, enterovirus → Aseptic meningitis

- H5N1 → influenza A virus/bird flu virus.
- Dengu Fever Diagnosis:

• Most sensitive and specific → Neutralization
• Most frequent – Haemoglutination inhibition.

- HANTA virus:

(Arbovirus) → Pulmonary syndrome is caused by inhalation of Rodent urine/faeces [Q]
HUS: Haemolysis uremia syndrome: It's a Coomb (–ve) hemolytic anemia [Q] HUS: ↓ • Hemolysis • Uremia • Thrombocytopenia

- POLIO:

Paralytic polio is not common.
Most of the cases are in apparent (90%)
Paralysis → Precipitates with physical exertion [Q]
Pulse polio immunization is given to all children <5 yrs of age [Q]

- RSV (Respiratory syncytial virus) ◉ Bronchiolitis (lower respiratory tract infection) in infants
- Measles:

SSPE (Sub Acute sclerosing Panencephalilis) → is a rare late complication of measles.

- Coxasackei virus inhabit the alimentary tract of children < 2yrs [Q]
- Negri bodies → Rabies
- prions:

<table>
<tr><td colspan="2">• Prions are infections proteins devoid of any nuclai acid (RNA/DNA)</td></tr>
<tr><td colspan="2">• Prion disease results from the accumulation of the abnormal prion protein Pr psc [Q]</td></tr>
<tr><td colspan="2">• Prion are most resistant to physical and chemical agents such as heat, irradiation and Antiseptics [Q]</td></tr>
<tr><td>Prion Diseases
Human
• CJD (Crentzfeldt jakob disease)
• Kuru
• Fatal familial insomnia</td><td>Animals
• Scrapie
• Bovine spongiform encephalopathy</td></tr>
<tr><td colspan="2">Hallmak of prion disease:
• The disease is confined to nervous system
• The basic features are new degeneration and spongiform changes
• The disease is always fatal
• The host shows No inflammatory response and No immune response → As agents do not appear to be antigenic No production of INF (interferon) There is no effect on host B cell or T cell function</td></tr>
</table>

LAST 5-YEAR QUESTIONS FROM THIS TOPIC

1. **Each of the following viruses possesses an outer lipoprotein envelope except:** *(KCET 12)*
   a. Varicella zoster
   b. Papilloma virus
   c. Influenza virus
   d. HIV

Ans. b

2. **Virus is usually cultured in:** *(AIPG 12)*

Ans. Embryonated hen eggs (Ref: Microbiology by naveen kango, 2010, p136)

3. **Dentist after suffering from jaundice due to hepatitis B has recovered since 3 months, but is not allowed to practice by medical board as he is a:** *(AIIMS Nov. 09)*

Ans. Convalescent carrier

4. **For 1° Herpes simplex the best diagnosis is made by:** *(AIIMS May 13)*

Ans. Flourescent stain for cytology (Ref: Burket oral medicine 10/e p53)

5. **For 1° Herpes simplex which is not commonly used:** *(AIIMS Nov. 12)*
   a. Culture with giemsa stain
   b. Culture with wright stain
   c. Routine cytology
   d. Flourescent stain for cytology

Ans. c

6. **Prions true is:** *(AIIMS May 12)*

Ans. have a long incubation period

7. **Oral polio vaccine, all are true except:** *(AIPG 11)*
   a. Killed vaccine
   b. Stored at sulezero temperature

c. Induces intestinal and humoral immunity
d. Residual neuro virulence is a problem

Ans. a (Ref: Harrison 17/e p1209)

8. Characteristic feature of retrovirus is: *(AIPG 10)*

Ans. Reverse transcriptase (Ref: Medical microbiology by jawetz, melnick and Adelberg 23rd p589-590)

9. Which of the following is true: *(AIPG 09)*

a. Hanta virus pulmonary syndrome is caused by inhalation of rodent urine and faces
b. Kyanasur forest disease is caused by bite of wild animal
c. Lyssa virus is transmitted by ticks
d. None

Ans. a (Ref: Ananthanarayan 7/e p533)

10. which of the following viruses produces both intranuclear and intra cytoplasmic inclusion bodies? *(COMED 09)*

Ans. Measles

11. The degradation of p 53 through ubiquitous – dependent proteolysis by the binding of high-risk HPV protein is: *(KCET 10)*

Ans. E6

12. Which is a DNA virus: *(COMEDK 11)*

Ans. Hepatitis B virus (Ref: Ananthanarayan 6/e p511)

13. Western blot test is a confirmatory test used for the diagnosis of: *(KCET 11)*

Ans. HIV (Ref: Textbook of microbiology by ananthanarayan 7/e p351)

14. Papulovesicular oral lesion are seen in: *(KCET 12)*

Ans. Herpangina

15. Presence of EBV in OHL can be demonstrated using following methods except: *(KCET 12)*

a. Tzank smear
b. PCR
c. In situ
d. Electron microscopy hybridization

Ans. a

16. Mumps is caused by which virus? *(KCET 12)*

Ans. paramyxo virus

PARASITOLOGY AND MISCELLANEOUS

- Dimorphic Fungi:

Ex- Candida albicans (Not Other candida), Blastomyces, Histoplasma
NB: Philaphora is Not dimorphic [Q]

- Parasitic disorder associated with billiary obstruction:

  - Clonorchis
  - Opisthorchis
  - Fasciola hepatica
  - Ascaries
  - Echinococceous

- Parasites causing Malabsorption:

Giardia, E-histolytica, Strongyloids, Cyclospora
Not by Ascaris [Q]

- Giardiasis → Causes Malabsorption + Diarrhea.
- E. histolytica – Investigation of choice for invasive amoebiasis/E. histolytica ◎ ELISA
- In amoebiasis flask shaped ulcer is seen.
- Chlamydia: Isolation of Chlamydia:

Tissue culture (Method of choice)	Yolk sac	Animal inoculation
McCoy cells and Hella cells	inoculation	

NOTE: The most sensitive test for diagnosis is NAAT (Nucleic acid amplification test) [Q]

- Chlamydia: "Obligate intracellular parasite"

Life cycle: Occurs in 2 forms (Biphasic)
- Elementary Body → Infective form Metabolically inactive. It is in this form Chlamydia exist extracellular.
- Reticular body → Derived from elementary body intracelluarly Reticular body grows in size within the cell and divides repeatedly by binary fission.
  – It metabolically active.

- Hydatid Disease:

Caused by Echniococcus/Dog tape worm
Man – Intermediate host, Dog → Definite host
NB: Man is the definitive host in most of the parasites infection except following where it is intermediate Host – Echinococcus, Plasmodium, Tanea Solium (Park tape work) and Toxoplasma gondi→ (Both definitive and Intermediate)

- Autoinfection: Taenia solium (Cystiearcosis), Strongyloids, Capillaria, Cryptosporidium
- Congenital toxoplasmosis:

• Not confirmed by IgG as can come from mother so, IgG is not diagnostic.
• IgM and IgA sed level diagnostic
• IgA more sensitive than IgM

- Multiple vesicles on hand and multiple eruption along lymphatic in Gardener → "Cutaneus sporotrichosis"
- Amoebic Meningoencephalitis:

Acute Amoebic M.E	Chronic
Nageleria [Q]	Acanthamoeba
Diagnosis → Trophozoites in CSF	

- Mycoplasma:

• Has no cell wall → so No 'L' form seen [Q] • L form is cell wall defective bacteria but in mycoplasma there is no cell wall • Is not inhibited by penicillin as it has no cell wall [Q] *(KCET 12)*
• Can grow in cell free media
• Requires sterols for growth
• Very small so does not produce turbidity in liquid media.
• No cell wall → so, resistant to penicillin
• Has an affinity for mammalian cell membranes they can pass through fitters of 450 nm pore size

- Histoplasmosis:

• Clinical presentation resembles TB [Q]
• Spores are infective not hyphal form [Q]
• No man to man transmission. (It is by inhalation of spores)

- Malaria:

Schuffner's dot → P. Vivax
Crescent shaped Gametocyte → P. Faliciparum

- Cryptococcus neoformans has significant predilection for CNS
- L.D. bodies are seen in kala-azar.
- Loeffer's syndrome:

Acute eosinophillic pneumonia caused by drugs/parasites except Giardia.

- Traveller's Diarrhea:

Most common → Enterotoxigenic E. Coli
M.C among viral → Rota virus, Norovirus
M.C. in South Asia → Campylobacter.

- Meningitis:

Septic	Aseptic
Bacterial cause	VIRUS (Ex-mumps)

- Weil felix Reaction used in the diagnosis of ricketessia.
- Heterophill antigen test:

Weil felix	Paul Bunnel	Forssman
Proteins Antigen used	Used in Infectius mononucleosis	Ag–Ab Reaction
For Ricktessia , Salmonella		

- Probiotics:

Example of probiotics to improve intestinal microbial balance: Bifidobacteria, Lactobacillus, Eubacterium, Certain yeast.

- Reynold's Brande phenomena:

Ability to form Germ tube.
It shown by Candida alibcans.

- Sabouraud's agar is used to identify C. alibicans
- Kaposi's sarcoma → Tissue of origin is → Vascular
- Kaposi's sarcoma is viral origin [Q]

LAST 5-YEAR QUESTIONS FROM THIS TOPIC

1. **All are dimorphic fungi, Except:** *(AIIMS May 11)*
   a. Histoplasma capsulatum
   b. Blastomyces dermatitidis
   c. Penicillium marreffei

d. Phialophora verrucosa

Ans. d (Ref: Harriison, 17/e p1242, 1266)

2. **Auto infection is seen with:** *(AIIMS May 11)*

Ans. Strongyloides (Ref: Harrison 17/e p1322)

3. **Which stage of P. vivax is infective to mosquito?** *(AIIMS Nov. 10, 09)*

Ans. Gametocyte (Ref: Sherman, Malaria p57-58)

4. **A young presented with UTI on urine examination, pus cells were would be test for culture?** *(AIIMS may 10)*

Ans. Mccoy culture (Ref: Ananthanarayan 7/e p425)

5. **Bacteria used in probiotics is:** *(AIPG 10)*

Ans. Bifido bacterium

6. **Most common organism associated with reactive arthritis:** *(AIPG 09)*

Ans. Chlamydia (Ref: Harrison 17/e p2113)

7. **Non septate hypae with a tendency to breanch at 90° angle is characteristic of:** *(KCET 09)*

Ans. Mucor (Ref: Lange microbiology by jawetz)

8. **Kvein–Siltzbach test is useful in the diagnosis of:** *(COMED 09)*

Ans. Sarcoidosis

9. **Which of the following parasites causes auto infection:** *(COMEDK 09)*

Ans. Taenia solium (Ref: Clarke general medicine 5/e p1123)

10. **Which one of the following does not present antigens?** *(COMEDK 10)*

a. NK cells
b. Dendritic cells
c. Langerhans cells
d. Macrophages

Ans. a

11. **Infective endocardictis is caused by:** *(KCET 10)*

Ans. Both bacteria and fungi

12. **The yeast which shows thick gelatinous capsule and positive for mucicarmine is:** *(KCET 10)*

Ans. Cryptococcus neoformans

13. **Durck granules are seen is:** *(COMEDK 11)*

Ans. Malaria (Ref: Malaria review by ashen I/e p68)

14. **Name the fungi which are ovoid/ spherical in morphology, produces budding cells and pseudohypae in culture media and in human tissues:** *(KCET 11)*

Ans. C. albicans (Ref: Texbook of microbiology by Ananthanarayan 7/e p592)

15. **Botulism toxin causes:** *(PGI Dec. 10, June 07)*

Ans. Bilateral cranial involvement (Ref: Ananthanarayan 7/e p283)

16. **LAD is associated with which chromosome number:** *(PGI 09)*

Ans. 21 (Ref: Net pubmed.com)

17. **Rapid evaluation of fungal hyphae/spores can be achieved with?** *(KCET 12)*

Ans. KOH wet mount

CHAPTER 15

Physiology

Topic

- General Physiology
- Respiratory System
- CVS
- GIT
- Reproductive System
- Excretory System
- CNS
- Endocrine System
- Miscellaneous

GENERAL PHYSIOLOGY

- Highest concentration of K ion – RECTUM/COLON
- Na and HCO_3 level is maximum in BILE.
- Normal range of serum osmolarity – 270-285 mosmol/kg.
- Histamine:

Histamine is mainly found within storage granules of mast cell but also found in other tissue
Mast cell histamine – mast cell and basophile.
Non mast cell histamine – Gastric mucosa.[Q]
ACTIONS: Gastric gland – histamine causes marked increase in gastric acid secretion. Smooth muscle – Vasodilatation and bronchoconstriction. Brain – Arousal. Sexual behaviour.
LEWIS TRIPLE RESPONSE: is caused primarily by the liberation of histamine and other related peptide. [Q]. Is characteristic 3 part response that develops when a pointed object is drawn firmly over the skin. • Red reaction – Direct vasodilating effect of histamine. • Flare reaction – Manifest in the form of spreading redness. Results from stimulation of axon reflex by histamine that causes vasodilatation indirectly. • Wheal – Manifest as swelling / localized oedema. Results from increased capillary permeability due to histamine.

- Physiological effects of smoking:

Depends on the number of cigarette smoked, smoking duration, the amount and type of smoke inhaled.
Nicotine in tobacco stimulates adrenal medulla, increasing plasma adrenaline and urinary catecholamine.
Plasma glucose concentration is enhanced within minutes after start of smoking.
Smoking increases the HR of smokers associated with increase of B.P and C.O. These changes are due to nicotine induced release of noradrenaline.

Chronic smoking is associated with increased serum cholesterol, reduced HDL ⟶ increases Risk and extent of advanced atherosclerosis.
Haematological changes – increases total RBC, leukocytes, fibrinogen causes alteration of platelets aggregation and survival that produce thrombosis
Smoking increases carboxyhaemoglobin. [Q]

- Turbulence:

Turbulence ∞ Re (Reynolds no) =ρDV/И
So increase in density → increases Re → increases turbulence [Q]

LAST 5-YEAR QUESTIONS FROM THIS TOPIC

1. **The most common cells in connective tissue are:** *(PGI Dec, June 09)*

Ans. Fibroblast (Ref: Inderbir singh histology)

2. **The most antigenic is:** *(PGI June 09)*

Ans. Proteins (Ref: Anantanarayan 7/e p80 – 81)

3. **Which of the following increases turbulence in blood flow?** *(AIPG 09)*

Ans. When diameter of blood vessel increases (Ref: Ganong 22/e p583)

4. **NOT a general compartment of body fluid is:** *(AIPG 12)*

Ans. Peritoneal fluid (Ref: Ganong 24/e p3)

5. **Ceruloplasmin is a protein containing:** *(KCET 11)*

Ans. Copper

6. **Ubiquitin is involved in:** *(COMEDK 11)*

Ans. Intracellular proteolysis

7. **Anaphylaxis refers to:** *(COMEDK 11)*

Ans. Severe reaction following re – injection of protein solutions in a sensitized individual

8. **Daily loss of iron/day in a healthy adult male is:** *(COMEDK 11)*

Ans. 0.6 mg

9. **The transmembrane adhesive molecules present in hemidesmosomes which specifically bind to basal lamina glycoprotein laminin are:** *(KCET 10)*

Ans. Integrin $\alpha6\beta4$

10. **The abundant glycoprotein in the basement membrane and has binding domain for both ECM and cell surface receptor is:** *(KCET 10)*

Ans. Laminin

RESPIRATORY SYSTEM

- NON respiratory function of lung:

• ACE synthesized by lung – Na balance.[Q]
• Fibrinolytic function – Pulmonary Endothelium is rich in PLASMIN activator.
• Heparin – Lung is rich in mast cells which secrete heparin.
• SURFACTANT – Synthesized by type 2 alveolar epithelial cells.[Q]

- **Factors maintaining pulmonary vascular resistance even during increased cardiac output (ex- exercise):**

• Recruitment – Increasing the number of open capillaries that were previously closed.[Q]
• GREATER DISTRIBUTION OF PULMONARY BLOOD VESSELS. Both are passive process and NOT regulated by SNS/PNS.

- Central chemoreceptor:

stimulated by change in pco2 in BLOOD.
stimulated DIRECTLY by Hydrogen ion.

- 2, 3DPG IN RBC:

Most abundant organic phosphate in RBC.
Lowers the oxygen affinity of Hb and allow increase delivery of oxygen to the tissue. → RIGHT SHIFT of oxygen dissociation curve.
Factors which increases the 2,3 DPG: • Hypoxia(high altitude) • Anaemia • Alkalosis • Exercise

- Foetal Hb has higher affinity for O_2 because HbF binds to 2, 3 –DPG less effectively than HbA (Adult Hb) [Q]
- Effect of O_2 on blood vessels:

Increased O_2– Vasoconstriction
Decreased O_2 – Vasodilatation.
OPPOSITE effect seen in pulmonary circulation.[Q]
Increased CO_2– vasodilatation

- Myocardial oxygen demand correlates with heart rate. [Q]

For Basal Metabolism – 25%
Associated with Muscle Contraction: • Internal cardiac work – 50% • External cardiac work – 25%

- Cyanosis:

Appears when the capillary content of reduced Hb > 5gm/dl.
Central cyanosis – caused by inadequate oxygenation of systematic arterial blood due to • Decreased arterial saturation – high altitude, impaired pulmonary function. • Haemoglobin abnormalities – methemoglobinemia (iron is in Fe 3+ state cannot bind oxygen. Central cyanosis is characterized by cyanosis affecting both mucous membrane and skin.
Perephderal cyanosis – is caused by slowing of blood flow. Causes – arterial and venous obstruction reduced cardiac output, cold exposure. Peripheral cyanosis is characterized by cyanosis of skin alone and sparing of mucous membrane.

- Cushing Triad: [Q]

HTN, Bradycardia and irregular respiration.
It's a protective reflex to overcome the CNS ischemic response due to increase in CSF pressure. → This reflex leads to increase in arterial pressure above the CSF and blood flows once again into B.V of brain to relieve ischemia. This increase in arterial pressure (hypertension) causes reflex BRADYCARDIA.

- 0Xygen Toxicity:

Occurs due to oxygen free radical effect.
CNS – convulsion, twitching
Respiration – pulmonary oedema.

Retinal damage – neonates on high oxygen progress to blindness due ANGIOGENESIS
CEREBRAL vasculature constricts in high pO_2. This is protective NOT toxic effect of increased pO_2. [Q].
Leads to decreased cerebral blood flow to protect brain.

LAST 5-YEAR QUESTIONS FROM THIS TOPIC

1. **Which of the following adaptations will be apt to increase the work capacity at high altitude?** *(AIPG 12, 10, AIIMS may 09)*

Ans. Decreasing workload, increasing duration of exercise (Ref: Ganong 22/e p657)

2. **Carbon monoxide has limited diffusion because:** *(AIIMS Nov 10, AIPG 12)*

Ans. It has high affinity for haemoglobin (Ref: rhoades and Bell. medical physiology: the principles for clinical Medicine p350)

3. **Stability of alveoli is maintained by:** *(AIIMS Nov. 10)*

Ans. Reduced surface tension by surfactant (Ref: Ganong 22/e p655)

4. **Hypercapnia results in:** *(AIPG 11, 10)*

Ans. Low blood pH (Ref: Ganong 22/e p692)

5. **Bronchial circulation is associated with:** *(AIPG 11, 10)*

Ans. Air conditioning (Ref: Levitzky. pulmonary Physiology 6/e p87)

6. **Pulmonary endothelium is NOT concerned with which of the following?** *(AIPG 11)*
   a. Lipoprotein lipase
   b. Plasminogen activator
   c. Thrombin
   d. Factor X

Ans. d (Ref: Pinsky. applied physiology in Intensive Care Medicine p221)

7. **CO poisioning causes:** *(AIPG 11, 10)*

Ans. Shift of oxygen dissociation curve to left (Ref: Ganong 22/e p661, 684, 690)

8. **An important non respiratory function of lung is:** *(AIPG 11)*

Ans. Sodium balance (Ref: Khurana. textbook of Medical physiology p401 – 402)

9. **Pulmonary circulation differs from systemic circulation in:** *(AIPG 09)*

Ans. Pulmonary vasoconstriction in hypoxia (Ref: Ganong 22/e p663 – 664)

10. **Cells that are NOT found in the lungs are:** *(AIPG 09)*
    a. Brush
    b. Clara
    c. Kulchitsky
    d. Langerhans

Ans. d (Ref: Gray's Anatomy 39/e p81 – 83. 1056 – 1058)

11. **Constituent of pulmonary endothelium cell wall is:** *(AIPG 12)*

Ans. Plasminogen activator (Ref: Journal of cell Sciences 110 (year 1997): 139 – 148)

12. **Function of carotid body is to measure:** *(AIPG 12)*

Ans. Pco_2 changes in venous blood (Ref: Ganong 24/e p661)

13. **A pulmonary disorder causes the alveoli to breakdown and coalesce into large air spaces.the lungs also loose elasticity and compliance is increased. a person who suffers from this disease will have.***(KCET 09)*

Ans. Increased dead air space

14. **The normal value of intrapeural pressure at the base of the lungs at the start of inspiration is:** *(COMEDK 09)*

Ans. -2.5 mm Hg

15. The approximate amount of air left in the lungs after maximal forced expiration in normal women is: *(KCET 12)*

Ans. 1.1 litre

16. Stimulation in baroreceptors result in: *(KCET 12)*

Ans. decrease in blood pressure

17. The work of breathing: *(COMEDK 10)*

Ans. Is inversely related to lung compliance

CVS

- Cardiac muscle – histologically similar to skeletal muscle and functionally similar to smooth muscle.
- Endothelium:

Is coated with Glycocalyx which repel clotting factor, thereby preventing coagulation in blood vessels.
The smoothness of endothelial cell surface also prevents coagulation in normal vascular system.

- Serum = plasma – clotting factors except factor 7
  So factor 7 is present in BOTH serum and plasma.[Q]
- Mean circulatory filling pressure:

Average circulatory filling pressure throughout CVS when heart stops beating.
Average = 7mmHg

- During cardiac imaging – phase of minimum motion of heart is – mid diastole. [Q]
- Phase of minimum motion of heart at increased Heart Rate (HR) (high) is late systole.
- Venous Return:

Gravity has no effect on venous return as both arterial and venous pressure increases in lower extremity so pressure gradient is not altered.

- Diastole vs. systole when HR is increased(exercise):

during exercise / increased HR diastole is shortened more than systole. [Q]
Duration of systole is much more fixed than duration of diastole when HR INCREASED(exercise).

- Effect of VAGUS on HR and FOC (force of contraction):

Vagus is distributed mainly on ATRIA so control HR (through SA node) and not much effect on ventricle so less effect on FOC (which is mainly dependent on ventricular muscle).
SNS – has strong effect on both HR and FOC.
Complete denervation of heart will cause an increase in HR (100/min).

- B.P:

VMC (VASOMOTOR CENTRE) and CVC(CARDIOVAGAL CENTRE) act TOGETHER to maintain blood pressure. [Q]

- Source of error in measuring B.P by sphygmomanometer:

especially in obese and elderly individual. [Q]
Small (narrower) cuff – leads to falsely high blood pressure.
large(wider) cuff – leads to falsely lower B.P recording.

- Local Metabolites:

Increasing blood flow during exercise.
Adenosine (mainly), k+, ATP, lactic acid, CO_2.

- With exercise blood flow to muscle increases Immediately [Q]

LAST 5-YEAR QUESTIONS FROM THIS TOPIC

1. Haemoglobin has: *(PGI Dec. 10)*

Ans. 4 heme molecules, 2 alpha and 2 beta

2. The RBC in beta thalassemia are typically: *(PGI Dec 10)*

Ans. Microcytic and hypochromic (Ref: shafer's 6/e p761)

3. The value of normal prothrombin time is: *(PGI Dec 10, 09, June 09)*

Ans. 11 – 15 secs (Ref: vinod kapoor 2/e p647)

4. The normal value of aPTT is: *(PGI June 09)*

Ans. 50 sec (Ref: KDT 5/e p557)

5. The main cause of increased blood flow to the exercising muscle is: *(AIIMS May 11)*

Ans. Vasodilatation due to local metabolites (Ref: Guyton 11/e p247)

6. The most common cause of pulmonary embolism is: *(AIPG 09)*

Ans. Thrombosis (Ref: Loscalzo. Thrombosis and Haemorrhage pg 356)

7. For 2nd heart sound true is: *(AIPG 10)*

Ans. Louder than the 1st heart sound (Ref: Ganong 22/e p569)

8. Fibrin degradation products are utilized in: *(AIPG 10)*

Ans. Disseminated intravascular coagulation (Ref: Davidson 20/e p1060)

9. Vit. K dependent clotting factors are:

Ans. 2, 7, 9,10

10. Excitation – contraction coupling in cardiac muscle: *(AIPG 10)*

Ans. Increases sarcoplasmic Ca2+

11. Differential leukocyte count is used for the diagnosis of: *(AIPG 11)*

Ans. Eosinophilia (NBDE Q)

12. Christmas disease occurs due to deficiency of: *(AIPG 11)*

Ans. Factor 9 (Ref: Ganong 20/e p522)

13. All of the following have defects in clotting mechanism EXCEPT? *(AIPG 11, 12)*

a. Christmas disease
b. Von Willebrand disease
c. Patients on brufen
d. Thalassaemia

Ans. d (Ref: Ganong's 22/e p545)

14. Life span of RBC is: *(AIPG 12)*

Ans. 100 days (Ref: Ganong 24/e p557)

15. One unit of packed RBC will increase the hematocrit by: *(AIPG 12)*

Ans. 3 – 5

16 Haemophilia A is due to deficiency of: *(KCET 09)*

Ans. factor 8

17. Embryonic haemoglobin is composed of: *(AIPG 12)*

Ans. Zeta and epsilon (Ref: Ganong 24/e p559 – 561)

18. Haemophilia B is caused due to deficiency of clotting factor: *(KCET 11)*

Ans. 9

19. Starling's law of the heart: *(COMEDK 09)*

Ans. Explains the increase in cardiac output that occurs when venous return is increased

20. Ivy technique is a test done to measure the: *(KCET 11)*

Ans. Bleeding time

21. The 1st heart sound is due to: *(KCET 11)*

Ans. Sudden closure of mitral tricuspid valves

22. The velocity of conduction in the purkinje fibres of the heart is: *(COMEDK 10)*

Ans. 1 to 4 m/sec

23. The vitamin K dependent protein C and S are characterised by their ability to inactivate factor: *(KCET 10)*

Ans. 7a and 5a

GIT

- Order of water absorptiom:

Jejunum > ileum > colon.

- Fe is actively absorbed in Duodenum andproximal jejunum.
- Cells of gastric gland:

• PO(Parietal/Oxyntic) – secretes HCl and CIF(Castle intrinsic factor)[Q]
• CP (Chief/peptic cell) – pepsinogen [Q]
• ECL – Histamin + serotonin.

- NO and VIP – causes relaxation of GIT smooth muscle and sphincters.
- Both CCK-PZ and GASTRIN secrete pancreatic juice rich in ENZYME.
- Secretin augments the action of CCK-PZ but secrete watery alkaline pancreatic juice.
- Thus both SECRETIN and CCK-PZ decreases gastric motility.
- OTHER action of CCK – contraction of gall bladder.
- Motilin – enhances gastric and intestinal motility.
- Highest Ph is of pancreatic juice of all secretions.
- GIT motility controlling factors:

• Mechanical – distension of gut
• Hormonal – cck-pz – increases motility of small intestine and colon (inhibits gastric emptying).
24. Neural: Parasympathetic/ cholinergic stimulation – enhances intestinal motility. Sympathetic stimulation – inhibits gastric and intestinal motility.
NOTE: intestinal motility is NOT independent of gastric motility. [Q]
PP(post prandial) contraction occurs maximally in DESCENDING COLON due to FAT component of food.

- Appetite Enhancers:

Appetite increasing	Appetite Decreasing
AGRP(agouti related peptide), MCH, Neuropeptide Y	MSH [Q]

- Orexins:

Synthesized in neurons located in lateral hypothalamus.
Orexins(neuropeptide)- control apatite and food intake.

- In Bile Salt synthesis:

7 – α hydroxylation of cholesterol is the 1st and rate limiting step.
Primary bile acid – cholic and chenodeoxycholic acid ↓ COLON BACTERIA ↓ Secondary bile acid - deoxycholic and lithocholic acid.
About 98 – 99 % bile is absorbed in terminal ileum.

- Vitamin D synthesis:

Enzymes involved – 25- hydroxylase in liver, 1α hydroxylase in kidney.

LAST 5-YEAR QUESTIONS FROM THIS TOPIC

1. Which is stable at acidic Ph?

Ans. pepsin (Ref: sembulingam 2/e p168)

2. Which of the following is NOT secreted by the neuro endocrine cells? *(AIIMS May 11, AIPG 10)*

Ans. Intrinsic factor (Ref: chaudhary 4/e p25, 113)

3. Chief cells are seen in: *(AIIMS Nov 09, May 09)*

Ans. Fundus

4. Intrinsic factor of castle is secreted by which of the following cells in gastric glands? *(AIIMS May 11)*

Ans. Parietal cells (Ref: Ganong 22/e p482 – 491)

5. If bile acid pool is small, recycling is: *(AIPG 11)*

Ans. Fast (Ref: Zakim. Hepatology A textbook of liver disease vol 1 3/e p387)

6. pH of Stomach is: *(AIPG 12)*

Ans. 4 – 5 (Ref: Ganong 24/e p459)

7. Which of the following is absorbed in stomach? *(AIPG 12)*

Ans. Alcohol (Ref: KDT 5/e p351)

8. Salivary flow rate is: *(PGI June 11)*

Ans. 5.3 ml/5 min

9. All the following cause the secretion of gastric juice during cephalic phase EXCEPT: *(KCET 09)*

a. Food in mouth
b. Sight of food
c. Food in stomach
d. Tought of food

Ans. c

10. The buffers of saliva maintain the oral ph at: *KCET 12)*

Ans. 7

11. The Ph of gastric acid is: *(KCET 11)*

Ans. 1

12. Decrease in salivary secretion is known as: *(KCET 11)*

Ans. xerostomia

13. Vit. B12 is absorbed in: *(COMEDK 09)*

Ans. Ileum

14. The most important action of secretin is to: *(COMEDK 10)*

Ans. increase secretion of bicarbonates by pancreas

REPRODUCTIVE SYSTEM

- Functions of Sertoli CellS:

Sertoli cells are specialized cells within the seminiferous tubule and are involved in the orchestration and coordination of all the key events of spermatogenesis including spermiogenesis. [Q]
Provide support and nutrition to developing spermatozoa.
Protect developing germ cells by forming BTB(blood testes barrier)
Secretion of ABP(androgen binding protein), inhibin, secrete MIS(mullerian inhibiting substance
Contain Aromatase- this convert testosterone to estrogen at peripheral tissue.
NOTE: Aromatase inhibitor – e.g.: letrazloe used in Gyanecomastia. [Q].
Have high affinity FSH receptor that bind FSH.
Play an important role in the final maturation phase of SPERMIOGENESIS which is characterized by shedding of excess/ residual cytoplasm of the spermatids.
Mature spermatozoa released by sertoli cells.[Q]

- Mature spermatozoa acquire motility in epididymis.[Q]
- Fertilization:

Occurs within few hours after ovulation NOT more than 24 hrs.
Implantation of blastocyst occurs within 5-7 days after fertilization [Q]
CAPACITATION and ACROSOMAL REACTION – occurs in female genital tract (ex –uterus) [Q]

- NOTE: Fallopian tube is lined by ciliated epithelium.
- FSH controls TIME of puberty – which is controlled by FSH regulatory peptide.
- FSH Regulatory peptide

Inhibition of FSH secretion	Activation of FSH secretion
(delay puberty)	(early puberty)
• Inhibin • Follistatin	Activin A.

- FSH and LH ReceptorS:

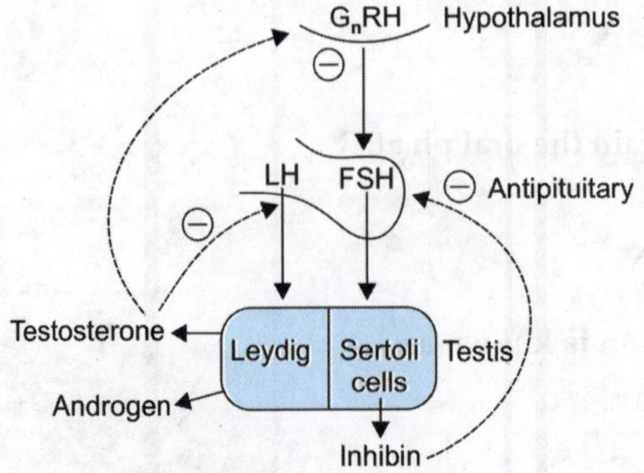

Fig. 15.1: FSH and LH receptors in male

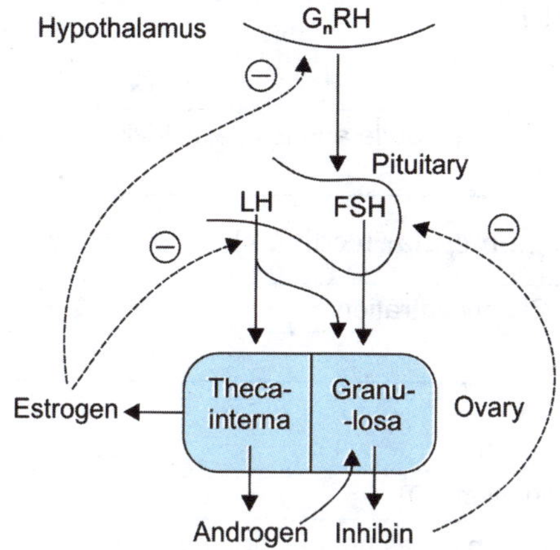

Fig. 15.2: FSH and LH receptors in female

- Effect of maternal glucocorticoid on foetal tissues:

• HPA (FOETAL) development
• Foetal thymic involution
• Foetal surfactant maturation

- NO effect of maternal glucocorticoid on thyroid development.

LAST 5-YEAR QUESTIONS FROM THIS TOPIC

1. **Inhibin B is secreted by:** *(AIPG 10)*

Ans. Sertoli cell activity (Ref: Ganong 22/e p432)

2. **Why do fetal cells continue to divide but terminally differentiated adult cells do NOT divide?** *(AIPG 09)*

Ans. There are many cyclin inhibitors that prevent cells to enter into S phase in adult (Ref: robbins Pathology 7/e p43, 91)

3. **The acrosome reaction occurs when the sperm:** *(KCET 11)*

Ans. Comes in contact with zona pellucida

4. **The male sex hormone testosterone is produced by?** *(KCET 11)*

Ans. Interstitial cells of leydig

EXCRETORY SYSTEM

- Kidney receives approx 25% of cardiac output [Q]
- Fluid entering DCT is always Hypotonic.
- Angiotensin 2 Action:

Increases thirst
Increases ADH secretion
Increases aldosterone.
It is the Most potent vasoconstrictor.

- Free Water Clearance:

Is regulated by ADH.
It is rate at which plasma is cleared of solute free water.

- Clearance greater than GFR of PAH
- Counter Current Multiplier System:

Objective is to produce HYPEROSMOTIC medulla and Primary driving force is reabsorption of Na and Cl ion in thick ascending loop. [Q]

- Function of Macula Densa (Tubulo glomerular feedback):

Macula densa senses change in NaCl concentration.
For autoregulation of GFR.

- Cutaneus shunt vessels:

Plays an important role in thermoregulation. [Q]
Nutritive function in skin is primarily of capillaries not of cutaneus shunts.

LAST 5-YEAR QUESTIONS FROM THIS TOPIC

1. **The tubuloglomerular feedback is mediated by:** *(AIPG 10)*

Ans. Sensing NaCl concentration in the macula densa (Ref: Ganong 22/e p700, 713)

2. **NOT a method of heat loss from body:** *(AIPG 12)*

Ans. Peripheral vasoconstriction (Ref: Ganong 24/e p319)

3. **The quantity of water lost in expired air each 24 hrs is about?** *(KCET 11)*

Ans. 400 ml

4. **Aldosterone secretion is increased when there is a fall in:** *(KCET 12)*

Ans. plasma Na^+

5. **Tubular maximum for glucose is:** *(COMEDK 10)*

Ans. 375 mg/min

CNS

- CSF:

Most of the CSF is formed by choroid plexus. [Q]
ARACHNOID VILLI absorb CSF into the venous sinuses. [Q]
CSF fills ventricle and subarachnoid space.
Volume – 150 ml
Rate of production – 550 ml/day
Chemical composition of CSF: Ph is slightly less than plasma. CSF contains NO neurtrophills. Lymphocyte – 60-70 % Monocyte – 30-50 % Neutrophills – none
CSF has protective function. It supports the brain. The importance of CSF in supporting the brain is illustrated by the pain produced after dural tap. [Q]. Removal of as little as 20 ml of CSF produces intense pain. This is because the brain hangs on the vessels and nerve roots, and traction on them in CSF deficiency stimulates pain fibres.

The pain can be relieved by intrathecal injection of sterile isotonic solution.
Causes of decreased CSF proteins – repeated lumbar puncture, psuedotumor cerebri, traumatic leaks, infants till 1 yr.
Causes of increased CSF proteins – hypothyroidism [Q]

- Crerbral Circulation:

The cerebral blood circulation is AUTOREGULATED and maintained at normal level when a person changes position from standing to lying down and during MODERATE EXERCISE. [Q]
CBF (cerebral blood flow) ∞ pco2 of arterial blood.
No effect of ions(ex- k ion) as they cannot cross BBB.
Positive Gravity (Black Out) - decreased C.O, Decreased Cerebral pressure.
Negative Gravity (Red Out) – Increased C.O, Increased cerebral pressure.

- Sensation transmitted by Posterior/Dorsal column:

Fine touch, fine pressure, vibration,joint pressure sense.

- Sensation transmitted by Antrolateral column/Spinothalmic tract:

Anterior Spinothalmic Tract	Lateral Spinothalmic Tract
Crude Touch, Crude Pressure [Q]	Pain, Temperature [Q]

- Spinocerebellar tract – regulates smooth and coordinated movements. [Q]
- Transection at mid pons level causes – APNEUSIS. [Q]
- PRE – Botzinger Complex:

Is cluster of interneuron in VL medulla
is pacemaker regulating rate of respiration. [Q]

- Regulation of sleep – by 3 important areas of hypothalamus:

• VLPO (ventrolateral preoptic area)
• TMN (tubero mammary neuron)
• SCN (suprachiasmatic nucleus) – maintain circadian sleep rhythm.

- Nrem and Rem Sleeps and Different Waves:

Different waves: order of frequency = TRICK: BAT – Dance B > α > theta > delta waves.
Stages of NREM sleep: Stage 1 – just as falling asleep – alpha rhythm. Stage 2 – unequivocal sleep – theta waves interspersed with sleep spindles and K complexes. [Q] Stage 3 – deep sleep [Q] – Theta waves - delta waves first appear. Stage 4 – very deep sleep – delta waves. [Q].
So DELTA waves are seen in DEEP and VERY DEEP SLEEP. [Q]
REM sleep – Dreaming, night mares, muscle atony [Q].

- Short term memory converted in HIPPOCAMPUS to long term memory and stored in Neocortex.
- Antegrade amnesia – lesion in hippocampus can lead to antegrade amnesia.

- Mechanism of Hearing and Memory:

Changes in the level of neurotransmitter of synapse.
Spatial reorganisation in synapse.
Increasing protein synthesis.
It does not depend on recruitment by multiplication of neurons.[Q]

- Memory:

• Immedite memory – seconds to minutes
• Recent memory – minutes to week upto month.[Q]
• Remote memory – month to years.

- Papez Cercuit – Concerned with expression of emotion.
- Nucleus – Anterior nucleus of thalamus. [Q]
  Connects limbic system to hypothalamus.
- Limbic System:

What consists of limbic system? Trick – CASH C – Cingulate gyrus A – Amygdala S – Septal nuclei H – Hippocampus formation.

- Transmission of signal through direct contact gap junction does not pass through ECF. [Q].
- Reflex:

Withdrawl reflex – 1st reflex to appear as spinal shock wears off in humans.
Withdrawl reflex is a polysynaptic reflex.
Monosynaptic reflex – ex: stretch reflex, knee jerk reflex.

- Substance P:

Is a neuropeptide.
It is present in nerve terminal.
Principle chemical mediator of pain impulse from peripheral nervous system to CNS.

- Weber – Fechner Law:

Interpreted signal strength is log of intensity of stimulus. [Q]

- Nerve Growth Factor:

Inhibits apoptosis in memory B cell. [Q], neurons and keratinocytes by preventing cyt C release, Bcl-2 protein phosphorylation and inactivation of p38.

- NOTE – Cortical representation of body in cerebrum is VERTICAL. [Q]

- Presynaptic Inhibition:

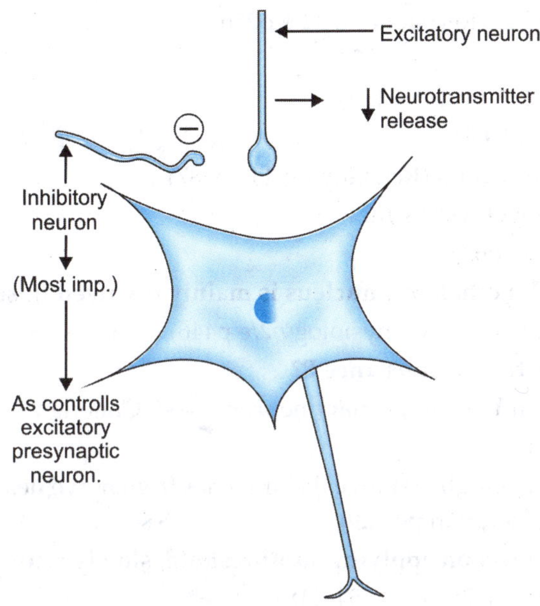

Fig. 15.3: Presynaptic inhibition

Inhibitory neuron produces inhibitory neurotransmitter (GABA) and inhibits the excitatory neuron with decrease in action potential at presynaptic nerve terminal which in turn decreases Ca ion entry and DECREASES THE AMOUNT OF NT (neurotransmitter) released. [Q]

- RODS and CONES:

There is no difference in their signal transduction.

- RESTING tremor – is seen in lesion of BASAL ganglion like like Parkinsonism NOT in cerebellar lesion (intentional tremor). [Q].
- Hyperkinetic features of HUNTINGTONS and PARKINSON'S disease:

Huntingtons – due to loss of GABA-ergic and cholinergic system.
Parkinson - due to loss of NIGROSTRIATAL dopaminergic system.

LAST 5-YEAR QUESTIONS FROM THIS TOPIC

1. The conversion of short term memory to long term memory is done in: *(AIIMS may 10, AIPG 10)*

Ans. Hippocampus (Ref: Guyton 11/e p723 – 726)

2. The mechanism of hearing and memory includes all EXCEPT: *(AIIMS may 10)*

a. Changes in level of neurotransmitter at synapse
b. Increasing protein synthesis
c. Recruitment by multiplication of neurons
d. Spatial reorganisation of synapse

Ans. c (Ref: Ganong 22/e p259 – 270)

3. Lesions of lateral cerebellum causes all of the following, EXCEPT: *(AIIMS Nov. 10)*

a. Incoordination
b. Intention tremor
c. Resting tremor
d. Ataxia

Ans. c (Ref: sembulingam 2/e p680)

4. The nucleus involved in the Papez circuit is: *(AIIMS may 10)*

Ans. Anterior nucleus of thalamus (Ref: Ganong 22/e p256

5. Delta waves are seen in: *(AIIMS may 10)*

Ans. Deep sleep (Ref: Ganong 22nd pg 195 – 196)

6. Broca's area: (AIIMS may 10, 09)

Ans. Is concerned with word formation (Ref: Guyton 11/e p687)

7. Transaction at mid pons level results in: *(AIIMS Nov. 10)*

Ans. Apneusis (Ref: Ganong 23/e p673)

8. Which of the following Hypothalamic nucleus is mainly involved in secretion of ADH? *(AIPG 11)*

Ans. Supraoptic (Ref: chowdhary. human physiology 2/e p446)

9. Which of the following is true of substance P? *(AIPG 11)*

Ans. It mainly mediates pain sensation at primary neurons. (Ref: Ganong 22/e p11)

10. Synaptic stripping: *(AIPG 10)*

Ans. Is that post inflammation microglia remove the branches from nerve near the damaged tissue (Ref: Geuna. Peripheral Nerve and Regeneration pg 429)

11. Increase in the threshold level on applying subthreshold, slowly rising stimulus is known as: *(AIPG 09)*

Ans. Accommodation (Ref: Ganong 20/e p53 – 54, 118)

12. Which of the following cranial nerve is likely to be damaged if direct / consensual light reflex are absent: *(AIIMS Nov. 12)*

Ans. Occulomotor (Ref: Guyton 11/e p649)

13. All of the following features are seen in cerebral dysfunction EXCEPT: *(KCET 09)*

a. Static tremor
b. Dysmetria
c. Scanning speech
d. Rebound phenomenon

Ans. a

14. Axon hillock is a part of the soma of neuron which: *(COMEDK 09)*

Ans. Has no nissl granules

15. Which of the following fibres are responsible for conduction of pain impulse: *(COMEDK 09)*

Ans. A delta

16. The absolute refractory period of an action potential is due to: *(COMEDK 09)*

Ans. Voltage inactivation of Na^+ - K^+ ATPase

17. In a nerve, the magnitude of the action potential overshoot is normally a function of the: *(COMEDK 11)*

Ans. Extracellular sodium concentration

18. Example of rapidly acting neurotransmitter is: *(KCET 10)*

Ans. Glycine

19. Which cells form the myelin sheath in the CNS? *(KCET 10)*

Ans. Oligodendrocytes

20. The contribution of operation of sodium – potassium electrogenic pump for the development of net – 90 millivot of resting membrane potential is: *(KCET 10)*

Ans. -4 millivolt

21. Epicritic perception of pain occurs at the level of: *(COMEDK 10)*

Ans. Area 3, 1,2

22. **Which of the following is used to measure pain intensity?** *(COMEDK 09)*

Ans. Visual analog scale

23. **Sudden loud sound is more likely to damage the chochlea than prolonged sounds because:** *(COMEDK 10)*

Ans. There is a latent period before the attenuation reflex can occur

24. **Which of the following is true regarding electric transduction of visual cycle?** *(AIIMS may 11)*

Ans. Hyperpolarisation (Ref: puri. textbook of medical biochemistry 3/e p392)

25. **The condition in which the person can see near objects but not the far objects is?** *(KCET 11)*

Ans. Myopia

26. **Which of the following events DO NOT occur in rods in response to light:** *(COMEDK 09)*

Ans. Opening of Na^+ Channels

ENDOCRINE SYSTEM

- Different receptors for hormones: [IMP.]

Mechanism and site	Hormone
A. At nuclear membrane →	Thyroid hormones
B. Cytoplasmic receptor →	Steroidal hormones e.g - glucocorticoid, mineralocorticoids, estrogen, progesterone.
So, intracellular receptors(transcriptional factor) are for thyroxine and steroidal hormones.	
C. Cell membrane receptors	
Tyrosine protein kinase →	Insulin, GH,IGF
Through IP3/DAG →	VASOPRESSIN, OXYTOCIN
Throgh cAMP →	Ant. Pituitary hormones(TSH,FSH,LH,PTH,ACTH), Adrenaline,glucagon
Through cGMP →	NO, ANF

- Mineralocorticoid receptors present everywhere except – LIVER.
- Catecholamine receptor:

Act through G protein coupled receptor (cAMP) which belong to super family of 7 pass transmembrane protein.

- Somatomedins:

Somatomedins are IGF (insulin- like growth factor) – have potent effect of increasing all aspects of bone growth.
Deposits chondroitin sulphate in cartilage. [Q]

- Insulin and Growth Hormone:

ACTION: GH – Na retention, decreased insulin sensitivity, lipolysis, protein synthesis, epiphyseal growth. IGF – insulin like activity, antilipolytic activity, protein synthesis, epiphyseal growth.

- Effect of hormones on insulin secretion:

All intestinal hormones stimulate insulin secretion.
Epinephrine – Net effect is INHIBITION of insulin secretion.[Q]

- Effect of insulin:

Increased glycogen synthesis
increase protein synthesis
increased lipogenesis
increased glycogen synthesis and increased glycolysis
decreased glucose output due to decreased gluconeogenesis
insulin prevents KETOGENESIS [Q]

- Estrogen, Progesteron, Insulin:

Estrogen promotes insulin dependent metabolic process while progesterone has opposite effect.

- Cacitonin:

Decreases serum Ca level by • Promoting bone absorption of Ca. • Promoting excretion of calcium. (Just opposite of PTH)
USE – Pagets, post menopausal osteoporosis.

LAST 5-YEAR QUESTIONS FROM THIS TOPIC

1. **All of the following are cause of adrenal deficiency EXCEPT:** *(AIPG 10)*
   a. Hypoglycaemia
   b. Hypocalcaemia
   c. Hypotension
   d. Hyponatraemia

Ans. b (Ref: Harrison 15/e p2009)

2. **All of the following use only c AMP as 2nd messenger, EXCEPT:** *(AIIMS Nov. 10)*
   a. Corticotrophin
   b. Dopamine
   c. Glucagon
   d. Vasopressin

Ans. d (Ref: norman and Litwack. Hormones, p124)

3. **Somatomedin mediates:** *(AIPG 11)*

Ans. The deposition of chondroitin sulphate (Ref: Ganong's 23/e p382)

4. **Glucose transporter in myocyte stimulated by insulin is:** *(AIIMS Nov. 10)*

Ans. GLUT – 4 (Ref: Champe. biochemistry, p95)

5. **Which of the following is NOT an endocrinal gland?** *(AIPG 12)*

Ans. Thymus (Ref: Ganong 24/e p323)

6. **Which of the following does NOT have a corresponding releasing hormone from hypothalamus?** *(AIPG 11)*
   a. FSH
   b. TSH
   c. ACTH
   d. Prolactin

Ans. d (Ref: Ganong 21/e p251)

7. **FSH, LH and TSH acts through which mechanism?** *(AIPG 10)*

Ans. Cyclic AMP (Ref: satyanarayan 2/e p471)

8. **Which is seen in acromegaly?** *(AIPG 09)*

Ans. Large tongue (Ref: Woolf. Pathology: Basic and Systemic pg 830)

9. **A patient with type 1 diabetes mellitus has a deficiency of insulin. Which cells secrete insulin?** *(KCET 12)*

Ans. B cells of pancreatic islets

10. **Parathormone in normal parathyroid gland is secreted by:** *(PGI Dec 11, COMEDK 10)*

Ans. Chief cells (Ref: Ganong 22/e p390)

11. **A positive chvostek's sign is suggestive of:** *(COMEDK 11)*

Ans. hypocalcaemia

12. **Parathyroid hormone:** *(KCET 11)*

Ans. Stimulates bone resorption

13. **Which of the following influence the ability of osteoclast to resorb bone matrix:** *(KCET 10)*

Ans. Cathepsin K and carbonic anhydrase

14. **Ultimobronchial body forms:** *(COMEDK 11)*

Ans. " C" cells of thyroid gland

15. **All the following hormones bind to cell surface receptors of the target tissue EXCEPT:** *(COMEDK 11)*
    a. TSH
    b. Glucagon
    c. Estrogen
    d. Epinephrine

Ans. c

MISCELLANEOUS

- BONE:

YOLK SAC, LIVER, SPLEEN – produces RBC prenatally.
From birth to 20 yrs both flat and long bone produces RBC.
After 20 yrs only FLAT bones produce RBC.

- Muscle spindLe and Golgi tendon:

Muscle spindLe – detects rate of change in muscle Length. [Q] Causes contraction of muscle by stimulating α – MOTOR NEURON. Muscle spindle acts through stretch reflex.
Golgi Tendon – Tension [Q] Causes relaxation of muscle by inhibiting α – MOTOR NEURON.Acts through inverse stretch reflex/autogenic inhibition/lengthening mechanism

- Reciprocal Innervation:

Relaxation of ANTAGONISTIC muscle when stretch reflex occur.
GOLGI BOTTLE NEURON(inhibitory interneuron) are involved.

- Isometric vs isotonic exercise:

In ISOMETRIC EXERCISE	ISOTONIC EXERCISE
Vascular resistance remains unchanged.(as length of vascular muscle fibre is constant)	Vascular resistance decreases.

- Addition of a.a (amino acid) in diet of a seriously ill patient:

Stimulate insulin release which has anabolic effect on metabolism.
It prevents breakdown of protein and also brings about protein synthesis.

KININ + PROSTACYCLINE – VASODILATOR
ENDOTHELIN – VASOCONSTRICTION.
BUT ALL are BRONCHOCONSTRICTOR.

- In myopathy and mysthenia gravis – small short duration polyphasic action potential seen.

LAST 5-YEAR QUESTIONS FROM THIS TOPIC

1. **Granularity of oncocytes is due to:** *(PGI June 11)*

Ans. Increase in number of mitochondria

2. **The site of RBC formation in a 20 year old healthy male is:** *(AIIMS May 10, AIPG 10)*

Ans. Flat bones (Ref: Guyton 11/e p420)

3. **Muscle spindle detects:** *(AIIMS May 11)*

Ans. Length (Ref: Ganong 22/e p130 – 134)

4. **Which of the following is true regarding the golgi tendon organ?** *(AIPG 09)*

Ans. It senses muscle tension

5. **True about recruitment and derecruitment of motor unit of muscles during increase and decrease of muscle force is?** *(AIPG 12)*

Ans. Motor unit recruited last is derecruited 1st (Ref: Ganong 24/e p109)

6. **Muscle spindles are present in striated muscle. The tension occurs after the stimulus of?** *(AIPG 12)*

Ans. Gamma fibers (Ref: Ganong 24/e p229 – 230)

7. **Decreased BMR is seen in:** *(AIPG 11)*

Ans. Obesity (Ref: Ganong 23/e p462)

8. **In an obese person, BMI is:** *(AIPG 09)*

Ans. > 30)

9. **Genes for sex determination is:** *(AIPG 10)*

Ans. SRY (Ref: Ganong 22/e p411 – 412)

10. **Which of the following is a vasodilator?** *(KCET 11)*

Ans. Bradykinin

11. **Contraction in smooth muscle is initiated when calcium binds to:** *(COMEDK 11)*

Ans. Calmodulin

CHAPTER

16 Pharmacology

Topic

- General Pharmacology
- Blood
- CVS and Respiratory System
- NSAIDS and Opiods
- CNS and PNS
- Chemotherapeutic Agents
- Endocrinology and Miscellaneous

GENERAL PHARMACOLOGY

- Zero order kinetics (Saturation kinetics):

Seen with–Trick–WATT
W–Warfarin
A–Alcohol + Antiepileptics (pheyntoin) + Aspirin
T–Tolbutamide
T–Theophylline

- Drugs undergoing high 1st pass metabolism:

TRICK: VP Singh Not Popular PM

V → Verapamil
P → Propanolol
Singh → Salbutamol
Not → Nitroglycerine
Popular → Propoxyphene
P → Pethidine
M → Morphine + methyltestesterone

- Hepatic Enzyme Inducer:

H–Habits (alcohol, cigarette, chloral hydrate, charcoal)
E–Epileptic drugs (Phenytoin, phenobarbitone, CMZ, Primidone)
I–INH, Rifampicin + Tetracycline + Chloramphenicol
NB: Amongst Antifungal drugs–Azoles are also Hepatic E. Inhibitor.

- Drugs causing hyperkalemia (Trick) K+ bank

K^+–Potassium sparing diuretics B–B blocker A–ACE inhibitors + Heparin and Cyclosporine N–NSAID's K–K^+ supplements

- List of prodrugs:

ACE inhibitors (except captopril and Lisinopril) Levodopa Ticlopidine Clopidogrel Mycophenolate Moftil INH Oxcarbamazipine Chloral hydrate Methyldopa etc.

- Drugs causing constipation:

$Al(OH)_3$, $CaCO_3$, $FeSO_4$ Opioids Phenothiazine (typical antipsychotic) TCA Verapamil [Q] NB: Mg → Diarrhea

- Drugs Acetylated: Trick–SHIP

S–Sulfohamides H–Hydralazine I–INH P–PAS (Para amino sulphuric acid)

- Drugs induced hirsutism:

Androgenic Drugs	Non-Androgenic Drugs
• Androgenic progestines (Norethisterone) (Danazol) [Q]	• Phenytoin [Q]
• Acetazolamide	• Minoxidil (Vasodilator)
• Anabolic steroids	• Cyclosporine
• Testesterone	

- Drugs causing gynaecomastia: Trick "disco"

D–Digoxin
I–INH
S–Spironolactone
C–Cimetidine + Clomephene Citrate
O–Oestrogen

- ED (Effective dose)/Potency vs efficacy

ED α Potency because (NEET-2013) Potency α dose dependent α ED
Efficacy is response related (maximum effects of a drug)

- Drug Affinity → Concentration of drug
- Drug specificity → Related to side effect of the drug
- Therapeutic index is used to assess drug Safety [Q]
- Drugs causing disulfuram like reaction: Trick: MSC (PMT)

M–**M**etronidazole
S–**S**ulfonamides
C–**C**ephalosporin (**C**efo**P**erazone, **C**efo**M**andole, **C**efo**T**etan)

- Causes of Drug induced aplastic anaemia:

  - Antibiotics–Chlormphenicol [Q]
  - NSAID's–Phenlybutazone [Q]
  - Antithyroid–Carbimazole, Methimazole
  - Antipsychotic–Chlorpromazine
  - Anticonvulsant–Phenytoin, CMZ, Valproate.
  - Cytotoxic drugs–Methotrexate, Vincristin

- Drugs causing HTN:

  - Cyclosporine → because ↓cytokinine (Vasodilators) release → so, vasoconstriction [Q]
  - Cocaine
  - NSAID [Q] → ↓Ses release of inflammatory mediators → ↓Vasodilatation
  - Erythropoietin [Q]
  - MAO inhibitors
  - TCA
  - Sympathomimetics

- Teratogenic drugs:

• Isotretinoin–Deafness, Cleft lip and palate, neural tube defect
• Lithium–Ebstein (Congenital) Anomaly
• Alcohol–Fetal alcohol syndrome
• Phenytoin–Fetal hydantoin syndrome (Microcephaly, cleftlip and palate)
• Warfarin–Craniofacial abnormality
• Barbiturates–Congenital Heart disease, cleft lip and palate
• Thalidomide–Phocomelia
• Valproate–Neural tube defect.
• Indomethacin–Premature closure of ductus arteriosus.

- Drugs that should be stopped before surgery:

• Lithium
• OCP (causes DVT)
• Aspirin
• Warfarin
• Oral hypoglycemic especially metformin (causes post of lactic acidosis) [Q]

- Drugs causing prolonged QT interval/Torsades de points:

Cisapride
Amiodarone
Amitryptylin (TCA)
Haloperidol
Terfenadine (2nd generation Anti histaminics), Erythromycin

- Drugs causing hepatic damage:

Granuloma (Hepatic) ↓ Allopurinol	Fatty liver ↓ Tetracyclin	Necrosis ↓ Paracetamol

- Luminal effect:

Absorption of drug affected by concurrently ingested drug e.g. tetracycline + Fe
Gut wall effect: drug can alter absorption by either altering motility (Anticholinergics, TCA, opioids and metoclopramide)/ Causing mucosal damage with neomycin, methotrexate and vinblastine

LAST 5-YEAR QUESTIONS FROM THIS TOPIC

1. **Drugs exhibit Ist pass metabolism are all except:** *(KCET 09)*
   a. Morphine
   b. Nitroglycerine
   c. Propanolol
   d. Salicylate

Ans. d

2. **Which among the following drugs is not used orally?** *(COMEDK 11)*
   a. Quinidine
   b. Verapamil
   c. Lignocaine
   d. Phenytoin

Ans. c (Ref: KDT 5/e p476)

3. **Which is not a prodrug:** *(AIPG 11, 10, 09)*
   a. Quinapril
   b. Fosinopril
   c. Benzopril
   d. Lisinopril

Ans. d (Ref: Satoskar 21/e p417)

Note: Also captopril

4. **Time required for a drug to reduce by 50% after termination of infusion is called:** *(AIPG 11)*

Ans. Context sensitive half life

5. **The following statements are true about i.v. route of drug administration except:**
   a. It is useful in emergencies
   b. Aseptic precautions are required
   c. Bioavailability is 100%
   d. Suspensions can be administered

Ans. d

6. **Loading dose depends upon:** *(NEET 13, AIPG 09, 10)*

Ans. Volume of distribution (Ref: KDT 6/e p34)

7. **Cross resistance of isoniazide is seen with** *(AIPG 10, 09)*

Ans. Ethionamide (Ref: Antimicrobial agents by bryskir I/e p111)

8. **Transient memory impairment can be caused by use of:** *(AIPG 10)*

Ans. INH

9. **Which of these drugs is Not acetylated:** *(AIPG 10, 09, AIIMS May 09)*
   a INH

b. Hydralazine
c. Dapsone
d. Metoclopramide

Ans. d (Ref: KDT 6/e p644)
Trick: SHIP
S–Sulphonamide, H–Hydralazine, I–INH, P–PAS

10. While prescribing a drug, The term "HS" indicates: *(AIPG 12)*

Ans. Taken at time of retiring (Ref: Ghom 2005, p74)

11. Sialogogue is: *(AIPG 12)*

Ans. Increases flow of saliva

12. Prolonged administration of INH causes deficiency of:

Ans. Thiamine

13. All of the following drugs causing SLE/SLE like reaction except: *(AIPG 12)*

a Isoniazid
b. Sulphonamide
c. Hydralazine
d. Penicillin

Ans. d

14. Which is a prodrug? *(AIIMS Nov 10. 09)*

Ans. Enalapril (Ref: KDT 6/e p23-24)

BLOOD

- Heparin:

A mucopolysaccharide
Acid (strongest organic acid present in the body)
Actions: • Anticoagulant action → By activating AT III (Antithromobin III) • Antiplatelet action → At higher doses → Inhibits platelet aggregation and prolongs B.T. (T/t-Lepirudin) • Lipemia clearing → Releases Lipoprotein lipase from the vessel wall
P/K: Doesn't cross BBB and placenta (Non teratogenic → Anticoagulant of choice during pregnancy [Q]
A/E: Bleeding, Thrombocytopenia, Alopecia, Osteoporosis
Inhibited by protamine sulfate → So, used in treating heparin Overdose [Q] *(AIIMS Nov. 10)*

- HIT (Heparin induced thrombocytopenia):

Is an important complication after heparin administration.
T/t: Lepirudin, Argobatran, Danaparoid, are the recommended alternative anticoagulant for patient with HIT.

- Drugs causing hemolytic anemia in G6PD deficiency/contraindicated in:

• Antimalarial • Sulfonamides (Dapsone, Cotrimoxazole) • Chlormphenicol • Analgesics (Aspirin) • Naldixic acid [Q] • Nitrofurantoin (ex-furazolidone) • Quinidine

- Management of bleeding due to over anticoagulation:

Guided by clinical feature and PT
PT is expressed as INR
INR–2–4.5 → Normal therapeutic range. INR–4.5-7 → Managed by withholding warfarin for 1-2 days and then reviewing the INR INR– > 7 → Withhold warfarin and give phytonadione but without bleeding 5 mg by slow i.v. infusion.
Bleeding threatening • Blood replacement • Reversal of anticoagulation: For rapid reversal–PT complex concentrate For Full reversal → Phytonadione

- Effect of oral anticoagulant during pregnancy:

↓ Sed effect seen as ↑sed clotting factor synthesis during pregnancy

- Tranexamic acid is a Antifrinolytic
- Vit K:

3 Forms of vit K are available for therapeutic use: Phytonadione, Menadione, Menaquinone.
To reverse the effect of overdose of oral anticoagulant phytonadione is the preparation of choice because its acts most rapidly.

- Warfarin:

It acts by inhibiting vit K dependent coagulation factor.

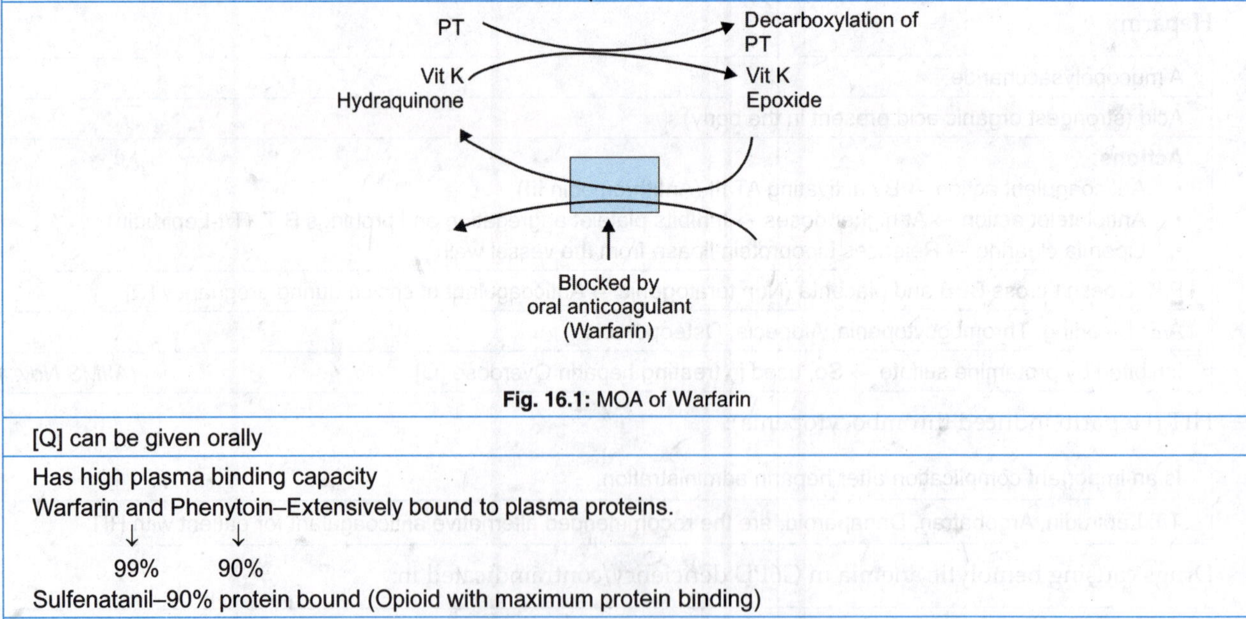

Fig. 16.1: MOA of Warfarin

[Q] can be given orally
Has high plasma binding capacity Warfarin and Phenytoin–Extensively bound to plasma proteins. ↓ 99% ↓ 90% Sulfenatanil–90% protein bound (Opioid with maximum protein binding)
Is added in rodenticide

- Drugs interacting with Warfarin: Trick "Academics" [Q]

A–Aspirin (or other NSAID's) → ↑ses P.T.
C–Cimetidine + Ciprofloxacillin → ↑ses P.T.
A–Aminodarone, Azaprazone → ↑ses P.T.

D–Dapsone → Ses P.T.	
E–Erythromycin → ↑ses P.T.	
M–Metronidazole → ↑ses P.T.	
I–Indomethacin → ↑ses P.T.	
C–Clofibrate + Other Hypolipidemics Ex-statins + Cholestyramine ses P.T. + Hepatic enzyme inducer	↓sec P.T.

- Drug Interaction of Pyridoxine

- Peripheral neuritis caused by INH can be reversed by pyridoxine [Q]
- Arachidonic acid pathway:

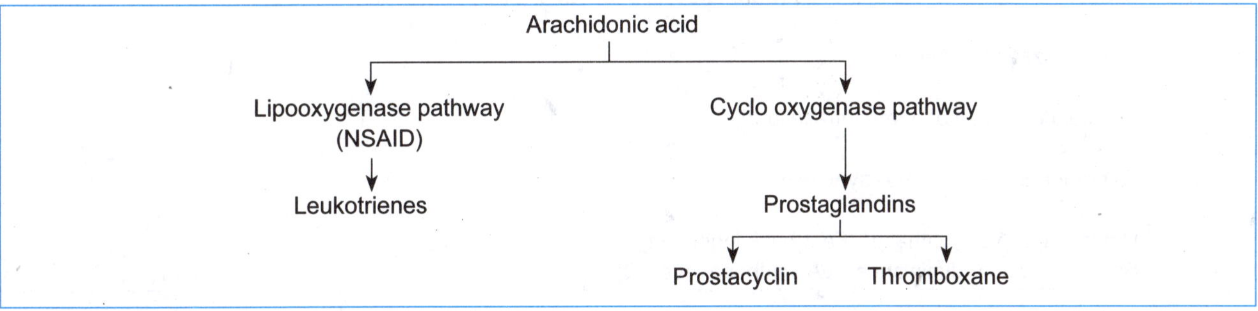

- Function of COX are:

- Antiplatelet drugs: Used in arterial thrombosis prophylaxis.

Salicylates	Anti ADP receptor on Platelet	GP II b/ III a receptor antagonist
TXA_2+COX Inhibitor	Clopidogrel	Trick–EAT E–Eptifibatide A–Abciximab T–Tirofiban
	Ticlodepine (Prodrug)	

- **Note:** (Triflusal–Antiplatelet drug)
- Nitrates:

• Relaxes all types of smooth muscle. The most prominent action is on the vascular smooth muscle.

• Nitrates are used in cyanide poisoning – Hb + Nitrates → Metahaemoglobin – Methamoglobin has a very high affinity for CN⁻and combines to form cyanomethaemoglobin → which is rapidly excreted from the body.

- Drug causes methaemoglobinemia:

N_2 drugs, LA + Sulfonamides
In methaemoglobinemia → Oxygen dissociation curve shifts towards left by remaining normal Hb [Q]

- Acute intermittent porphyria:

• Group of disease in which derangement of synthesis of heme occurs.
• ALA (Aminolevulonic acid → Immediate precursor of heme ↑ ALA synthase
• Drugs like hepatic enzyme induce (Barbiturates, phenytoin, CBZ) ↓ ↑Ses utilization of heme ↓ ↓se concentration of heme intracelluarly ↓ To compensate ↑sed ALA synthesis ↓ Diminishes "ALA synthase" (Feedback inhibition) So, H.E. inducer diminishes ALA synthase level [Q]

LAST 5-YEAR QUESTIONS FROM THIS TOPIC

1. **Which of the following is preferred in an elderly women having macrocytic anemia with early signs of neurological deficit:** *(KCET 10)*

Ans. Hydroxycobalamine

2. **Nitrates are not used in:** *(AIPG 11)*

Ans. Renal colic (Ref: KDT 6/e p524-530)

3. **Drug binds to activate the receptor in same fashion which directly/indirectly brings effect is:** *(AIIMS Nov 12)*

Ans. Agonist (Ref: KDT 6/e p41)

4. **Filgastrin is:** *(AIPG 10)*

Ans. Used in neutropenia

CVS AND RESPIRATORY SYSTEM

- Antiarrythmic Drugs:

Classification: MBA college M–Membrane stabilizing (Class I) B–B- blocker (class–II) A–Action potential widening agent College–Calcium Channel blocker.
Membrane stabilizer (class-I) Ex-Quinidine, Lignocaine, Phenytoin, Propafenone.

Drugs used for supra ventricular arrhythmia: ABCO A–Adenosine B–B-blocker C–CCB ex-verapamil D–Digoxin
Drugs for ventricular arrythmia–Lignocaine (No effect on SA node, AV node)
Drugs for both supra ventricular and ventricular arrhythmic Quinidine, procainamide, propafenone,
Aminodarone • ↑ses C.O. (Cardiac output) → systolic B.P. no effect on diastolic B.P • Maintains tissue perfusion → used in shock → Class I → Amiodarone: is the drug with prominent action. A–Antiarrythmis M–Multiple actions i.e, block K+, Na+, Ca+ channel and B-receptor I–Iodine containing (so may interfere with thyroid function) O–Orally used mainly D–Duration of action is very long A–ADP (Action Potential duration) and ERP (effective refractory period increases AF, VT and Recurrent VF O–on i.v injection myocardial depression and B.P. ↓ses. On prolonged use–Pulmonary fibrosis. N–Neuropathy E–Eye: Corneal microdeposits may occur. Photosensitization + Dry Cough (Not productive cough)

- ACE inhibitors:

• Severe hypotension may results in patients taking diuretics so omission of prior diuretic dose may reduce postural HTN [Q]
• ACE inhibitors should be given to all patients with impaired left ventricular systolic dysfunction.
• Reduces overall mortality in MI.
• ACE I in chronic renal failure–Delays the progression of renal disease
Diabetic Nephropathy → Prevent end stage renal failure in type I and Type II DM
A/E of ACEI: Hypotension–Ist dose hypotension
Enalapril → use mainly for hypertensive emergency
→ t½ life of warfarin–36–48 hrs. [Q]

GTN → Venodilator > Arterial dilator Hydralazine → On arteriole

- Hydralazine + Nifedepine → Arteriodilator
- Nitrates–Venodilator > Arteriolar
- Sodium Nitroprusside–Both Arteriolar and Venodilator
- Drugs given during hypertensive pregnancy:

Better–B-blocker Mother–Methyl dopa (D.O.C.) Care–Clonidine During–Disophyridine CCB (Nifedipine) Hypertensive–Hydralazine (D.O.C. in hypertensive pregnancy) Pregnancy–Prazosin NB: ACE inhibitors are absolutely C/I in pregnancy.

- Verapamil vs Nifedepine:

Verapamil	Nifedepine
Cause vasodilation as well as marked Cardiac depression	Marked vasodilatation and direct depression of heart is minimal
Marked Bradycardia A-V block, Cardiac arrest And hypotension	Reflex tachycardia by reflex sympathetic Stimulation
May worsen heart failure	Aggravates MI due to reduced coronary Flow.
	Rapid and short acting. So, used in hypertensive Emergency.
	Worsens angina
	Replaced by slow and long acting Amlodipine

- **Note:** Nimodipine relaxes cerebral vasculature used in subarachnoid hemorrhage
- Digoxin vs Digitoxin

Digoxin	Digitoxin
Highly polar so excreted Unchanged through kidney So, toxicity precipitated by renal failure	Hepatic metabolism seen as most lipid soluble. So, Toxicity precipitated by liver failure.

- Interaction of digoxin:

Quindine, Thiazide, CCB (Verapamil, Deltiazem), B-blocker, cholestyramine

- Drugs which increase No: N_2 drugs (GTN, Na nitroprusside), hydralazine
- In case of renal failure, the clearance of calcium channel blockers (CCBs) is not affected by heamodialysis (AIIMS Q)
- Anti IgE antibody:

"Omalizumab" [Q]
used for asthma

LAST 5-YEAR QUESTIONS FROM THIS TOPIC

1 **Which one of the following is Not true of ACE inhibitor?** *(KCET 09)*

a. May cause Hyperkalemia in diabetic patient
b. Contraindicated in pregnancy
c. Contraindicated in diabetic nephropathy
d. NSAIDS may impair its hypotensive effect

Ans. c (Ref: Goodman and Gillman 11/e p415)

2. **Most common oral change in patients on CCB is:**

Ans. Gingival enlargement

3. **Felypressin is:** *(KCET 11)*

Ans. Vasoconstrictor, predominant effect on venous system (Ref: Malamed's LA 5/e p52)

4. **True about ACE inhibitor:** *(AIPG 11)*

a Adverse effect is hypokalemia
b. Secondary hyperaldosterism and K+ loss due to diuretics
c. Rebound hypertension on withdrawal
d. Used safely in asthmatics

Ans. d (Ref: Goodman and Gillman 11/e p415)

5. **Which of the following is not used in heart failure** *(AIPG 11)*

Ans. Trimetazidine (Ref: Harrison 7/e p227.4 table)

Note: Trimetazidine is an antianginal drug

6. Drug most commonly used to treat hypertensive crisis is *(AIIMS Nov 12)*

Ans. Sodium Nitroprusside (Ref: KDT 6/e p554)

NSAID'S AND OPIODS

- Aspirin: Pharmacological actions

• As analgesic–300-600 mg • Anti inflammatory dose–3-5g Irreversible inhibition of COX at this dose • In MI–60-100 mg → Reduces the incidence of MI by inhibiting platelet aggregation – Aspirin is C/I in pregnancy because → delay labor, crosses placenta, premature closure of PDA – Aspirin on prolonged use causes ↓sed synthesis of clotting factors hypoprothombinemia
Duration of action of aspirin depends on fresh newly synthesized platelets/Cyclo oxygenase

- NSAID:

• Oxicams → Enterohepatic circulation → long duration of action (piroxicam, meloxicam)
• Acute Gout → Strong anti inflammatory NSAID's Ex-indomethacin, piroxicam
• Nimesulide → is a safe NSAID that can be given to asthmatics (Preferential COX-2 inhibitor)

- Opioid withdrawl:

Symptoms are:
Lacrimation
Sweating
Mydriasis
Diarrhoea + weight loss → Opposite to morphine effects

- Pharmacological actions of Morphine:

  - CNS → Analgesia + sedation + Euphoria + Respiratory depression + suppression of cough+ Nausea and Vomiting
  - CVS → Vasodilatation
  - GIT → Constipation
  - Biliary colic
  - Bronchoconstriction
  - Urinary urgency + difficulty in micturition

- Morphine:

  - ↓ses pulmonary congestion so used in left ventricular failure
  - As bronchoconstrictor → So. C/I in Asthma

- NSAID's: phenylbutazone causes → Marked agranulocytosis (Banned)
- Piroxicam: only NSAID's undergoing enterohepatic circulation [Q]
- Drugs acting on Opioid receptors:

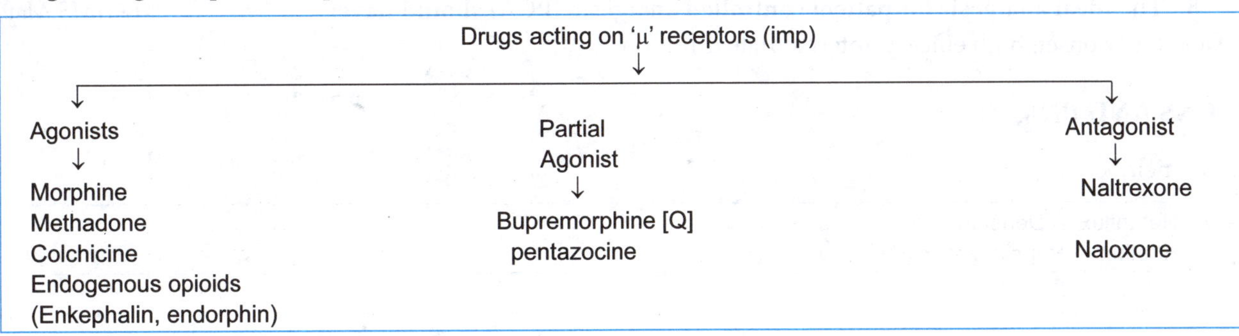

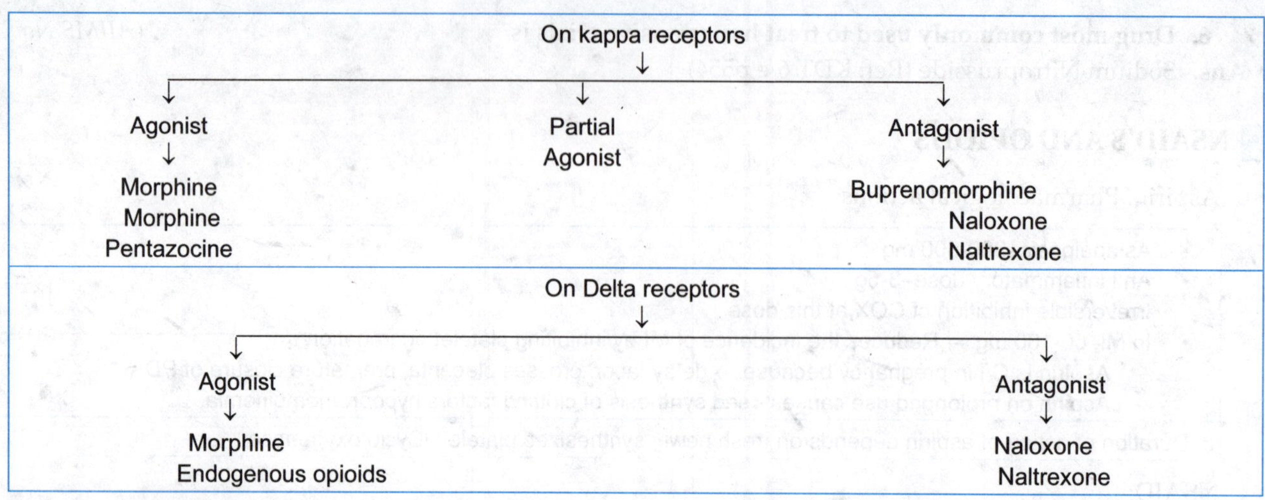

- Opioid antagonist:

Naloxone	Naltrexone	Nalfemine
Oral bioavailability Low (Short D.O.A.) ↓ So used for opioid induced Constipation	Long D.O.A ↓ Used in Alcohol withdrawal	Long D.O.A. ↓ Used in alcohol withdrawal

- (D.O.A = Duration of action)
- Opioid withdrawal is Not precipitated as low oral bioavailability

QUESTIONS FROM THIS TOPIC IN LAST 5 YEARS

1. **All of the following statements about ketorolac are incorrect except:** *(KCET 10)*
   a An effective analgesic for mild to moderate post operative dental pain
   b. Like morphine it interacts with opioid receptors
   c. Administered only by i.v. route
   d. Safe even in chronic use

Ans. a

2. **Which of the following drugs is better analgesic for patient who is undergoing orthodontic tooth movement?** *(KCET 11)*

Ans. Acetaminophen (Ref: Profit p281)

3. **Most important factor for calculating dose for NSAIDS in children?** *(NEET 13, AIPG 11, 09)*

Ans. Body weight of child (Ref: KDT 5/e p52-53)

4. **Which NSAIDS shows enterohepatic cycling:** *(AIPG 10)*

Ans. Piroxicam

5. **The ideal analgesic for patient controlled analgesia (PCA) should have:** *(AIIMS May 11)*

Ans. Early onset, high efficacy, intermediate duration

CNS AND PNS

- Remember:

Na^+ Influx → Depolarizaton K^+ eflux → Repolarization [Q]

- Status epilepticus:

Drugs used–1°–Diazepam, Clonazepam
2°–Phenytoin, Phenobarbitone, Thiopentone sodium (GA) Not CMZ (Carbamazepine)

- Antiepileptics: A/E of valproate: (Trick) is valproate

V–Vomiting
A–Alopecia
L–Liver toxicity (Idiosyncratic Reaction)
P–Pancreatitis (rare)
R–Rashes
O–Oedema (weight gain) [Q] (topiramate causes weight Loss)
A–Ataxia
T–Teratogenic (neural tube defect)
E

- Antiepileptics associated with interference of folate leads to megaloblastic absorption: Trick–3P's

3P–Phenytoin, Phenobarbitone, Primidone [Q]

- Sodium Valproate:

Under antiepileptic drugs → As sodium valproate acts by all 3 mechanism so it interacts with phenobartibone, Diazepam (GABA cl^-) and Phenytoin (Na^+ Channel) and may precipitate absence seizure

- Phenytoin: Adverse effect (A/E)–phenytoin

P H – Hirsutism , hyperglycemia (↓Insulin release) E N Y T O – Osteomalacia I – Interfere with folate absorption → Megaloblastic anaemia N – Neurological manifestation at higher dose

- Hallucinogen–LSD, Mescaline, Phenylcyclidine
- Peripheral decarboxylase inhibitors in parkinsonism:

Ex-Carbidopa, Benserazide.
They are used with levodopa in parkinsonism to prevent peripheral decarboxylation of levodopa [Q]

- Drugs used in prophylaxis of migraine:

–Propanolol, Topiramate, methlsergide, Valproate, flunarizine.

- S/E of TCAs: (S/E = Side effect)

Trick is TCAS
T–Tremor
C–CVS side effect
A–Anticholinergic side effect (so not given with rivastigmine in alzheimer) → Cholinergic
S–Sedation + Seizure

- Anxiolytics: 3 B's (Trick)

B–BZD
B–Buspirone (5HT1A agonist)
B–β–Blocker (Propanolol)

- BZD:

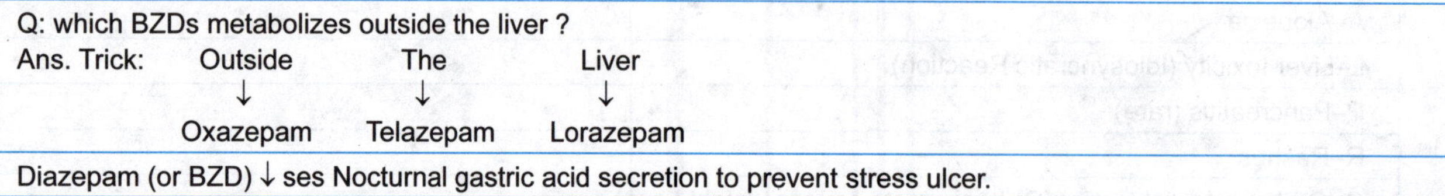

Diazepam (or BZD) ↓ ses Nocturnal gastric acid secretion to prevent stress ulcer.

- BZD Metabolizing outside the liver can be given safely in pregnancy
- BZD's at higher concentration is safer than other hypnotics
- i.v. diazepam administration:

Cause Verill's sing (Drooping of upper eyelids).This shows correct administration of correct dosage of diazepam
Midazolam EVE's sign is more reliable indicator for Endpoint of midazolamm (patient is unable to touch his/her nose with forefinger)

- Fluoxetine:

SSRI
GIT disturbance (loose stools) are most common side effect of fluoxetine [Q]

- Symptoms of Li toxicity: Trick–Lithuium

LI → Leukocytosis increased
T → Tremor
H → Hypothyroidism
IU → Increased urination
M → Moms beware (Teratogenic → Cardiac Anomaly (M.C.) [Q]
T/t: • Amiloride–D.O.C. (K-sparing diuretic) • Thiazide For IU (Increased urination)

- Classificatoin of Antipsychotic drugs

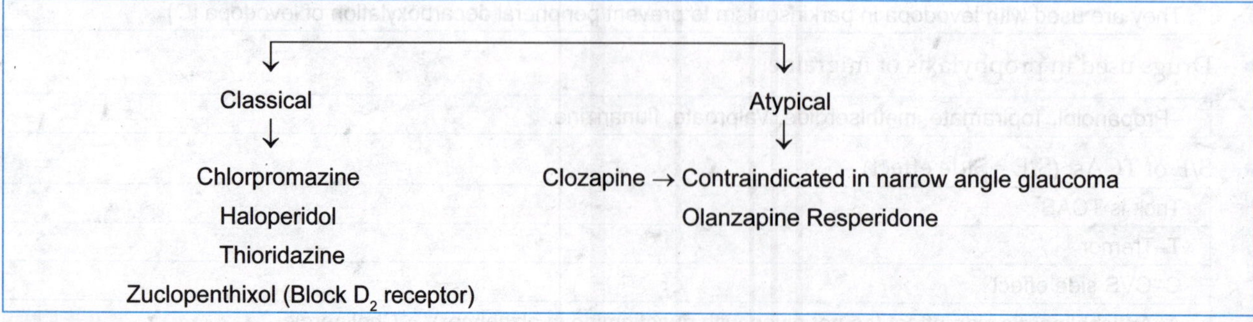

- Antipsychotic Drugs:

Have anticholinergic side effect which is marked with atypical antipsychotic. Ex-Clozapine → Minimal extrapyramidal side effect ↓ Marked anticholinergic side effect → So C/I in acute narrow angle glaucoma *(AIPG 2009)*
Opposite effect in typical antipsychotic Ex-prothiazine–Chlorpromazine, • Fluphenazine • Haloperidol → Marked extrapyramidal side effect

- MAO inhibitors potentiate the actin of epinephrine norepinephrin, dopamine and serotonin (AIIMS Q)
- NMS (Neurolept malignant syndrome):

life threatening idiosyncratic reaction to neuroleptics
occurs with all drugs affects Dopaminergic system.
Both agonist (Amantadine) and Antagonists (D_2–Blocker–Except Domperidone → Can't cross BBB)

- Antipsychotic drugs and oculogyric crysis:

Oculogyric crisis–Acute ocular dystonia due to antipsychotic drugs
Antipsychotic drugs ↓ ↓ Inhibition of dopaminergic system ↓ Unopposed over activity of Cholinergic system ↓ Variety of dystonia including Oculogyric crysis, Parkinsonism

- Guanethidine and Betrylinium → Inhibits the release of NA
- Reserpine–Inhibits the granular reuptake of NA → depletion of NA
- Bladder selective anticholinergic: Trick "Dot"

D–Darifenacin O–Oxybutynim T–Tolteroxine } Used to relieve bladder spasm detrusor instability
Duloxetin → Used in stress incontinence by ↑sing sphincter tone

- Atropine → used for the treatment of bradycardia [Q]
- Anticholoinesterase poisoning
- Treatment: specific antidote

Atropine	Cholinesterase reactivators
For both organophosphates and Carbamates	Ex-Pralidoxime [Q]
Atropine however doesn't reverse peripheral Muscular paralysis	For only organophosphate poisoning (Melathion, parathion)

- Atropine poisoning: Neostigmine can't cross BBB so physostigmine is used

- Catecholamines:

Agonist	Antagonist
α1–Phenylephrine (C/I in erectile dysfunction)	α Non selective– Phenoxybenzamine, Phentolamine used for pheachromocytoma
α2–Chlonidine/Abraclonidine	α1 - Prazocin, Terazocin
β1–Dobutamine	α2–Yohimbine
β2–Terbutaline	
Central sympatholytics–Clonidine, methyldopa (D.O.C. in pregnancy for HTN [Q])	

- Clonidine causes postural hypotension [Q] it is α2 receptor agonist [Q]
- B_2 Agonist:

• Relaxation of smooth muscles.
• Metabolic effects–Hyperglycemia, Lipolysis, Hypokalemia
• Contraction of skeletal muscle (Tremor)

- Long acting β_2 agonist:

↓	↓
Slow acting Ex-salmetrol	Rapid acting Ex-Formoteral (Fast)

- Classification of B-blockers:

Non Selective B-Blocker	Cardioselective B-blockers (B_1)
Ex-Propanolol, Pindolol, Timolol, Nadolol.	Ex-Atenolol, Esmolol, Metoprolol

Non Selective B-blockers with additional actions (vasodilation)	Selective B-blocker With additional actions
Carvidelol, Cartelol, Labetalol [Q]	Ex- Betaxalol [Q]

- Drugs used for Rx of B-blocker induced excessive bradycardia:

Dopamine, calcium chloride, Glucagon, Epinephrin, Amrinone, Mg. Not Dobutamine (AIIMS Q)

- Loading dose of aminophylline → 5-6 mg/kg
- Tolazoline–Non selective blocker (uses as vasodilator)
- Skeletal Muscle relaxants:

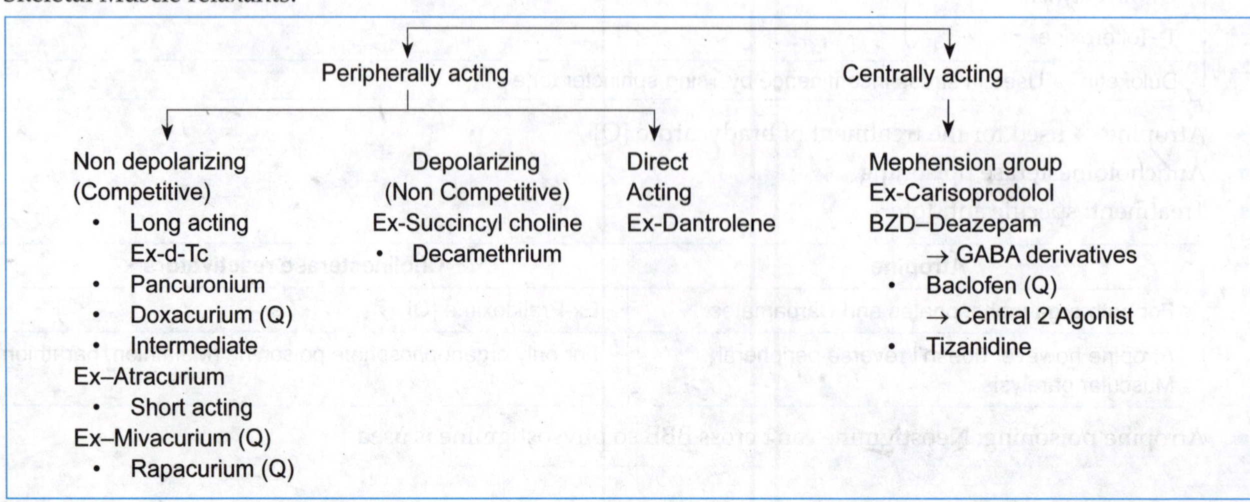

- Skeletal muscle relaxant:

Curare (d-Tc) poisoning: Reversed by Anticholine esterase (Edrophonium) ↓ Skeletal muscle paralysis
Curare acts by mast cell degranulation → So causes hypotension

- Octreotide:

Somatostain Analogue: Route–i.v, i.m, s.c , Non oral preparation		
Actions:		
↓Ses Gastric motility	↓Ses Hormonal Secretion (GH, Insuline)	Vascular smooth muscle Contraction
Use-Secretary diarrhea	Use + Pituitary adenoma Acromegaly, Gastrinoma	Portal blood flow Use–Variceal bleeding

- Penile erection is mediated through parasympathetic while ejaculation is sympathetic mediated.
- Drug used in treatment of Impotence: Trick: Penile

P–Phosphodesterase inhibitor ex-sildenafil. P–Papaverine P–Phentolamine P–Prostaglandins
Priapism–painful penile erection, is the side effect of above drugs. ↓ Rx- Phenylephrine.

- The 2 most common drug cause of impotence: B-blocker and Thiazide [Q]
- Tocolytics → Inhibit uterine contraction Ex-B2 agonist
- Antiobesity Drugs:

Nor adrenergic	
• PPA (Phenyl propanolamine) S/E–Hemorrhage stroke	Orlistat
• Serotonergic Fenfluramine Dexen fluramine	Olestra
• Both non adrengic and Serotonergic Sebutramine	Neuropeptide Y–Antagonist

- Serotonin syndrome:

Refers to a dangerous/potentially fatal syndrome caused by excess synaptic serotonin levels due to the uses of serotonin potentiating drugs.
Drugs causing are: Tryptophan → enhanced serotonin synthesis Cocaine + Amphetamine → Enhanced Serotonin release Buspirone, Li → Serotonin agonists MAO Inhibitors → Inhibit Serotonin catabolism TCA: Mepiridine/Pethidine Pentazocine → Inhibit serotonin Re-uptake

LAST 5-YEAR QUESTIONS FROM THIS TOPIC

1. **Atropine is used in preanesthetic preparation to?** *(PGI Dec 11, 10, 09 June 07, June 10)*

Ans. Decrease salivary secretions and depress vagal reflex (Ref: K.D. Tripathi 5/e p346)

2. **What is the metabolism product of chloral hydrate which is responsible for its CNS effects:** *(PGI June 11)*

Ans. Trihydrate ethanol (Ref: Goodman and Gillman's pharmacology 2/e p345)

3. **B-blocker with additional Blocking property is:** *(KCET 09)*

Ans. Labetalol (Ref: Goodman and Gillman 11/e p248)

4. **Which among the following would be most effective in absence seizures?** *(COMEDK 09, KCET 09)*

Ans. Valproic acid

5. **All of the given drug are positively ionotropes except:** *(COMEDK 11)*

a. Dopamine b. Dobutamine
c. Digoxine d. Doxepin

Ans. d

Note: Doxepine is TCA

6. **The beneficial effect of drug neostigmine in the treatment of myasthenia gravis is due to the action** *(KCET 10)*

Ans. It inhibits the action of cholinesterase

7. **Which of these drugs can be given safely to a patient with renal disease?** *(KCET 11)*

Ans. Diazepam, (Ref: KDT 5/e p365)

8. **The most common adverse effect associated with phenytoin is** *(KCET 11)*

Ans. Gum hypertrophy (Ref: KDT 6/e p404)

9. **Morphine withdrawal is characterized by all except** *(KCET 11)*

a. Miosis b. Yawning
c. Lacrimation d. Diarrhoea

Ans. a (Ref: KDT 6/e p457)

10. **Drug used in treatment of malignant hyperthermia is**

Ans. Dantroline (Ref: KDT 5/e p316)

11. **Drug used for prophylaxis of migraine is** *(AIPG 11)*

Ans. Both propranol and topiramate

12. **All are α_2 blockers except** *(AIPG 11)*

a. Yohimbine b. Phentolamine
c. Prazoan d. Sibutramine

Ans. c

13. **Which of the following does not cause sedation** *(AIPG 11)*

a. Buspirone b. Diazepam
c. Chlordiazepoxide d. Zolpidem

Ans. a (Ref: KDT 5/e p400, 401, 366)

14. **Dopamine acts on D2 Receptors that have an inhibitory effect on prolactin secretion. Now if D2 receptors are blocked, Which of the following effects will not be seen** *(AIPG 11)*

Ans. Visual disturbance

15. **Benzodiazepine antagonist** *(AIPG 10, 09, AIIMS May 09)*

Ans. Flumazenil (Ref: KDT 6/e p399)

16. **Which drug can be given safely in a patient with renal diseases?**

Ans. Diazepam

17. **D.O.C. for anaphylactic shock is**

Ans. Adrenaline

18. Long acting B-2 agonist *(AIPG 10, 09)*

Ans. Salmeterol (Ref: KDT 6/e p218)

19. Which statement is true about carbamezapine *(AIPG 09)*

Ans. Used in trigeminal neuralgia (Ref: KDT 6/e p407)

20. Buprenorphine is *(AIPG 09)*

Ans. Partial agonist (Ref: KDT 6/e p464)

21. Ist drug to be used in absence seizures *(AIPG 09, AIIMS May 10)*

Ans. Valproate (Ref: KDT 6/e p408)

22. When midazolam and diazepam are compared for their efficacy, midazolam is all except *(AIPG 12)*

a Less thromophlebitis due to low solubility in H_2O
b. Better Anxiolysis and amnesia
c. More potent than diazepam
d. Binds to BZD receptors with 3-4 times more avidly

Ans. a (Ref: KDT 6/e p376-380)

23. All of the following are atypical antipsychotic drugs, except *(AIIMS May 10)*

a. Olanzapine
b. Clozapine
c. Risperidone d
Thioridazine

Ans. d (Ref: KDT 6/e p424-425)

24. Antiepileptic that is not associated with congenital malformation when used in pregnant women is *(AIIMS May 10)*

Ans. Phenobarbitone (Ref: CMDT p200/799)

CHEMOTHERAPEUTIC AGENTS

- Antiviral drugs:

Use of RIBAVARIN R → Respiration infection I B → Influenza B A → Arena virus
Amantadine → Influenza – A (Dopamine fascillator → so used in parkinsonism)

- Antiretroviral agents for HIV: (very imp.)

Reverse transcriptase inhibitors			Protease inhibitors
Nucleoside analogues (NRTI)	Non Nucleoside (NNRIT)	Nucleoside Analogue	Trick–drugs end with "VIR" (Except–Abacavir) Saquinovir Ritonavir Nelfinavir etc.
• Zidovudine • Dibanosine • Stavudine • Lamivudine • Abacavir	• Nevirapine • Efavirenz	• Tenofovir	
3rd category of drug is: Fusion inhibitor→ Raltegravir)			

- Zidovuidine:

Non teratogenic used in pregnancy to prevent transmission of AIDS from mother to fetus [Q]

- All protease inhibitors are → Inhibitors for CYP 3A except sequinavir (least)
- S/E of anti retroviral drugs:

Dibanosine	Stavudine
Pancreatitis (Most serious) peripheral neuropathy	Peripheral neuropathy (Maximum seen with stavudine)

- Thalidomide:

Worst teratogen known in the history of medicine.
Clinical use: AIDS related apthous ulcers [Q] AIDS related wasting syndrome Multiple myeloma Prevention of GVHS (Graft versus host disease) after transplantation Rheumatoid Arthritis Ankylosing spondylitis Crohn's disease and Behcat syndrome [Q]

- M.O.A. (Mechanism of action)

• Sulfonamide → Inhibit bacterial folate synthease [Q]
• Fluoroquinolones → Inhibits bacterial DNA gyrase [Q] • Tetracyclin → Binds to 30s ribosome [Q]
• Chloramphenicol → Binds to 50s ribosome
• Clindamycin [Q] → Inhibits protein synthesis by binding to 50s ribosome
• Streptomycin → binds to 30s ribosome other aminoglycosides [Q] → bind to both 30s and 50s ribosome
• Vancomycin + Teicoplanin + Penicillin + [Q] Cephalosporin [Q] } → Inhibit all wall synthesis
• Polymyxin B+ colistin → Form pseudopore in cell membrane

- Bactericidal drugs: Trick–Pacca Mango

P–Penicillin A–Aminoglycosides C–Cephalosporin C–Ciprofloxacin M–Metronidazole

- Folic acid metabolism interfered by:

Proguanil + pyrimethamine + sulphonamides + 3P (phenytoin + phenobaribitone + primidome) [Q]

- Chemoprophylaxis: for common diseases

Cholera–Tetracycline Diphtheria–Erthromycin Influenza A–Amantadine Meningococcal meningitis–Sulphadiazine Pneumonic plague–Tetracycline

- Antiamoebic drugs:

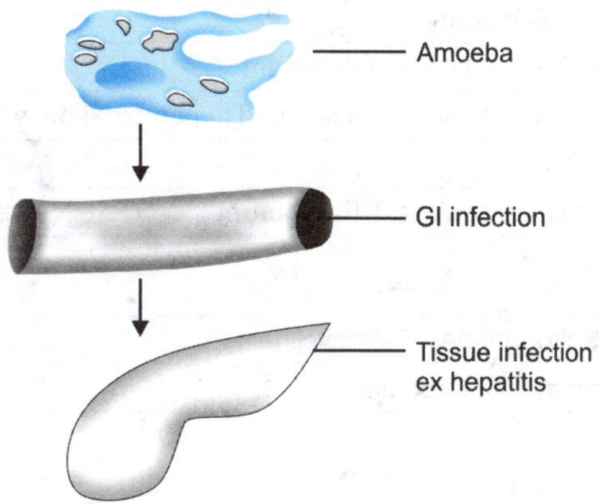

Fig 16.2: Path of action of amoeba

• G.I. luminal amoebicide only: ex-Diloxanide • Tissue amoebicide only: Amoebic liver abscess Ex-Chloroquin • Both G.I. and Tissue infectious ex-metronidazole, Tinidazole – Metronidazole is the D.O.C. for Amoebiasis
Clinical use of Metronidazole: Anerobic infection, Giardiasis, Trench Mouth (ANUG) Adverse Effect: A → Anorexia, Abdominal cramps alcohol intolerance G → Glossitis and Giddiness T → Taste–Metallic, Thrombophlebitis (i.v), Teratogenic potential

- Antifungal drugs:

• For topical infections: Like candidiasis, Ring Worm → Ist choice–Fluconazole, Itraconazole "Azoles" → Can use both topically and Systemically → Ketoconazole
• For systems infections: Like, Mucormycosis, Aspergillosis, Blastomycosis, Cryptococcosis. Amphotericin B is the D.OC. but fluconazole and Itraconazole can also use. Amphotericin–B → Most effective drug for systemic mycosis and is gold standard antifungal therapy. But because of higher toxicity of AMB, The "AZOLES" Antifungals are now preferred in condition where there efficacy approaches to AMB. → So ketoconazole came → Now fluconazole and Itraconazole have replaced it because of their efficacy and fewer S/E **NOTE:** for Mucormycosis → Only AMB Azoles are H.E.I. (Hepatic enzyme inhibitor) Resistance becoming a significant clinical problem. The drug also inhibits human gonadal and Adrenal steroid synthesis.

- Antifungal agents mostly act on cell membrane except griseofulvin (acts by interfering mitosis)
- Antifungals:

Flucytosine (5 FC)–is an antimetabolic, anticancer and Anti fungal drug used with AMB (Amphotericin B.to lower their toxicity

- Azoles:

Are not effective in candida krusi and Mucormycosis
candida krusi → Rx: Variconazole
Mucormycosis → Rx: AMB

- Antimalarial drugs:

Artesunate → D.O.C for severe falciparum.
Artemether + Lumenfantine → Treatment of P. falciparum
Pyrimethamine → Slow acting so can't use alone so used in combination with any sulfonamides
Clinical care–chloroquine
Artesunate is not used in prophylaxis against P. Falciparum

- Antimalarial drugs:

Slow acting–Pyrimethamine, Sulfonamides, Tetracycline
Fast acting–Artemether, Artesunate, Chloroquine

- Antihelminthics:

• Intestinal worms → (round worms, hook Worms, pin and Whip worms)	Antihelminthic of choice: Imidazoles Ex-Albendazole, mebendazole, ivermectin
• Platyhelminthes → (tape worm)	Praziquantel

- Filaria:

• 1st line of drug → DEC (Diethyl carbamazine)
• Ivermectin

- Nephrotoxicity caused by aminoglycosides → Reversible
- Diptheria:

Penicillin G. 1200 mg for treatment
Erythromycin → for Prophylaxis

- Penicillin:

Effective against all cocci + gram +ve bacilli
Majorities of Gram (–)ve bacilli are insensitive to penicillin except–E.coli, proteus
Chlamydia, Ricketessia, TB are all resistant
• Pencillins: Are one of the safest antibiotics. However they have following adverse effects: Tricks ADR A → Allergic reaction Ex–Angioneurotic edema and Anaphylactic shock D → Diarrhea (due to opportunistic infection) R → Rare toxicity: Dose Related [Q] Acute high dose → Convulsion Chronic high dose → Anemia and Neutropenia

- Methicillin causes Interstitial nephritis [Q]
- MRSA (Methicillin resistant staphylococcus aureus)

• Due to altered PBP–2A (localized on cell membrane) encoded on a Mec A gene.
• Mec A gene transmits resistance. (And Not via plasmid)
PBP = Pen Binding protein

- Drugs commonly used in MRSA (Methicillin resistant Staph. Aureus)

Vancomycin	Teicoplanin	Linezolid
↓	↓	↓
MRSA	MRSA + VRE	MRSA + VRE (Vancomycin resistant enterococci)+ VRSA (Staph aureus)

- Aminoglycosides:

Are highly ionized → neither absorbed nor destroyed in GIT. So, volume of distribution nearly equal to extracellular volume.
Among the aminoglycosides → Streptomycin is least teratogenic.
Aminoglycosides (Streptomycin): Inhibits the release of Ach at NMJ and also ses the sensitivity of motor end plate to Ach. → So, 1) precipitate Myaesthenia weakness • Streptomycin should not be used with d-Tc → Causes prolonged Apnea
Aminoglycoside causes: Ototoxicity + Nephrotoxicity + NMJ blockade but not cardiotoxicity *(AIPG 08)*
Aminoglycosides (AMGS) → Are C/I during pregnancy

- Macrolides: Erythromycin, Azithromycin, Clarithromycin

Clinical use: Trick: Remember vaccines of National immunization
DPT, Measles, Polio, BCG
D–Diptheria (in prophylaxis)
P–Pertusis
T–Tetanus
M–Mycoplasma
P–Penicillin Alternative in Penicillin Allergic patients.
B–Bacterial diarrhea
C–Chacroid caused by H. Ducreyi
G–Genital infections as caused by chlamydiae.

- Erythromycin–is the safest drug can used during pregnancy *(COMEDK 07)*
- Fluoroquinolones undergoing "Non" renal excretion: Trovofloxacin, Grevofloxacin, Pevofloxacin, Nalidix acid
- Enterococci are resistant to penicillin, Aminoglycosides, Cephalosporin, vancomycin
- MDR: Multiple Drug resistance

Seen in cancer chemotherapy → ↑MDR gene expression → Causes efflux of drugs [Q]

- Cephalosporin:

Ist generation–Trick "Cepha/cefa" Except "Cefaclor" which is under 2nd generation Ex-Cephalothin, Cefazolin, Cephalexin, Cefdroxil Active against Gram + ve Cocci.
2nd G → Cefaclor, Cefuroxime, Cefoxitin, Cefuroxime → More against gram – ve Some activity against gram + ve organism.
3rd G → Trick "t" Present Ceftriaxone, ceftazidime, Cefoperazone, Cefixime, Cefotaxime. 3rd G → Cefoperazone and cefitazidine → Antipsuedomonal → High activity against gram –ve organism → Less active against gram+ve cocci and anaerobes.
4th G → Cefepime 4th G → No activity against anaerobes
Remember: No cephalosporin is active against → E. Ficalis, MRSA, Listeria M.

- Cephalosporin:

Cefoperazone + Cefiuiramide → Excreted through bile [Q]

- Actisite–25% Tetracycline
- Atridox–10% Doxycycline
- Ledermix Paste–Demeclocycline + Triamciline → For subsiding pain in irreversible pulpitis
- Glycopeptide antibiotics:

Antibacterial	Antineoplastic
Vancomycin [Q]	Bleomycin
Teicoplanin [Q]	

- Macrolides (Erythromycin) → binds with motilin receptor and increases gastric motility.
- Antileprotic Drug: Trick–CDE

C–Clofazimine–Cutaneus discoloration D–Dapsone–Degradation of RBC E–Ethionamide–Emesis

- Jarish Herxheimer reaction: Seen In

• Lepra reaction → Due to release of Ag from killed bacilli
• Occurs when penicillin is given in syphilitic patient. Due to sudden release of Spirochaetal lytic product
T/t for lepra reaction → Clofazemine Other → Thallidomide, Chloroquine

- Tetracycline, Clindamycine are Broad spectrum

  ↓

  Superinfection with clostridium difficle

  ↓

  Psuedomembrane Colitis [Q]
- D.O.C. for neurosyphillis:

Ist line → Aqueous Or crystalline penicillin
Alternative → Procaine penicillin

- Amikacin → is reserve drug for hospital acquired pneumonia (Psuedomonas)
- D.O.C. (drug of choice):

For meningococcal meningitis → penicillin
If allergic to penicillin → chlormphenicol is D.O.C.

- Drug of choice for psuedomonas:

1st choice → Imipenem + Amikacin Antipsuedomonal pen. + Aminoglycosides.

- Uricosuric (For GOUT) → Probenecid , sulfinphrozone
- Linezolid:

Causes bone marrow thrombocytopenia (most common) depression.
Used for Rx of resistant G+ve Cocci and Bacilli [Q]

- Antitubercular Drugs:

First line drugs: F → Field defect causing drug ie, Ethambutol. I → INH R → Rifampicin S → Streptomycin T → Twice a day given drug ie, pyrozinamide
Adverse effects of 1st line Antitubercular Drugs: INH → I (Insanity i.e, psychosis), N (Neuritis), H ((Hepatitis) Rifampicin: R (Red discoloration of urine), I (induction of liver enzyme), F (Flu like symptoms on intermittent dose) Pyrazinamide–Pain in the joint due to hyperuricemia Ethambutol–Eye toxicity (Optic neuritis) [Q] Streptomycin–Similar to other AMGs
• Streptomycin → Only the Ist line Antitubercular drug given parentally (Highly ionized)
Second line drugs: S–Salicylates like PAS E–Ethionamide C–Cycloserine O–Old drug–Thiacetazone N–New drugs–Quinolones–Ciprofloxacin, Ofloxacin –Macrolides–Clarethromycin, Azelhromycin D–Drugs rarely used–Aminoglycosides–Amikasin, Kanamycine

- S/E of Thalidomide–Constipation + Sedation
- Vancomycin:

Is nephrotoxic
RED Man syndrome *(KCET 2012)*
Is given at an interval of 72 hrs in a patient with creatinine clearance of < 10

- Anticancer Drugs (very imp.)

Cell cycle specific agents	Non cell cycle specific agents
• 5 phase specific agents – Antimetabolites – Methotrexate [Q] – 6MP – 6 TG – 5 FU – Cyatarabine → Cerebellar toxicity – Azathioprine → VZ infection	• Alkylating: – Cyclophosphamide → Hemorrhagic Cystitis Ifosfamide Chlorambucil Busulphan → Pulmonary fibrosis Cisplatin → Causes 2° Leukemia → Ototoxicity → Nephrotoxicity → Amifostine A Cytoprotective agent used for the reduction of renal toxicity associated with cisplatin – Carmustine–Sustained neutropenia (AIIMS 08) (Carmustin > Methotrexate) Miscellaneous: Actinomycin D–Antibiotic used as anti-Cancer agent Mitomycin → Acts on Hypoxic cell

	L–Asparginase → Hypercoagulabity Doxorubicin (Adriamycin) → Leomyosarcoma MOPP–Regimen (KCET) M–Mechlorethamine O–Oncovin P–Procarbazine P–Prednisolone
• G2 Phase specific – Bleomycin → causes hyperplasia of type II Pneumocyte (Q) – Etoposide → Topoisomerase II (Q) – Topatetan, Iridotecan } → Topoisomerase I (Q)	
• M phase specific: Vincristin Vinblastin Paclitaxel/Docetaxel → Antimicro–Tubule agent. Stabilizes microtubule [Q]	

- Sustained neutropenia caused by carmustine > Methotreaxate > Doxarubicin [Q]
- Busulfan + Bleomycin + Methotrexote cause pulmonary fibrosis. Methylsergide also causes pulmonary fibrosis to some extent
- Melphalan is used in the treatment of multiple myeloma [Q]
- Newer agents for cancer chemotherapy targeting HER1 (EGRF) and HER 2 Receptors:

HER 1	HER 2	HER 1 + HER 2
Remember examples of HER2 and HER1 + HER 2 .(Rest are HER 1)	Trastuzumab (Herception) Breast cancer	Lapatinics [Q] Breast cancer
Ex-cetuximab SCC of head and neck		

- Anticancer drugs:

Mitomycin C: Is antibiotic group of drug effective against hypoxic cells Potent radiosensitizer Highly toxic → used mainly in resistant cases of stomach, colon and cervix cancer

- Imatinib + Sunitinb:

TK inhibitor
Use–GIST, CML, H and N Cancer

- Cytarabin (Ara–c) → AML
- Immunosuppressants:

Cyclosporine, Tacrolimus, Mycophenolate mofetil → Is a prodrug, which doesn't cause Nephrotoxicity

- L–Asparginase cause hypercoagulability side effect due to deficiency in synthesis of protein C and S in normal tissues.
- Major problem with Cancer chemotherapy → Development of drug resistance
- Hand foot syndrome → Capacitabine > Cisplatin
- Imiquimod → is Immunomodulator used in Genital warts

- S/E of high dose methotrexate → Reversible and transient oligospermia
- Methotrexate toxicity: Leucoverin/Folinic acid given with methotrexate to reduce their toxicity [Q]
- Immunosuppressants:

Tacrolimus (FK-506)	Cyclosporine
• All toxicities are higher (More potent, more toxic)	
• No gum hypertrophy and hirsutism	• But hirsutism and Gum hyperplsia only here
• No Ototoxicity	• No ototoxicity
• Inhibits calcineurin	• Inhibits calcineurin

- Mycophenolate mofetil (Immunosuppressant):

Mechanism: Inhibits purine synthesis Via IMDH (Inosine monophosphate dehydrogenase)

- Anticancer drugs act by hypomethylation: Decitabine, Azacytidine.
- Anticancer drugs excreted by lung–5 FU [Q]
- Anticancer drugs: MESNA can be given orally/i.V. along with cyclophosphamide to se nephrotoxicity
- Hormonal treatment of breast cancer:

• Aromatase inhibitor–letrozole, Amastrazole, Exmestane (AIIMS)
Prevents peripheral conversion of testosterone → Estrogen so used in breast cancer (at extra ovarian site like breast)
NOTE: (Tamoxifen citrate + clomiphene citrate → used in breast cancer)

- Clomiphene citrate:

Pure estrogen antagonist, prevent (–)ve feed back at hypothalamus by estrogen ↓ So ↑LH and FSH ↓ Ovulation
Use–Anovulation fertility

- Q: Which of the following drugs require dose adjustment in patients during radiotherapy in order to prevent radiation toxicity ?
  Ans. The drugs which are "Radiosensitizer" ex-Actinomycin, Mitomycin, Dactinomycin

LAST 5-YEAR QUESTIONS FROM THIS TOPIC

1. Antibiotic prophylaxis is recommended before dental treatment for: *(PGI Dec 11)*

Ans. Patient with liver disease (Ref: Cessentials of oral pathology and oral medicine 8/e p378)

2. All are ureidopenicillin except: *(PGI Dec 11, 10)*

a. Piperacillin
b. Azlocillin
c. Maziocillin
d. Flucloxacillin

Ans. (d) (Ref: KDT 6/e p702)

3. Which antibiotic can be given safely throughout pregnancy? *(PGI June 11)*

Ans. Penicillin (KDT 5/e p634)

4. Which of the following does not require antibiotic prophylaxis? *(PGI June 10)*

Ans. Child under 15 years

5. Which of the following statements about azoles is false? *(KCET 09)*

a. They are fungi static
b. They are hepatotoxic
c. Resistance to the drug is common such as cyclosporine

d. They effect the metabolism of drugs

Ans. d (Ref: Lippincott pharmacdogy 2/e p342)

6. The most preferred acute emetic for emesis induced by anticancer drugs is: *(KCET 09)*

Ans. Ondasetron (Ref: Pharmacology by Goodman and Gillman 11/e p647)

7. Combination of ampicillin and gentamicin is an example of: *(COMEDK 09)*

Ans. Synergism (Ref: Lippincott's illustrated pharmacology 2/e p301)
(Note: Same Q was asked in AIPG-12 for Amoxicillin + Clavulanic acid)

8. Ethambutol causes: *(KCET 11)*

Ans. Optic neuritis (Ref: KDT 5/e p421)

9. Ipratropium bromide is used for: *(KCET 11)*

Ans. Optic neuritis (Ref: KDT 5/e p97)

10. Which among the following antibiotics should be avoided in pregnancy: *(COMEDK 09, 12)*

a. Erthromycin
b. Tetracyclin
c. Cephalexin
d. Amoxicilin

Ans. b (Ref: Pharmacology by Goodman and Gillman 11/e p1102)

11. The drug which has antabusive effect when alcohol is ingested is: *(COMEDK 10)*

Ans. Metraonidazole

12. Which among the following is a cell cycle specific anti-neoplastic drug? *(COMEDK 10, AIPG 07)*

Ans. Methotrexate

13. Pseudomenbranous colitis is an adverse effect following the long-term use of: *(COMEDK 10, AIIMS Nov 12, AIPG 13)*

Ans. Clindamycin
Note: Tetracycline also does the same

14. Among the drugs given below, which is least likely, to be implicated in drug induced hepatitis: *(COMEDK 11)*

Ans. Streptomycin

15. Which among the drugs given below, does not act by protease inhibition? *(COMEDK 11)*

Ans. Zanamivir

Note: Zanamivir is anti-influenza drug

16. Which among the following is the drug of choice for clostridium difficile induced colitis? *(COMEDK 11)*

Ans. Metronidazole

17. Each of the following statements is correct about metronidazole except that it: *(KCET 10)*

a. Is a broad spectrum antiprotozoal drug
b. Active against bacteroids and clostridium
c. An effective alternative for infection caused by aerobic gram positive cocci.
d. May cause peripheral neuropathy on prolonged use

Ans. c

18. Which among the following anti–HIV drugs is also used to treat viral hepatitis B?

Ans. Lamivudine
Note: Rx includes INF + Lamivudine + Famcyclovir

19. During the cell cycle, Colchicine is known to act in *(COMEDK 11)*

Ans. M phase

20. Which of the following ATT drug is bacteriostatic. *(COMEDK 11)*

Ans. Ethambutol

21. Which among the following is used as an immunosuppressant *(COMEDK 11)*

Ans. Cyclosporine

22. A replacement drug used as substitute for cyclosporine exhibiting less severe gingival enlargement is:

Ans. Tacrolimus

23. An antibiotic that achievers high concentration in hard tissue, because of its molecular size is? *(KCET 11)*

Ans. Clindamycin (Ref: Topazian 4/e p120)

24. A replacement drug used as a substitute for cyclosporine exhibiting less severe gingival enlargement is: *(KCET 11)*

Ans. Tacrolimus (Ref: Carranza's clinical periodontology 10/e p378)

25. Which is the preferred drug in patient with vancomycin resistant infection: *(AIPG 11)*

Ans. Linezolid (Ref: KDT 5/e p691-692)

26. A female patient on oral contraceptive was given rifampicin. After some time, she becomes pregnant what is the probable cause? *(AIPG 11)*

Ans. Rifampicin activate hepatic enzyme which metabolizes oral contraceptives *(AIPG 11)*

27. Which of the following is true about penicillin: *(AIPG 11, AIIMS Nov 10, 09)*

a. Acid resistant
b. Excreted mainly through kidney
c. More concentrated in prostatic fluid
d. Is a broad spectrum antibiotic

Ans. b (Ref: KDT 5/e p654)

28. Which cephalosporin has anti-pseudomonal action:

Ans. Cefoperazone (AIPG 11, 10, AIIMS Nov 10)

29. Which of the following drug inhibit cell wall synthesis:

Ans. Cephalosporin

30. All are true about aminoglycosides except: *(AIPG 10)*

a. Are bacteriostatic
b. Distributed only extracellularly
c. Are teratogenic
d. Excreted unchanged in urine

Ans. a

31. The incidence of allergy to pencillin among various population ranges from:

Ans. 1% to 10%

32. Which of the following is not true about penicillin G: *(AIPG 10, 09)*

a. Very active against sensitive gram positive cocci
b. Destroyed by gastric acid
c. More concentrated in prostatic secretions and intraocular fluid
d. Used for treatment of meningococcal meningitis

Ans. c (Ref: KDT p654, 655)

33. Antibiotic coverage for extraction in a prosthetic mitral valve patient is: *(AIIMS Nov 12)*

Ans. 2 mg amoxicillin 1 hr before the surgery (Ref: Neelima malik I/e p106)

34. Redman syndrome is side effect of:

Ans. vancomycin

35. Which drug does not cross BBB? *(AIIMS Nov 11, 12)*

Ans. Netlimicin (Ref: Net sources)

36. Drug not used in H. pylori infection: *(AIPG 09, AIIMS May 09)*

Ans. Mosapride (Ref: KDT 6/e p637)

37. Amphotericin B is used for treatment of: *(AIPG 12)*

Ans. Fungi

38. Which of the following drugs is not useful for MRSA? *(AIIMS Nov 09)*

Ans. Cefaclor (Ref: KDT 6/e p706)

Note: Also Cefixime

39. All of the following causes hypoglycaemia, except: *(AIIMS May 11)*

a. Natiglinide
b. Glimepiride
c. Insulin
d. Acarbose

Ans. d (Ref: Mogenson pharmacology of diabetes p87-90)

40. Which of the following is Not true of exenatide? *(AIIMS May 11)*

a. Glueoregulatory actions similar to GLP-1
b. Suppressed inappropriate glucagon secretion
c. Helps slow down gastric emptying
d. Used in type 1 diabeties mellitus subcutaneously

Ans. d (Ref: Poretsky principles of diabetes mellitus p64)

41. All of the following are true about ifosfamide alkylating agent except: *(AIIMS May 11)*

a. Acetaldehyde conversion to chloroacetaldehyde.
b. It is a nitrogen mustard
c. It is metabolized by CPY
d. It causes less neurotoxicity than cyclophosphamide

Ans. d (Ref: Coleman Human drug metabolism p92)

42. Which of the following uphalosporins done need dose modifications even in the presence of raised levels of GFR? *(AIIMS May 11)*

Ans. Cefoperazone (Ref: KDT 6/e p706)

43. If bacteria were susceptible to both pencillin and erythromycin, then it would not be appropriate to treat the patient with both the antibiotics at the same time, because *(AIIMS Nov 10)*

Ans. Pencillin acts only on growing bacterial population (Ref: KDT 6/e p677)

ENDOCRINOLOGY AND MISCELLANEOUS

- Both estrogen and Antipsychotic drugs ↑ses prolactin level by inhibiting → PIF (Prolactin inhibiting factor) of hypothalamus
- HPA axis and adrenal gland suppression seen with → 20-25 mg/kg of hydrocortisone or 5 mg of prednisolone
- Oral hypoglycemic:

Oral hypoglycemic
Sulfonyl urease → ↑ses insulin secretion from pancreas
Metformin (Biguanides): Don't cause insulin release Major action is suppression of hepatic glueoneogenesis Adverse effect: • lactic acidosis • B_{12} Deficiency
Sitagliptin and vildagliptinn: DPP–4 inhibitors → ↑ses GLP → ↑ses insulin

- Insulin preparation:

Insulin preparation
• Rapid acting human insulin analogs – Insulin Lispro – Insulin Aspart – Insulin Glulisine
• Short acting Insulin – Regular insulin

• Intermediate acting – NPH insulin
• Long acting – Glargine [Q] → It gets deposited as micro precipitates after s.c injection and provides a low continuous level of circulating insulin. Its action is thus peakless (Peakless insulin) It is an acidic insulin Usually administered once daily.

- Acarbose:

Is a glucosidase inhibitor and thus it prevents the postprandial digestion and absorption of starch and disaccharide
• Ide and the postprandial rise in plasma glucose is blunted
• Reduces postprandial plasma glucose level in type I and II DM
• Acarbose improves fibrinolytic activity in patient with impaired glucose tolerance.

- Prostaglandins analogues: Clinical use:

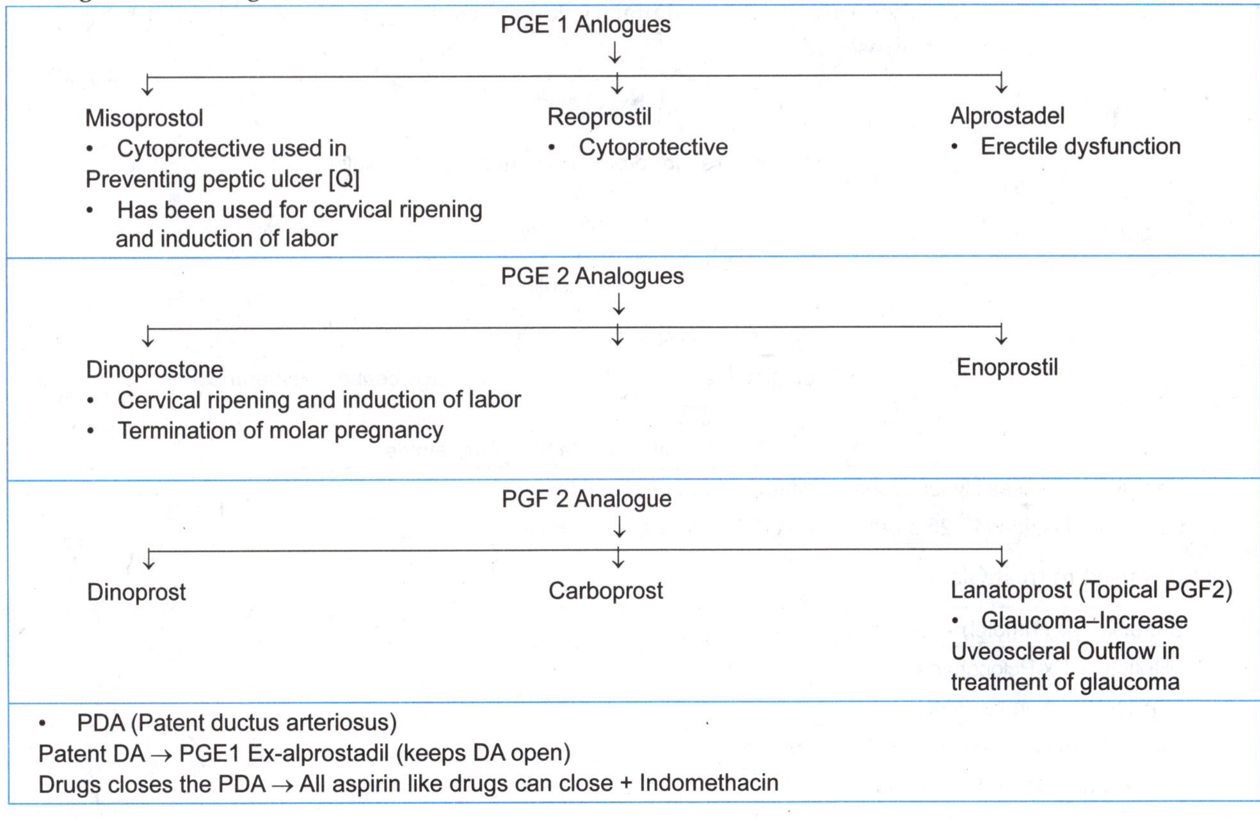

- Donesumab:

Fully humanized monoclonal Ab.
Used in Osteoporosis → Acts against RANKL receptor which is present on osteoclast [Q]

- Diuretics:

Carbonic Anhydrase inhibitors: Acetazolamide
• Inhibition of HCO_3 (Metabolic acidosis) P Na^+ reabsorption + hypokalemia • Adjunct to antiepileptic drugs: As raises CO_2 level in brain ↓ ↓pH → raising seizure threshold.

- Zolamide (Ex–Aceta zolamide, Brunzolamide):

Are sulfonamides derivatives so contra indicated in sulfonamide allergic patients.
They are carbonic anhydrase inhibitors (weak/adjunct diuretics)

- Site of actions of Diuretics: Tricks coltp

C – Carbonic anhydrase Inhibitor (At the proximal convulating Tubule) O – Osmotic diuretic (Loop of Henle) L – Loop diuretics (At the ascending loop) T – Thiazide (at DCT) P – Potassium sparing (At the collecting tubule)

- K–Sparing diuretics:

Direct Acting	Aldosterone Antagonist
Ex-Amiloride, Triamterene	Ex-spironolactone [Q]

- Furosemide–is used i.V. only is case of acute pulmonary edema (as ses systemic vasodilatation)
- Thiazide (High dose) and furosemide:

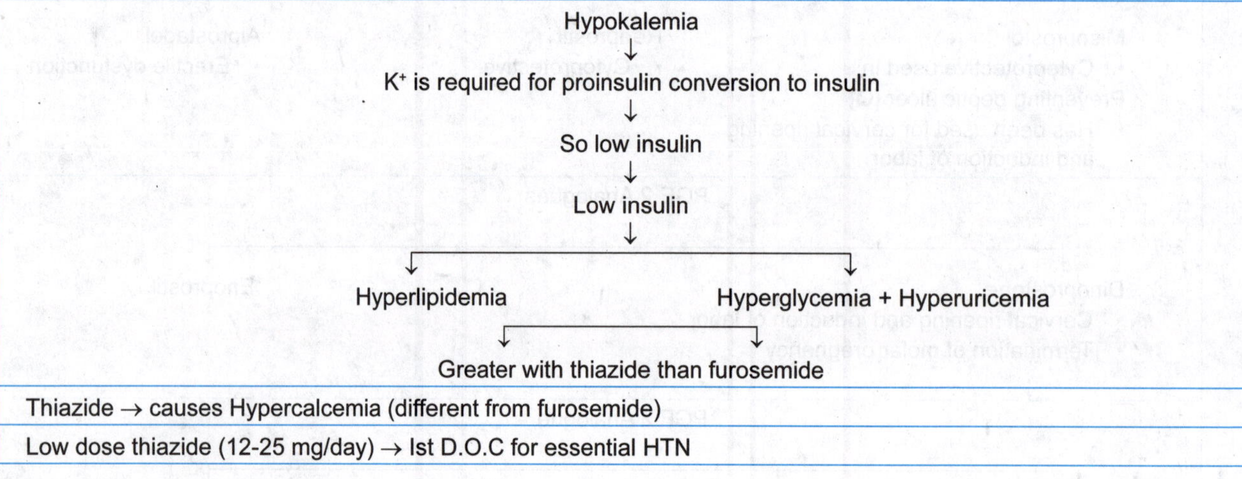

Thiazide → causes Hypercalcemia (different from furosemide)
Low dose thiazide (12-25 mg/day) → Ist D.O.C for essential HTN

- Drugs used to treat Glaucoma:

B-blocker → (Timolol) → Ist choice
Mitotics → Ex-Pclocarpine
α–Agonist–Phenylephrine
Carbonic Anhydrase inhibitor → Acetazolamide
PGE2 (Lanatoprost) → ses outflow

- Corticosteroids:

Long acting–Dexamethasone, Betamethasone Inhalation → Beclomethasone Systematic → Hydrocortisone, Prednisolone, Dexamethasone
Steroids based on Action: • 1° Glucocorticoid action → Mostly (Dexamethasone, Betamethasone) • Only mineralocorticoid action → DOCA (Deoxycorticosterone acetate) • 1° Mineralocorticoid action → Fludrocortisone aldosterone

- Asthma → Leukotriene antagonist and Ipratropium bromide are mainly used for regular prophylactic use. Not for acute attack
- AT II (Angiotensis II) is the most potent Vasoconstrictor of the body
- Papavarin → Originally extracted for but devoid of narcotic property
- Siadh:

Associated with hyponatremia is "Euvolumic"
Rx–Demedocycline/Lithium

- Causes of siadh:

Anticancer drugs–vincrestin, Vinblastin, cyclophosphamide , CNS drugs, Oxytocin (Dimag wale drugs)
Rx–Demeclocyclin

- Domperidone → used in levodopa induced emesis
- Isotretinoin:

Is retinoic acid
Teratogenic. Deafness (Characteristic) cleft lip and palate.

- Antihistaminic classification:

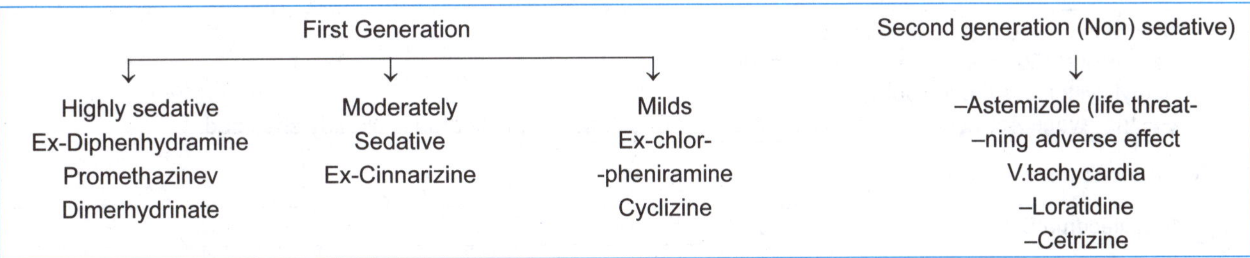

- Trick for 2nd generation antihistaminics: Red flame

Rupatadine Fexofenadine Loratadine/Levocetrizine/Levocabastine Acrivastine/Azelastine Mizolastine Ebastine

- 5HT3 Antagonists → Highest affinity for 5HT3 → Palonosetron
- Potential drug interaction that decrease the effectiveness of OCP (oral contraceptives)

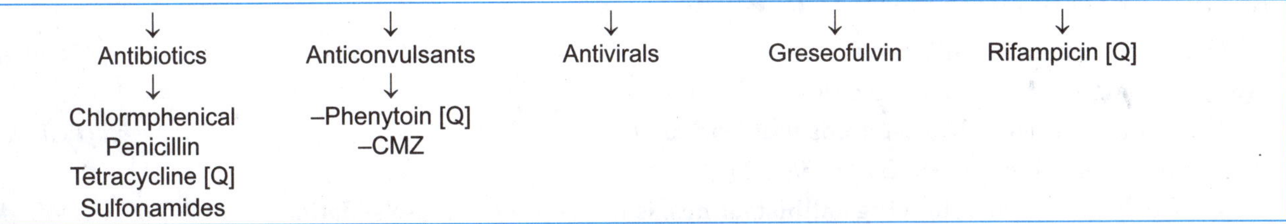

- Medications used in alcohol withdrawal:

• Alcohol withdrawal including for seizures–BZD (Diazepam) is preferred D.O.C.
• Rehabilitation of alcoholics: Naltrexone, Disulfiram, Acamprosate.

- Opioid withdrawal:

• Methadone–Synthetic opioid Used as substitute therapy in opioid dependence
• Alternative medicines for maintenance: Buprenorephine–Partial agonist of 'μ' receptor Opioid antagonist–Naltrexone.
• Clonidine in opioid withdrawal: Mimics opioid effects.

- Drugs used in heavy metal poisoning:

Mercury toxicity → BAL
Cu toxicity (Wilson disease) → Penicillamine + Trientine (In is very important)
Fe toxicity (Wilson disease) → Defuroxamine (only i.v), Deferiprone (oral)
Arsenic toxicity → BAL
Lead toxicity: DMSA if Pb < 70 → No CNS symptoms. EDTA if Pb > 70 → CNS symptoms (Seizure)

- Paracetamol poisoning:

NABQI is the metabolite which is toxic Large dose 150 mg/kg or, > 10 g in an adult Acetyl cysteine is the Antidote Gastric lavage/Activated charcol is not effective if duration > 4 hrs. as drug is already absorbed.

- Methanol poisoning:

(Papilledema/Discedema)
T/t: • Fomepizole: by inhibiting alcohol dihydrogenase • Folate therapy–Reduces formic acid level by enhancing its metabolism

- Iron preparation vs Route

Iron preparation	Route
Iron dextran	i.m/i.v
Iron sorbitol	i.m
Iron sulphate + Iron gluconate	Oral

LAST 5-YEAR QUESTIONS FROM THIS TOPIC

1. **Fe requirement of children is:** *(PGI Dec 11)*

Ans. 20–25 ug/kg (Ref: K.D.T. 5/e p546)

2. **Prolonged use of corticosteroids will lead to:** *(PGI Dec 11)*

Ans. Adrenal insufficiency (Ref: KDT 5/e p265)

3. **Which among the following antihistamines, is least likely to cause sedation?** *(AIPG 09, COMEDK 09)*

Ans. Loratidine

4. **Stimulation of receptors of ANP (Antineuritic peptide) leads to increase in concentration of which of the following:** *(PGI Dec 10)*

Ans. Guanyl cyclase (Ref: Hypertension 1995, 26: 628-633)

5. **All of the following glucocorticoids can be given by inhalation except:** *(KCET 09)*
   a. Dexamethasone
   b. Beclomethasone
   c. Budesonide
   d. Fluticasone

Ans. a (Ref: Goodman Gillman 11/e p466)

6. **In the physiologic system, nitric oxide is known to act through:** *(COMEDK 09)*

Ans. Cyclic GMP (Ref: Pharmacology by Goodman and Gillman 19/e p123)

7. **Inhaled general anesthetic with low blood gas partial coefficient is characterized by:** *(COMEDK 12)*

Ans. Rapid induction and quick recovery from anesthetic (Ref: Principles of pharmacology: the pathophysiologic basis of drug therapy by David E. Golan 1/e p252)

8. **Which of the following is also called "Peakless unsulin" analog:** *(COMEDK 11)*

Ans. Insulin glargine (Ref: Goodman and Gilman's II/e p1047)

9. **Which among the following is not used for surface anesthesia?** *(COMEDK 10)*

Ans. Procaine (Trick: Liberty)

L–Lignocaine

B–Benzocine

T–Tetracaine

10. **Hyperthyroidism can be caused by:** *(COMEDK 10)*

Ans. Amiodarone

11. **All the following drugs reduce the gastric acid secretion except:** *(KCET 10)*
    a. Ranitidine
    b. Sucralfate
    c. Misoprostol
    d. Pantoprazol

Ans. b

12. **Success factor for intraligamentary anesthesia:** *(KCET 10)*

Ans. Injection under strong back pressure

13. **All are tocolytic agents except:** *(AIPG 11)*
    a. Ritodrine
    b. Isoxsuprine
    c. Phenobaritone
    d. Atosiban

Ans. c

14. **All are true about "Sitagliptin" except:** *(AIPG 11)*
    a. Is not give alone, always with sulfonylureas
    b. Major side effect is respiratory depression and pharyngitis
    c. Increases insulin secretion
    d. Inhibits DPP4 and decrease the metabolism of GIP

Ans. c

15. **Which of the following is mismatch:** *(AIPG 11)*
    a. Paraquat–Herbiside
    b. Naloxone–TCA
    c. Cholestyramine Colestipal–Warfarin
    d. Acetylcystine–Paracetamol

Ans. b (Ref: Goodman–Gillman 10/e p1896)

16. Role of corticosteroid in inflammation can be suggested by all except: *(AIPG 11)*

a. Decrease in number of neutrophil
b. Decreased ICAM-I release from inflammatory cells
c. Alteration in thromboxane A2 Synthesis
d. Decreases production of inflammatory cytokine

Ans. a (Ref: KDT 5/e p258)

17. Which is not a 2nd generation antihistaminic: *(AIPG 10, 09, AIIMS May 09)*

Ans. Cyclizine (Ref: KDT 6/e p156)

18. All are true about metformin except: *(AIIMS Nov 12)*

a. Inhibits cellular respiration in mitochondria
b. Excreted unchanged in urine
c. Reduce hepatic glucose production
d. Used in decompensated heart failure

Ans. d (Ref: KDT 6/e p269)

19. Alkaptonuria an inherited metabolic disorder is due to deficiency of:

Ans. Homogentisate oxidase

20. Progestin compound that does not alter lipid profile is:

Ans. Gestodene

21. Which drug is used in morphine withdrawal: *(AIPG 10, AIIMS May 10)*

Ans. Methadone (Ref: KDT 6/e p399)

22. Oral hypoglycemic which should be stopped prior to surgery under GA is: *(AIIMS Nov 12)*

Ans. Metformin (Ref: Goodman and Gilman p1053)

23. For propofol, all are true, except: *(AIIMS Nov 09)*

a. It has a rapid recovery rate
b. It is used for induction and maintenance of anesthesia
c. It causes vomiting after use
d. It causes sedation

Ans. c (Ref: Sateskar 18/e p101)

24. Sildenafil is a selective inhibitor of: *(AIIMS Nov 09)*

Ans. PDE–5 (Ref: Satoskar 18/e p958)

25. Antiemetic is: *(AIIMS May 09)*

Ans. Propofol

26. Which of the following is a LT receptor antagonist: *(AIPG 10)*

Ans. Monteleukast

27. Finasteride is a: *(AIPG 09)*

Ans. 5-x reductase inhibitor

28. Which of the following drugs is both antiresorptive and bone formative? *(AIIMS May 11)*

Ans. Strontium ranelate (Ref: Bartl, Frisch and bartl, Osteoporosis: Diagnosis, Prevention, therapy, 2009 p152)

29. Which of the following is associated with thiazide diuretics? *(AIIMS Nov 10)*

Ans. Impotence (Ref: KDT 6/e p566-67)

30. First L.A. to the used clinically was: *(AIIMS Nov 10, 09)*

Ans. Cocaine (Ref: Katzung 10/e p412)

CHAPTER

17

General Medicine

Topic

- General Medicine
- CVS
- Hematology and Immunology
- Respiratory System
- Digestive System
- Excretory System
- Neuro Endocrinology

GENERAL MEDICINE

- SIRS (Systemic inflammatory response syndrome):

• Hyperthermia/hypothermia
• Leukocytosis/leucopenia
• Tachypnea/tachycardia

- Remember: Viral meningitis is rarely seen in elderly Patients.
- Strawberry tongue → Scarlet, Kawasaki
- DNA viruses vs RNA viruses

DNA Viruses	RNA Viruses
• Pox viridans (largest) Ex. Small pox	• Piconaviridae (Smallest) Ex. polio
• Herpesviridae	• Paramyxoviridae • Ex. Measles, mumps
• Adenoviridae	• Orthomyxoviridae Ex. influenza
• Hepadnaviridae–Hepatitis B.	• Toga viridae
	• Rhabdoviridae (Rabies virus)
	• Flaviviridae (Hepatitis C)
	• Calciviridae (Hepatitis E)

- Incubation periods:

Measles–1-2 weeks (AIPG 2012)
• Mumps Rubella Chicken Pox } 2-3 weeks
• Cholera-2-3 hr
• Hepatitis B–1-6 month
• TB–Months–years
• Leprosy–2-5 yrs.

- Classification of AIDS:

Class I → Prodromal symptoms Seroconversion (2-6 wks)
Class II → Asymptomatic
Class III → Persistent generalized Lymph adenopathy (> 500 CD4)
Class IV → AIDS syndrome (Opportunistic infection)

- Flow cytometry: Classifies cell types in leukemia and AIDS
  ↓
  [Q] CD4: CD8
- Teratogenic viruses: Trick–torch

T–Toxoplasmosis
O–Other agents → Syphillis + Varicella (Limb defect)
R–Rubella
C–CMV
H–HSV (Note: NOT HIV)

- Monocytes:

↑ses in: [Q]	↓ses in:
• Chronic infection–TB, Brucellosis sarcoidosis, SABE	• Acute infection
• Parasitic infection	• Aplastic anemia
• Malignancy–Leukemia, Lymphoma	• Hairy cell leukemia [Q]

- HIV binds to macrophages having CD4, CCRS, CXCR4
- For the microbiological assays of vit B12:

Lactobacillus leishmanni is used.

- Tumor lysis syndrome:

Features: Hyperuricemia, Hyperphosphatemia, Hyperkalemia
This Hyperphosphatemia causes → Reciprocal "Hypocalcemia"

- The characteristic feature of Rheumatoid arthritis (RA) is sparing of → Distal interpharyngeal joints
- Urea breath test: Test of choice to see the eradication of H. Pylori after treatment (prognosis)
- Behcat's → Bilateral conjunctival hypopyon(Purulent)
- Kawasaki → Bilateral conjunctival congestion (Non Purulent)

- Leprosy:

Female genital tract is rarely involved in leprosy. If involved it is ovary. Uterus is not involved.

- Iron+Folate deficiency → Due to inadequate dietary intake
- Cobalmine deficiency → Due to Malabsorption
- Neutropenic colitis → Lower abdominal pain is associated with chemotherapy
- Non Erosive arthritis → SLE + Reiter's syndrome. [Q]
- Fluoride doesn't cause osteoporosis But causes osteosclerosis
- T. Pallidum: Can be found in CSF in 1° and 2° syphilis while CNS and CVS manifestation seen in 3° syphilis.
- Biocompatibility Test:

• Cytotoxicity test → TB test (Trypan blue test)	
• Test that measure metabolic/other cell function → MTT test.	
• Mutagenic test (Test that measures effect on genetic material)	
Ame's test (AIPG)	Style's test (KCET)
Bacterial test	Mammalian test

Mycotic Aneurysm	Mycotic abscess	Mycoses fungoides
Misleading term ↓ Results from infected aneurysm ↓ In either intravascular or Extra vascular source ↓ Most commonly arises as a result of embolisaton from I.E. [Q]	Fungal infection	Cutaneus T-cell Lymphoma

- Chronic regional pain syndrome: Pain + swelling + Osteoporosis + hyperhydrosis
- HELLP syndrome:

Group of syndrome occurring in pregnant women.
H → Hemolysis, EL → Elevated liver enzyme, LP → Low platelet

- Angioneurotic edema vs Anaphylaxis

Angioneurotic edema	Anaphylaxis
Recurrent episodes of edema of face and larynx	Presence of intense pruritis
Pruritis and Urticarial lesions are characteristically absent.	Evidence of vascular collapse (Hypotension) in the presence of angioedema (Swelling of face and Lips)
Cause: Deficiency of C1 esterase inhibitor ↓ ↑ Activity of bradykinin and Kinase	

- Behcet's syndrome:

Chronic multisystem relapsing vascular inflammatory disease of unknown origin.
Associated with HLA-B5 positive

Diagnostic criteria → Essential criteria plus two of the non essential criteria for diagnosis.	
Essential criteria	Non-Essential criteria
Recurrent oral ulceration (Hall mark) [Q]	• Recurrent hypopyon [Q] • Recurrent genital ulcers. • Positive pathergy test
NOTE: Pathergy refers to hyperactivity to skin to any intracutaneous injection/needle stick positive pathergy is characteristic of Behcet's	

- Causes of clubbing:

• Pulmonary: – Bronchogenic CA – Lung abscess – Bronchietasis – Tuberculosis
• Cardiac – I.E. – Cyanotic congenital heart disease –Trick 'T' – T-Tricuspid atresia, Tetralogy of fallot – Pulmonary A-V Fistula
• Alimentary: – Ulcerative colitis – Crohn's disease
• Endocrine – Myxedema – Thyroid acropachy

- Methotrexate → In high doses used for Osteosarcoma
- Metal toxicities:

Metal	Deficiency	Toxicity
Zn	Growth retardation, Alopecia, Gonadal atrophy	Pulmonary fibrosis
Se	Endemic cardiomyopathy (Keshan disease)	
Ca	Osteoporosis	Milk alkali syndrome (Renal insufficiency)
Iodine		Acne like eruption

- In leukemic patient, gingival bleeding occurs during oral prophylaxis because of platelet disorder.
- Neck flexion results in physiologic dead space decrease
- Chemo therapeutic drugs cause both necrosis and apoptosis
- Familial retinoblastoma is AD in inheritance
- Cross–matching is not required for cryoprecipitate
- Unit used for Ringer's lactate–MEq/L (K)
- PAS stains:

Glycogen, fungal cell wall BM of human (Not of bacteria)
BM = Basement Membrane

- Remember: Formaldehyde and Glutaraldehyde → Both are active against spores
- Low reticulocyte associated anemia → Nutritional anemia (Fe deficiency anemia, folate deficiency anemia, vit. B12 deficiency anemia)
- Arsenic poisoning → Predominately sensory
- Lead poisoning → Purely motor
- H. pylori causes ulcer in antral portion of stomach
- In childhood AIDs → Kaposi sarcoma not seen
- Causative organism for Meningitis:

Pneumococcus > meningococcus > H pylori.

- Osteosarcoma and Osteoclastoma → Pulsatile tumor of long bone.
- It is β carotene/Provitamine A which is Antioxidants (Not Vit. A/Retinoic acid.)
- Tocolytics:

B2 Agonist CCB $MgSO_4$
Atosibam → Drug of choice as tocolytics in cardiac pts.

- Chances of congenital malformation is greater if infection is acquired during Ist trimester *(AIPG 2012)*
- Chances of Transmission of infection from mother to fetus are maximum when infection occurs during 3rd trimester.
- Most common childhood tumor → leukemia
- Retinoblastoma:

Most common inherited childhood tumor → retinoblastoma (40% hereditary)
Tumor is not associated with leukemia [Q] but associated with coarctation of Aorta

- Stones:

Most radio-opaque → Cysteine [Q]
Stone resistant to lithotripsy → Cysteine > Ca oxalate [Q]

- Site of Bone tumor:

Epiphysis → Osteoclastoma [Q] *(AIPG 2013)*
Metaphysis → Osteomylitis + Osteosarcoma [Q]
Diaphysis → Ewing Sarcoma [Q]

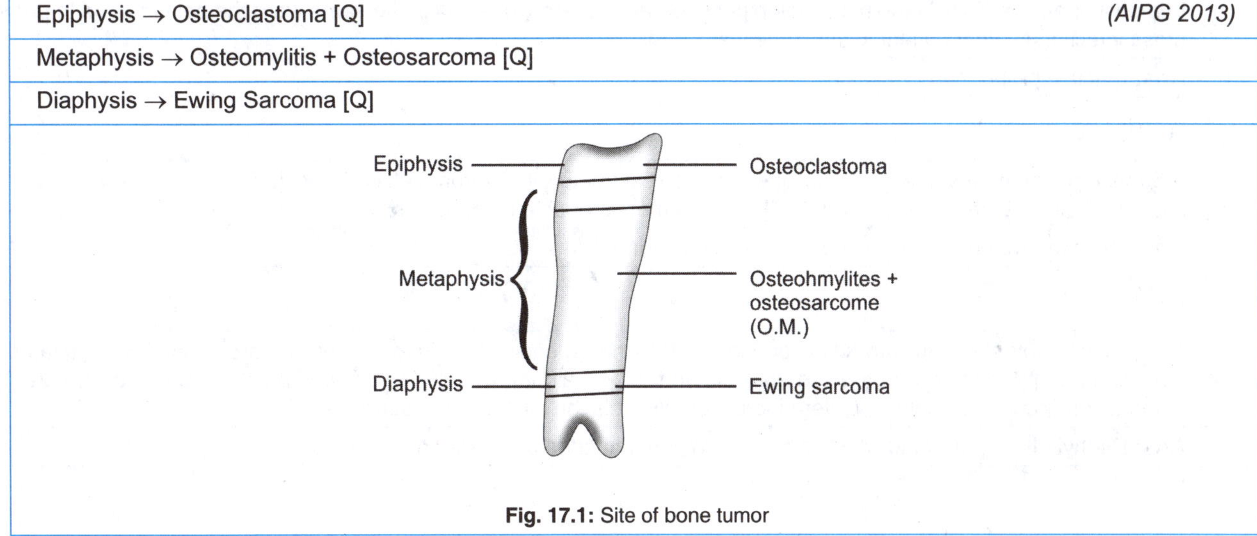

Fig. 17.1: Site of bone tumor

- Neonates: Can't produce heat by shivering [Q]
- Susceptibility of cell cycle to radiation:

G2M > G2 > M > G1 > Early S > Late S [Q]

- Tuberculous Osteomyelitis:

Periosteal Reaction is minimal
Sequestras are very uncommon

- HBV is too large to cross placenta
- Measles:

Koplic spot occurs 1-3 days before onset of rash, i.e. during prodromal phase.

- Metastasis:

Most common site of metastasis: Regional lymph nodes
2nd most common site of metastasis → liver

- Tetracychine + clindamycin → cause Colitis
- Enterocolitis is a major problem with clindamycim
- ALP (Alkaline phosphatase):

Produced from both liver and bone
↑Ses In → Bone disorder → Rickets, paget's disease, HPT, fibrous dysplasia, CA bone → Liver disease → Cholestasis, infective hepatitis, liver cirrhosis.
↓Sed ALP → Hypophosphatasia, Celiac sprue, Milk alkali syndrome.

- Case-I:

38 Children consumed eatables procured from a single source, 20 children develop abdominal cramps followed by vomiting and watery diarrhea 6-10 hrs after party .etiology is:
Ans: Clostridium perfringes infection. A case of food poisoning.

- Case-II:

In a post operative ICU, 5 patients develop post operative wound infection in the same ward the best method to prevent cross infection in other patient in the same ward is to:
Ans: practice proper hand washing

- Case-III:

A 50 year old man presented with multiple pathological fracture his serum calcium was 11.5 mg/dl, phosphate was 2.5 mg/dl and alkaline phosphatase was 94 IU/dl. The most probable diagnosis is:
Ans: Multiple myeloma as alkaline phosphatase is normal

- Case IV:

A 2 year old boy presents with fever for 3 days, Which responded to administration of paracetamol 3 days later, he developed acute renal failure, marked acidosis and encephalopathy, his urine showed plenty of Oxalate crystals. The blood anion gap and osmolal gap were increased. What is the most likely diagnosis:
Ans: Diethyl glycol poisoning which is present in contaminated paracetamol.

LAST 5-YEAR QUESTIONS FROM THIS TOPIC

1. **Hepatitis–E virus cause:** *(AIIMS Nov 12)*

Ans. Acute liver failure (Ref: Davidson 18/e p711)

2. **Untrue about fungal infection is:** *(PGI Dec 11)*
   a. Necrotic foci are common
   b. Indolent growth is a characteristic feature
   c. Less virulent in pathogenicity
   d. More common in immune compromised individuals

Ans. a (Ref: Ananthanarayan 7/e p610)

3. **Algorithm of life saving does not include?** *(PGI June 11)*

Ans. Blood pressure (Ref: Bailey's and love 23/e p273)

4. **Which of the following is the Ist marker seen in hepatitis B?** *(PGI June 11)*

Ans. HBs Ag (Ref: Bailey's and love 23/e p111)

5. **Antibiotic prophylaxis is mandatory in case of:** *(PGI Dec 09)*

Ans. Open reduction of fractured mandible (Ref: Peterson's 3/e p362)

6. **In SIRS there is** *(PGI Dec 09)*

Ans. B.P. > 110/70 (Ref: Internal sources)

7. **HIV binds to the macrophages having:** *(PGI June 09)*

Ans. CD4 and CCR5 molecules (Ref: ananthnarayan 6/e p543)

8. **A patient suffering from malaria taking primaquine reports to emergency with crisis. The patient may be deficient in:** *(AIPG 12)*

Ans. Glucose 6 phosphate dehydrogenase

9. **A lady delivers a neonate who has congenital phocomelia of limbs. The lady during her pregnancy might have taken:** *(AIPG 12)*

Ans. Thalidomide (Ref: Color atlas of embryology by Draws 1995 p363)

10. **In a pregnant lady the chances of rubella causing cardiac abnormalities is most probable in:** *(AIPG 12)*

Ans. Ist trimester (Ref: Donald school atlas of fetal anomalies by kurjak, chervenak, Carrera 2007, p315)

11. **All of the following are symptoms seen in SIRS except:** *(AIIMS May 11)*
    a. Oral temperature > 38°C in the mouth
    b. Infectious/non infectious etiology
    c. Leukocytosis
    d. Thrombocytopenia

Ans. d (Ref: Harrison 17/e p1696)

12. **Leukemia is not seen in:** *(AIPG 11)*
    a. Down syndrome
    b. Bloom syndrome
    c. Ataxia telegectasia
    d. Turner

Ans. d

13. **Fulminant hepatitis in pregnant woman is most commonly caused by:** *(AIPG 11)*

Ans. Hepatitis E (Ref: Parks 17/e p165)

14. **Prostate specific antigen is a:** *(AIPG 11)*

Ans. Tumor marker (Ref: Harrison 17/e p483)

15. **Gout is disorder of:** *(AIPG 11)*

Ans. Purine metabolism (Ref: Harrison 17/e p244)

16. Which of these is not included in parenteral therapy: *(AIPG 11, 10)*

Ans. Fibers

17. A 6 year old child is suffering with chronic pyogenic meningitis. Biochemical analysis of his CSF sample shows No change in glucose and protein, little/No change in neutrophil count and a marked increase in lymphocyte count. The most probable cause of meningitis is: *(AIPG 11)*

Ans. Viral (Ref: Robbins 7 p1370)

18. In human preterm birth refers, to the birth of a baby of less than: *(PGI June 12)*

Ans. 37 weeks gestational age.

19. Risus sardonicus of facial muscles is seen in: *(AIPG 10)*

Ans. Tetanus (Ref: Davidson's medicine 20/e p1232)

20. In falciparum malaria, all of the following are causes of anemia except: *(AIPG 10)*

a. Hemolysis
b. Malabsorption
c. Spleen sequestration
d. Bone marrow depression

Ans. b (Ref: Davidson's medicine p342-348)

21. Chronic carrier state is seen in all except: *(AIPG 10)*

a. Measles
b. Diphtheria
c. Typhoid
d. Gonorrhea

Ans. a

22. RDA recommendation for dietary modification in case of type 2 diabetes mellitus includes: *(AIPG 10)*

Ans. Increased dietary fiber (Ref: Harrison's 16/e p2171)

23. True about polio: *(AIPG 09)*

a. Paralytic polio is most common
b. Spastic paralysis is seen
c. Increased muscular activity leads to increased paralysis
d. Polio drops given only in < 3 years.

Ans. c (Ref: Harrison 17/e p1208)

24. Higoumenaki's sign is seen in: *(KCET 12)*

Ans. Syphilis

25. "Kissing lesion" is representive of: *(KCET 12)*

Ans. Candidiasis

26. Kolmer test is screening test done for: *(KCET 12)*

Ans. Syphilis

27. The following are the stigmata of late congenital syphilis (Hutchinson's classic triad) Except: *(KCET 12)*

a. Interstitial keratitis
b. Dysarthria
c. Hutchinson's teeth
d. 8th nerve deafness

Ans. b

28. Predisposing factors for urinary tract infection are: *(KCET 09)*

Ans. Pregnancy + Obstruction to urinary tract + vesicourethral influx disorder (Ref: Cecil textbook of medicine p112)

29. Recurrent epidydimitis is a feature of following infection: *(KCET 09)*

Ans. Wuchechereia bancrofti

30. The histologic criterion for diagnosis of acute appendicitis is neutroplilic infiltration of: *(COMEDK 09)*

Ans. Muscularis propria

31. Pre auricular sinus: *(COMEDK 09)*

Ans. Recurrence after excision is common (Ref: Greenfled's surgery)

32. All of the following viruses are capable of causing human cancers except: *(COMEDK 09)*

a. Papilloma virus
b. HBV
c. EBV
d. Parvovirus B-19

Ans. d

33. Which virus given below is not a teratognenic virus: *(COMEDK 10)*

a. Rubella
b. Cytomegalovirus
c. Herpes simplex
d. Measles

Ans. d

34. In case of anaphylactic reaction, the emergency treatment is: *(COMEDK 10)*

Ans. Adrenaline 0.5 to 1 ml of 1:1000 s.c/.i.m.

35. Following are criteria for SIRS except: *(KCET 12)*

a. Hypothermia < 36°c
b. Hyperthermia > 38°c
c. Tachycardia > 90/min
d. Respiratory rate < 20/min

Ans. d

36. MCS classification done for: *(KCET 10)*

Ans. Medical risk assessment

37. While performing a procedure, a resident doctor injures herself with a suture needle that has been used to stitch a patient with HIV infection for 11 years. He has been complaint with therapy for several years and has recently changed his tablets because of alteration in his appearance. His last CD4 count was 360 cells/mm. The doctor is offered post exposure prophylaxis. Which regimen should she take? *(KCET 12)*

Ans. Zidevudine + lamivudine + Indinavir.

38. At which stage congenital defects are more pronounced, especially when certain teratogenic agents interfere during development of embryo? *(KCET 10)*

Ans. 4 to 8 weeks

39. A 30 year old patient developed high fever of sudden onset. Peripheral blood smear showed crescent shaped gametocytes. Malaria pigment was dark brown in color. Which of the following malarial parasites is the causative agent? *(KCET 10)*

Ans. Plasmodium falciparum

40. General paresis in neurosyphilis is a feature of: *(KCET 12)*

Ans. 3° Syphilis

41. A young man presents with jaundice and itching. His viral serology showed active hepatitis E infection. Which of the following is true about hepatitis E? *(KCET 11)*

Ans. Transmission is by faeco-oral route (Ref: Ananthanarayan 7/e p559)

42. **A patient presents with jaundice. Physical examination reveals an enlarged nodular liver CT of the abdomen shows a cirrhotic liver with a large mass. CT guided biopsy of the mass demonstrates a malignant tumor derived with which of the following viruses would most directly relate to the development of this tumor?** *(KCET 11)*

Ans. HBV (Ref: Robbins 7/e p327)

43. **A 60 year old male presents with a 2 day history of a severe left ear ache with a burning sensation in the ear and loss of taste. There is left sided weakness of both upper and lower facial muscles. Facial sensation is normal. A few vesicles are seen in pharynx. What is diagnosis?** *(KCET 11)*

Ans. Ramsay hunt syndrome (Ref: Shafer 5/e p482)

44. **Case Report** *(COMEDK 12)*

A 41 year old man presented to the emergency department with a 9 month history of cough, exertional dysponea, nocturnal diaphoresis (profuse sweating) and weight loss of 10 kg. The physical examination revealed painless, massive, discrete, rubbery cervical, supraclavicular and axillary lyphadenopathy. Plain radiography of the chest showed bilateral hilar lymphadenopathy. The serum calcium was elevated at 16.2 mg/dl; serum parathyroid hormone is within normal range.

a. **The probable diagnosis of the above condition is**

Ans. Hodgkin's lymphoma

b. **Urgent treatment to be instituted for his would be**

Ans. C.V. Normal saline and a bisphosphonate

c. **A diagnostic investigation was performed on him**

Ans. Excisional biopsy of axillary node.

d. **The treatment of choice:**

Ans. Chemotherapy of doxorubicin, bleomycin, vinblastine and dacarbazine

45. **The classical karyotype of klinefilter:** *(KCET 11)*

Ans. 47, XXY

46. **An 18 year. Old lady presents with severe sore throat, fever and malaise. She has cervical lymphadenopathy, splenomegaly and scattered petechiae on the soft palate with enlarged tonsils covered with white exudates. Which of the following investigations is most likely to help guide for managements:** *(KCET 11)*

Ans. Heterophil antibody test (Ref: Shafer's 5/e p1065-1068)

47. **The vaccine currently used against HBV infection is:** *(COMEDK 12)*

Ans. Recombinant

48. **A 20 year male complains of recurrent attacks of sore throat since 2 years. The TLC was 1000/dl. A differential count revealed severe neutropenia. The diagnosis is:** *(COMEDK 12)*

Ans. Agranulocytosis (TLC < 2000)

Note: Drugs with highest risk to cause Agranulocytosis are macrolides and antithyroids

CVS

- S_3 heart sound heard in: [Q]

Physiological	Pathological
High cardiac output conditionst	
• Athletes • Fever • Thyrotoxicosis • Pregnancy • A–V fistula	• Left to right shunt i.e. Acyanotic heart Disease ex-ASD, VSD, PDA • Constructive pericarditis

- S_4 heart sound:

Physiologic	Pathological condition
Old age	HOCM
	HTN
	MR

- Clinical spectrum of HOCM:

Asymptomatic patient/Sudden death (Ist clinical manifestation)/Symptomatic pt.
Symptoms: Dysponea, Angina, Syncope Double/Triple pericardial Impulse, Brisk carotid upstroke
Sign 4th Heart Sound Systolic murmur

- Rx for MI (Acute MI):

PCI (percutaneus intervention) → Angiography and 1° Angioplasty thrombolytic therapy
PCI > Thrombocytic

- HTN is most common cause of left ventricular hypertrophy
- Ventilation to perfusion Ratio:

High for Apex.
Changes with standing to lying down.

- The Jones criteria of rheumatic fever:

Major criteria:

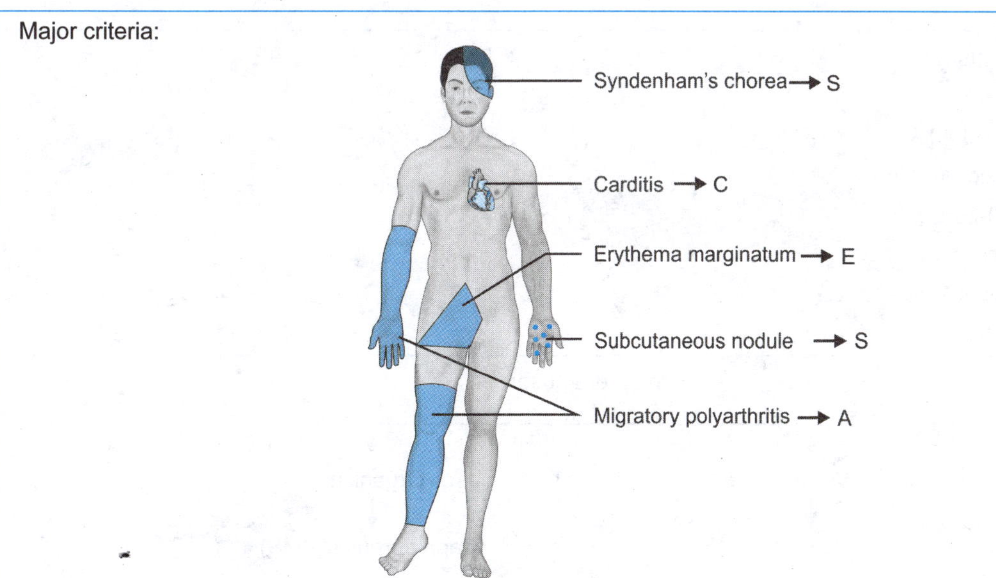

Fig. 17.2: Jones criteria of rheumatic fever

Trick for major criteria: "CASES"
Carditis (2) → 'C'
Migratory polyarthritis (3) → 'A'
Sydenhem's chorea (1) → 'S'
Erythema marginatum (5) → 'E'
Subcutaneous nodules (4) → 'S'

NOTE: *Aschoff's nodule is the characteristic of rheumatic fever (AIPG 2012)
Pulmonary valve → is least commonly involved in Rheumatic fever.
Minor criteria: Fever, Athralgia Plus ASO titer > 300 (Children) ASO titer > 200 (Adult)

- The duke criteria for I.E.

Major criteria: • Positive blood culture • Positive echo cardiographic finding of vegetations.
Minor criteria: Cardiac failure Pyrexia i.v. drug abuse Embolic phenomenon vasculitic phenomenon Splinter hemorrhage Hematurea (60-70%) Osler's nodes Roth's spot in fundi Digital clubbing
Causative organism • Streptococci – Viridans–30-40% – Enterococci–10-15% – Other–20-25% • Staphylococci – S. Aureus–9-27% • HACEK group
I.E. in i.v. drug user:

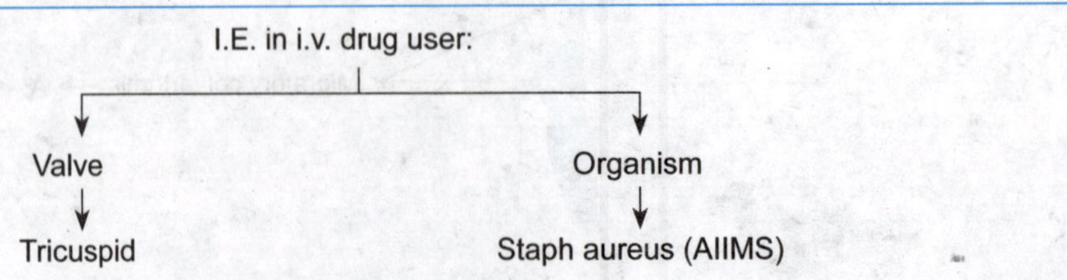

- I.E. (Infective endocarditis):

Risk factors: • High Pressure areas (Left side of heart) • Patients with Valvular incompetence (regurgitation) than those with stenosis so, MR >> MS. MR, prosthetic heart valve + congenital heart disease except ASD

- JVP:

Chamber of interest
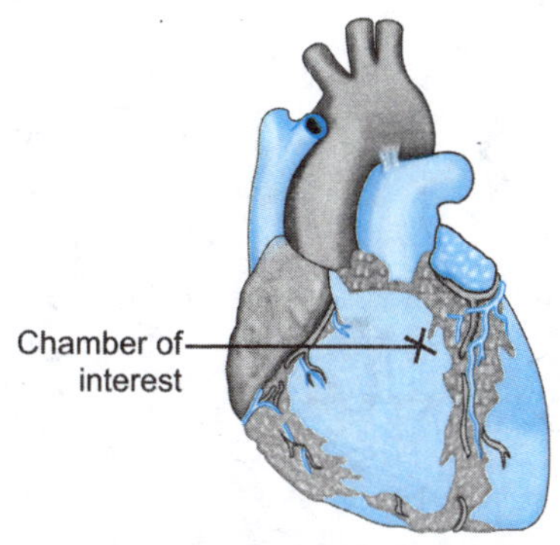 **Fig. 17.3:** JVP chamber of interest
• Arterial systole: Giant a = Forceful contraction of Right Auricle – Seen in TS – Against stiff ventricle RVH → (Right ventricular hypertrophy) Pulmonary HTN → leads to RVH
• C-wave → seen with bulging of tricuspid valve into RA (right auricle) [Q]
• V-wave → Due to venous filling of RA Giant v → 'TR' [Q]

- Intracranial hemorrhage:

Intra cerebral	Sub Arachnoid
Most common reason: Basal ganglion	2nd most common Berry Aneurysum

- If pressure > 10 mm Hg → Portal HTN
- Murmur:

Are due to vibrations produced by the turbulent flow at: • The region of the valve • Near the valve • Abnormal communication within the heart
Early systolic murmur: Murmur begins with the Ist heart sound. Ex-MR, TR
MID-systolic murmur: MVP (Mitral valve prolapse) [Q]
PAN systolic murmur: MR, TR and VSD [Q]

- During operation non selective β blocker are not given to control HR (As causes further cardiac depression)
- Pregnancy:

Hyperdynamic circulation ↓ Stroke volume, C.O (Cardiac output)

LAST 5-YEAR QUESTIONS FROM THIS TOPIC

1. **The Ist heart sound is loud in all of the following except:** *(KCET 09)*
   a. Mitral stenosis
   b. Short PR interval
   c. Tachycardia
   d. Mitral valve calcification

Ans. d

2. **False about risk factor for stroke:** *(KCET 09)*
   a. Diabetes
   d. Anemia
   c. Heart failure
   d. Alcohol

Ans. b (Ref: Cecil text book of medicine p65)

3. **Pan systolic murmur seen in all of the following except:** *(PGI June 12)*
   a. MS
   b. Atrial septal defect
   c. VSD
   d. TR

Ans. a

4. **Most important drug used in the treatment of coronary artery disease is:** *(KCET 09)*

Ans. Aspirin (Ref: Cecil textbook of medicine p71)

5. **Giant 'V' wave on examination of the JVP is suggestive of:** *(COMEDK 10)*

Ans. Tricuspid incompetence

6. **When PR interval in bipolar limb lead electrocardiograph prolongs beyond 0.20 seconds the patient has:** *(KCET 10)*

Ans. Ist degree incomplete block

7. **The Ist heart sound is loud in all the following except:** *(KCET 12)*
   a. MS
   b. Short PR interval
   c. Tachycardia
   d. Mitral valve calcification

Ans. a

8. **The following are recognized cause of neutropenia except:** *(KCET 12)*
   a. Corticosteriod therapy
   b. Typhoid fever
   c. Aplastic anemia
   d. Viral infection

Ans. b

9. **An elderly man develops syncope. He is known to have IHD. Peripheral pulse are absent, BP is not recordable and ECG revealed wide complex tachycardia, immediate management consists of which of the following?** *(KCET 12)*

Ans. DC cardioversion

10. **A young woman is seen in OPD and is found to have loud Ist heart sound, an early diastolic sound followed by mid diastolic murmur. What is her likely diagnosis?** *(KCET 12)*

Ans. MS with mobile leaflets

11. A 64 years old gentleman is brought with severe central chest pain radiating to the left arm for the last 30 min. He is profusely sweating and is in agony. Which of the following disease he is likely to be suffering from? *(KCET 12)*

Ans. Acute MI

12. Mural thrombi are thrombi in: *(KCET 12)*

Ans. Heart chamber

13. The dominant histologic feature of infarction is: *(KCET 12)*

Ans. Coagulative necrosis

14. Differential diagnosis of stroke include all except: *(KCET 10)*

a. Cerebral tumors
b. Subdural hematoma
c Myocardial infarction
d. Encephalitis

Ans. c

15. Treatment of torsade de pointes is i.v.: *(COMEDK 11)*

Ans. Magnesium (Ref: Davidson 19/e p411-412)

16. Which one of the following is indicative of cardiac tamponade? *(COMEDK 11)*

Ans. Pulsus paradoxus (Ref: Davidson 20/e p526-645)

17. Acute rheumatic fever usually follows an infection with: *(COMEDK 11)*

Ans. Streptococcus pyogens (Ref: Davidson 20/e p616)

18. You are managing a cardiac arrest. Which drug is to be given for ventricular fibrillation after unsuccessful defibrillation: *(KCET 11)*

Ans. 1 mg epinephrine (Ref: Davidson 18/e p557)

19. A patient presents with CCF with depressed ejection fraction. Which drug may be effective in reducing mortality? *(KCET 11)*

Ans. Enalapril (Ref: KDT 5/e p468)

20. A 30 year old lady, previous rheumatic heart disease presents with 3 month history of fatigue, weight loss, night sweats and dysponea on exertion. She is pyrexial with evidence of mitral regurgitation and splint hemorrhage ECHO confirms vegetation, blood cultures are taken and a diagnosis of infective endocarditis is made. What is the most likely infective organism in this case? *(KCET 11)*

Ans. Streptococcus viridians (Ref: Davidson 19/e p464)

21. The dicrotic notch on aortic pressure curve is caused by: *(COMEDK 12)*

Ans. Closure of aortic valve

22. The most common organism associated with SABE: *(AIPG 11)*

Ans. Streptococcus viridians (Ref: Robbin's 7/e p596)

HEMATOLOGY AND IMMUNOLOGY

- Antinuclear antibodies in auto immune disease:

• Anti dsDNA → SLE
• Anti histone antibodies → Drug induced lupus erythematosis
• Anti Sm antibody → SLE
• SSa (RO) and SSb (La) → Sjogren syndrome
• Anti DNA topisomerase antibody (SCL70) → Systemic sclerosis
• Anti Centromere Ab → CREST syndrome
• Anti mitochondrial Ab → 1° billary cirrhosis

- Fanconi's Anemia:

Is a form of inherited a plastic anemia → AR
Sed risk of malignancy (AML)
Congenital anomalies of all system seen → Solid tumors (SCC of heads neck)

- Coomb's test:

Heterophil agglutination test used in – Blood transfusion Spherocytosis (Immune mediated) [Q] Hemolytic anemia Brucellosis

Warm Antibody	**Cold Antibody**
Hemolytic Anemia	
E.g: Cell (B cell type) SLE Drug–Methyl dopa	E.g: Mycoplasma infection Infection Mononucleosis

- Deficiency of all clotting factors is associated with AR except VIII and IX
- Auto Immune hemolytic Anemia is associated with:

• B cell CLL
• Non Hodgkins lymphoma

- DIC:

Is associated with important endocrine syndromes: • Pituitary → Sheehan's syndrome • Adrenal → Fredrich Hausen syndrome

- Kawasaki:

Immune mediated systemic vasculitis
So, t/t → I.v. Ig.

- Anemia of Chronic disease:

Seen in TB, RA
Microcytic hypochromic anemia.
This anemia is characterized by Ample storage of Iron.

- Cytokinine:

Inhibitory effect on CFUE → Anemia
Stimulation of hepicidin (Synthesized in liver) → Inhibits the release of iron from the anemia stored pool

- Arteritis:

Giant cell Arteritis	Takayasu/Non specific aorto Arteritis
Temporal Arteritis	
Age > 50 yrs	< 50 yrs
Precipitates with combing	Aortic aneurysm

- Giant cell Arteritis (Temporal Arteritis):

Large vessel vasculitis. Mostly affects temporal artery. Granulomatous inflammation.
Elderly > 55 years, woman > men.
Lab feature → ESR, Anemia
Typical presentation • Headache (Most commonly localized over temporal region) patients present with typical pain in scalp when they comb or brush their hair. • Jaw claudication → most specific symptoms. Typically present with pain in the masseter muscle on prolonged chewing. • Visual blindness

- Thunder clap headache:

Most commonly due to subarachnoid hemorrhage age > 50 yrs.

- TTP:

Absent ADAMTS B enzyme (VWF metalloproteinase)
↓
Accumulation of VWF
↓
↑Sed platelet aggregation
↓
Thrombus
(Composed mainly of platelets, No fibrin, Normal complement)

- Wiskott–Aldrich syndrome:

• Immunodeficiency with thrombocytopenia and Eczema.
• X-linked
• Mutation of WASP gene.
• IgM
• IgE → (ECZEMA)

- Wegner's Granulomatosis:

Though it is called granulomatous vasculitis, Granuloma is seen only is respiratory tract.
Other organs demonstrate → Necrotizing vasculitis

- Wegner's granulomatosis vs Allergic branchopulmonary:

Wegner's Granulomatosis	Allergic Branchopulmonary Arthritis
Weight Loss	No Weight loss/oligoarthritis
Oligoarthritis	

- Tolosa Hunt syndrome vs cavernous sinus thrombosis:

Tolosa Hunt Syndrome	Cavernous Sinus Thrombosis
Chronic inflammation of cavernous sinus	Thrombosis
Dilation of Sinus Not thrombosis	Opthalmoplagia

- Hemolysis in GGPD is caused by all quinine derivatives.

- Bernald Soulier syndrome vs Glanzmann's Thrombasthenia:

→ Deficiency of GPIb → platelets can't adhere by vWF	→ Deficiency of GP II b/IIIa, platelets can't aggregate by fibrinogen. (Inter platelet aggregation abnormal)
→ Ristocetin → No aggregation	→ Ristocetin Aggregation: Normally to ristocetin
→ Platelet → Number → ↓ ses Thrombocytopenia → Size–Large	→ Both → Normal
→ B.T	→ ↑ B.T.

- Fanconi's syndrome:

Characterized by triad of: • Cystinosis • Wilson disease • Hereditary fructose intolerance

- ECG changes:

Hypokalemia	Hyperkalemia
• ST depression	• ↑sed 'T' Wave amplitude
• Prolong P-R interval	• Prolonged P-R
• Flattened or inverted 'T' wave	• Prolonged QRS duration
• Prominent 'V' wave	

Hypocalcemia	Hypercalcemia
Prolonged QT	Decreased QT

- TB:

• Pulmonary artery aneurysm in tuberculosis cavity → Rasmussen's Aneurysm
• The Aneurysm responsible for massive Hemoptysis in TB Cavity → Bronchial artery aneurysm.

- Stress ECHO:

Stress + Echocardiography.
Used for coronary artery disease to judge the severity of ischemia.
Initially echocardiography was used, now the combination of stress testing + Echocardiography is used. • Exercise stress testing • Pharmacological stress testing → It is done by infusion of dobutamine to se myocandial O_2 demand.

- Vasculitis:

Granulomatous	Necrotizing
Wegner's	PAN
Takayasu	Good pasture syndrome
Temporal	Chrug–strauss.

- Major "Indicator" for coronary heart disease → HDL
- Major "Risk factor" for coronary heart disease → LDL

- Anti TNF:

Used in all types of arthritis (RA + seronegative arthritis) + Crohn's (NOT SLE) [Q]

- Good pasture syndrome:

Auto antibody against basement of kidney and Lung.
Kidney → Rapidly proliferating Glomerulonephritis
Lung → Pulmonary hemorrhage (Hemoptysis)
T/t → Plasmapheresis + Corticosteroid

- VWD:

Rx:
Antidiuretic

↓
Desmopressin
↓
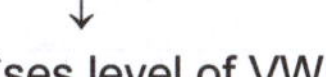
↑ses level of VWF

- LAP (Leukocyte Alkaline phosphatase):

Screening test used to distinguish CML from other myloproliferative disorder because LAP ↑ ses in all myeloproliferative disorder except CML
↓
So ↑ses in polycythemia, myelofibrosis.

- Hereditary hemosiderosis → AR with incomplete penetrance.
- Bone marrow biopsy is absolutely indicated in hairy cell leukemia because aspiration can't be done
- DIC:

B.T, C.T., PTT, PT (All) ↑sed
FDP (Fibrin degradation product) [Q]
Most common site of DIC → Brain (for thrombus formation)

- Bone scan → Least useful in diagnosis of multiple myeloma
- In stored blood → citrate chelates with both Ca and Mg → causes Hypocalcaemia and Hypomagnesaemia
- In Aneurysm → Tunica media in Affected
- Crush Injury → Acute renal failure [Q], DIC
- Streptokinase/urokinase, (i.e. thrombolysin):

Absolute C/I → malignancy
Relative C/I → Peptic ulcer patients on anticoagulant

- Cardiac tamponade:

Acute heart failure due to deposition of fluid around pericardium
Beck's triad of cardiac tamponade: • Hypotension • Soft/absent heart sounds • JVP

- Erythropoesis:

Intra uterine 3 wk to 3 month → Yolk sac 3 month to 5 month → Liver + spleen > 5 Month → Red bone marrow
Birth to 20 yrs → Flat + long bones
> 20 yrs → Flat bone

- Most common site of peripheral aneurysm → popliteal artery
- Polycythemia vera:

RBC, WBC and Blood volume ↑ ses B.T. and C.T → Normal Lap score ↑ sed

- All clotting factor except factor VIII are synthesized by liver
- Severe hypertensive emergency: (Ex-pre echlampsia)

• Hydralazine, Labetalol [Q]

- ASD, VSD, PDA → All are common in female
- Common coagulation pathway:

1, 2, 5, 10, 13 factors

- Migraine Prophylaxis:

Trick: Very Volatile Pharma Agent For Migraine Prophylaxis
V → Verapamil V → Valproate P–Pizotifen A → Amitryptilline F→ Flunarazine M → Methylserzide P–Propanolol.

- Evan syndrome:

Auto immune destruction of RBC and Platelets
so combination of ITP and Auto immune hemolytic anemia seen.

LAST 5-YEAR QUESTIONS FROM THIS TOPIC

1. **In hemophilia treatment includes:** *(PGI Dec 09)*

Ans. Factor 8 replacement

2. **A Patient is on anticoagulant therapy then there must be prolonged:** *(PGI Dec 09)*

Ans. Prothrombin time (Ref: Vinod kapoor 2/e p647)

3. **General lack of bone marrow activity is seen in which anemia:** *(PGI June 12)*

Ans. Aplastic anemia

4. **Which of the following investigations should be done immediately to best confirm a non matched blood transfusion reaction:** *(AIIMS Nov 10)*

Ans. Direct coomb's Test (Ref: Harrison 17/e p710)

5. **Monocytes are seen in TB, Monocytic leukaemia, typhoid and:** *(AIIMS Nov 10)*

Ans. SABE (Ref: Shafer 5/e p1066)

6. **A 9 year old girl after tonsillectomy presents with uncontrolled bleeding with laboratory findings of prolonged a PTT, normal PT anda normal ptalelet count. What could be the deficiency?** *(AIIMS Nov 09)*

Ans. Von-willebrand disease

7. **Test for 1° homeostasis is** *(KCET 09)*

Ans. Bleeding time (Ref: Kecil text book of medicine p251)

8. **Hemoptysis is caused by:** *(KCET 09)*

Ans. Leukemia + heaemophilia + anticoagulant therapy

9. **Kaposi's sarcoma usually occurs when CD4 lymphocyte counts are:** *(COMEDK 09)*

Ans. Below 200

10. **Commonest mode of inheritance of von willibrand disease is:** *(COMEDK 09)*

Ans. AD

11. **A 3 year-old child presented with progressive anemia, jaundice and failure to thrive. O/E pallor, splenomegaly + peripheral smear showed normoblasts and small round intensely stained red cells. The likely diagnosis is:** *(COMEDK 09, 12)*

Ans. Hereditary spherocytosis

12. **"Auer roods" are seen in:** *(COMEDK 10)*

Ans. Myeloblast

13. **Spontaneous mouth petechiae and gingival bleeding occur typically at platelet levels:** *(COMEDK 10)*

Ans. Between 20,000–30,000/mm^3

14. **Hair on end appearance is not seen:** *(PGI June 12)*
    a. Thalassaemia
    b. Sickle cell anemia
    c. Paget's disease
    d. Cooley anemia

Ans. c (Ref: Naville p542)

15. **In during blood transfusion, transfusion reaction occurs inform of incompatibility the Ist thing to be done is:** *(KCET 11)*

Ans. Stop the transfusion (Ref: Davidson 19/e p915)

16. **Slow ESR is usually seen in:** *(COMEDK 12)*

Ans. Congestive heart failure

Note: ESR sed in–Infection, MI, connective tissue disorder, inflammatory disease, malignant lymphoma, oral contraceptive use,

ESR ced in–Sickle cell anemia, allergy, jaundice

RESPIRATORY SYSTEM

- Bacterial pneumonia associated with cavitation:

Staph. aureus, Kliebsiella, pseudomonas + 2° TB

- Acidosis (Metabolic and respiratory):

Causes both hyperkalemia + hyperphosphatemia

- Lung disease:

Obstructive lung disease: Trick–ABC	Restrictive lung disease
A= Asthma B = Bronchictactis C =Cystic fibrosis, COPD	Sarcoidosis.

- Hypocapnea causes vasoconstriction, Hypercapnea causes vasodilatation–Both are contraindication in head injury.
- Lung CA:

• Adeno carcinoma is the most common type
• SCC variant is central in location + cavitatory.
• Large cell → cavitatory
• Small cell (Oat) → central
• Adeno carcinoma is just opposite of SCC so peripheral in location and Non cavitatory.

- Most common site for metastatic calcification → Alveoli wall of lung.
- Obstructive vs Restrictive lung disease:

Obstructive	Restrictive
$\frac{FEV1}{FVC}$ = ↓Sed	$\frac{FEV1}{FVC}$ = Normal (very Imp.)

- COPD:

Emphysema → Pink puffer
Chronic bronchitis → Blue bloater

- Wheezing/Rhonchi seen in → Asthma/COPD (Obstructive lung disease)
- Stony dull note → Pleural effusion
- DVT vs Embolism:

The most common site for DVT is calf muscle but most common site pulmonary embolism is pelvic/femoral vein. (large leg vein)

- Normal diameter of chest wall:

A-P: Lateral = 5: 7
↑Ses in COPD [Q]

- Katagener' s syndrome:

Cilliary dysfunction syndrome of respiratory epithelium, sperm and other cells characterized by recurrent sinusitis, bronchiectasis, dextrocardia and infertility

- Emphysema: Though obstructive lung disease but diffusion capacity decrease (Like restrictive lung disease)
- Ca2+ is present in surfactant
- Pectus carinatum/pigeon chest → Severe Asthma and Rickets
- Cor pulmohate: In pulmonary HTN secondary to RVH (Right Ventricular Hypertrophy)
- Adam's stroke attack: is recurrent syncope associated with ventricular arrhythmia
- Pulse paradoxus:

The dramatic fall in B.P. during inspiration
It is characterized by tamponade severe airway obstruction.
The phenomenon is exaggeration of normal

- Hemodynamic effect of respiration:

Inspiration → B.P. falls due to reduction of blood flow to the heart.
Expiration → B.P. rises due to rise in venous return to the left heart.

- PAD (Peripheral artery disease):

Intermittent claudication → brought on by exercise/walking due to mild to moderate arterial occlusion.
Critical limb ischemia → Rest pain. Severe arterial Occlusion ex-gangrene, ischemic ulcer.

LAST 5-YEAR QUESTIONS FROM THIS TOPIC

1. Paradoxical movement of chest in a patient who has suffered trauma is called: *(AIPG 11)*

Ans. Flial chest

2. Most common mode of treatment of a 1 year old child with asthma: *(AIPG 09)*

Ans. Inhaled short acting B-2 against (Ref: Ghai 6/e p358, 359)

3. All the following are features of acute severe asthma except: *(KCET 09)*

a. Respiratory rate > 25
b. Heart rate > 110
c. PEF < 50% of normal/predicted
d. Temperature > 102° F

Ans. d (Ref: Cecil textbook of medicine p101)

4. In lobar pneumonia, the presence of fibrino suppurative exudates with disintegration of red cells are seen in the stage of: *(COMEDK 10)*

Ans. Grey hepatization

5. All of the given drugs may be given in acute exacerbation of bronchial asthma except: *(COMEDK 10)*

a. Cromolyn sodium
d. Hydorcortisone
c. Salbutamol
d. Ipratropium

Ans. d (Ref: Katzang 7/e p154)

6. The beneficial effect of O_2 therapy in histotoxic hypoxia is about: *(KCET 10)*

Ans. 0%

Note: In this type of hypoxia tissues are unable to utilize O_2, so O_2 therapy is of no use.

7. Risk factors of TB include: *(KCET 10)*

Ans. HIV + Type, diabetes mellitus + chronic renal failure

8. Mantowx test is done for diagnosis of: *(KCET 11)*

Ans. TB

9. 2° Amyloidosis is seen most commonly in: *(COMEDK 12)*

Ans. TB

10. Which of the following disease cause damage of vertebral body and inter vertebral space: *(AIIMS Nov 12)*

Ans. Tuberculosis (Ref: Harrison's 16/e p497)

DIGESTIVE SYSTEM

- Crohn's disease:

May be caused by C. Difficle, Shigella, Salmonella, Campylobacter.

- Obstructive Jaundice → Dark color urine + clay stool
- "D-Xylulose test" is indicator of mucosal function of GIT (Absorbed completely without pancreatic enzyme)
- Organism causing invasive diarrhoea: Shigella, Salmonella, Y. enterocolitica, listeria, Amoeba

- Clinical features of cirrhosis:

• Hepatomegaly
• Ascitis
• Spider telangectasia
• Epistaxis
• hepatic encephalopathy
• Gynaecomostia
• Portal HTN:
  – Splenomegaly
  – Variceal bleeding (KCET 2012)

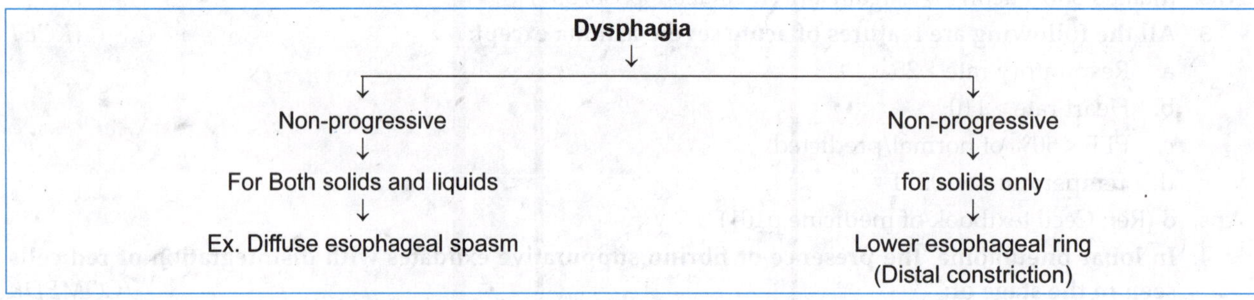

- Flask shaped ulcer seen in → Amoebiasis
- Cystic fibrosis:

Characterized by • Liver cirrhosis • Pancreatitis

- Gastric CA → Hypochlorhydria/Acholhydria (HCL)
- Alcohol → reduces thermo genesis (Vasodilatation)
- Case III:

A 5 year old boy passed 18 loose stools in last 24 hrs and vomited twice in last 4 hrs. He is irritable but drinking fluids. The optional therapy for this child is:
Ans: Oral rehydration fluids as he is able to drink fluids.

LAST 5-YEAR QUESTIONS FROM THIS TOPIC

1. Lesions caused by Entameoba histolytica predominantly involve: *(COMEDK 10)*

Ans. Caecum and large intestine

2. Syndrome associated with jaundice include all except: *(KCET 10)*

a. Gilbert's syndrome
b. Dubin–Johnson syndrome
c. Gardner's Syndrome
d. Rotor's Syndrome

Ans. c

3. Factors precipitating hepatic encephalopathy include all except: *(KCET 10)*

a. Infection
b. Magnesium trisilicate therapy
c. Hpokalaemia
d. Gastrointestinal bleeding

Ans. b

4. **Which of the following is the right choice of Rx for portosystemic encephalopathy?** *(KCET 12)*

Ans. Lactulose

5. **In a patient with liver cirrhosis, which one of the listed feature is characteristic of portal hypertension:** *(KCET 12)*

Ans. Esophageal varices

EXCRETORY SYSTEM

- Nephrotic syndrome:

Hypercoagualability (Due to ↑ sed loss of inhibitors of coagulation Antithrombin, protein C, S)
Hypercholestrolemia (High risk of Atherosclerosis)

- Quantifying proteinurea [Q]

< 30 mcg → Normal
30–300 → Micro albuminurea
> 4g → Nephrotic Range

- Electrolytic imbalance in Renal failure:

Hyperkalemia	Hyponatremia
Hypermagnesemia	Hypocalcemia (Due to ↓ sed vit. D synthesis)

- In coagulation disorder → only PTT ↑ ses not PT
- PT ↑ sed in:

Warfarin therapy, Vit k deficiency [Q]

- aPTT is ↑ sed in heparin and Hemophilia [Q]
- 1° Gouty arthritis is mainly due to ↓sed renal excretion of uric acid not due to over production
- Jaundice:

For the excretion of bilirubin in kidney i.e bilirubinurea bilirubin has to be conjugated in liver.
Hemolytic jaundice: ↓ Excess breakdown of RBC ↓ So excess amount of bilirubin is produced liver ↓ can't conjugate all bilirubin (Although liver can function 6 times more) ↓ So ↑sed urobillinogen in urine) [Q] ↓ So presence of unconjugated bilirubin in blood → Hyperbilirubinemia But unconjugated bilirubin can't excreted through urine so, NO hyperbilirubinurea [Q] ↓ Obstructive jaundice: ↓ Conjugation occurs in liver ↓ But because of obstruction can't go to intestine ↓ So, NO urobilinogen in urine ↓ But as conjugate → so can execrate in urine → Bilirubinurea.

- Hereditary hyperbilirubinemia [Q]:

Unconjugated	Conjugated
Crigler Najjar syndrome	Dubin Johnson syndrome
Gilbert syndrome	Rotor's syndrome

- Ascending loop of Henle is impermeable to water → Hypotonic urine
- PCT → Isotonic urine
- Diabetes insipidus → Rx Demeclocyline (Anti ADH action)
- Wilm's tumor → most common neoplasm of kidney *(AIPG 12)*
- Causes of spleenomegaly:

Trick–CHINA
C–Congestion/cellular infiltrate H–Haematological (Hemolytic/SCA) I–Infection/Infraction (Malaria, CMV) N- Neoplasm (CML, Lymphoma) A–Auto immune

LAST 5-YEAR QUESTIONS FROM THIS TOPIC

1. **Dehydration is the common concern in early edentulous patients because of:** *(COMEDK 09)*

Ans. Reduced ability to sense thirst (Ref: Evans textbook of geriatric medicine p22)

2. **Mg⁺ level in blood increases in:** *(COMEDK 09)*

Ans. Kidney failure

3. **Nephrotic syndrome is characterized by:** *(KCET 10)*

Ans. Proteinuria + edema + serum albumin < 30 g/dl

4. **A 50 year old female with end stage renal disease (ESRD) develops pulmonary TB which drug should be used in a reduced dose?** *(KCET 11)*

Ans. Ethambutol (Ref: KDT 5/e p699-701)

5. **A 30 year old known SLE female presents with ankle swelling. Her BP is 170/100 mm Hg and she has marked lower limb edema. Urine dip stick discloses 4+ proteins with no haematuria. Plasma creatinine is 1.4 mg /dl, albumin is 1.5g/dl and urine protein excretion rate was 6g for 24 hrs. What is the cause for this presentation?** *(KCET 11)*

Ans. Class V Lupus nephritis (Ref: Harrison principles of internal medicine 14/e p1548)

NEURO ENDOCRINOLOGY

- DM (Diabetes mellitus):

Is associated with
• Coronary artery disease • Peripheral artery disease • Stroke Not with DVT

- LMN (Lesion of VII nerve) vs UMN:

LMN	UMN
• Bell's palsy (VII nerve palsy) • Herpes zoster	• Tumors • Cerebrovascular accident
Presentation • One half of the face is involved on the same side • Inability to close the ipsilateral eye and drooling of saliva is characteristic of VII nerve palsy. • Deviation of mouth towards opposite side. • Comes normal with smile	• Contra lateral lower half of the face is involved whereas the upper half of the face is spared as it has bilateral innvervation
→ Reflexes: Both superficial and Deep lost	→ Reflexes: Superficial → Lost Deep → Exaggerated *(PGI 12)*

- Lambert Eaten myasthenia Syndrome vs Myasthenia gravis:

Lambert Eaten myasthenia Syndrome	Myasthenia gravis
• Presynaptic disorder antibodies to Ca^{2+} channels ↓se in presynaptic release of Ach at N-M junction is the fundamental defect	• Post synaptic disorder antibodies against ACH receptors. Decrease in number of ACH receptors at post synaptic muscle membrane is the fundamental defect.
• Proximal limb muscles >> Extraocular and • Limb Muscle (Involved)	• Extra ocular and lib muscles > proximal limb muscle
• No fatigability/Incremental response	• Fatigability/Decremental response
• Repeated stimulation causes ↑sed muscle strength	• Repeated stimulation causes ↓sed muscle strength
• Reflex-Hyporeflexia/Assent reflexes	• Reflexes → Intact
• Autonomic changes	• No associated autonomic changes
• Diagnosis: – Repeated nerve stimulation: Incremental response [Q] – Tensilion test/Endrophonium • Neostigmine → Characteristically positive [Q] • Note: Edrophomium/Tensilon test is more specific for M. graves than repeated nerve stimulation [Q]	• Diagnosis: – Repeated nerve stimulation: Decremental – Tensilion test/Endrophonium • Neostigmine: Negative

- Men (Multiple Endocrinal neoplasia):

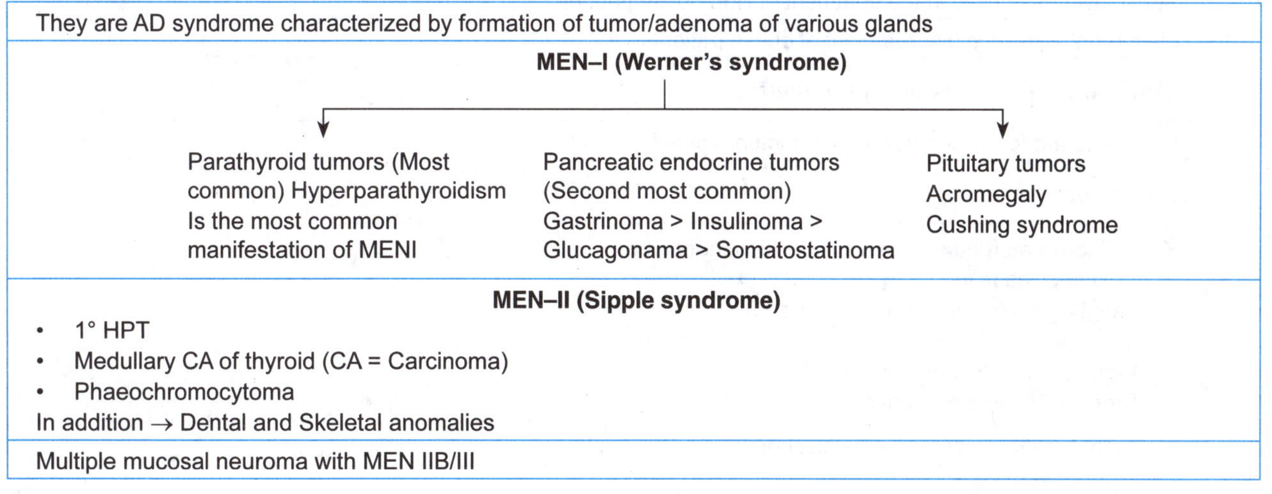

They are AD syndrome characterized by formation of tumor/adenoma of various glands

MEN–I (Werner's syndrome)

Parathyroid tumors (Most common) Hyperparathyroidism Is the most common manifestation of MENI

Pancreatic endocrine tumors (Second most common) Gastrinoma > Insulinoma > Glucagonama > Somatostatinoma

Pituitary tumors
Acromegaly
Cushing syndrome

MEN–II (Sipple syndrome)

- 1° HPT
- Medullary CA of thyroid (CA = Carcinoma)
- Phaeochromocytoma

In addition → Dental and Skeletal anomalies

Multiple mucosal neuroma with MEN IIB/III

- Progressive multi focal encephalopathy:

• By J.C. virus
• Most commonly associated with AIDS
• MRI is used for the diagnosis

- Inflammatory myopathy:

Sparing of extra ocular muscle
CK is diagnostic
• Polymyositis → No rash • Dermataomyositis → with rash (Proximal muscle weakness) • Inclusion body myositis → Distal muscle weakness

- Mono neuritis multiplex:

It is a painful asymmetric peripheral neuropathy involving 2 or more separate nerves.
The most common cause in INDIA → Leprosy.

- Brain biopsy:

Diagnostic of PRION liver biopsy
Gold standard for Wilson disease.

- Causes of Adrenal insufficiency:

1° Causes	2° causes (ACTH)
• Primary hypoaldosterism (Addison's disease)	
• 1° Adrenocortical failure ↓ So ↓sed Aldosterone and Cortisone ↓ So ↑sed ACTH ↓ ↑In Melanin pigmentation	Improper withdrawal of glucocorticoid therapy ↓ HPA axis suppression ↓ So, ↓ACTH

- Diabetes:

Sulphonylurease used in the treatment of Non obese patients.
Metmorfin → used in the treatment of obese patients.

- DXA (Dual energy X-ray absoptionmetry):

Gold standard for osteoporosis Area–lumbar spine hip.

- Cerebral hemisphere:

• Left lobe/caterogorical hemisphere /dominant lobe: → Defect leads to Languages (Aphasia) + Dyscalculia [Q] ↓ Wernicks ↓ Empty meaningless [Q] Broca' is reverse of Wernick's
• Right lobe/Representative hemisphere

- CNS:

Disorder of Cortex → Alzheimer
Disorders of basal ganglia → • Parkinson's disease → Destruction of dopominergic fibers. • Wilson disease • Chorea–Abnormal involuntary jerky movements. • Athetosis–Slow rhythmic and Twisting movements • Hemiballismus → violent involuntary abnormal movements on one side of the body

- Polymyositis:

• Seen in old age
• Diagnosed by process of exclusion: should not have – Rash – Involvement of extraoccular and facial muscles.

- Hypergonadotropic hypogonadism → Kleinfilter (most common), Viral orchitis, Noonan syndrome
- Hypogonadotropic hypogonadism → Kallman's syndrome
- Thymona → is most commonly associated myasthaenia gravis
- Carpel tunnel syndrome:

DM (diabetes mellitus) + Acromegaly + Hypothyroidism and Hyperparathyroidism NOT Addison's [Q]

- Psuedohypoparathyroidism:

Features of hypoparathyroidism with ↑ PTH [Q]

- Psuedohyponatremia:

Low serum Na with normal or high plasma osmolarity [Q]

- Cushing Disease vs Cushing syndrome:

Cushing Disease	Cushing syndrome
Pituitary microadenoma is the cause	All causes including pituitary microadenoma
↑ACTH, ↑cortisol	Ao, either ACTH increase so, either ACTH increase

- Midbrain and Pontine syndrome:

Midbrain syndrome Trick: BWNC B → Benedikt's syndrome W → Weber's Syndrome N → Nothangel's syndrome C → Claude's syndrome
Pontine Syndrome Millard gubler syndrome Foville Syndrome Raymond Syndrome → (+TN (Vth CN) Palsy

Spinal cord hemisection

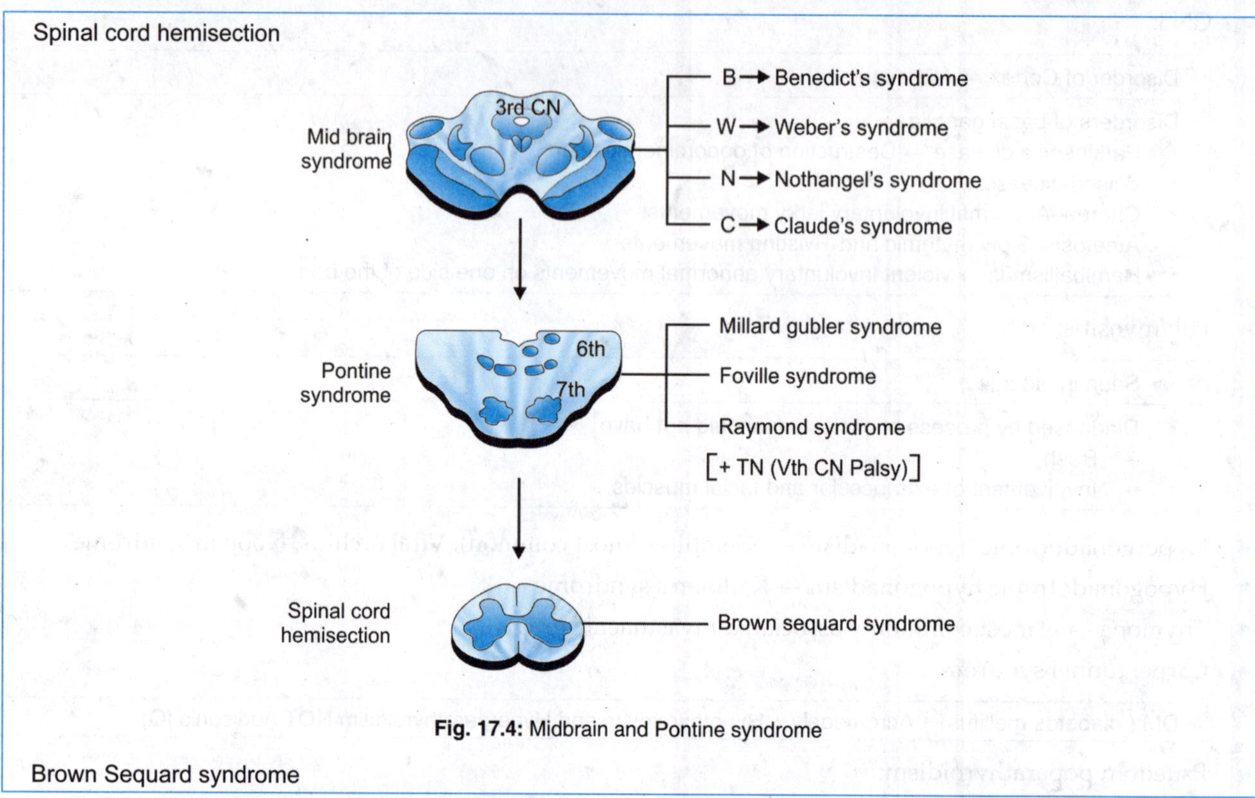

Fig. 17.4: Midbrain and Pontine syndrome

Brown Sequard syndrome

- Neurofibromatosis "AD" Condition [Q]:

NF-I	NF-II
• Peripheral neurofibromatosis	• Central neurofibromatosis (Bilateral acoustic neurofibromatosis)
• Von recklinghausen's syndrome	Acoustic neuroma (Bilateral) [Q]
• Diagnose when any of 2 present: – Six or more cafe-an-lait macule over 5mm in greatest diameter(Café-audait spot occurs shortly after birth) – Axillary/Inguinal freckling – Iris lisch nodule – Optic glioma – Scoliosis	Juvenile posterior subcapsular opacity (Cataract)
Cafe-an-lait spot + axillary frecking → Pathognomic of NF–I [Q]	

- GBS (Gullian Berry) → Predominately motor syndrome
- Delirium is seen with drugs and alcohols
- Glycosylated Hb:

< 7 → Good diabetic control (KCET-12)
7-8 → Moderate Diabetic control
> 8 → Need to improve

- Cerebrum:

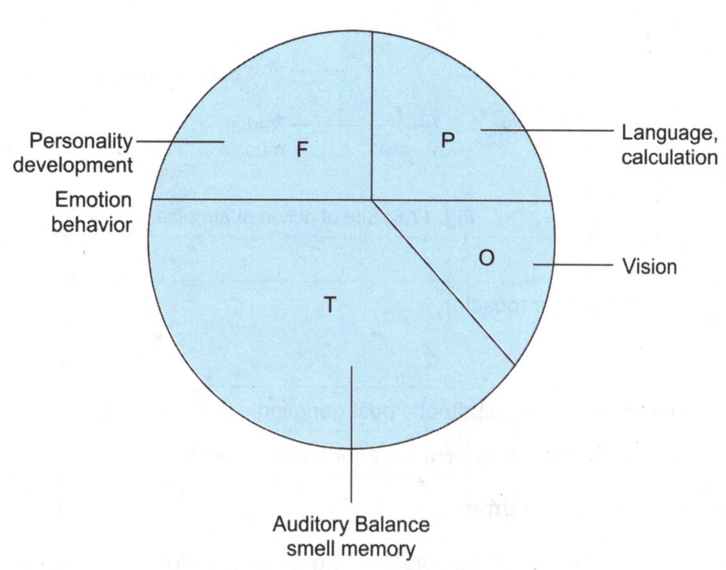

Fig. 17.5: Functions associated cerebrum

F–Frontal lobe-Personality development Emotion behavior

P–Parietal lobe-Language, Calculation

O–Occipital lobe-Vision

T–Temporal lobe-Auditory balance smell memory

- "Pretibial myxoedema":

Seen in Graves disease
NOTE: Graves's disease is distinguished from other form of HPT by preitial myxoedema and opthalmopathy.

- Non Reacting pupils → Botulism
- Diabetic neuropathy: isolated 3rd nerve palsy and papillary spearing is a characteristic feature of diabetic neuropathy with involvement of 3rd nerve.
- Radial nerve: High nerve repair capacity.
- Ulnar nerve: Most common nerve for monitoring during anesthesia.
- IDDM mother: Most common anomaly in fetus are

  - Cardiac anomaly
  - Macrosomia

- Hemithyroidectomy:

  Preservation of parathyroid gland → So, No hypocalcemia

- Both type I and II Lepra Reaction + ENL (Erythema Nodosum Leprosum) → Steroid is the D.O.C
- Spinal cord terminate at L1 [Q]
- Spinal anesthesia given at L2–L4
- ACE inhibitors: Can be safe in diabetics and Asthmatics

- Atropine:

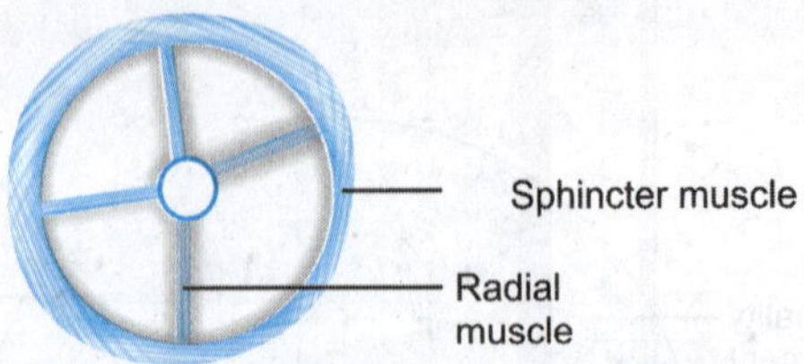

Fig. 17.6: Site of action of atropine

Muscarinic Antagonist
Action on sphincter papillae (Circular muscle) ↓ Relaxation (mydriasis)
Sphincter muscle → supplied by parasympathetic post ganglionic from ciliary ganglia
Radial muscle → By post ganglionic fibres from superior cervical ganglion [Q]

- Effects of Nor Adrenaline and Adrenaline:

• Both nor Adr + Adr → act Through B1 receptor → ↑ Force and rate of contraction of heart → thus both raises SBP In Excess amount → causes Cardiac arrhythmia
• Nor adr. → α1 Receptor → Vasoconstrictions in most organs but Adr through β2 receptor causes vasodilatation of skeletal and liver blood vessels and vasoconstriction elsewhere and total PR drops (↓) (PR-Perepheral resistance) So, As Adr. raises SBP (β1) and decreases DBP → Causes "widening of pulse pressure" [Q] Adr → (H.R. +C.O.) ↑ses [Q]
• Nor Adr. infused → Both S.B.P. + D.B.P raises ↓ HTN ↓ Stimulate the baroreceptors ↓ Reflex bradycardia [Q] ↓ That overrides the β1 Cardioaccelatory effect of Nor A. Consequently Cardiac output (C.O.) ↓ ses ↓ So, Nor A. → (H.R. + CO.) ↓ ses [Q]

- Midazolam:

3 times more patient than diazepam.
Dose of midazolam → • Child → Oral–0.25 to 1 mg/kg wt i.m. → 0.1 to 0.15 mg/kgwt • Adult → 2-5 mg **Note:** Dose of Diazepam = 5–10 mg (Adult) → For status epilepticus → given 10mg to i.v. followed by fractionated dose every 10 min.
Midazolam → D.O.C. for status epilepticus.
It is water soluble compared to limited solubility of diazepam
Midazolam can be given i.m. i.v., oral or intra nasal **Note:** diazepam–i.v. only

- Cerebral edema:

Results in herniation of the brain from foramen magnum + sed intracranial pressure.
It is a result of ced lymphatic drainage + and increase in plasma protein concentration.

LAST 5-YEAR QUESTIONS FROM THIS TOPIC

1. A patient reported in emergency with symptoms of tachycardia, bronchodilation, increased temperature and constipation. Me may be suffering from poisoning with: *(AIPG 12)*

Ans. Atropin poisoning

2. In uncompensated diabetic ketoacidosis: *(AIPG 12)*

Ans. HCO_3 decrease

3. Hyperparathyroidism in a growing child presents all of the following features except: *(AIPG 12)*

a. Increase in plasma Ca
b. Increase in plasma phosphate
c. Serum alkaline phosphate increases
d Withdrawal of minerals from bone

Ans. b

4. Tremor in proximities while movement is seen in: *(PGI June 12)*

Ans. Cerebellar lesion

5. Regarding UMN palsy true is: *(PGI June 12)*

Ans. Contra lateral paralysis of lower side

6. Self biting tendency is seen in: *(PGI June 12)*

Ans. Lyschnyn syndrome.

7. Lesions of the lateral cerebellum cause all of the following, except: *(AIIMS Nov 10)*

a. In coordination
b. Intention tremor
c. Resting tremor
d. Ataxia

Ans. c

8. Transection at mid pons level results in: *(AIIMS Nov 10)*

Ans. Apneusis (Ref: Ganong 23/e p673).

9. A patient is wide eyed, very nervous with an increased systolic pressure (with widening of pulse pressure), increased pulse rate, fine skin and hair and loss of body weight. He is probably suffering from: *(AIIMS Nov 10, AIPG 09)*

Ans. Hyperthyroidism (Ref: 5/e p898)

10. Lesions of midline cerebellar region causes all, except: *(AIIMS Nov 10)*

a. Uncoordinated posture and gait
b. Nystagmus
c. Decomposition of coordinated movement
d. Titubation of head and/trunk

Ans. c (Ref: Conn, neuroscience in medicine p241)

11. Obesity is associated with all except: *(AIIMS Nov 09)*

a. Growth hormone deficiency
b. Hypothyroidism
c. Diabetes mellitus
d. Estrogen deficiency

Ans. d

12. Increased intracranial tension causes all, except: *(AIIMS Nov 09)*

a. Nausea and vomiting
b. Headache
c. Paraperesis
d. Visual blurring

Ans. c (Ref: Davidson medicine 18/e p1016-17)

13. Broca's area is concerned with: *(AIIMS May 09)*

Ans. Word formation (Ref: Harrison 17/e)

14. Exopthalmos, nervousness, tachycardia, heat intolerance and hypertension are indicative of:

Ans. Hyperthyroidism (Ref: Harrison 17/e) *(AIIMS May 09)*

15. Patient suffering from prolonged decreased carbohydrate lead to: *(PGI June 12)*

Ans. Ketoacidosis

16. Glycated hemoglobin checked before pdl surgery in: *(PGI June 12)*

Ans. Controlled diabetes mellitus + uncontrolled diabetes mellitus + pre screening diabetes

17. Diabetes insipidus result from lesion of which hypothalamic nuclei: *(AIPG 11)*

Ans. Supraoptic (Ref: Khurana p703)

18. Autism is characterized by: *(AIPG 11, 09)*

Ans. Incapacitating emotional and mental disturbance (Ref: Kaplan and saddock comprehensive psychiatry 8/e p3164)

19. The type of epilepsy is specially seen in children which has no aura phase is: *(AIPG 10)*

Ans. Petit mal epilepsy (Ref: Harrison's 16/e p2358)

20. All of the following statement are true about Benedict's syndrome except: *(AIPG 09)*

a. Contra lateral tumor
b. 3rd nerve palsy
c. Involvement of penetrating branch of basilar artery
d. Lesion at level of pons.

Ans. d (Ref: Harrison 16/e p174)

21. In Millard Gubler syndrome all are involved except: *(AIPG 09)*

a. 5th cranial nerves
d. 6th cranial nerve
c. 7th cranial nerve
d. Contra lateral hemiplegia

Ans. a (Harrison 16/e p175)

22. Thyrotoxicosis is characterized by: *(KCET 09)*

Ans. Exopthalmos (Ref: Cecil textbook of medicine p270)

23. All of the following are features of cerebellar disease except: *(COMED 09)*

a. Resting tremors
b. Past pointing
c. Nystagmus
d. Ataxic gait

Ans. a

24. Which neurofibroma is potentially threatening? *(COMEDK 09)*

Ans. Acoustic neuroma (Ref: Cecil textbook of medicine p554)

25. All of the following are adverse effects of long term corticosteroids except *(COMEDK 09)*

a. Hypoglycemia
b. Psychosis

c. Peptic ulcers
d. Osteoporosis

Ans. a (Ref: Goodman and Gilman 11/e p1603)

26. The triad of cirrhosis, haemochromatosis and diabetes are referred to as: *(COMEDK 10)*

Ans. Bronze diabetes

27. Type I diabetes mellitus is associated with: *(COMEDK 10)*

Ans. Islet cell auto antibodies (Ref: Clark medicine 5/e p1103)

28. Addison's Disease is caused by: *(KCET 10)*

Ans. Tuberculosis + HIV + Metastatic carcinomas

29. The treatment of Tic douloureux include: *(KCET 10)*

Ans. Carbamazepine administration in all patients

30. Cause of 1° Hyperparathyroidism: *(KCET 12)*

Ans. Parathyroid carcinoma

31. Serum calcitonin is a marker of: *(KCET 12)*

Ans. Medullary carcinom

32. A 34 year old male presents with a history of thirst, polyuria and a recent 3.2 kg weight loss. His urine contains a small amount of ketones. Which of the following would suggest he is most likely to have type 2 diabetes rather than type 1? *(KCET 12)*

Ans. High circulating insulin level

33. Good diabetic control is said to be present when glycosylated hemoglobin is: *(KCET 12)*

Ans. 7-9%

34. The stimulus for parathyroid hyperplasia in secondary hyperparathyroidism is: *(KCET 11)*

Ans. Chronic hypocalcaemia (Ref: Davidson 19/e p718)

35. Hb/AC/glycohemoglobulin > 9% indicates:

Ans. Poor diabetes control. (COMEDK 12)

36. A 70 year old male is admitted to the hospital with a left hemiparesis and altered consciousness he is on aspirin 75 mg OD atrovastatin 10 mg OD and glibenclamide 15 mg daily. His wife says he has been unwell for a couple of days and he has been off food. He has however still been giving him all his medications. Which of the following tests is going to be most useful in finding an immediately reversible cause for his symptoms: *(KCET 11)*

Ans. Blood glucose level (Ref: KDT 5/e p248)

CHAPTER

18

Community Dentistry

Topic

- Biostatistics and Epidemiology
- Diseases
- Levels of Prevention
- Health Education and Communication
- Finance
- Fluorides
- Indices
- Dates and Years
- Miscellaneous

BIOSTATISTICS AND EPIDEMIOLOGY

- Formulas:

$$\text{Sensitivity} = \frac{\text{true positive}}{\text{true positive + false negative}} \times 100$$

Most important Parameter for SCREENING. [Q]
Identify those who have the disease (true positive)

- $$\text{Specificity} = \frac{\text{true negative}}{\text{true negative + false positive}} \times 100$$

  Identify those who do not have the disease [TRUE NEGATIVE] *(AIPG 2009)*
  Increase specificity decreases false positives. [Q]
  Radiograph in diagnosis of periodontal disease are more specific and less sensitive.[as 30 to 40 bone loss is required]. [COMED K 10]
  ELISA is more sensitive while western blot is more specific.

- Predictive value- Diagnostic power of the test. [Q]
  In addition of sensitivity and specificity , performance of a screening test is measured by PREDICTIVE VALUE which reflects its diagnostic power.

  $$\text{Positive predictive value(PPV)} = \frac{\text{true positive}}{\text{true positive + false positive}} \times 100$$

  $$\text{PPV} = \frac{S \times p}{S \times P + (1-\text{SPECIFICITY})(1-p)}$$ [Q]

  Where s = sensitivity, p = prevalence

  $$\text{Negative predictive value (NPV)} = \frac{\text{true negative}}{\text{true neivegative + false negative}} \times 100$$

- Positive predictive value depends on Sensitivity as true positive is numerator in both PPV and sensitivity
  Negative predictive value depends on specificity as true negative is denominator in both NPV and specificity.

- Prevalence (P):
  Although referred to as a rate, prevalence is actually a RATIO (NEET 13)

  $$P = \frac{\text{Total no. of individuals having a disease}}{\text{poulation at risk of developing the disease}}$$

  Prevalence affects predictive value.
- P = ID (duration)
  Prevalence is zero for 'suicide" as have a zero duration.
  Prevalence is NOT ideal to measure/study disease etiology because it depends on incidence and duration of disease while incidence reflects causal factor. hence incidence rate should be used in formulating and testing hypothesis.

- $n = \frac{4pq}{L2}$

  Where n = sample size,
  p = approximate prevalence
  q = 1-p [Q]
  L = permissible error

- DEGREE OF FREEDOM = (r – 1) (c – 1)
  Where r = no of rows, c = no of column.

- $\chi 2 = \frac{\varepsilon(O - E)^2}{E}$

  Yates correction = $\frac{\varepsilon(O - E - 0.5)^2}{E}$ { YATES CORRECTION in chi square – when cell frequency cell than 5 } [Q]

  Where O = observed value
  E = expected value

- S.D (standard deviation) = $\sqrt{\frac{(X - X1)^2}{\eta}}$

  Where X – X1 is deviation from mean
  η is sample size
  η – 1 taken in denominator if sample size is less than 30

- S.D = $\sqrt{VARIENCE}$ (AIPG 12)

- Coefficient of variance = $\frac{S.D}{X} \times 100\ \% \propto$ VARIABILITY (used to compare variability) (AIPG 12)

- Standard error (S.E) of MEAN = $\frac{S.D}{\sqrt{\eta}}$

- S.E of difference of mean = $\sqrt{\frac{\sigma 1^2}{\eta 1} + \frac{\sigma 2^2}{\eta 2}}$ where σ stands for S.D

- S.E of proportion = $\sqrt{\frac{pq}{\eta}}$ *(AIIMS)*
- S.E of difference of proportion = $\sqrt{\frac{p1q1}{\eta 1} + \frac{p2q2}{\eta 2}}$

- Correlation coefficient (r) = – 1 to + 1. [Q]

- Confidence limits = mean ± margin of error
  mean ± ZS.E.
  If precision increases confidence level becomes narrower (i.e with Increase of sample size and decrease of variability of sample precision increases.)

- MMR = $\frac{\text{Total no. of female death due to pregnancy/child birth within 42 days of delivery in an area in a year}}{\text{total no. of live birth}}$
- NOTE: Still birth NOT included *(AIPG 2011)*

- NMR (neonatal mortality rate) = $\frac{\text{total no of death in 28 days}}{\text{total live birth per yr}}$
- SO in both MMR and NMR denominator includes ONLY LIVE BIRTH.

- ARI (annual rate of infection)of TB – 1.7%
  1 ARI corresponds to 50 new cases of smear +ve TB/ YEAR for 1,00,000 population. [Q]

- NRR (net reproductive rate) – average no. of girls (daughter) a new born girl will bear is NRR.
- NRR of 1 = equals to child norm → GOAL of 2006 if 60 of population are practising family planning.

PREVALENCE(P)	INCIDENCE(I)
Total no. of individuals affected by a disease in a given population is prevalence. [AIIMS12]	No. of new cases seen in a given population.
Both new and old cases	incidence should be calculated per 1000 population. [Q]
Caries prevalence – its a RATIO. *(NEET 2013)*	caries incidence – it's a RATE e.g –YEARLY [Q]

- Prevalence (p) vs incidence (i)
- Mortality Rate:

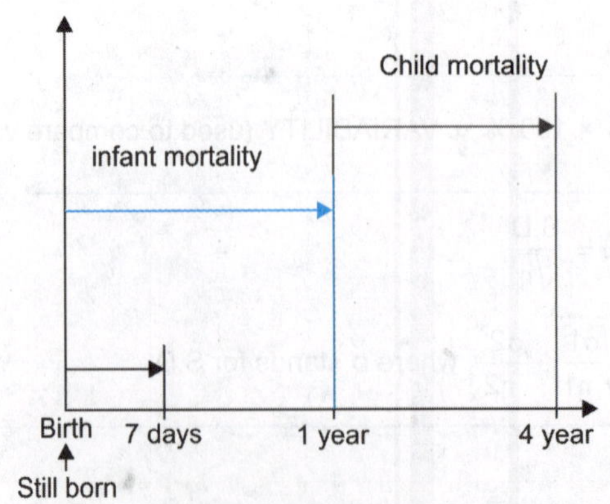

Fig. 18.1: Mortality rate

- Variables:

Independent variable	Dependent variable
E.g-Cause, predisposing factor, risk factor	Outcome, result, effect
Can be manipulated [Q]	Cannot be controlled or manipulated

- Characteristics of a normal distribution curve:

Bell shaped.
symmetrical
continuous
Asymptotic – The two tails never touches the X-axis.
Standard deviation= variance
Mean = median = mode = 0 (COINCIDE) *(AIPG 09)*
Standard deviation=

- Measure kf Central Tendency *(Very Imp. For NEET/AIIMS)*

• MEAN – most commonly used in biostatistics. Most of the value in data spread along the mean. *(PGI)*
• MEDIAN – BETTER indicator of central tendency *(PGI)* Maximum Observation are concentrated around median • If EXTREME VALUEs are recorded then mean can't be used. Use median. [Q]
• MODE – Rarely used. A series can have - no mode, 1 mode or, multiple mode.

- Measure of dispersion variability:

• Variance
• Standard deviation
• Range
• Interquartile range

- Null hypothesis:

• Is rejected when $p<0.05$, meaning the difference is unlikely to have occurred by chance. [Q] • TYPE 1 ERROR- null hypothesis is rejected when it is true. [Q] • TYPE 2 ERROR – OPPOSITE of type 1 error.

- Screening test vs diagnostic test:

SCREENING TEST	DIAGNOSTIC TEST
Less accurate, less expensive	More accurate, more expensive.

- Criteria of screening test:

Reliability/repeatability – test must give consistent result when repeated. [Q]
Validity- refers to what extent the test accurately measures which it is suppose to measure (same as in index). [Q]
Yield –is the amount of previously unrecognised disease that is diagnosed as a result of screening.

- Index case

The case that 1st comes to the knowledge of investigator. May or may not be the primary case *(AIPG 2010)*

- Sampling Methods:

Sampling Methods
Simple random sampling – applicable when the population is small, homogenous. In random sampling chances of being picked up is SAME and KNOWN. *(NEET 2013)* Done by lottery method or, a table of random numbers.
• Multistage sampling – large country survey. *(PGI 09)* Multistage sampling – sample procedure is carried out in several stages using simple random technique. [AIPG 2012] ONLY 'MULTISTAGE" method. Examples - farmers in India may be grouped into various states, then into districts, then into talukas, further into villages within talukas and then farmers within villages.
• Multiphase- sampling done in different phases- e.g. - TB survey.
• SUBGROUP means 'STRATA' → Mentioned in Stratified sampling. Stratified sampling – used when population is heterogeneous. The population under study is 1st divided into homogenous group/classes called strata and then the sample is drawn from each stratum at random in proportion to its size such as selecting sample from defined areas, classes, religions, ages or sexes.
• NATURAL HABITAT e.g.-village/region → used in cluster sampling. Cluster sampling – used when units of population are natural groups or clusters such as village, schools etc. – Both stratified and cluster is 2 stage sampling methods. – The main difference b/w them is that in cluster sampling the cluster is treated as sampling unit so analysis is done on a population of cluster while in stratified sampling the analysis is done on elements within strata. The main objective of cluster sampling is to reduce cost by increasing sample efficiency. This contrast with stratified sampling where the main objective is to INCREASE PRECISION. Cluster sampling gives a high standard error.

- Types of data:

Types of data
Nominal – qualitative category can't be quantified. No implication of order or ratio. Ex-urban/rural, male/female.
Ordinal – qualitative category, can't be quantified. Data can be placed in meaningful order. E.g. - student ranked in order as 1st, 2nd and 3rd. Interval – can be measured or quantified. Data can be placed in meaningful order. Ratios of scores are not meaningful. E.g.- temperature In order – 90 0C ,100 0C, 120 0C
Ratio – can be measured or quantified. Data can placed in meaningful order and ratios of scores are meaningful. E.g.: - pulse rate/min – 90/min.

- Presentation of data:

<table>
<tr><td>

- **For Quantitative data:**
  - Histogram –variables on x- axis is called 'abscissa" and frequency marked on y- axis is called 'ordinate".
  - Frequency polygon – indicated when sets of data to be elicited on same diagram.
    Bell/normal curve is the most common type of frequency polygon. It resembles a smooth curve.
  - Line diagram
  - Scatter /Dot/correlation diagram – shows the nature of correlation between 2 variables. If the dots cluster around a straight line , it shows a linear relationship.

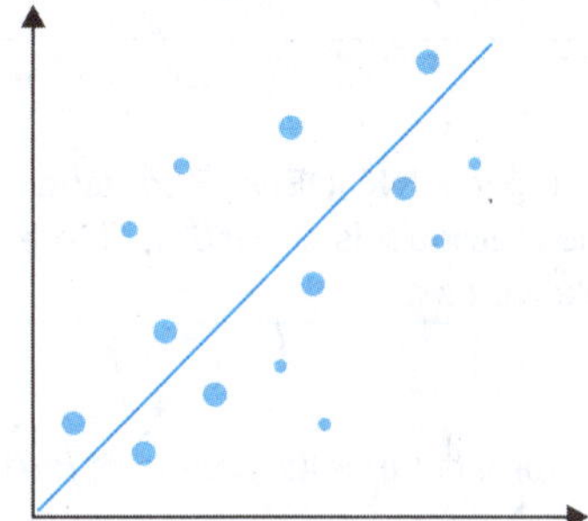

Fig. 18.2: Scatter/dot/correlation diagram

</td></tr>
<tr><td>

- **For qualitative data:**
  - Bar diagram
  - Pie diagram

</td></tr>
</table>

- Data:

QUALITATIVE - Only frequency varies (ex-counting the individuals) NO notion of magnitude. CHI SQUARE is used. [Q]
QUANTITATIVE – BOTH magnitude (HEIGHT, WEIGHT, SERUM cholesterol, B.P) and frequency varies. E.g. 1. No. of person with height 150 cm may be 20 while no of person with height 154 cm may be 30 2. B.P , SERUM CHOLESTEROL –as have magnitude

- Qualitative data vs Quantitative data

CHI SQUARE is used.	e.g. - INTERVAL, RATIO etc.
To find association between two variables	STUDENT –t test: variable should be normally
to examine difference between TWO FREQUENCY	Test used to find significance of difference between TWO MEAN – t – test. [Q]
For LARGE sample	FOR SMALL SAMPLE. [Q]
	Ex- B.P, Serum cholesterol Comparison of serum cholesterol before and after ingestion of hamburgers on A SINGLE group ↓ PAIRED t - test used
	MORE than one group – UNPAIRED t test used.

- Anova

When multiple groups are studied in terms of only ONE factor – ONE way ANOVA *(AIIMS 2012)*
When multiple groups are studied in terms of TWO factors – TWO way ANOVA

- Confounding factor:

One which is associated With BOTH exposure and disease and is distributed UNEQUALLY in study and control group.
It is itself a RISK FACTOR for the disease. [Q]
e.g. - study of coffee drinking and lung cancer – if coffee drinker is also a cigarette smoker then this cigarette smoking is a confounding factor. Confounding factor can be neutralized by MATCHING.

- Studies:

Cohort study:
it is a PROSPECTIVE STUDY
Risk factor present → disease will occur gives INCIDENCE so used in estimation of relative risk [Q]
It is a LONGITUDIONAL study so same individual is studied at different ages. E.g. Ram is studied at 6yr. 12 yr,18yr.
- Cohort study/ incidence study - relative risk.

Case control:
A RETROSPECTIVE STUDY
Risk factor is to be identified ← disease present [useful in case of rare diseases]
[Q] GIVES odd – ratio.
Best method to study RARE disease – Case control study. [Q]
NESTED case control study -is a case control study nested within COHORT study so it is a PROSPECTIVE stu dy [Q]

Cross-sectional:
Gives PREVALENCE.
Studies one point at a time (One point study). Different individual of SAME age group ,studied only once - 1 point study
Is very important in Study of SUDDEN OUTBREAK OF DISEASE. [Q]

- **ESTIMATION OF RISK IN STUDIES:**

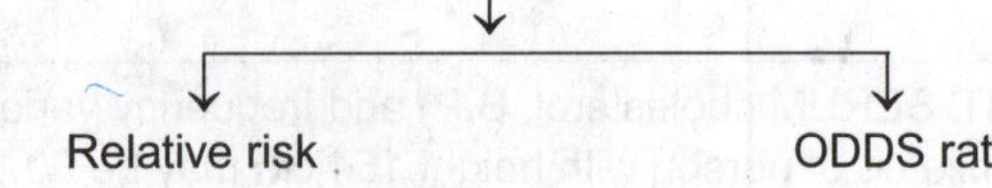

Relative risk

$$= \frac{\text{incidence exposed}}{\text{incidence among non exposed}}$$

Calculated by COHORT studies only as incidence rate is provided by ALSO ATTRIBUTABLE RISK.
A Case control study can't provide incidence rate from which relative risk can be calculated

ODDS ratio

Case control studies only provide ODD ratio ,which is a measure of strength of the association. risk factor and outcome(disease).
ODD ratio 1= Strong association
=1 =NO association

(PGI 2011)

NOTE:
Interpretation of odds ratio: if odd ratio >1 and confidence interval doesn't include 1 then → STRONGER ASSOCIATION.

- Bias:

Berkesonian bias - It is a type of selection bias. Arises because of different rate of admission to hospital. [Q]
Admission rate bias.
BERKESONIAN bias(admission rate bias) – occurs in study of hospitalized pts. [Q]

Confounding bias- especially when a disease has multiple risk factors which are related to each other.

Memory/recall bias

selection bias

Interviewer bias
Pygmalion effect – researcher's beliefs affect outcome can be eliminated by double blinding.

- Epidemiological study:

DEFINITION:
- MacMahon – 'the study of the distribution and determinants of disease frequency in man". *(KCET 2012)* TRICK – (small definition.)
- John M. Last – 'The study of the distribution and determinants of health related states or, events in specified populations, and application of this study to the control of health problems."

Most commonly used definition.

- Demographic cycle: Has 5 stages:

First (high stationary) – High birth rate and high death rate.
Second (early expanding) – Death rate decline but birth rate remains unchanged.
Third phase (Late expanding) – Death rate declines more than birth rate. India has entered this phase. [Q]
Fourth phase (low stationary) – Low birth rate low death rate Zero growth rate – Austria
Fifth phase (declining) – birth rate lower than death rate Seen in Germany and Hungary.

LAST 5-YEAR QUESTIONS FROM THIS TOPIC

1. **Before declaring that a patient is HIV positive ELISA is confirmed BY Western BLOT:** *(AIPG 08)*

Ans. To reduce chance of false positive.

2. **A TEST has high false positive rate in community. True is:** *(AIIMS 11)*
   a. Low prevalence
   b. High specificity
   c. High prevalence
   d. Low prevalence

Ans. d

3. **Most important epidemiologic factor while deciding sample size:** *(AIPG 10)*

Ans. Expected prevalence of disease.

4. **True positive and true negative indicates:**

Ans. Sensitivity and specificity respectively.

5. **Negative predictive value 0.75 means:** *(AIPG 2011, 12)*

Ans. 75% chances that disease will not be present if test is negative.

6. **In a data set when the mean is highest and mode is least , the distribution of data will be:** *(AIPG 11)*

Ans. Positively skewed.
NOTE: Negatively skewed when mean < mode.

7. **In a study done for the evaluation of prevalence of caries in a given population, the ratio of its standard deviation to the mean of data will be called:** *(AIPG 2011, 12)*

Ans. Coefficient of variance

8. **If the incidence of a disease is high and prevalence is low ,it means:** *(AIPG 2011, 12)*

Ans. Disease is either cured easily or is fatal.

9. **Reliability of screening test means:** *(AIPG 2011)*

Ans. Gives same value on repeated testing.

10. Detection of undiagnosed cases from a general population is called:

Ans. Screening.

11. In statistics, value of p=0.4 means: *(AIPG 2012)*

Ans. Probability of no significant difference is 40% and significant difference is 60%. Or, probability of significance by chance is 40%.

12. After applying a statistical test, an investigator gets the p value of as 0.01. it means that: *(AIIMS Nov. 2011)*

Ans. The difference is not significant 1% times % significant 99% times.

13. About MMR which is not true: *(AIPG 2011)*

Ans. Denominator includes still birth.

14. In India the leading cause of Maternal mortality is:

Ans. Haemorrhage.

15. Measure of relative variability. *(AIPG 2009)*

Ans. Coefficient of variance.

16. ALL are measure of dispersion except:

a. Mean
b. SD
c. Variance
d. Range

Ans. a

17. An investigator want to know the similarity of the mean peak flow of expiratory rate in non smokers, light smokers, moderate smokers, andheavy smokers, which is statically test of significance:

a. One way ANOVA
b. Two way ANOVA

Ans. a

Note: As here multiple groups are studied in terms of only one factor that is mean peak flow expiratory rate.

18. A researcher attempted to find the ALT levels in cirrhotic patients. In a series of 100 patients, the mean levels of ALT were 70 IU/L with a standard deviation of 25 IU/L. What is the 95 % confidence interval for estimated ALT?

Ans. 20 – 120 IU/L

19. SAMPLING unit represents: *(AIPG 2009)*

Ans. Every individual in sample.

20. In a school survey, the prevalence of dating habit was studied. For the survey schools were randomly selected. Within each school a section was randomly selected. Within each section students were randomly selected. This type of selection criteria is called: *(AIPG 2012)*

Ans. Multistage sampling.

21. Age used to determine child mortality: *(AIPG 08)*

Ans. 1 to 4 yrs.

22. Recently two methods of cPAP: conventional and bubble cPAP were compared. In the conventional method 90 out 160 showed extubation while 40 out of 160 showed extubation failure in the bubble method. Which test would be the best to compare the statistical significance between the rates of extubation failure in the two tests: *(AIPG 2012)*

a. Paired t test
b. Chi square

c. Student t test

d. ANOVA

Ans. b (as here only frequency varies, no notion of magnitude so here the data is qualitative and among the option only chi square is qualitative test).

23. Yearly increase in carious lesion in mouth of a patient is called: *(AIPG 2010)*

Ans. Caries incidence

24. If incidence is 50 cases per 1000 population and mean duration of disease is 5 yrs , the prevalence in 5 yrs is: *(AIPG 08)*

Ans. 250 [p = 50 * 5]

25. In a study in UK, an association was found between sale of antiarrythmic drug and an increase in death due to asthma. This is an example of: *(AIPG 09)*

Ans. Ecological study [Ref: Park 19/e p58]

26. Sequence in planning a randomized control trial: *(AIPG08)*

Ans. Protocol, selection of subjects, randomization, intervention, follow up and assessment. *(Ref: Park 19/e p76).*

27. Rural and Urban differences in prevalence is seen in all of the following disease except:

Ans. Tuberculosis.

28. The prevalence of dental caries in a population in the year 2000 and 2003 was 18% and 38% respectively. Incidence of the same population in 3 yrs would be: *(AIPG 08)*

Ans. 20% [38 – 18 = 20]

DISEASES (VERY IMPORTANT FOR AIPG)

- EMPORIATRICS – Science of health of travellers. [Q]
- Disease transmitted by mites and ticks: *(Very Imp.)*

• 1SOFT TICK- Q fever, relapsing fever [Q] Q fever- NO arthropods involved –no vectors in humans. Extra human vectors are there. [Q]
• HARD TICK – tick typhus, viral encephalitis, viral hemorrhagic fever, KFD, tularaemia.
• LOUSE borne - EPIDEMIC typhus (R. Prowazeki), EPIDEMIC relapsing fever (B. Recurrentis), trench fever. [TRICK – EPIDEMIC word is associated with louse born.]
• Thromboculid mite → scrub typhus [Q] → Orentia tsutsugamushi [Q]
• Reduvid bug – Chagas disease (American sleeping sickness caused by Trypanoma cruji).
• Tse-Tse fly- African sleeping sickness. • Rat flea – bubonic plague, endemic plague, endemic typhus. *(AIPG)*
• Mosquito: Anopheles – Malaria Culex – Filaria, Japanese encephalitis,west nile fever Aedes – Yellow fever, dengue, dengue hemorrhagic fever, Chickengunya fever. All 3 can cause FILARIA. [Q] Aedes + anopheles survive in clean water Culex survive in dirty water
• Sandfly – Kala Azar Oriental sore [Q]

- Biological transmission:

• PROPAGATIVE- the agent merely multiplies in the vector but there is no development or change in form.
• CYCLODEVELOPMENTAL- only development but no multiplication in vector E.g.- Filarial parasite *(AIPG 09)*
• CYCLOPROPAGATIVE- both development and multiplication in vector. E.g - Malaria parasite

- Carriers: 3 types

Incubatory carrier– shed infectious agent during incubation
Convalescent carrier– shed the infectious agent during the period of covalence (during recovery from illness). [Q] Pose a serious threat to the unprotected household members.
Healthy carrier –those who have developed carrier state without suffering from overt disease. **Note:** Chronic carrier- more important source of infection than cases.

- Disease and Isolation:

• Some disease where isolation is strictly recommended-diphtheria , cholera, pneumonic plague [Q]
• Some disease where isolation is unlikely to be effective: – Measles, mumps, typhoid, polio, hepatitis A [Q]

- SAR (secondary attack rate):

Communicability of disease in exposed person following exposure to primary case. [Q]
Chicken pox – 90%, whooping cough -90 %,mumps- 86%,measles- 80 %, Small pox- 35-40%.
NOTE: The period of communicability for measles is approximately 4 days before and 5 days after the appearance of rash.

- **HERPETIC WHITLOW:** Caused by hsv-1/hsv2. It's an example of Autoinoculation.
- **HERD IMMUNITY:** Immunity of a community against a particular disease. If herd immunity is sufficiently high the chances of epidemic is low. Herd immunity may lead to elimination of disease.
- Disease control → disease elimination → disease eradication

  ↓ ↓

  Interruption of transmission of disease. (Smallpox) [Q]

  e.g. - polio and measles

Chemoprophylaxis for common diseases:

Cholera, pneumonic plague – Tetracycline
Diphtheria, conjunctivitis(bacterial) - Erythromycin.
Influenza – Amantadine
Meningitis – sulfadiazine.

- India aims to eliminate disease:

  Malaria, kala azar, TB – BY 2010

  Filaria - by 2015. *(AIPG 11)*

Who clinical staging system for HIV:

Clinical STAGE 1 – asymptomatic, persistent generalized lymphadenopathy (PGL) [Q]
STAGE 2 – Weight Loss < 10% , minor mucocutaneous changes.
STAGE 3 – Weight Loss >10% Oral candidiasis [Q] Oral hairy leukoplakia [Q] Pulmonary tuberculosis Unexplained chronic diarrhoea and unexplained prolonged fever > 1 month.

STAGE 4 – CD4 <50.
HIV wasting syndrome (Weight Loss >10% + Unexplained Chronic diarrhoea and unexplained prolonged fever > 1 month) Pneumocystic carinii pneumonia [Q] Toxoplasmosis Cryptococcosis CMV KAPOSI Sarcoma [Q] Atypical mycobacteriosis.

- Modes of transmission of HIV:

Blood transfusion – >90% [Q]
Tissue organ transplant – 50-90%
Mother to baby – 30% [Q]
Injection/injuries – 0.5-1%.
Sexual intercourse – 0.1-1%

- Treponemal infection:

Veneral	Non-veneral
Syphilis: T.pallidum	YAWS: T. pertenae
	PINTA: T. Carateum
	Endemic syphilis: T.endemicum

- Food borne diseases and associated TOXINS:

Food Borne Disease	Toxins
lathyrism	BOAA found in seeds of pulse lathyrus sativa (khesari dal)
Epidemic dropsy	Sanguinarine [Q]
ENDEMIC ASCITIS	Pyrolizidine alkaloids

- Transmission of infectious agent:

Transovarian	Trans Stadial (trick - stages) [Q]
infectious agent is transmitted Vertically from infected female → to her progeny.	transmission of infectious agent/disease from one stage to other.
Ex- p.vivax	

- Common Occupational Cancer: [Q]

Skin cancer (75%) > lung
Liver cancer LEAST associated with occupation
Breast cancer NOT associated with occupation *(AIPG 09)*

- **POLIO:** Clinician must follow all cases of AFP (acute flaccid paralysis) for minimum of 60 days to check for residual paralysis. [Q]
- WHO definition of vision:

Low vision - 6/18 with best possible refractive correction.
Blindness - 3/60 with best possible refractive correction.

- **Vaccination:**

Live Vaccine	Killed Vaccine	Toxoids
OPV (Sabin),BCG,MMR	e.g. DPT, HBV, RABIES	Diphtheria toxoid *(PGI 12)*
No booster is required in live vaccine except OPV		
Live vaccines are Contraindicated in pregnancy		
Live vaccine requires proper refrigeration to retain their effectiveness. Inadequate refrigeration has caused serious failure of measles and polio immunization. [Q]		

- WHO EPI (immunisation schedule):

AGE	VACCINE
birth	BCG+OPV
6wks	DPT+OPV
10wks	DPT+OPV
9mo	measles(MMR – not included in EPI) *(AIPG 10)*

Note: Interval between two doses should not be less than 1 month.
BOTH measles and Tetanus are highly efficacious vaccine. [Q]
Toxic shock syndrome is caused by contaminated measles vaccine. [Q]

LAST 5-YEAR QUESTIONS FROM THIS TOPIC

1. **Lice is a vector of all of the following except:**
   a. Q fever
   b. Relapsing fever
   c. Epidemic typhus
   d. Trench fever

Ans. a

2. **Man is the principle reservoir for which of the following enteric pathogen:**

Ans. E. Histolytica

3. **Most common factor for death in south Asian population:** *(AIPG 12)*

Ans. Infection.

4. **MODE of transmission most difficult to control is:** *(AIPG 10)*

Ans. Air borne.

5. **Mass chemoprophylaxis in endemic areas is recommended for all of the following except:** *(AIPG 11)*

Ans. Leprosy [Ref: Park 20/e p236, 287]

6. **Most effective route for HIV transmission is:**

Ans. Blood borne

7. **National AIDS control program has following components except:**
   a. Serosurvillance
   b. Screening of blood and blood products
   c. Health education and information
   d. Banning of sexual contacts with foreigners.

Ans. d

8. **Least common occupational cancer:**

Ans. liver carcinoma

9. ADJUVANT used in DPT vaccine: *(AIPG 09)*

Ans. Aluminium [Ref: Park 18/e p135]

LEVELS OF PREVENTION: [VERY IMPORTANT]

- Health belief model – individual behaviour regarding preventive health. [Q]
- Levels of prevention:

CONCEPT: while solving questions based on level of prevention, go to the basic definition of these level of preventions.
• PRIMORDIAL – prevent the emergence of risk factor. *(AIPG 08)* • Aims at prevention of CHRONIC DISEASES. [Q]
• PRIMARY – caries activity test, oral prophylaxis, space maintainers. *(AIPG 2012)* Examples of specific protection – immunisation, use of specific nutrients (e.g. VIT. A [Q]), chemoprophylaxis, protection from specific carcinogen/accidents. Primary prevention includes the concept of positive health. [Q] • IODINE CONTROLL PROGRAM: • Can be estimated by NEONATAL HYPOTHYROIDISM (Neonatal thyroxin level) [Q]
• SECOMDARY – Screening of oral diseases so, biopsy , oral cytology are under secondary prevention. PRR PULP CAPPING *(KCET 09)* Scaling and root planning. Largely the domain of clinical medicine. It is more expensive and less effective. The health programme initiated by government is usually at the level of secondary prevention.
• TERTIARY: {IMPAIRMENT – ANY loss/ abnormality of psychological/ anatomical/functional /physiological is impairment.} Disability limitation and rehabilitation. e.g. PULPOTOMY, RCT, EXTRACTION, ,Deep curettage , root planning, RPD, FPD.

- IDEAS, STEPS and ICF:

IDEAS: Indian disability evaluation and assessment scale. For mental disorder. A scale for measuring and quantifying disability in mental disorder.
STEPS – WHO STEPS: Step wise approach for surveillance of risk factor for NON COMUNICABLE disease.
ICF – (International classification of functioning, disability and health) *(2001)* Earlier it was ICIDH (international classification of impairment ,disability and handicap).

- Health education and communication
- BOTH attitude and belief are extremely difficult to change. Practice or Habit is associated with emotional value and most likely to be influenced by motivation. [Q]
- Committes and their respective works:

ALMA ATA committee – PHC (1978) [Q].
BHORE committee – Comprehensive health care (1946)
SHRIVASTVA committee – Medical education and support manpower.

- Different missions:

Rural health scheme -1977 (Local dai)
National health policy -1983(health for all)
ICDS (integrated child development scheme) – Aganwadi worker.
NRHM (national rural health mission)- 5th April 2005 (ASHA) *(PGI 11)*

- Asha

Posted at village level under NRHM. *(VERY IMP)*
1 ASHA =deployed for 1000 people. *(AIPG 10)*
Non ASHA State – North east.

- Health education:

Principles of health education: • Credibility-it is the degree to which message is perceived as trustworthy by the people. [Q] • Interest • Participation • Motivation • Comprehension • Reinforcement • Learning by doing • Known to unknown • Setting an example • Good human relation • Feedback • Leadership
• Well known approaches to health education: *(AIIMS 11)* – Regulatory – Service – Health educational – Primary health care
• Comprehensive School Health Education – All students to be productive learner about health decisions. (Not Programme)

- PHC – essential components of PHC are (given by ALMA ata declaration): [Q].

• Education about health problems and their preventive and controlling methods.
• Adequate supply of safe water and basic sanitation.
• Provision of essential drugs.
• Promotion of food supply and proper nutrition.
• Maternal and child health care, including family planning.
• Immunisation against infectious disease.
• Prevention and control of endemic diseases.

- NUMBER of centres per unit population:

SUB CENTER – 5000.(1 sub centre per 5,000 population) [Q]
PHC – 30000 (1 PHC per 30,000 population)
CHC – 120000 (1 CHC per 1,20,000 population)

- SOAP notes –subjective objective assessment plan- classify patients' Problems. *(KCET)*
- Soil – people, seed –health facts, sower- media [Q].
- Health promotion at genetic level:

EUGENICS: Science which aims for improvement of human genetic endowment. *(AIPG 08)*
EUTHENICS – Science which deals with environmental manipulation for providing better environment so that DESIRABLE GENE can EXPRESS themselves thus improving health of the individual.

- Medical ethics in genetic counselling:

AUTONOMY
NON-MALEFICENCE
BENEFICENCE
INFORMED CONSENT

- Health communication:

Types of Communication: • ONE WAY – DIDACTIC *(PGI 12)* • TWO WAY – DILECTIC/SOCRATIC *(KCET 12)*
SYMPOSIUM – there is no discussion among members. SERIES OF SPEECHES on a selected subject.
GROUP DISCUSSION – most commonly employed method because the experts can exchange and discuss their views. No public participation 6 – 12 people are involved.
PANEL DISCUSSION – 4 – 8 people and public participation is there.

LAST 5-YEAR QUESTIONS FROM THIS TOPIC

1. dental health education is considered successful if the patient: *(AIPG 08)*

Ans. Take appropriate action to improve oral health.

2. Primary prevention of dental disease can be done by:

Ans. Wearing gloves and sterilization of instruments.

3. Medical ethics in genetic counselling involve all except: *(AIPG 12)*

a. Beneficence
b. Confidentiality
c. Informed consent
d. Directive guidance

Ans. d

4. In a health education programme 10 people are planning to speak on topic of common interest. The best educational approach for this would be:

Ans. Group discussion.

FINANCE

- Deductible/front end payment – stipulated flat sum that the patient must pay toward the cost of treatment before benefits of the program go into effect. [Q]
- Co-insurance or copayment – patient pays a percentage of the total cost of the treatment. [Q]
- Fee schedule – a list of charges established or agreed by a dentist for specific dental services. [Q]
- Table of allowance – a list of covered services.
- UCR – usual, customary and reasonable fee as their preferred method for reimbursement for dentist in prepayment plan.
- Non Proffit health service corporation:

Delta dental plans – almost exclusively use the UCR concept. The participating dentists are paid 90th percentile of the fee The non participating dentists are paid 50 th percentile of fee. *(COMED K 13)*
Blue cross/ blue shield [Q] – limited dental coverage as a part of medical policies.

FLOURIDES [VERY IMP. FOR PGI, KCET]

- History:

Mc KAY – Discovered Colorado stains in 1901. Called it MOTTLED enamel. [Q]
DEAN – Shoe leather survey(1931). Told water fluoridation is associated with decreased dental caries.
CHURCHILL – discovered FLUORIDE in 1931 in BAUXITE CITY.
1st water fluoridation – Grand Rapids -1945 and Muskegon was control. *(PGI)*
100% Water fluoridation in – HONKONG and SINGAPORE. *(PGI June12)*

- MILK fluoridation – Zeigler. *(PGI)*
- SALT fluoridation – Wespi *(PGI)*
- BIBBY – in 1942 told that repeated application of Na/K fluoride results in reduction in caries prevalence. *(KCET 12)*
- F^- in body is carried by plasma (Mainly)and RBC.
- 1ppm F = 1mg F in 1 L/Kg of H2O. [PGI Q]
  Normal fluoride concentration in drinking water. [Q]
- Fluoride mouth rinse:

0.02%/0.05% -ONCE DAILY
0.2% – FORTHNIGHTLY/monthly twice/per week [PGI Q]

- ACCRETION – In highly fluoridated bone /teeth fluoride replaced HCO_3-.This is called accretion. So bone/teeth have less HCO_3- content.
- Fluoride inhibits following –
- ENOLASE enzyme of glycolysis [Q], bacterial phosphatases and potassium transport of bacteria.
- For maximum benefit, F^- supplementation should begin at birth. [Q]
- Distribution of fluoride to foetus:

Placenta acts as PARTIAL barrier/COMPLETE BARRIER/placenta only acts as a barrier where there is a sudden increase in maternal plasma F^- level. *(AIPG 2012)*
Primary teeth are less prone to develop fluorosis as placenta act as barrier.

- Cariostatic effect of F^- on developing teeth:

Initially that is just before calcification , the enamel is very porous and absorb F^- preferentially. So highest amount of fluoride in enamel is found just before enamel begins to calcify rapidly. So, CARIOSTATIC LEVEL of F^- is manifested in CALCIFICATION STAGE of tooth development. [Q]

- F Concentration:
- cementum> dentin> enamel. [Q]
- Fluoride content:

F^- Concentration in dental plaque – 15-64 ppm *(PGI)*
In dried tea leaves – 98 ppm [Q]. The maximum amount of fluoride is present in dried tea leaves. [AIIMS 06] 2nd in Sea fish. [Q]
IN human milk - 6-12 µg/ml. [Q]

- Recommended daily dose of fluride: *(Very Imp. For PGI)*

Level of water F^- → Supplement of Fluoride ↘ AGE of child ↓	0.3 ppm	0.3-0.7ppm	>0.7ppm
Birth to 2 yrs	0.25 mg	0	×
2 – 3 yrs	0.50 mg	0.25 mg	×
3 – 14 yrs	1 mg	0.5 mg	×

- Supplemental fluoride depends on AGE of child and F^- level in water.

Below 4 years fluoridated dentifrices not recommended
Below 2 years F^- tablets not recommended.
Below 6 yrs F^- mouthwash not recommended.
If F^- concentration of community water is > 0.7 ppm, NO need of any F^- supplement at any age.

- Topical Preparation of fluoride:

SnF: Freshly prepared mix has PH of 2 [Q] and increases to 7. Tin Hydroxy Phosphate → responsible for metallic taste after Topical application *(AIPG 12)*
APF: GEL has ph 0f 4-5 and sol of 3 *(KCET 12)* APF acts by formation of DCPD + CaF2+ FLUROAPATITE *(COMED K 12)* ↓ (Dicalcium phosphate dehydrate)
2% NaF – neutral , ph=7 [PGI 12]
Best compound for mouth rinse is NaF BUT most effective topical F^- is APF gel.(most commonly used in clinic)
As NaF is neutral – causes no pigmentation so used with porcelainand silicate restoration. APF and SnF2 not used.
APF gel – it has thixotropic property [Q] due to sodium Carboxymethyl cellulose. Composition =NaF + HF + orthophosphoric acid.

- Fluoride varnish:

Duraphat – 2.26%F^- = 22600 ppm *(PGI 11)* It's the 1st fluoride varnish. [developed in GERMANY]
Fluor protector – 0.7%F^-= 7000 ppm (silane fluoride)
Carex -1.8% F^-
ALL other than fluor protector are NaF based. [Q].

- Fluoridated dentrifrice:

NaF BASED. Contains 800-1000ppm F^- and free available F^- is 500-600ppm *(PGI)*

- Systemic fluoridation acts on smooth surface [Q] NOT on pit and fissure.
- Fluoride tablets:

Fluoride chewable tablets – provide both topical and systemic effects.
Used in area where fluoride is NOT available.
F^- Tablet releases half fluoride of their weight. That is 1mg of tablet releases 0.5mg of fluoride.
Note: Topical F^- is given even if fluoride is present in water because there effect is ADDITIVE.

- Water fluoridation:

Water fluoridation depends on TEMPERATURE in that area and BODY Weight
Galgan formula for fluoride: Ppm of F^-= - 0.038 +0.0062 Temperature in Ferenhite [Q]
Variation of ppm of F^- with Temperature: >26 0C = 0.5 -0.7 ppm 18- 26 0C = 0.8 -1 ppm <18 0C = 1.1 -1.3ppm
Water fluoridation system:

Type of fluoridation system	Component used
Saturator system	4% NaF saturated solution
Dry feeder system	NaF or silicofluoride
Solution feeder system	Hydrofluorosilicic acid. [Q].

In school water fluoridation 3-4 times MORE fluoride than community water is used(1ppm F^- in community water).
Community water fluoridation decreases incidence of caries by 50-65%.
CARIOSTATIC level of F^- IN DRINKING WATER - 1ppm [Q].
fluorspar is CaF2 [Q] is also used in water fluoridation.

- Fluoride toxicity:

Safety recommended dose – above 3 yrs old child is 1mg/day – adult 1.7 – 3.3 = 2.2 approx. [Q]
STD(safety tolerated dose) – 8to16 mg F /kg wt
CLD (certain lethal dose) – 32 to 64 mg F/kg wt(4 times of STD) = 5-6g [Q]
PROBABLE lethal dose = 5mg/kg wt. *(PGI)*
Nephrotoxicity due to Fluoride is at 850 ng/ml [Q]
Plasma level of fluoride > 2μg – causes DENTAL fluorosis.
SKELETAL fluorosis → 10–25 mg F^-/days to 10–25 yrs. ↓ (crippling fluorosis) → H_2O level > 8ppm. [Q]
ACUTE toxicity of fluoride – vomiting most common feature because HF is gastric irritant. Death by blocking normal cellular metabolism – respiratory and cardiac failure. T/t – induce vomiting, oral Ca, milk, cardiac monitoring.

- Genu valgam:

Newer form of fluorosis reported from A.P and T.N
Seen in people whose staple diet was jowar
Characterized by osteoporosis and GENU VALGAM.

LAST 5-YEAR QUESTIONS FROM THIS TOPIC

1. Best way to prevent caries by APF gel application in patient with high caries index: *(AIPG 09)*

Ans. 2 times per year

2. Absorbed fluoride is eliminated mainly by:

Ans. Kidney.

3. In community water fluoridation process, which of the following sequence is correct: *(AIPG 08)*

Ans. Dental decay → fluoride content in water→ central water Community approval supply.

Note: The first step starts with identifying problem i.e., diagnosis of dental caries. Then preventive measure one of which is water fluoridation. The last step is taking community approval.

4. **A pregnant lady uses fluoridated water drinking water. All of the following are true regarding exposure of the foetus to fluoride except:** *(AIPG 12)*
   a. Placenta act as regulator and reduces the concentration of fluorides reaching the foetus.
   b. Placenta acts as a regulator and increases the concentration of fluorides reaching the foetus.

Ans. b

INDICES

- Ideal requisite of an index:

TRICK: C V Raman A Qualified Scientist
C → Clarity
V → Validity (VALIDITY-the index should measure what it is intended to measure. *(KCET 12)*
Raman → Reliability (RELIABILITY- the index should measure consistently the SAME at all times and all places.[Q])
A → Acceptability
Qualified → Quantifiability
Scientist → Sensitivity

- Dean's flurosis index: *(AIPG, KCET 07)*

SCORE	CRITERIA
Normal (0)	Normal enamel
Questionable (0.5)	Enamel discloses white flecks to occasional white spots.
Very mild (1)	White opaque area involving 25% of tooth.
Mild (2)	White area 25-50% *(KCET 2007)*
Moderate (3)	All enamel surfaces are affected.
Severe (4)	Marked hypoplasia, pitting with widespread brown stains. The general form of tooth is affected with a corroded like appearance.

- Gingival bleeding index:

Aim of index is to DIAGNOSE the GINGIVAL HEALTH NOT to measure/quantify gingival bleeding. So GINGIVITIS > gingival bleeding. *(PGI)*
bleeding on probing – tell states of gingival health ON DAY OF EXAMINATION. [Q]

- OHI-S (simplified oral hygiene index):

Greene and Vemillion – 1964
Teeth examined – 6 1 6 6 1 6
Criteria – tooth should be fully erupted and in occlusion.
Interpretation: Good – 0 – 1.2 Fair – 1.3 – 3 Poor – 3.1 – 6

- Php index (patient hygiene performance index):

Used to score the patient before and after oral hygiene instruction. *(AIPG 10)*
Developed by Podishadley and Haley (TRICK: one of the scientist's name has iPod in reverse order.)
Selection of teeth – same as in OHI-S.
SCORE = 0 TO 5

- PLAQUE index:

Silness and loe 1964.

Purpose – to assess the thickness of plaque only at gingival surface.

Selection of teeth – whole mouth basis (entire dentition)

Selected mouth basis – 6 2 4
4 2 6

Score criteria:

SCORE	FINDING
0	no plaque in the gingival area
1	a film of plaque may be recognized only after application of disclosing agent or by running a probe.
2	Moderate accumulation can be seen by naked eye.
3	Abundance of deposition.

Interpretation: Good – 0
Fair – 0.1 – 0.9
Poor – 1 – 1.9

- Gingival Index – Loe and Sillness 1963:

(TRICK: As 'G' of gingival index is before 'P' of plaque index so LOE is before SILNESS in gingival index)

Selection of teeth – same as in Plaque index.

Score:

Score	Criteria
0	Normal gingiva
1	Mild inflammation, slight changes in colour, slight oedema no bleeding on probing.
2	Moderate inflammation, bleeding on probing (b.o.p)-moderate. Gingivitis. *(KCET 2013)*
3	Severe inflammation, marked redness and hypertrophy, ulceration, spontaneous bleeding.

Interpretation – Mild gingivitis – 0.1 – 1
Moderate – 1.1 – 2
Severe – 2.1 – 3

- Periodontal index: Russell

Purpose – to assess and score the periodontal disease status of population and in EPEDEMIOLOGICAL studies.

Assess the severity of periodontitis in epidemiological studies of a large population. *(AIPG 2009)*

Only mouth mirror and light source used.

Selection of teeth – entire dentition:

Score	Criteria	Radiographic feature
0	Negative- no inflammation, nor loss of function due to destruction of supporting tissue	Normal
1	Mild gingivitis: inflammation in the free gingiva which does not circumscribe the tooth.	
2	Gingivitis: inflammation completely circumscribes the tooth.	
4	Used only when radiographs are available	Notch like resorption of alveolar crest
6	Gingivitis with pocket formation	Horizontal bone loss
8	Advanced destruction with loss of masticatory function	Advanced bone loss

Russell's rule – when in doubt, assign the lower score."

Interpretation:

Clinical condition	Individual PI score
Clinically normal supportive tissue	0 – 0.2
Simple gingivitis	0.3 – 0.9
Beginning destructive periodontal disease	1 – 1.9
Established destructive periodontal disease	2 – 4.9 [Q]
Terminal disease	5 – 8

- Cpitn:

Corresponds to – 'COMMUNITY PERIODONTAL INDEX OF TREATMENT NEEDS" *(KCET 13)*

(Ainamo et. Al. For the joint working committee of WHO and FDI, 1982)

CPITN/WHO probe/TRS (technical recording series):
Purposes – 1.to measure the pocket depth
2.to detect sub gingival calculus
5 gms in weight

CPITN –E: black marking starting at 3.5 mm and ending at 5.5 mm

Disadvantage –partial recording
exclusion of some important signs of past periodontal breakdown notably attachment loss.

Selection of teeth – sextant [Q]
Index teeth upto 19 yrs – 6 1 6
6 1 6
Index teeth aged 20 yrs or more – 2nd molar also included.

Codes and criteria:

Code	Criteria
0	Healthy
1	Bleeding observed after probing
2	Calculus detected during probing.
3	Pocket 4-5mm (black band visible).
4	Pocket 6mm or more(black band not visible)
X	Excluded sextant(less than two teeth present.
9	Not recorded

Treatment needs:	
TN-O	For code 0 or X and need for treatment.
TN-1	A CODE OF 1 or higher indicates a need for improving the personal oral hygiene
TN-2a	A code of 2 or, higher indicates need for professional cleaning and removal of plaque.
TN-2b	For code 3, same treatment as for code 2
TN-3	A CODE OF 4 INDICATES complex t/t like deep scaling ,root planning and more complex surgical procedure.

- CPI (Community Periodontal Index):

Modification of the CPITN by inclusion of measurement of attachment loss and elimination of treatment needs category.

CPI probe – used to measure overjet and overbite and open bite also.
Selection of teeth – same as CPITN index.

Codes and criteria: -
Same as CPITN.

Loss of attachment:
Note – loss of attachment should not be recorded for children under the age of 15.

Score	Criteria
0	Loss of attachment 0-3 mm
1	4-5 mm(CEJ within the black band.)
2	6-8 mm (CEJ between the upper limit of the black band and the 8.5mm ring)
3	9-11 mm (CEJ between 8.5 and 11.5 mm rings)
4	4 - 12mm or more (CEJ beyond the 11.5 mm ring)
X	Excluded sextant
9	Not recorded (CEJ neither visible nor detectable).

- Dmft index:

Purpose – to determine the prevalence of coronal caries.
Selection of teeth – All 28 teeth are examined. Teeth not included are: • 3rd molar • Unerupted teeth • Congenitally missing teeth and supernumerary teeth. • Teeth removed for reason other than dental caries such as orthodontic treatment or impaction. • Teeth restored for reasons other than dental caries such as trauma, bridge abutment etc. • Primary tooth is never evaluated in this index.
Who modification of dmf index: • All 3rd molars are included • Temporary restorations are considered as decayed. • Only carious cavities are considered as decayed. Initial lesions are considered as sound.
Limitations: • Dmf values are not related to the number of teeth at risk. • Can be invalid in older adults b/c teeth can be lost for various reason other than caries. • Little use in studies of root caries.

- Def index:

Gruebbel		
Caries index for primary dentition.		
Age specific index. [Q]		
D=decayed teeth,	e = extracted teeth,	f = filled teeth

LAST 5-YEAR QUESTIONS FROM THIS TOPIC

1. **Index used to assess the severity of periodontitis in large population is:** *(AIPG 11)*

Ans. Periodontal index [Ref: Soben peter 2/e p151, 153]

2. **Which of the following plaque indices does not use disclosing agent?** *(AIPG 11)*

Ans. Debris component of simplified oral hygiene index. [Ref: Hiremath 2/e p200]

3. **The following plaque index divides each tooth surface into into 9 areas.** *(AIPG 11)*

Ans. Modified navy plaque index

4. **The PHP index describes.** *(AIIMS May 11)*

Ans. Performance of oral hygiene by patient after brushing for self evaluation. [Ref: Soben peter 2/e p141]

DATES AND YEARS

- 1946 –IDA
- 1948 – DENTIST ACT (29th march), WHO (7th April)
- 1949 – DCI (12th April)
- 1964 – 1st fluoridated dentifrice + 1st fluoridated varnish [Q]
- 1975 – India became SMALL POX free.
- 1st April 1976 – The CIGARETTE ACT of 1975' was introduced by the government of India on. *(KCET 06)*
- 1977-Rural health scheme. [Q]
- 1981 – 1ST Reported case of AIDS *(AIIMS Nov 12)*
- 1982 – NCRP (The national cancer registry programme) was initiated by Indian council of medical research in the year. [KCET 11]
- 1983 – 1st human immunodeficiency virus detected. *(AIIMS 12)*

- 2003 – Cigarette and other tobacco product act' TO prohibit the advertisement. *(KCET 11)*
- Important days:

30TH Jan – antileprosy day
31st may – world no tobacco day.
1st July – doctor's day
11th July – population day.
1st dec –anti AIDS day
11th dec – UNICEF day.

MISCELLANEOUS

- Waste disposal (Very Important):

Yellow bag: Anatomical waste, microbiology and biotechnology waste, solid waste + clinical waste of hospital. *(KCET 11)*
Red bag – microbiology and solid waste.
Blue /white bag – sharp waste [Q]
Black bag - cytotoxic drugs , non infectious waste(office paper, kitchen waste, plastic wrapper of surgical syringe. [Q]

- Category of wastes:

Category 1 – anatomical waste	*(KCET 12)*
Category 4 – sharp waste	*(KCET 13)*
Category 5 – cytotoxic drug	
Category 6 – solid waste contaminated with blood	
Category 9 – incinerated ash	

- Different methods of waste disposal:

DUMPING: most unsanitary method. [Q]
CONTROLLED TIPPING(sanitary landfill) - most satisfactory. [Q]
INCINERATION: Best method for disposal of HOSPITAL waste. [Q] NO or limited manure value.

- Composting: The compost has considerable manure value.

Bangalore method – anaerobic method of composting. [Q]
Mechanical method – aerobic method.

- Hardness of water:

Temporary hardness due to CO_3^{-} and HCO_3^{-} Removed by simple heating.
Permanent hardness due to SO_4^{--}. Removed by addition of $Na_2(CO_3)$ OR, by permutit process (Base Exchange process)

- Purification of water:

SLOW Sand Filter	RAPID Sand Filter
Biological filter	Filtration is rapid ,so can meet the demand of cities– so the IDEAL CHOICE.
Rate of filtration- 0.1-0.4 /hr/	Filtration is rapid ,40-50 times of slow sand filter (5-15/ hr)
Vital layer/zoogleal layer are the heart of slow sand filter. The formation of vital layer is called RIPENING of filter.	
Total bacterial count is reduced By 99.99%.	
	Large sand grain size.

- Residual chlorine: 0.5mg /lit after 1hr. [Q]
- Pasteurisation:

Is tested by: Phosphatase test, standard plate count, coliform count and Methylene blue reduction test. [Q]
METHODS of pasteurisation: • Holder method – 63-66 0C For at least 30 min. [Q] • Flash method -72 0C for 15 secs. [Q]

- Planning and survey:

Goals are not measurable while Target and objective are measurable. [Q]

- Criteria used in EVALUATION of dental services:

EFFECTIVENESS – A measure of the accuracy/success of services. To evaluate its USEFULLNESS. *(AIIMS O5)*
EFFICACY – The extent to which a treatment achieves its intended purpose.
EFFICIENCY – Cost in relation to the output of the programme.

- Osha guidelines:

Category 1 – tasks that involve exposure to blood , body fluids or tissues. Most tasks performed by the dentists. *(COMED K 05)*
Category 2 – do not involve routine exposure to blood, body fluids or tissues. Workers who help clean up the office.
Category 3 – no exposure to blood/body fluids/tissues. e.g. Receptionist
NOTE: OSHA guidelines advise that all dental office staff in category 1and 2 and dentists should be trained in infection control to protect themselves and their patients.

- ART:
- Indication – Small cavities, in those cavities accessible to hand instrument, public health programme.
- Vitamins:

Vit. D and B12 are found only in foods of animal origin.
Halibut fish liver oil → richest source of vit Aand D.
Vit A – ANTICARCINOGENIC *(AIPG 12)*

- FATTY acids:

n-3 FA – linolenic acid.
n-6 FA – linoleic acid.
Ideal fat has PUFA: SATURATED FA = 0.8 to 1 and n6 to n3 = 5-10 in total diet.
Flax seed oil is richest source of n3.
Groundnut and corn oil is rich in n6 PUFA. [Q].
Order of saturated fatty acids content: [imp] Coconut oil>butter>palm oil>groundnut>soybean>sun flower [Q]

- Cholesterol:

Normal level should be < 200 mg/dl *(KCET 13)*
Daily dietary intake < 300mg/day.
Rich sources – egg, beef, milk and milk products, poultry. EGG is the richest source. No cholesterol in plant.
HDL – major indicator for CHD(chronic heart disease) [Q]
LDL – major risk factor for CHD. [Q]

- Fish:

Contains EICOSAPENTANOIC acid [Q], rich in vit Aand D. **NOTE:** Breast milk – docosahexanoic acid [Q].
Fish bones are excellent source of ca, po4, F^-.
Fish provides quality protein and mineral and has no carbohydrate.

- Breast milk:

Maximum Output at 5-6 month.
Milk content of Fe is low but its bioavailability is HIGH.
The coefficient of Fe uptake is 70% where as it is only 30% in cow milk.
Docosahexanoic acid present. *(AIPG 12)*
Human and cow's milk – only sugar content (lactose) is HIGHER in human milk compared to cow milk so increased chances of caries.
milk is a good source of all vitamins except vit C + (poor source of Fe) [Q]

- Egg protein:
- Is the reference protein but human milk is the reference protein for infants.
- Criteria for indian reference man and woman:

Particulars	Man		Woman
Age	20-39 yrs [Q]		20-39 [Q]
Weight	60 kg		50 kg
Daily activities	8hrs in bed		8hrs in bed
Energy requirements: Light work Moderate Heavy	 2400 2900[Q] 3800	 trick (-)600	 1900 2200 2900
Protein	1gm/day		1gm/day
Fat intake	20gm/day		20gm/day

- BMI:

BMI = weight(kg)/height
Normal = 18 – 25
Overweight = >25
Obese => 30 [AIPG 09]

- Assessing malnutrition:

WEIGHT FOR AGE – common to BOTH acute and chronic malnutrition. *(AIIMS 12)*
HEIGHT FOR AGE – for chronic malnutrition.
WEIGHT FOR HEIGHT – acute malnutrition

- Insecticide:

Anti adult measure – DDT [Q], pyrethrum.
Melathion – both larvicidal and antiadult.

- Antiseptics:

Savlon = Cetrimide + CHX
Dettol = Chloroxylenol
Dakin's solution = NaOCl [COMED K 13] + boric acid dissolved.
Eusol = Chlorinated lime +boric acid
Dakin's solution and eusol dissolves necrotic tissue and pus so used in cleaning infected wounds.

- Common disinfectants for Hospital use:

Phenol – It not readily inactivated by organic matter Not sporicidal. Halogen – Recommended for disinfection of equipment soiled with blood (because of hepatitis risk) BUT rapidly inactivated by organic material. [Q].
Alcohols – Water must be present for bacterial killing i.e., 70% ethanol is best. [Q]
Aldehydes – Gluteraldehyde – SPORICIDAL, more active, less toxic than formaldehyde. Disinfection of endoscopes and bronchoscopes. [Q]
HCHO – Fumigation of operation theatre.

- Union minister of HEALTH and FAMILY welfare:

Union list	Concurrent list
TRICK - does Big works	TRICK = 'does small works'
Ex- regulation and development Of medical profession[Q]	

LAST 5-YEAR QUESTIONS FROM THIS TOPIC

1. In India government expend how much of GDP in healthcare:

Ans. 1.2%

NOTE: and aim is 2 %.

2. In PHC, which anticoagulant is used to send the blood sample for blood glucose:

Ans. Potassium oxalate + sod. fluoride

3. Glycemic index is least in: *(AIPG 08)*

Ans. Ice cream

Note: Order of glycemic index in order of from LOWEST:
brown rice > ice cream >soyabean=groundnut. (Ref: Park19/e p514.)

4. n-3 PUFA is present in ALL of the following EXCEPT:

a. Mustard oil
b. Fish oil
c. Corn oil
d. Ground nut oil

Ans. Ground nut > corn oil

5. Highest amount of PUFA is found in:

Ans. Soybean

6. HIGHEST Amount of saturated fatty acids is present in: *(AIPG 08)*

Ans. Palm oil.

7. Incineration is not done for: *(AIPG 10)*

Ans. Sharp infected waste.

Questions from Recent Exams

1. Auriculotemporal nerve encircles which artery? *(AIIMS Nov. 14)*

a. Superficial temporal artery
b. Superficial temporal vein
c. Middle meningeal artery
d. Deep temporal

Ans. c

2. All of the following are anti flux agents except: *(AIPG 14)*

a. Boric acid
b. Graphite
c. Iron oxide
d. Calcium carbonate in alcohol

Ans. a

3. A male child with extra x chromosome is most likely to have: *(AIIMS May 14)*

a. Cheesy molars
b. Taurodontism
c. Dens evagellatous
d. Dilaceration

Ans. b

4. Which is a measure of dispersion: *(AIIMS May 14)*

a. Measure of central tendency of data
b. Measure of standard deviation
c. Value repeating frequently
d. Measure of variation around mean

Ans. b

5. A pregnant lady uses fluoridated drinking water. All of the following are true regarding exposure of the fetus to fluoride except: *(AIIMS May 14)*

a. Placenta acts as regulator and reduces the concentration of fluoride reaching the fetus
b. Placenta act as regulator and increases the concentration of fluoride reaching the fetus
c. Placenta has no role in fluoride regulation to fetus
d. Placenta acts as a barrier to fluoride ions

Ans. b

6. Highest water solubility is seen in: *(AIPG 14)*

a. Zinc phosphate
b. Zinc oxide eugenol
c. Zinc Silicophosphate
d. Zinc polycarboxylate

Ans. c

7. Which test of hepatitis tells about most infective stage? *(AIIMS Nov. 14)*

a. HBeAg
b. Anti HBsAg

c. Anti HBcAg
d. None

Ans. a

8. Most common cause of incomplete casting when using a centrifugal casting machine: *(AIPG 14)*

a. Narrow sprue
b. Increase porosity of the investment
c. Large reservoir
d. Hollow sprue

Ans. a

9. Wavelength of ND-YaG laser used in dentistry is: *(AIPG 14)*

a. 1.06 μm
b. 10.60 μm
c. 0.6 μm
d. 300 μm

Ans. a

10. Bilateral mandibular involvement is seen in: *(AIIMS May 14)*

a. Cherubism
b. Lichen planus
c. Central giant cell granuloma
d. Osleoma

Ans. a

11. Millennium development goal was adopted in which year? *(AIIMS May 14)*

a. 1977
b. 2000
c. 1984
d. 2004

Ans. b

12. World no tobacco day: *(AIIMS May 14)*

a. 31st May
b. 1st November
c. 1st April
d. 7th April

Ans. a

13. Which of the following is a group 1 functional appliance: *(AIIMS May 14)*

a. Activator
b. Bionator
c. Oral screen
d. Twin block

Ans. c

14. Most common cyst associated with adjoining vital teeth? *(AIIMS May 14)*

a. Dentigerous cyst
b. Globulomaxillary cyst
c. Periapical cyst
d. Lateral periodontal cyst

Ans. a

15. **During the cap stage of tooth development, signaling for the cusp formation is largely controlled by which of the following:** *(AIPG 14)*
    a. Inner enamel epithelium
    b. Dental follicle
    c. Dental papilla
    d. Enamel knot

Ans. d

16. **Calcification of permanent teeth begins at:** *(AIPG 14)*
    a. 1 year
    b. 2 year
    c. At birth
    d. 4 months

Ans. c

17. **For wound healing which minerals helpful?** *(AIIMS Nov. 14)*
    a. Calcium
    b. Selenium
    c. Magnesium
    d. Copper

Ans. d

18. **Minimum number of lobes for tooth development:** *(AIPG 14)*
    a. 2
    b. 3
    c. 4
    d. 5

Ans. c

19. **Which of the following is an example of a centric holding cusp?** *(AIPG 14)*
    a. Mesiopalatal cusp of maxillary first molar
    b. Mesiobuccal cusp of mandibular first molar
    c. Palatal cusp of maxillary 1st molar
    d. Distolingual cusp of maxillary 1st molar

Ans. a

20. **Universal immunization programme of government of India does not include:** *(AIIMS May 14)*
    a. BCG
    b. MEASLE
    c. HPV
    d. DPT

Ans. c

21. **Lee way space is due to:** *(AIPG 14)*
    a. Space difference between deciduous canine and molar to their succedaneous permanent teeth
    b. Space difference between deciduous incisors and their succedaneous permanent teeth
    c. Difference between deciduous and permanent maxillary canine
    d. None

Ans. a

22. **Dontrix is:** *(AIIMS May 14)*
    a. A plier to give orthodontic bends
    b. A spring that measure force of orthodontic wire

c. measure strength of wire
d. measure wire distortion and deformation

Ans. b

23. Which of the following cysts is associated with a vital tooth? *(AIPG 14)*

a. Glubulomaxillary cyst
b. Lateral cyst
c. OKC
d. Dentigerous

Ans. a

24. Condition in which tongue is attached to the floor of the mouth by a small frenum is called: *(AIPG 14)*

a. Labial frenum
b. Lingual frenula
c. Ankyloglossia
d. Tongue tie

Ans. c

25. In statistics data represent: *(AIIMS May 14)*

a. Whole sample
b. Individual unit in a sample
c. The unit in which sample is given (kg, mm etc)
d. Observations

Ans. d

26. Which of the following is not present in posterior triangle of neck? *(AIIMS Nov. 14)*

a. Phrenic nerve
b. Subclavian nerve
c. External jugular vein
d. Hypoglossal nerve

Ans. d

27. Involucrum is: *(AIPG 14)*

a. New bone forming in the dead space within the bone
b. Dead bone lying within a bony cavity rejected by the body
c. Newly forming bone surrounding dead bone
d. Newly forming bone surrounding a dead space inside a bone

Ans. c

28. In a patient with angular chelitis, the histologic examination of a smear from the lesion would most probably reveal: *(AIPG 14)*

a. HSV-1
b. Tubercle bacilli
c. Candida
d. Spirochetes

Ans. c

29. Bending orthodontic wire at room temperature is an example of: *(AIIMS May 14)*

a. Strain hardening
b. Annealing
c. Suctility
d. Strain flexure

Ans. a

30. **Amongst the following conditions: syphilitic glossitis, hepatitis A, Plummer Vinson syndrome and Pagets disease, which 2 are predisposing conditions to development of squamous cell carcinoma?** *(AIPG 14)*
   a. Syphilitic glossitis, hepatitis A
   b. Hepatitis A, Plummer Vinson syndrome
   c. Syphilitic glossitis, Plummer Vinson syndrome
   d. Syphilitic glossitis and Pagets disease

Ans. c

31. **A 5-year-old child developed a fibrous verrucous growth on the lower lip which was non mobile, pedunclated, hyperkeratotic and exophytic. The histologic examination showed finger like projections of epithelium running deep into the connective tissue. The examination of the hands of the child revealed papillomatous growth on his left thumb which was larger than the right thumb. What could be the probable diagnosis?** *(AIPG 14)*
   a. Papilloma
   b. Keratoacanthoma
   c. Carcinoma in situ
   d. Squamous cell caricinoma
   e. Pemphigus

Ans. a

32. **Least amount of mercury is required in:** *(AIIMS May 14)*
   a. Admixed alloy
   b. Spherical
   c. Hybrid
   d. Lathe cut alloy

Ans. b

33. **Thick muscular labial frenum is because of:** *(AIIMS Nov. 14)*
   a. Septal muscle
   b. Orbicularis oris
   c. Buccinator
   d. Nasopalatine muscle

Ans. b

34. **Discoloration of a tooth due to hyperbilirubinemia during tooth development is called:** *(AIPG 14)*
   a. Onchronosis
   b. Chlordontia
   c. Leong's tooth
   d. Pink tooth of mummery

Ans. b

35. **Changes in size, colour and texture of gingiva are seen in which stage of gingivitis:** *(AIPG 14)*
   a. I
   b. II
   c. III
   d. IV

Ans. c

36. **Mother of a 3-year-old child is worried about small yellowish white nodular eruptions along the mid palatine raphe that have formed in the child's mouth. The child is normal and does not seem to have any adverse signs or symptoms. What is the possible diagnosis:** *(AIPG 14)*
   a. Epstein pearls
   b. Eruption cyst

c. Premature teeth
d. Keratoacanthoma

Ans. a

37. A patient has multiple epidermoid cysts, intestinal hamartomas, osteomas of skull and multiple impacted teeth. He is most probably suffering from: *(AIPG 14)*

a. Gorlin-Goltz syndorme
b. Gardner's syndrome
c. Neurofibromatosis
d. Osteosarcoma

Ans. b

38. Method for plaque control on concavities of root: *(AIIMS Nov. 14)*

a. Tooth pick
b. Interdental brush
c. Dental Floss
d. Tooth brush

Ans. b

39. Which of the following conditions have maygnant potential: *(AIPG 14)*

a. Pagets disease and fibrous dysplasia
b. Pagets disease and osteopetrosis
c. Fibrous dysplasia and osteopetrosis
d. Pagets disease and cherubism

Ans. a

40. To differentiate between hemifacial hypertrophy and unilateral fibrous dysplasia of the maxilia, evaluation of which of the following would be most useful: *(AIPG 14)*

a. Comparison of size of jaws and teeth on both sides
b. Shape of face
c. Shape and sized of soft palate
d. Distance of soft tissue landmarks from mid palatine rahbe

Ans. a

41. Taurodontism occurs because of: *(AIPG 14)*

a. Failure of fusion of dental papilla with inner enamel epithelium
b. Failure of Hertwig's epithelial sheath diaphragm to invaginate at the proper horizontal level
c. Premature destruction of the cervical loop.
d. None

Ans. b

42. Bilateral mandibular involvement is seen in which of the following conditions? *(AIPG 14)*

a. Osteoma
b. Lichen planus
c. Central giant cell granuloma
d. Cherubism

Ans. d

43. The characteristic feature seen during the histologic examination of a Langerhans Cell Histiocytosis lesion is: *(AIPG 14)*

a. Granuloma formation
b. Histiocytes
c. Birbecks granules
d. Eosinophils

Ans. c

44. When collecting oral tissues by scraping for diagnosis of oral cancer, all of the following are considered true except: *(AIPG 14)*

a. Deeper layers constitute cells with more diagnostic information
b. It is not an accurate diagnostic test
c. Keratin can interfere with staining and make it difficult to interpret the result
d. Transepithelial cells can be obtained

Ans. c

45. A 45yr old known diabetic patient reports to emergency in subconscious state. What will you do as first step for management of this patient? *(AIIMS Nov. 14)*

a. I.V 5% Dextrose
b. I.V Insulin
c. I.V dexamethasone
d. Blood test to monitor the blood glucose

Ans. d

46. When collecting oral tissues by exfoliative cytology for diagnosis of oral cancer, all of the following are considered true except: *(AIPG 14)*

a. Deeper layers constitute cells with more diagnostic information
b. It is not an accurate diagnostic test
c. Keratin can interfere with diagnosis and make it difficult to interpret the result
d. Transepithelial cells can be obtained

Ans. d

47. Nowadays swine flu is in news, it is considered as: *(AIIMS May 14)*

a. Pandemic
b. Epidemic
c. Endemic
d. Seasonal variation

Ans. a

48. Burning sensation in mouth is caused by all except: *(AIPG 14)*

a. Pernicious anemia
b. Iron deficiency
c. Diabetes mellitus
d. Ranula

Ans. d

49. The wavelength of conventional light cure unit is: *(AIIMS May 14)*

a. 400–500
b. 200–300
c. 600–700
d. 20–50

Ans. a

50. Tooth within a tooth seen in: *(AIPG 14)*

a. Mandibular 1st premolar
b. Mandibular lateral and central incisor
c. Maxillary Lateral incisor
d. Maxillary and mandibular lateral incisor

Ans. c

51. Gingival lesions are usually not found in: *(AIPG 14)*

a. Herpes
b. Recurrent apthae

c. Erythema Multiforme
d. Pyogenic granuloma

Ans. b

52. The purpose of pulpotomy in young permanent tooth: *(AIIMS May 14)*

a. Prevent tooth fracture
b. To induce root formation
c. Formation of hard base to support restoration
d. To minimize infection

Ans. b

53. The most common oral lesion in HIV infected patients is: *(AIPG 14)*

a. Oral hairy leukoplakia
b. Oral candidiasis
c. Kaposi's sarcoma
d. Oral hyperpigmentation

Ans. b

54. PDL does not have: *(AIIMS Nov. 14)*

a. Mature elastic fibers
b. Angioblasts and undifferentiated mesenchymal cells
c. Myelinated nerve fibers
d. Fibroblasts

Ans. a

55. Riga fede disease associated with: *(AIPG 14)*

a. Taurodontism
b. Aspirin therapy
c. Multiple impacted teeth
d. Natal teeth

Ans. d

56. The property which make a restoration to withstand occlusal forces: *(AIIMS May 14)*

a. Resistance form
b. Retention form
c. Convenience form
d. Outline form

Ans. a

57. Herpes zoster caused by: *(AIPG 14)*

a. Herpes simplex
b. CMV
c. Varicella
d. EBV

Ans. c

58. PHC in hilly areas include: *(AIIMS May 14)*

a. 20000 population
b. 30000 population
c. 50000 population
d. One lakh population

Ans. a

59. Cyst derived from stellate reticulum and grows in place of lhe affected tooth is called: *(AIPG 14)*

a. Dentigerous cyst
b. OKC
c. Primordial cyst
d. Radicular

Ans. c

60. Shade matching should be done within _____ seconds to avoid fatigue of eyes to colour. *(AIPG 14)*

a. 5
b. 10
c. 15
d. 20

Ans. a

61. Which ceramic is based on lithium disilicate? *(AIPG 14)*

a. IPS empress
b. IPS empress 2
c. In Ceram
d. Captek

Ans. b

62. Not responsible for chronic gingival inflammation: *(AIIMS Nov. 14)*

a. Neutrophil
b. Macrophages
c. T -lymphocytes
d. Plasma cells

Ans. a

63. Which of the following is a shrink free ceramic? *(AIPG 14)*

a. Emax
b. Dicor
c. Dicor MGC
d. Cerestore

Ans. d

64. Paresthesia of lower lip is most common in fracture of: *(AIIMS May 14)*

a. Body of mandible
b. Condyle
c. Coronoid
d. Symphysis

Ans. a

65. The main component of most denture cleaning powders is: *(AIPG 14)*

a. Sodium perborate
b. Detergents
c. Alkali agents
d. Hydrogen peroxide

Ans. a

66. When we try to find out significance of difference in height of children between 2 classes in a school, which test is used? *(AIIMS May 14)*

a. Unpaired test
b. Anova

c. Chisquare
d. Cofficient of variance

Ans. a

67. Kennedy bar connector is a type of: *(AIPG 14)*

a. Lingual bar
b. Lingual plate
c. Double lingual bar
d. Labial bar

Ans. c

68. Rabies vaccine not to be given in case of: *(AIIMS Nov. 14)*

a. Rat bite
b. Cat bite
c. Dog bite
d. Monkey bite

Ans. a

69. In a bilateral distal extension situation, all of the following clasps used engage undercut close to the edentulous area except: *(AIPG 14)*

a. Bar clasp
b. Embrasure clasp
c. Reverse circlet
d. Combination clasp

Ans. d

70. Schielder Principle: *(AIIMS May 14)*

a. Minimal enlarged canal
b. Shape of the canal can be changed
c. Use of 3–5 times larger than first binding file
d. Original canal curvature should be altered to make it compatible with obturating material

Ans. a

71. Metal oxides used in porcelain: *(AIPG 14)*

a. To improve strength
b. To improve bonding with porcelain
c. Impart colour
d. All of these

Ans. c

72. An upper central incisor in a 7-year-old child has an open apex and needs to undergo root canal treatment. The best way to determine the working length in this case is by: *(AIPG 14)*

a. Using an apex locator
b. Radiographic determination using IOPA X-ray
c. Paper point method
d. Tactile method

Ans. c

73. Most radiosensitive tissue is: *(AIIMS Nov. 14)*

a. Mucosa
b. Neurons
c. Salivary gland
d. Basal layer cells

Ans. d

74. Time of application of glutaraldehyde pellet to pulp stump in glutaraldehyde pulpotomy is: *(AIPG 14)*

a. 30 seconds
b. 4 minutes
c. 2 minutes
d. 5 seconds

Ans. b

75. In a patient with acute pulpitis, it is difficult for the patient to locate the pain. This is because: *(AIIMS May 14)*

a. No nociceptors are present in the pulp
b. Less proprioceptors are present in the pulp
c. Patient cannot speak
d. Patient is not cooperative

Ans. b

76. Second generation apex locators work on the principle of: *(AIPG 14)*

a. Electrical resistance
b. Electrical conductance
c. Electrical impedance
d. Circuit breaker

Ans. c

77. Latest technique by which bone graft is obtained without damaging vital structures, vessels/veins is based on: *(AIIMS Nov. 14)*

a. Piezoelectric vibration
b. Osteotome
c. Ultrasonic/soft lasers
d. Electrocautery

Ans. a

78. Irrigant of choice in a tooth with an acute pulpal abscess is: *(AIPG 14)*

a. Sodium hypochlorite
b. Hydrogen peroxide
c. Normal saline
d. EDTA

Ans. c

79. Rigafede disease is associated with: *(AIIMS May 14)*

a. Natal teeth
b. Permanent incisors
c. Multiple impacted teeth
d. Primary incisors

Ans. a

80. The most important aspect of irrigation is: *(AIPG 14)*

a. Volume of irrigant used
b. Chelating action of solution
c. Lumen of needle
d. Aspiration of solution

Ans. a

81. When using bioactive substances for the repair of a root perforation, which of the following zones will not be seen: *(AIPG 14)*

a. Zone of necrosis
b. Zone of proliferation

c. Zone of hard tissue formation
d. Zone of stimulation

Ans. a

82. Which of the following are primary colonizers of gingival plaque? *(AIIMS Nov. 14)*

a. Gram positive aerobes
b. Gram positive facultatives
c. Gram -ve anaerobes
d. Gram+ve anaerobes

Ans. b

83. Fiber reinforced composite can be used for all of the following except: *(AIPG 14)*

a. Obturation of deciduous teeth
b. As a space maintainer
c. As a splint
d. As a post in teeth with crown fractured due to trauma

Ans. a

84. A 40 year old woman has ameloblastoma, histomorphic features will be: *(AIIMS May 14)*

a. Peripheral pallisading cellular strand with central loose stellate reticulum
b. Peripheral pallisading with central stromal retraction artefact
c. Peripheral pallisading cellular strand with peripheral loose stellate reticulum
d. Central loose stellate reticulum shows marked nuclear atypia and numerous mitotic figures

Ans. a

85. In case of pulpitis a patient is not able to locate the exact offending tooth. This because: *(AIPG 14)*

a. The patient cannot speak
b. Lack of proprioceptors in the pulp
c. The pulp lacks nociceptors
d. Patient cannot understand the question

Ans. b

86. Beta - hemihydrate calcination true is: *(AIIMS Nov. 14)*

a. In presence of air
b. In absence of air
c. In presence of $Cacl_2$ (3%]
d. Under steam pressure in autoclave

Ans. a

87. A 16-year-old boy reports with a history of traumatic injury 3 hours back leading to the avulsion of the upper permanent incisor. The tooth is present with the patient. Which of the following should be the line of treatment? *(AIPG 14)*

a. Wash the tooth with normal saline, clean, replace the tooth in the socket, check with a radiograph and splint
b. Scrape the periodontal ligament curette the socket replace and splint
c. Seal the apex of the tooth with retrograde amalgam restoration and replace the tooth
d. Clean the tooth, autoclave, replace and splint

Ans. a

88. Orthodontically treated midline diastema is best retained by: *(AIIMS Nov. 14)*

a. Not required
b. Hawley's appliance for 6 months
c. Hawley's appliance for 12 months
d. Lingual bonded retainer

Ans. d

89. A tooth with acute pulpitis will give what kind of response to pulp testing: *(AIPG 14)*

a. Lower reading compared to adjacent normal tooth
b. Lower reading to adjacent and opposing tooth
c. Higher reading compared to adjacent normal tooth
d. Similar reading as the adjacent tooth

Ans. b

90. Which of the following is true microdontia of lateral incisor? *(AIIMS May 14)*

a. Peg lateral
b. Hutchinson tooth
c. Mulbery tooth
d. Cheesy tooth

Ans. a

91. A 16 year old boy suffered traumatic injury to his upper central incisors a few years back. On percussion the incisors reveal dull metallic sound. The type of injury that the teeth may have suffered is: *(AIPG 14)*

a. Lateral luxation
b. Hitrusion
c. Extrusion
d. Subluxation

Ans. a

92. While placing orthodontic bracket in fluorsed teeth, acid etching is done with? *(AIIMS May 14)*

a. Hydrotluoric acid
b. Phosphoric acid
c. Nitric acid
d. Hydrochloric acid

Ans. d

93. A 29-years-old woman with a pregnancy of 17 week has a 10 years old boy with down syndrome, she does not want another down: syndrome kid; best advice to her is: *(AIIMS Nov. 14)*

a. No test is required now as her Age is below 35 years
b. Ultra sound at this point of time will definitely tell her that next baby will be down syndromic or not
c. Amniotic fluid samples plus chromosomal analysis will definitely tell her that next baby will be down syndromic or not
d. Blood screening at this point of time will clear the exact picture

Ans. c

94. Increased ANB angle is seen in: *(AIIMS May 14)*

a. Maxillary protrusion
b. Mandibular protrusion
c. Mandibular re trusion
d. Deep bite

Ans. a

95. The most physiologic medium to transport an avulsed tooth is: *(AIPG 14)*

a. Viaspan™
b. Normal saline
c. Cold milk
d. Hanks balanced salt solution

Ans. a

96. Median rhomboid glossitis is due to: *(AIIMS May 14)*

a. Non fusion of mesodermal thickening and retraction of tuberculum impar
b. Atrophy of filli form papilla
c. Ectodermal covering with absence of mucosa
d. Absence of fungiform papilla

Ans. a

97. Preventive resin restoration is indicated in: *(AIPG 14)*

a. Noncavitated pit and fissures
b. Deep caries to prevent progress of lesion
c. Cavitated fissures which require restoration
d. Wide cavity to prevent cusp fracture

Ans. c

98. Not true about NRHM: *(AIIMS Nov. 14)*

a. Appoint ASHA
b. Strengthen institutional delivery under JSY
c. Health and family welfare societies
d. State and district health mission

Ans. c

99. For etching of teeth with fluoros is for the purpose of orthodontic bonding, which acid should be used: *(AIPG 14)*

a. Hydrofluoric acid
b. Phosphoric acid
c. Acetic acid
d. Hydrochloric acid

Ans. b

100. Which of the following model analysis would be useful in planning extractions for a 14 year old boy with severe Class II division 1 malocclusion: *(AIPG 14)*

a. Ashley Howe analysis
b. Ponts analysis
c. Peck & Peck analysis
d. Bolton's analysis

Ans. a

101. A 50 year old epileptic patient prescribed carbamazepine for epilepsy, true statement: *(AIIMS Nov. 14)*

a. It does not cause Agranulocytosis
b. No correlation between serum concentration and control of epilepsy
c. Serum cone. > 40 g/ml is fatal
d. Nephrotoxic

Ans. c

102. Which of the following is a solid solution: *(AIIMS May 14)*

a. Amalgam
b. Cobalt-chromium
c. Silver-palladium
d. Gallium-silver

Ans. c

103. The importance of proximal caries in deciduous 1st molar for an orthodontist is: *(AIPG 14)*

a. Reduction in arch length due to growth of mandible
b. Loss of arch length

c. Class I occlusion
d. Flush terminal plane malocclusion

Ans. b

104. Following a bilateral parasymphysis fracture of mandible in the canine region. The anterior segment of mandible is displaced posteriorly by the action of? *(AIIMS May 14)*

a. Anterior belly of digastric muscles, geniohyoid and genioglossus
b. Thyrohyoid, genioglossus and hyoglossus
c. Mylohyoide, genioglossus and geniohyoid
d. Mylohyoide, geniohyoid and thyrohyoid

Ans. a

105. Increased ANB angle signifies: *(AIPG 14)*

a. Retrognathic maxilla
b. Retrognathic mandible
c. Prognathic mandible
d. Bimaxillary protrusion

Ans. b

106. A 3 year and 7 month old child with history of traumatic intrusion of 51, iopa reveals foreshortening. The treatment is? *(AIIMS May 14)*

a. Immediate reposition and splinting of 51
b. Wait and watch
c. Orthodontic extrusion
d. Immediate extraction

Ans. b

107. Adams clasp is formed from which gauge of stainless steel wire? *(AIPG 14)*

a. 23 mil
b. 22 mil
c. 24 mil
d. 28 mil

Ans. d

108. Lingually placed mandibular posteriors will cause all except: *(AIIMS Nov. 14)*

a. Gagging
b. Speech difficulties
c. Excessive pressure on ridge
d. Tongue interference

Ans. c

109. A patient with maxillary midline diastemma which has been closed orthodontically requires what kind of retention: *(AIPG 14)*

a. Fixed palatal retainer
b. Begs retainer for 6 months
c. Begs retainer for 1 year
d. No retention

Ans. a

110. Retarder in PMMR to prevent polymerisation is: *(AIIMS May 14)*

a. Hydroquinone
b. Polyacrylic acid
c. Benzoylperoxide
d. Dibutyl phthalate

Ans. a

111. In a stainless steel crown on a deciduous molar with overhanging margins, gingival pain and inflammation occurs due to: *(AIPG 14)*
  a. Plaque retention
  b. Excess cement
  c. Crown margins causing irritation
  d. Engaging undercut

Ans. a

112. Space maintainers are categorised in to which level of health protection? *(AIIMS May 14)*
  a. Specific protection
  b. Health promotion
  c. Disease limitation
  d. Tertiary protection

Ans. a

113. Maximum Lip thickness is seen at what age in males: *(AIPG 14)*
  a. 10 years
  b. 16 years
  c. 18 years
  d. 21 years

Ans. b

114. A 40 year old woman has Ameloblastoma, Histopathologic picture is? *(AIIMS Nov. 14)*
  a. Peripheral pallisading strand with central stellate reticulum
  b. Peripheral pallisading strand with central stromal retraction artifact
  c. Peripheral pallisading strand with peripheral stellate reticulum
  d. Central loose stellate reticum shows marked nuclear atypia and numerous mitotic figure

Ans. a

115. Specific plaque hypothesis state that: *(AIIMS May 14)*
  a. All plaque is pathogenic
  b. Only specific micro-organisms are responsible for pathogenicity of plaque
  c. Only specific microbes cause caries
  d. Plaque is pathogenic only when signs of associated disease are present

Ans. d

116. Skeletal classification of malocclusion was first given by: *(AIPG 14)*
  a. Salzman
  b. Angle
  c. Kratz
  d. Moyers

Ans. a

117. Christmas disease is due to deficiency of? *(AIIMS May 14)*
  a. Plasma thromboplastin anticedent
  b. Plasma thromboplastin component
  c. Hageman factor
  d. Platelets

Ans. b

118. Begg's bow is: *(AIIMS May 14)*
  a. Canine to canine
  b. 1st premolar to 1st premolar
  c. 1st molar to 1st molar
  d. 2nd premolar to 2nd premolar

Ans. c

119. Most common dental problem associated with cleft lip and palate is: *(AIPG 14)*
- a. Rotation of central incisor
- b. Anterior deep bite
- c. Unilateral or bilateral posterior cross bite
- d. Anterior open bite

Ans. c

120. Nasal epistaxis occurs due to: *(AIIMS May 14)*
- a. Anastomosis between two arteries in anterosuperior part of nasal septum
- b. Anastomosis between two arteries in anteroinferior part of nasal septum
- c. Anastomosis between two veins in anteroinferior part of nasal septum
- d. Anastomosis between vein and artery at anteroinferior part of nasal septum

Ans. b

121. The dimensions of the inner bow of the face bow used in orthodontics is: *(AIPG 14)*
- a. 0.4 mm and 0.6 mm
- b. 0.90" and 1.62"
- c. 0.045" and 0.125"
- d. 0.045" and 0.051"

Ans. d

122. Which inflammatory mediator involve in intracellular killing of microbes? *(AIIMS Nov. 14)*
- a. Catalase
- b. Oxidase
- c. Lysozyme
- d. IL6

Ans. c

123. Which among the following are associated with increased incidence of osteosarcoma? *(AIIMS May 14)*
- a. Cherubism and osteopetrosis
- b. Paget and polystotie fibrous dysplasia
- c. Paget and cherubism
- d. Polystotic fibrius dysplasia and cherub ism

Ans. b

124. A 5 year and 4 months old child has a retrusive chin with reduced lower facial height. On intraoral examination, full cusp distal step molar relation is seen. The cephalometric parameters reveal a normal SNA but a reduced SNB. What should be the line of treatment: *(AIPG 14)*
- a. Frankel II
- b. Twin Block
- c. Review at 6 years
- d. Bionator

Ans. c

125. The cribriform plate connects: *(AIIMS May 14)*
- a. Nasal cavity and anterior cranial fossa
- b. Nasal cavity and orbit
- c. Nasal cavity and oral cavity
- d. Anterior cranial fossa and orbit

Ans. a

126. Interincisal angle is increased in: *(AIPG 14)*
- a. Class I malocclusion with bimaxillary protrusion
- b. Class II division I malocclusion

c. Class 11 division 2 malocclusion
d. Class I type 2 malocclusion

Ans. c

127. Oro-antral fistula in maxillary 3rd molar region is best/commonly treated by: *(AIIMS May 14)*

a. Buccal mucoperiosteal flap
b. Palatal mucoperiosteal flap
c. Palatal island flap
d. Bridge flap

Ans. c

128. A 3 year old child suffered traumatic lateral luxation injury to his upper central incisor. The tooth is not mobile and does not interfere in occlusion. What should be done: *(AIPG 14)*

a. Reposition the tooth and splint
b. Reduce the affected tooth
c. Reduce both the affected and the opposite tooth
d. Wait and watch

Ans. d

129. Delayed transfusion reaction involves all except: *(AIIMS Nov. 14)*

a. Positive DAT
b. Spherocytes positive
c. Haemoglobinuria
d. Reduced haemoglobin

Ans. b

130. Baker's anchorage is also known as: *(AIPG 14)*

a. Intramaxillary anchorage
b. Intraoral anchorage
c. Extraoral anchorage
d. Intermaxillary anchorage

Ans. d

131. Among the syphilic glossitis, plummer-vinson syndrome, mickuliz disease and hepatitis A, which of the following is/are associated with squamous cell carcinoma? *(AIIMS May 14)*

a. Syphilitic Glossitis, Plummer-Vinson syndrome
b. Mickuliz disease and Plummer-Vinson syndrome
c. Hepatitis A , Syphilitic Glossitis. Mickuliz disease
d. Plummer-Vinson syndrome and hepatitis A

Ans. a

132. Regarding oropharyngeal throat pack all are true except: *(AIIMS May 14)*

a. It is given in awake patient
b. Should be given after general anesthesia
c. Prevent ingress of oropharyngeal secretions to trachea
d. Prevent Soiling of trachea

Ans. a

133. In a mouth breather, tonicity of upper lip is: *(AIPG 14)*

a. Increased
b. Decreased
c. Slightly affected
d. No change

Ans. b

134. Transient Bell's palsy during mandibular nerve block after injection of local anesthesia occurs due to needle piercing in to: *(AIIMS May 14)*

a. Maxillary artery
b. Parotid
c. Buccinator
d. Temporal muscle

Ans. b

135. The undesirable side effect most commonly associated with use of finger spring to tip the crown of the tooth is: *(AIPG 14)*

a. Pain
b. Gingival inflammation
c. Tendency for the tooth to intrude
d. Tendency of the root apex to move in the direction opposite to the crown

Ans. d

136. Study model with mounted base and trimmed height is: *(AIIMS Nov. 14)*

a. 55mm
b. 70mm
c. 60mm
d. 90mm

Ans. b

137. Gingival involvement is unusual finding in: *(AIIMS May 14)*

a. Pyogenic granulotna
b. Erythema multiforme
c. Primary herpes
d. Recurrent apthae

Ans. d

138. Nasotracheal intubation is contra indicated in: *(AIIMS May 14)*

a. Maxillary fracture
b. Ethmoid fracture
c. Condyle fracture
d. Mandibular fracture

Ans. b

139. Which of the following organism is associated with Juvenile Periodontitis: *(AIPG 14)*

a. A. acetemcomitans
b. S. Sanguis
c. Prevotella
d. B. forsythus

Ans. a

140. Which facial bone is most prone to fracture? *(AIIMS May 14)*

a. Mandible
b. Nasal
c. Zygoma
d. Frontal

Ans. b

141. Drug most effective in treatment of refractory periodontitis including localized juvenile periodontitis: (AIPG 14)

a. Amoxicillin + metronidazole
b. Tetracycline

c. Ciprofloxacin
d. Penicillin G

Ans. a

142. Which of the following is not a secondary colonizer of dental plaque? *(AIPG 14)*

a. P. gingivalis
b. Bacteroides
c. S. sanguis
d. Fusobacterium

Ans. c

143. Phagocytes combine with lysosomes to form phagolysosomes, they kill intracellular bacteria by: *(AIIMS Nov. 14)*

a. Catalase
b. NADPH oxidase
c. Peroxidase
d. Superoxide dismutase

Ans. a

144. Typical periodontal disease associated with AIDS is: *(AIPG 14)*

a. Acute necrotizing gingivitis
b. Necrotizing ulcerative gingivitis
c. Linear gingival erythema
d. Acute ulcerative gingivitis

Ans. c

145. Diameter of bristles used in soft tooth brush is: *(AIPG 14)*

a. 0.007 inches
b. 0.012 inches
c. 0.014 inches
d. 0.0 10 inches

Ans. a

146. Ideal ratio of nose length to width is: *(AIPG 14)*

a. 62.5%
b. 66%
c. 65%
d. 70%

Ans. d

147. Office personnel who are at higher risk of NO toxicity, to prevent them the most sensitive test for nitrous oxide detection: *(AIIMS Nov. 14)*

a. Lamilar flow
b. Dosimeter
c. Infrared spectrophotometer
d. High suction speed

Ans. c

148. Oronasal intubation is not indicated in: *(AIPG 14)*

a. Le Fort I fractures
b. Le Fort II and III fractures
c. Parietal bone fractures
d. Mandibular fractures

Ans. b

149. A child suffers from trauma which causes intrusion of primary central incisor. The tooth is not in occlusion and does not cause any interference, what should be done: *(AIIMS May 14)*

a. Allow passive and spontaneous re-eruption
b. Orthodontic extrusion and splinting
c. Reduce opposing tooth
d. Be interacted

Ans. a

150. A 30 year old female reported with a mild swelling and pain of the mandible on the right side in the region of tooth #46. The cortex showed mild elevation without perforation. The CT scan of the mandible showed onion skin appearance of the underlying bone. What is the probable diagnosis? *(AIPG 14)*

a. Osteosarcoma
b. Ewing's sarcoma
c. Chronic osteomyelitis
d. Fibrous dysplasia

Ans. b

151. Metal oxides are added in porcelain provide all except: *(AIIMS May 14)*

a. Strength
b. Improve bonding
c. Cosmetic
d. Impart colour

Ans. a

152. A patient presents with mild pain in the mandibular 1st molar area associated with a carious tooth. X-ray reveals presence of hyperdense bone surrounding the tooth, endosteal sclerosis and widening of mandibular canal with mild elevation of the cortex. What is the most probable diagnosis: *(AIPG 14)*

a. Acute suppurative osteomyelitis
b. Chronic non suppurative osteomyelitis
c. Garre's osteomyelitis
d. Chronic proliferative periostitis

Ans. c

153. A boy age 11 year with grossly carious right side lateral incisor, LA is given, complains of burning sensation in right eye, swelling in right eyelid, best statement to explain this condition: *(AIIMS Nov. 14)*

a. Middle meningeal artery has tortuous course
b. LA reaches the eyelid via infraorbital foramen
c. Reaction is due to preservative in the LA , it will subside in some time
d. Pain will subside in few minutes

Ans. c

154. Check point in the reduction of zygoma during management of maxillary complex fractures is: *(AIPG 14)*

a. Symmetry at the infraorbital rim
b. Symmetry at the frontozygomatic suture area
c. Symmetry of the zygomatic arches
d. Alignment at the zygomatic maxillary buttress area

Ans. c

155. The type of strain develop when force is applied perpendicular to surface: *(AIIMS May 14)*

a. Compressive strain
b. Tensile strain
c. Shear stress
d. Tensile stress

Ans. a

156. Inferior alveolar nerve paresthesia is most commonly associated with which of the following mandibular fractures: *(AIPG 14)*

a. Condylar
b. Coronoid
c. Body
d. Symphysis

Ans. c

157. Best medium to transport/store an avulsed tooth, which is not to be reimplanted immediately? *(AIIMS May. 14)*

a. Viaspan
b. Hanks balanced salt solution
c. Coconut water
d. Milk

Ans. a

158. In bilateral parasymphyseal fractures of mandible the symphysis falls back due to the action of: *(AIPG 14)*

a. Geniohyoid and anterior belly of digastric
b. Geniohyoid and mylohyoid
c. Geniohyoid and masseter
d. Geniohyoid and temporal is

Ans. a

159. Infant mortality rate does not include: *(AIIMS Nov. 14)*

a. Still birth
b. Early neonatal death
c. Late neonatal death
d. Post neonatal death

Ans. a

160. Percentage of carbon in carbon steel hand instruments is: *(AIIMS May 14)*

a. 1-1.2 %
b. 10-12%
c. 0.6 to 0.8%
d. 6 to 8 %

Ans. a

161. Transient Bell's palsy during mandibular nerve block after injection of local anesthesia occurs due to needle piercing into: *(AIPG 14)*

a. Maxillary artery
b. Buccinator muscle
c. Temporalis muscle
d. Parotid gland

Ans. d

162. Following metal alloy help in reducing hardness of orthodontic wires: *(AIIMS May 14)*

a. Chromium
b. Cobalt
c. Silicon
d. Carbon

Ans. b

163. Technique not used for surgical repair of cleft lip is: *(AIPG 14)*

a. Le Mesurier
b. Von Langenback
c. Millard's
d. Tennison- Randall

Ans. b

164. Spheno-occipital synchondrosis fuses by what age? *(AIIMS May 14)*

a. Three years
b. Nine years
c. Thirteen years
d. Sixteen years

Ans. d

165. Most stable correction of anterior open bite can be achieved ' using which of the following surgical procedures: *(AIPG 14)*

a. Inverted L osteotomy
b. Bilateral sagittal split osteotomy
c. Intraoral subsigmoid osteotomy
d. Le Fort I osteotomy

Ans. d

166. Not true about vibrio cholera is: *(AIIMS Nov. 14)*

a. Increase water and sodium loss by debilitating diarrhea
b. Toxic protein is cholera protein
c. Activate Adenylcyclase
d. Gram positive

Ans. b

167. An adult female on chronic steroid treatment needs removal of multiple decayed teeth. Which of the following should be given prior to extraction? *(AIPG 14)*

a. Antihypertensives to prevent shock
b. Antihistaminics
c. Antibiotics
d. Atropine to prevent vasovagal attack

Ans. c

168. A child of 2 month age is having rootless tooth like structure in lower front region at the level of gingiva, treatment, of choice: *(AIIMS May 14)*

a. Extraction immediately under LA
b. Reassure the patient, root will develop later
c. Extraction under GA
d. None

Ans. b

169 According to composite resection criteria proposed by Gold, Upton and Marx, hard tissue jaw tumors should be removed using which approach: *(AIPG 14)*

a. Excision of bone along with tumor
b. Resection of tumor along with the affected side of the jaw
c. Resection of tumor' along with a large amount of normal tissue
d. Resection of" tumor with preservation of the marginal bone

Ans. c

170. True about conversion of monomer to polymer is: *(AIIMS Nov. 14)*

a. Density changes from 1.19gl cm3 to 0.9 and volume shrinkage is 21 %
b. Density changes from 1.19gl cm3 to 0.9 and volume shrinkage is 7%
c. Density changes from 0.9gl cm3 to 1.19 and volume shrinkage is 21 %
d. Density changes from 0.9gl cm3 to 1.19 and volume shrinkage is 7%

Ans. c

171. A patient comes with the complaint of acute pain and discomfort in jaw. He reveals a history of tooth extraction 3 days back. On examination, the socket is found to be extremely tender, foul smell and fetid discharge emanating from the socket. The patient had no lymph node enlargement in the cervical area or fever. What treatment should be done? *(AIPG 14)*

a. Curettage of the socket and search for broken roots
b. Mild irrigation of the socket followed by placement of a medicated dressing in the socket
c. Mild irrigation of the socket followed by placement of a medicated dressing and suturing.
d. No treatment is indicated

Ans. d

172. Role of plasticizer in synthetic resins in dentistry is: *(AIIMS May 14)*

a. Increase smoothness
b. To increase bulk
c. To prevent polymerisation shrinkage
d. To reduce softening and fusion temperature

Ans. d

173. A patient with acute infection of upper left lateral incisor comes diffuse with swelling on the left side of face. There is associated palatal swelling also which is tender and rebounds on pressure. The patient is febrile and in visible discomfort. What should be the treatment? *(AIPG 14)*

a. Intraoral incision and drainage
b. Antibiotics, heat and fluids
c. Antibiotics therapy only
d. Heat application

Ans. a

174. Ocular fibrous histiocytomif involves most commonly: *(AIIMS Nov. 14)*

a. Eyelid
b. Epibulbar
c. Intraocular
d. Orbit

Ans. d

175. Dental care under local anesthesia is usually feasible in: *(AIPG 14)*

a. Mentally retarded
b. Adults
c. Psychological disorder
d. Children

Ans. b

176. Condensation reaction occurs in: *(AIIMS May 14)*

a. Agar
b. Alginate
c. Polysulfide
d. ZOE

Ans. c

177. Which is not a theory of TMJ ankylosis? *(AIPG 14)*

a. Condylar burst
b. Fracture with deviation causing increased distance between condyle causing it to fuse with zygomatic arch
c. Synovial fluid leakage attracting calcium ions
d. Calcification around the joint

Ans. c

178. 3 year old girl having delayed milestones, playing with himself, difficulty in learning is likely to be suffering from: *(AIIMS May 14)*

a. Mental retardation
b. Autism
c. Specific Learning Disorder
d. ADHD

Ans. b

179. Most common cause of TMJ ankylosis: *(AIPG 14)*

a. Infection
b. Trauma
c. Hereditary
d. Idiopathic

Ans. b

180. Inheritance of cleft lip and palate is: *(AIIMS Nov. 14)*

a. Monogenic
b. Polygenic
c. Multifactoral
d. Sex linked

Ans. c

181. Discrepancy between centric relation and centric occlusion is: *(AIIMS May 14)*

a. 0.15 to 0.2 mm
b. 0.20 to 0.40 mm
c. 0.50 to 1.5 mm
d. 1-2 mm

Ans. c

182. Patient with prosthetic valve is under surgery to avoid infective endocarditis which regimen should be given: *(AIPG 14)*

a. 2 mg amoxicillin 1 hour before surgery
b. 2 gm amoxicillin 1 hour before surgery
c. 500 gm penicillin 1 hour before surgery
d. 1 gm amoxicillin 2 hour before surgery

Ans. b

183. An avulsed tooth is replanted, loss of lamina dura radiographically, dull sound on percussion means: *(AIIMS May 14)*

a. Internal resorption
b. External resorption
c. Replacement resorption
d. Cervical resorption

Ans. c

184. Recommended dose of prednisone for the treatment of desquamative gingivitis is: *(AIPG 14)*

a. Daily dose of 40 mg to 50 mg reduced to daily maintenance dose of 5 to 10 mg
b. Daily dose of 30 to 40 mg reduced to daily maintenance dose of 5 to 10 mg
c. Daily dose of 30 to 40 mg reduced to daily maintenance dose of 10 to 20 mg
d. Daily dose of 50 to 60 mg reduced to daily maintenance dose of 10 to 20 mg

Ans. b

185. To increase radiopacity of composite: *(AIIMS May 14)*

a. Aluminium oxide is added
b. Ferric chloride is added
c. Sodium chloride is added
d. Iron oxide

Ans. a

186. Permanent deformation following strain in compression in increasing order for elastomers: *(AIIMS Nov. 14)*

a. Addition silicone, condensation silicone, polyether, poly sulfide
b. Poly sulfide, poly ether, addition silicone, condensation silicone
c. Poly sulfide, poly ether, condensation silicone, addition silicone
d. Polyether, poly sulfide, addition silicone, condensation silicone

Ans. a

187. Which of the following is true regarding exposure to radiation exposure: *(AIPG 14)*

a. Young rapidly dividing cells are least affected
b. In adult cells the changes are short term which revert back quickly
c. All biologic cells are not altered structurally by radiation
d. Only the central beam is important in evaluation of radiation exposure

Ans. c

188. Alginate at 20 deg. gel is formed in: *(AIIMS May 14)*

a. 3-4 mins
b. 6-8 mins
c. 15-16 mins
d. 1-2 min

Ans. a

189. Amount of radiation exposure during recording of an IOPA radiograph is: *(AIPG 14)*

a. 5 μSv
b. 25 μSv
c. 200 μSv
d. 5000 μSv

Ans. a

190. C-factor is associated with: *(AIIMS May 14)*

a. Condensing force for amalgam
b. Cavity preparation factor for amalgam
c. Root curvature
d. Polymerisation shrinkage in composite

Ans. d

191. Radiograph of a tooth shows appearance of a 'halo' around the root. It may be indicative of: *(AIPG 14)*

a. Horizontal root fracture
b. Widening of the periodontal ligament

c. Root caries
d. Periapical periostitis

Ans. d

192. Prolonged spatulation of gypsum products increases? *(AIIMS May 14)*

a. Increase hygroscopic expansion
b. Decrease setting time
c. Final hardness
d. Compressive strength

Ans. a

193. Hanging drop appearance in the maxillary sinus is indicative of: *(AIPG 14)*

a. Nasolith
b. Antrolith
c. Blowout of orbit
d. Nasal polyp

Ans. c

194. IOTN includes all except: *(AIIMS Nov. 14)*

a. Bimaxillary protrusion
b. Cleft lip & palate
c. Aesthetic component
d. Dental Health Component

Ans. a

195. Radiation dose administered during radiotherapy is measured in: *(AIPG 14)*

a. Curie
b. Sieverts
c. Grays
d. Hertz

Ans. b

196. Which of the following does not corrodes the metal surface in oral cavity? *(AIIMS May 14)*

a. Chlorides
b. Oxides
c. Sulfides
d. Carbonates

Ans. d

197. Which of the following is the least radiosensitive tissues? *(AIPG 14)*

a. WBC, bone cells, epithelial cells
b. Muscle cells, nerve cell, bone cell
c. Connective tissue cell, endothelial cell, Muscle cell
d. RBC, muscle cell, nerve cell

Ans. d

198. Preventive resin restorations are indicated in: *(AIIMS May 14)*

a. Non-cavitated pit and fissures
b. Deep caries to prevent progress of lesion
c. Cavitated fissures which require restoration
d. Wide cavity to prevent cusp fracture

Ans. c

199. An adult patient was treated for a tumor in the right parietal region of the brain 4 years back with radiation and chemotherapy. He returns with a complaint of severe headache, nausea, vomiting and pain in the right side of head. The best investigation for diagnosis of the problem is: *(AIPG 14)*

a. Dual phase CT with digital subtraction angiography
b. 99mTc HDPO PET
c. Gadolinium enhanced MRI
d. FDP SPECT

Ans. c

200. Vertical height of face is not measured by: *(AIIMS May 14)*

a. Boos bimeter
b. Boleys gauge
c. Vernier
d. Wills

Ans. a

201. Pediatric patient planed for costochondral graft for TMJ ankylosis is intubated best by: *(AIIMS Nov. 14)*

a. Topical anesthesia plus sedation
b. General anesthesia
c. Awake fibreoptic intubation
d. Tracheostomy

Ans. c

202. All of the following investigations can be done for investigation of the coronary artery except: *(AIPG 14)*

a. Contrast Echocardiography
b. Intravascular Ultrasonography
c. Invasive angiography
d. CT scan

Ans. a

203. If accidental injection LA with adrenaline goes in to the blood vessel what will happen? *(AIIMS May 14)*

a. Hypotension plus bradycardia
b. Hypertension plus bradycardia
c. Hypertension plus tachycardia
d. Hypotension plus tachycardia

Ans. c

204. Linear accelerators used in medical radiology produce which types of particles? *(AIPG 14)*

a. Electrons and photons
b. Photons and neutrons
c. Electrons and neutrons
d. Neutrons and protons

Ans. b

205. In biopsy true about formalin as fixative is all except: *(AIIMS Nov. 14)*

a. To prevent autolysis
b. To make tissue rigid
c. To kill micro organisms
d. 2% formaline is used

Ans. d

206. Who was associated with second Amalgam war? *(AIIMS Nov. 14)*

a. G V Black
b. Charles ben
c. Huggins
d. Alfred stok

Ans. d

207. Which of the following is not used as disinfectant? *(AIIMS Nov. 14)*

a. 1-2% cetrimide
b. 100% alcohol
c. 2% Lysol
d. 5% chloroxylene

Ans. b

208. Which of the following drugs does not acts through competitive inhibition? *(AIIMS Nov. 14)*

a. Methotrexate
b. Statin
c. DFP disoprppylfluoro phosphate
d. Sulphanilamide

Ans. c

209. Nausea and vomiting postoperatively can be because of all except: *(AIIMS Nov. 14)*

a. Blood ingested
b. N_2O
c. Opioid
d. Acetaminophen

Ans. d

210. Dolichocephalic facial pattern is: *(AIIMS Nov. 14)*

a. Long and narrow arches
b. Long and broad arches
c. Broad and narrow arches
d. Short and wider arches

Ans. a

211. A 12 year old child complains of recurrent pain over right maxillary posterior tooth but clinically no caries can be found. He also reports of cold and fever speells. What should be advised to the patient? *(AIIMS Nov. 14)*

a. Extract the primary retained tooth i.e., 54, 55
b. Extract the tooth 16,54,55
c. Refer to physician for the evaluation of maxillary sinus
d. Do nothing

Ans. c

212. Animal test to check the biocompatibility of dental material are all except: *(AIIMS Nov. 14)*

a. Buehler test
b. Implantation test
c. Ame's test
d. L850

Ans. c

213. Among the following which is most mucostatic impression material: *(AIIMS Nov. 14)*

a. Impression compound
b. Plaster of paris

c. Zinc oxide eugenol paste
d. Dental wax

Ans. b

214. DPT vaccine is not contraindicated in? Gelation temperature of hydrocolloid impression material is: *(AIIMS Nov. 14)*

a. Progressive neurological disorder
b. Severely immunocompromised patient
c. High allergic response to 1st dose
d. Severe convulsions in a patient

Ans. b

215. True about enameloma: *(AIIMS May 14)*

a. A globule like structure usually found on root due to misplaced ameloblast
b. True neoplasm of ameloblast
c. Tumor resembling enamel present on gingival
d. Tumor of ameloblast which fail to differentiate terminally

Ans. a

216. Gelation temperature of hydrocolloid impression material is: *(AIIMS Nov. 14)*

a. 25-35
b. 18-30
c. 35-37
d. 37-38

Ans. d

217. School based dental health care for whole country is adopted by which of the following country? *(AIIMS Nov. 14)*

a. USA
b. NewZealand
c. Sweden
d. Australia

Ans. b

218. Microorganisms responsible for rapid progressive periodontitis: *(AIIMS Nov. 14)*

a. A. Actinomycetemcom itans, Porphyromonas gingivalis
b. Porphyromonas gingivalis and T.forsythus
c. Capnocytophaga and Porphyromonas gingivalis
d. A. actinomycetemcomitans and capnocytophaga

Ans. a

219. Microorganism responsible for acute necrotizing ulcerative gingivitis: *(AIIMS Nov. 14)*

a. Parvotella, Spirochete, fusobacterium
b. Staphylococcus, streptococcus, T. forsythus
c. Capnocytophaga, spirochete, staphylococcus
d. Fusobacterium, staphylococcus, Porphyromonas gingivalis

Ans. a

220. Which is true for a prosthetic valve patient requiring gingival surgery? *(AIIMS Nov. 14)*

a. Antibiotic prophylaxis is not recommended
b. 0.2% chlorhexidine mouth wash is only required
c. No specific measures
d. Antibiotic prophylaxis is recommended

Ans. a

221. Autoinnoculation is seen with: *(AIIMS May 14)*

a. Ameloblastoma
b. Papilloma
c. Benign pemphigoid
d. Leukoplakia

Ans. b

222. A young male present with loose motions and intermittent abdominal pain over the past 1 year. Wet mount stool specimen showed the presence of multiple ova which are more than 10011 in diameter. The causative organisms for the disease shall not include? *(AIIMS Nov. 14)*

a. Fasciola gigantic
b. Gastrodiscoideshominis
c. Echinostimaileocaanum
d. Opistoorchis viverini

Ans. d

223. All of the following can be categorized under a problem village except when the: *(AIIMS Nov. 14)*

a. Underground depth of water is more than 15mtr
b. The dis Lance for safe water is more than 1.6 km
c. When there is excess of mineral ions like heavy fluoride saline iron
d. Water infested with guinea worm

Ans. d

224. The theory behind TENS (transcutaneous electric nerve stimulation) can be explained on the basis of: *(AIIMS Nov. 14)*

a. Allodynia
b. Referred pain
c. Central pain
d. Gate control theory

Ans. d

225. Which is responsible for adhesion of platelet on exposed collagen fibril after an injury? *(AIIMS Nov. 14)*

a. Von willibrand factor
b. Factor 8
c. Factor 9
d. Fibronectin

Ans. a

226. TNM means *(AIIMS Nov. 14)*

a. Tumor necrosis metaplasia
b. Tumor node metastasis
c. Teratoma necrosis metaplasia
d. Tumor necrosis metastasis

Ans. b

227. If accidental injection of LA with adrenaline goes in to the blood vessel what will happen? *(AIIMS Nov. 14)*

a. Hypotension + bradycardia
b. Hypertension + bradycardia
c. Hypertension + tachycardia
d. Hypotension + tachycardia

Ans. c

228. Mid palatal split following Le-Fort I osteotomy is done by moving the maxilla in which direction? *(AIIMS Nov. 14)*

a. Superior
b. Inferior
c. Antero- posterior
d. Transverse

Ans. d

229. Which of the following nonaqueous elastomeric impression materials has the least shelf life? *(AIIMS Nov. 14)*

a. Poly ether
b. Addition silicone
c. Condensation silicone
d. Polysulphide

Ans. a

230. Which of the following orthodontic wire has least modulus of elasticity? *(AIIMS Nov. 14)*

a. NiTi
b. Beta titanium
c. Stainless steel
d. Co-Cr-Ni

Ans. a

231. If you are going to restore lower molar with amalgam which is having cavity with proximal box wide buccolingually, which wedging technique will you use? *(AIIMS Nov. 14)*

a. Double wegding
b. Wedge wedging
c. Single wedging
d. Piggy wedging

Ans. a

232. Study design that is most commonly affected by recall bias: *(AIIMS Nov. 14)*

a. Cohort
b. Case control
c. Cross sectional
d. RCT

Ans. b

233. Reed Sternberg cells in Hodgkin's Lymphoma are derived from: *(AIIMS Nov. 14)*

a. Macrophages
b. N K cell
c. T cell
d. B cell

Ans. d

234. All of the following can be used to differentiate primary teeth from permanent teeth except: *(AIIMS Nov. 14)*

a. Cervical ridge is less prominent than permanent on labial aspect
b. Lighter in colour
c. Roots are long and narrow as compared to the permanent teeth
d. Crown is wider mesiodistally than the crown length

Ans. a

235. Not seen in classical triad of megaloblastic anemia: *(AIIMS Nov. 14)*

a. Howell-jolly bodies
b. Reticulocytosis
c. Hypersegmented neutrophil
d. Macro-ovalocytes

Ans. b

236. Structure that is formed by 2nd branchial arch: *(AIIMS Nov. 14)*

a. Muscles of facial expression
b. Masticatory muscles
c. Condyle
d. Mandible

Ans. b

237. Regarding type l impression compound not true: *(AIIMS Nov. 14)*

a. Incomplete kneading leads to incorporation of water that increases flow of impression compound
b. Even when needed in small quantity it is not heated over flame
c. Is softened in water bath
d. Also called as type j compound according to ADA

Ans. a

238. Which of the following is not true about *H. influenza*? *(AIIMS Nov. 14)*

a. Rarely presents as meningitis in children less than 2 months of age
b. Capsular polypeptide protein is responsible for virulence
c. Requires factor V and X for growth
d. M.C invasive disease of H influenza is meningitis

Ans. b

239. Localised shrinkage porosity can be due to: *(AIIMS Nov. 14)*

a. Rapid solidification
b. Entrapment of the air bubble
c. Incomplete elimination of Wax and incomplete investing
d. Excessive heating of the alloy

Ans. a

240. During which stage of tooth formation the size of the tooth is determined: *(AIIMS Nov. 14)*

a. Apposition
b. Histo differentiation
c. Morpho differentiation
d. calcification

Ans. c

241. Characteristic Histopathological featnre of basal cell carcinoma is: *(AIIMS Nov. 14)*

a. Nuclear palisading
b. Keratin pearls
c. Psammoma bodies
d. Foam cells

Ans. a

242. In normal growing child, the expected increase in weight on the first birth day as compared to birth weight is? *(AIIMS Nov. 14)*

a. 100%
b. 200%

c. 300%
d. 50%

Ans. b

243. Which is not true about phenotype? *(AIIMS Nov. 14)*

a. It is modified with the passage of time
b. It is the appearance of an individual
c. It is genetic sequence of an individual
d. It is influenced by genotype

Ans. c

244. A patient comes to a dentist with decade mandibular 1st molar including mesiobuccal and distobuccal cusp, restoration of choice is: *(AIIMS May 14)*

a. Intermediate restoration
b. Composite
c. Cast metal
d. GIC

Ans. c

245. Which of the following is not true for incubation period? *(AIIMS Nov. 14)*

a. For determining isolation period of a disease
b. To prevent infection among contacts
c. For quarantine of disease
d. To differentiate among secondary cases and co-primary cases

Ans. a

246. A children 10-11 years of age cannot follow the demonstration of tooth brushing technique when he has IQ Level below? *(AIIMS Nov. 14)*

a. 36-51
b. 90-110
c. 70-75
d. 52-68

Ans. a

247. Hox gene is responsible for: *(AIIMS Nov. 14)*

a. Holoprocencephaly
b. Axenfeld-feiger syndrome
c. Gorlin syndrome and
d. Synpolydactyly

Ans. d

248. Which of the following metal ion also acts as a second messenger? *(AIIMS Nov. 14)*

a. Calcium
b. Magnesium
c. Sodium
d. Potassium

Ans. a

249. Minimum concentration of oxygen needed in NO analgesia: *(AIIMS May 14)*

a. 10%
b. 20%
c. 30%
d. 40%

Ans. c

250. True about the common property of amalgam and ceramic: *(AIIMS Nov. 14)*

a. Increased compressive strength and decreased tensile strength
b. Increased compressive and tensile strength
c. Decreased compressive strength and increased tensile strength
d. Increased setting and working time

Ans. a

251. A one year old child, who is earlier normal, is suffering from copious nasal discharge, coarse facial features, large tongue, bulging head and flattened nose. He is also having enlarged spleen and liver. What may be the cause? *(AIIMS Nov. 14)*

a. Hypothyroidism
b. Beckwith widman syndrome
c. Proteussyndrome
d. Hurler syndrome

Ans. d

252. A novel acidic non amelogenin enamel protein which helps in mineralization: *(AIIMS May 14)*

a. Enamelin
b. Tuftelin
c. Sheathlin
d. Amelogenin

Ans. b

253. Bone sounding done in modern times is performed by which method? *(AIIMS Nov. 14)*

a. RVG
b. Probing
c. CBCT
d. Radiovisiography

Ans. c

254. Which combination forms day care anesthesia? *(AIIMS Nov. 14)*

a. Fentanyl, propofol, Isoflurane
b. Pethidine, Propofol, Isoflurane
c. Thiopental pethidime, Halothane
d. Thiopentane, isoflurane fantanyl

Ans. a

255. Most common sign of airway obstruction is: *(AIIMS May 14)*

a. Slow pounding pulse
b. Strenuous breathing
c. Increase pulse rate
d. Decrease pulse rate

Ans. b

256. Most biocompatible elastomeric impression material is: *(AIIMS Nov. 14)*

a. Polysulfide
b. Polyether
c. Addition silicone
d. Condensation silicone

Ans. a

257. Monitoring and diagnosis after completion of H. pylori treatment is done through: *(AIIMS Nov. 14)*

a. Gastric acid test
b. Urea breath test

c. Bacterial culture of stool

d. Sodium chloride test

Ans. b

258. The pattern of change of disease trends of mortality and morbidity where the pandemics of infection are replaced by degenerative and manmade disorders as the main cause of morbidity and mortality is known as: *(AIIMS Nov. 14)*

a. Epidemiological transition

b. Demographic transition

c. Paradoxical transition

d. Reversal of transition

Ans. a

259. Centric holding cusp is: *(AIIMS May 14)*

a. Mesiobuccal cusp of maxillary 1st molar

b. Mesiolingual cusp of mandibular first molar

c. Distolingual cusp of mandibular 1st molar

d. Mesiopalatal cusp of maxillary 1st molar

Ans. d

260. Nasal RAE, intubation true is: *(AIIMS Nov. 14)*

a. Can be done in case of basilar skull fracture

b. Keeps patient intubated in post op period

c. Is used to perform cleft palate surgery

d. Keeps surgical field free during surgery

Ans. d

261. Throat pack is used in: *(AIIMS Nov. 14)*

a. Endotracheal tube without cuff

b. After LMA intubation

c. Endotracheal tube with cuff

d. In all oral surgical intubations

Ans. d

262. A study was done where the sale of anti-asthma drug was recorded and the number of deaths because of asthma was measured over a period of 15 years (1975 - 1990). This is which type of study: *(AIIMS Nov. 14)*

a. Ecological

b. Case reference

c. Experimental

d. Psephology

Ans. a

263. A patient is not responding even after undergoing multiple platelet transfusion. Which of the following will be the best treatment for him? *(AIIMS Nov. 14)*

a. A random platelet donor

b. B single platelet donor

c. C HLA matched platelet

d. Irradiated platelets

Ans. c

264. Regarding oropharyngeal throat pack all are true except: *(AIIMS Nov. 14)*

a. It is given in awake patient

b. Should be given after general anesthesia

c. Prevent ingress of oropharyngeal secretions to trachea
d. Prevent soiling of trachea

Ans. a

265. The fourth canal in maxillary first molar is commonly located in: *(COMEDK 14)*

a. Distobuccal
b. Palatal
c. Mesiobuccal
d. Distolingual

Ans. c

266. The occupational Safety and Health Administration (OSHA) has set a threshold limit value as the maximum amount of mercury vapor allowed in a workplace. This value is: *(COMEDK 14)*

a. 0.05mg/m3
b. 0.5mg/m3
c. 1.5mg/m3
d. 4mg/m3

Ans. a

267. Acquired, symmetric hyper pigmentation of the sun exposed skin of the face & neck which is strongly associated with pregnancy & use of oral contraceptives is called as: *(COMEDK 14)*

a. Melanoma
b. Café-au-lait spots
c. Freckle
d. Melasma

Ans. d

268. The suckling reflex and infantile swallow normally disappear by the: *(COMEDK 14)*

a. First year
b. Second year
c. Sixth year
d. Eight year

Ans. a

269. Id, ego and super ego are part of: *(COMEDK 14)*

a. Piaget's theory
b. Freud's psychoanalytical theory
c. Stone and Churchill's theory
d. Erickson's theory

Ans. b

270. The number of fibroblasts in the periodontal ligament ____________ with age. **(COMEDK 14)**

a. Increase
b. Decrease
c. Remains same
d. May increase or decrease

Ans. b

271. Most common lesion in Mucous membrane pemphigoid is: *(COMEDK 14)*

a. Esophageal ulcer
b. Symblepharon
c. Ulcer of Soft palate
d. Desquammative gingivits

Ans. d

272. When the time of exposure is doubled? *(COMEDK 14)*

a. The number of Photons generated is doubled
b. The energy of Photons generated is doubled
c. The velocity of photons is doubled
d. The mass of photons is doubled

Ans. a

273. While making impression of flabby fibrous tissues on maxillary ridge for complete denture prosthesis, care is taken to: *(COMEDK 14)*

a. Use mucostatic impression technique
b. Use selective pressure technique of impression making
c. Use a close fitting tray
d. Follow normal procedures

Ans. a

274. Cricothyroidotomy is contraindicated in: *(COMEDK 14)*

a. Age below 5 years
b. Age between 15-20 years
c. Age between 20-30 years
d. Age between 30-40 years

Ans. a

275. The ideal crown height space needed for a fixed implant prosthesis should range between: *(COMEDK 14)*

a. 4-6mm
b. 6-8mm
c. 8-12mm
d. 15-16mm

Ans. c

276. Which among the following antibiotics should be avoided in pregnancy? *(COMEDK 14)*

a. Erythromycin
b. Tetracycline
c. Cephalexin
d. Amoxicillin

Ans. b

277. Most commonly used treponemal text in diagnosis of syphilis is: *(COMEDK 14)*

a. TPI (Treponema pallidum immobilisation)
b. TPIA (Treponema pallidum immune adherence)
c. TPHA (Treponema Pallidum Haemagglutination)
d. FTA ABS (Fluorescent treponemal antibody absorption test)

Ans. c

278. Which of the following is a DNA virus? *(COMEDK 14)*

a. Hepatitis A virus
b. Hepatitis B virus
c. Hepatitis C virus
d. Hepatitis D virus

Ans. b

279. Glucose transporters present in the β cells of the Islets of Langherhans is: *(COMEDK 14)*

a. GLUT1
b. GLUT2

c. GLUT3
d. GLUT4

Ans. b

280. Ludwig's angina is caused due to pus collection in: *(COMEDK 14)*

a. Submandibular region
b. Parotid region
c. Cardiac muscle
d. Nasal cavity

Ans. a

281. Best treatment for large cyst involving vital structures: *(COMEDK 14)*

a. Enucleation with primary closure
b. Enucleation followed by chemical cauterization
c. Marsupialization followed by enucleation
d. Marsupialization

Ans. c

282. Which of the following are stress bearing areas? *(COMEDK 14)*

a. Buccal shelf area, incisive papilla and palatine rugae
b. Slopes of residual ridge, palatine rugae and midpalatine raphe
c. Incisive pailla, slope of the residual ridge and crest of the residual ridge
d. Slope of residual ridge, buccal shelf area and hard palate

Ans. d

283. In Anterior mandibular occlusal projection, the central x-ray beam enters the patient's face through the: *(COMEDK 14)*

a. Tip of the chin
b. Tip of the nose
c. Floor of the mouth
d. Below the chin

Ans. a

284. Most common cause of clicking: *(COMEDK 14)*

a. Disc displacement with reduction
b. Disc displacement without reduction
c. Hypermobility
d. Loose articular bodies

Ans. a

285. Gingival enlargement is associated with: *(COMEDK 14)*

a. Anemia
b. Hyperpingmentation
c. Leukemia
d. Hyperthyroidism

Ans. c

286. Clinician should avoid using cow-horn forcep for extraction of primary molars because: *(COMEDK 14)*

a. It has poor grip due to peculiar morphology of primary molars
b. It cause damage to gingival tissues
c. It poses great possibility of injury to the crypt of the permanent tooth
d. Greater chances of splitting the concerned tooth while extracting

Ans. c

287. The least favourable form of attempted repair of the root fracture is: *(COMEDK 14)*

a. Healing with calcified tissue
b. Healing with interposition of connective tissue
c. Interposition of bone and connective tissue
d. Interposition of granulation tissue

Ans. d

288. Which of the following orthodontic appliance allows "Passive Expansion"? *(COMEDK 14)*

a. Transpalatal arch
b. Quad helix
c. Frankel
d. Rapid maxillary expansion

Ans. c

289. Which of the following shows 'Inverted pear' shaped radiolucency in Radiographs? *(COMEDK 14)*

a. Globulomaxillary cyst
b. Stafne cyst
c. Median palatine cyst
d. Lateral periodontal cyst

Ans. a

290. Which of the following is likely to have bifurcated roots? *(COMEDK 14)*

a. Mandibular Canine
b. Maxillary Canine
c. Mandibular Incisor
d. Maxillary Incisor

Ans. a

291. Incipient caries consists of opaque, chalky white areas that appear when the tooth surface is dried, this is referred as: *(COMEDK 14)*

a. White spot
b. Hot spot
c. Translucent zone
d. Body of lesion

Ans. a

292. The most likely cause of fluctuating jaundice in a middle aged or elderly man is: *(COMEDK 14)*

a. Periampullary carcinoma
b. Liver fluke
c. Choledochal cyst
d. Carcinoma of head of pancrease

Ans. a

293. Which of the following diagnostic techniques is most specific for pulmonary embolism? *(COMEDK 14)*

a. Pulmonary angiography
b. Ventilation lung scanning
c. Perfusion lung scanning
d. Arterial blood gas analysis

Ans. a

294. A full course of immunization against, Tetanus with 3 doses of Tetanus toxoid, confers immunity for how many years? *(COMEDK 14)*

a. 5
b. 10

c. 15
d. 20

Ans. b

295. Malignant ulcer is differentiated from benign by: *(COMEDK 14)*
a. Heaping up of margins
b. Fibrous scars radiating from crater
c. Induration of base
d. Clean base

Ans. a

296. The reservoir of protozoal infection caused by toxoplasma gondii in children is usually: *(COMEDK 14)*
a. Cats
b. Sheep
c. Dogs
d. Rats

Ans. a

297. The predominant immunoglobulin found in GCF *(COMEDK 14)*
a. IgG
b. IgA
c. IgM
d. IgE

Ans. a

298. The following condition is associated with brown skin pigmentation, hypoplasis of kidney and spllen, absent or hypoplastic thumb or radius, microcephaly mental and sexual retardation: *(COMEDK 14)*
a. Aplastic anemia
b. Pernicious Anemia
c. Sickle Cell Anemia
d. Megaloblastic Anemia

Ans. a

299. The Hinge axis is an imaginary line passing through or near the: *(COMEDK 14)*
a. Center of the external auditory meatus
b. The coronoid process
c. Center of the condylar fossae
d. The center of the condyle

Ans. d

300. Gow-Gates L.A. Block refers to: *(COMEDK 14)*
a. Mandibular Block
b. Posterior Superior Alveolar Block
c. Infra Orbital Block
d. Auriculo Temporal Block

Ans. a

301. The plasma coating of a Titanium Dental Implant (TPS) is done to: *(COMEDK 14)*
a. To increase its acceptance is bone
b. To make the Implant Biocompatible
c. To avoid implant anchorage power in bone
d. To improve implant anchorage power in bone

Ans. d

302. Narrow, high arched plate, prolonged retention of deciduous teeth and failure in the eruption of permanent teeth is a characteristic feature of: *(COMEDK 14)*

a. Pagets disease
b. Cherubism
c. Cleidocranial Dysplasia
d. Osteogenesis imperfect

Ans. c

303. When the dental plaque is allowed to accumulate in the absence of any plaque control procedures, it results in gingivitis within? *(COMEDK 14)*

a. 1 to 3 Days
b. 7 to 21 Days
c. 2 Months to 3 Months
d. 24 hours to 48 hours

Ans. b

304. Negative space with respect to buccal corridors is an infication for: *(COMEDK 14)*

a. Intrusion of maxilla
b. Distalization of molar
c. Expansion of arches
d. Constriction of arches

Ans. c

305. Most commonly occurring neoplasm in AIDS patients is: *(COMEDK 14)*

a. Fibrosarcoma
b. Verrucous carcinoma
c. Kaposi's sarcoma
d. Angiosarcoma

Ans. c

306. Type of Ceementum located in the furcation areas of multi-rooted teeth is: *(COMEDK 14)*

a. Cellular Extrinsic fiber Cementum
b. Cellular Intrinsic fiber Cementum
c. Cellular Mixed Stratfied Cementum
d. Acellular Intrinsic fiber Cementum

Ans. c

307. Which of the following materials SHOULD NOT be used as liner or base under composite restorations? *(COMEDK 14)*

a. Resin Modified Glass Ionomers
b. Flowable composite
c. Zinc Oxide Eugenol
d. Compomer

Ans. c

308. According to the American Dental Association, examining the oral cavity by tongue depressor and available illumination is: *(COMEDK 14)*

a. Type-I examination
b. Type-II examination
c. Type-III examination
d. Type-IV examination

Ans. d

309. Indicator of viral replication in Hepatitis B infection is: *(COMEDK 14)*

a. HbsAg
b. HbeAg
c. IgM anti HBc
d. Anti Hbe

Ans. b

310. Combination of sulfamethoxazole and trimethoprim is synergistic due to: *(COMEDK 14)*

a. Enhanced entry into bacteria
b. Sequential blockade in folate metabolism
c. Inhibition of drug inactivating enzymes
d. Inhibition of drug efflux

Ans. b

311. Microscopic examination of a pus sample shows a filamentous organism which is Acid fast with 1% sulphuric acid. Which of the following organisms could it be? *(COMEDK 14)*

a. Actinomyces israeli
b. Nocardia brasiliensis
c. Streptomyces somaliensis
d. Blastomyces dermatitidis

Ans. b

312. The first plasma protein to be generated after severe protein deficiency is: *(COMEDK 14)*

a. Albumin
b. Globulin
c. Fibrinogen
d. Thrombin

Ans. c

313. Epinephrine should NOT be combined with one of the following local anesthetic: *(COMEDK 14)*

a. Cocaine
b. Lignocaine
c. Procaine
d. Mepivacaine

Ans. a

314. Ethical principles that requires health professionals to fully inform their patients and protect their confidentiality is the principles of: *(COMEDK 14)*

a. Justice
b. Autonomy
c. Veracity
d. Beneficence

Ans. b

315. Major drawback of porcelain is: *(COMEDK 14)*

a. High compressive strength
b. Brittleness
c. Transluscency
d. Hardness

Ans. b

316. Instrument used for lateral condensation of gutta perch along the canal wall: *(COMEDK 14)*

a. Barbed broach
b. Plugger

c. Reamer

d. Spreader

Ans. d

317. Test tube retepegs are seen in the microscopic section of: *(COMEDK 14)*

a. ANUG

b. Inflammatory gingival hyperplasia

c. Gingival enlargement due to Dilantin solution

d. Plasma cell gingivitis

Ans. c

318. Typically rapid palatal expansion is done with a jack screw that is activated at the rate of: *(COMEDK 14)*

a. 1.0 to 2.0 mm/week

b. 1.0 to 2.0 mm/day

c. 0.5 to 1.0 mm/week

d. 0.5 to 1.0 mm/day

Ans. d

319. Genetic factors, Age, Gender & Socioeconomic status are also known as: *(COMEDK 14)*

a. Risk Indicators

b. Risk Determinants

c. Risk Markers

d. Riak Factors

Ans. b

320. A radiographic film to dark and fogged could be because of: *(COMEDK 14)*

a. Increased Exposure time

b. Thin patient tissues

c. Poor film storage

d. High developer concentration

Ans. c

321. SUNARY OR SUN BURST radiographic pattern is seen in: *(COMEDK 14)*

a. Osteogenic Sarcoma

b. Osteogenic Carcinoma

c. Ameloblastoma

d. Fibrous Dysplasia

Ans. a

322. Absorbable suture is: *(COMEDK 14)*

a. Cat Gut

b. Nylon

c. Silk

d. Linen

Ans. a

323. Overall optimum degree of taper of tooth preparation for maxillary anterior tooth is: *(COMEDK 14)*

a. 6°

b. 10°

c. 14°

d. 19°

Ans. b

324. Glucose concentration in gingival crevicular fluid is: *(COMEDK 14)*

a. 2-3 times greater than in serum
b. 2-3 times lesser than in serum
c. 10 times greater than in serum
d. 10 times lesser than in serum

Ans. a

325. In children below age of 8 year, high level of cranio-facial disjunction of Lefort III classification is rarely seen because: *(COMEDK 14)*

a. Children in that age group really get affected by such traumatic incidence
b. Facial skeleton is covered with thick soft tissue
c. There is lack of poorly developed ethmoidal & sphenoidal sinus
d. The line of demarcation between medullary & cortical bone is less evident

Ans. c

326. To minimize the effects of diffusion hypoxia during N2O–N2 analgesia, the patient should be oxygenated for: *(COMEDK 14)*

a. 30 second to 1 minute
b. 3 to 5 minutes
c. 10 to 30 minutes
d. 30 to 45 minutes

Ans. b

327. Among the following which one is considered as pathologic problem when planning treatment in orthodontics: *(COMEDK 14)*

a. Tendency of lower jaw & teeth to be behind upper
b. Deep Overbite
c. Minimal attached gingival in lower anterior
d. Decalcification

Ans. c

328. In hypodentia, the most commonly affected tooth is: *(COMEDK 14)*

a. Permanent third molar
b. Permanent secnd permolar
c. Permanent lateral incisor
d. Permanent Canine

Ans. a

329. The best bio-compatible dental casting alloy is: *(COMEDK 14)*

a. Co-Cr
b. Ni-Cr
c. Titanium alloy
d. Gold

Ans. c

330. Instruments used for removal of lingual shoulder and enlarge orifices of a root canal are: *(COMEDK 14)*

a. Gates Gliden drills
b. Peeso reamers
c. Compactor
d. H File

Ans. a

331. A two-way process of exchanging or shaping ideas, feelings and information is called as: *(COMEDK 14)*

a. Education
b. Communication
c. Interview
d. Suggestions

Ans. b

332. Heparin therapy is best monitored by which of the following given test? *(COMEDK 14)*

a. Prothombin time
b. Bleeding time
c. Activated Partial Thromboplastin Time
d. International Normalised Ratio

Ans. c

333. The presence of Heinz bodies in erythrocytes indicates: *(COMEDK 14)*

a. Malarial infection
b. Haemoglobin abnormalities
c. Oxidative stress
d. Degraded bacterial forms

Ans. c

334. Which one of the following is seen in facial palsy? *(COMEDK 14)*

a. Dropping of eyelid
b. Loss of taste sensation in anterior 2/3 of tongue
c. Excess of saliva secretion
d. Loss of general sensation in cheek

Ans. b

335. The objective of the access cavity preparation is to gain direct access to: *(COMEDK 14)*

a. Pulp chamber
b. Canal orifice
c. Apical formen
d. Middle third of the canal

Ans. c

336. According to FDI tooth numbering system the number 45 refers to: *(COMEDK 14)*

a. Deciduous mandibular right second molar
b. Mandibular right second premolar
c. Mandibular right second permolar
d. Deciduous maxillary right second molar

Ans. b

337. The unalloyed form of titanium used to form dental implants in the: *(COMEDK 14)*

a. Beta form
b. Alpha form
c. Gamma form
d. Delta form

Ans. b

338. The schilling test is used detecting: *(COMEDK 14)*

a. Presence of intrinsic factor
b. Deficiency of riboflavin
c. Excretion of Folic acid
d. Capillary fragility

Ans. a

339. In a preadolescent child mximum midline diastoma that will be closed spontaneously after canine eruption: *(COMEDK 14)*

a. 1 mm
b. 2 mm
c. 4 mm
d. 5 mm

Ans. b

340. Cyclic neutropenia is an autosomal dominant condition in which the individuals are at risk for opportunistic infection at intervals of: *(COMEDK 14)*

a. 25 days
b. 21 days
c. 45 days
d. 31 days

Ans. b

341. The principle consideration in cases of surgical obturators during initial healing period is to gain maximum: *(COMEDK 14)*

a. Esthetics
b. Phonetics
c. Accuracy in fit of the defect
d. Stabilization

Ans. d

342. The maximum lidocaine dose with vasoconstrictor: *(COMEDK 14)*

a. 4.9 mg/kg
b. 7 mg/kg
c. 3.6 mg/kg
d. 7.4 mg/kg

Ans. b

343. The amino acid which undergoes most significant hepatic oxidative determination which is used for urea synthesis is: *(COMEDK 14)*

a. Glutamine
b. Glutamate
c. Asparate
d. Arginine

Ans. b

345. Which one of them is not a measure of dispersion: *(COMEDK 14)*

a. Range
b. Mean Deviation
c. Standard Deviation
d. Mean

Ans. d

346. At what age does calcification of the primary dentition begin? *(COMEDK 14)*

a. 6–10 week in utero
b. 13–19 weeks to utero
c. 22–26 weeks in utero
d. 30–34 weeks in utero

Ans. b

347. The term Localized acute Alveolar Osteomyelitics is also used to describe: *(COMEDK 14)*

a. Dry Socket
b. Garre's Osteomyelitis
c. Selerotic cemental masses
d. Florid osseuous dysplasis

Ans. a

348. Primary tumors of the posterior third of the tongue are best treated by: *(COMEDK 14)*

a. Radium implants
b. External beam radiotherapy
c. Surgery
d. Chemotherapy

Ans. b

349. Tram line is seen in: *(COMEDK 14)*

a. CSF Ottorhoea
b. CSF Rhinorrhoea
c. Condylar fracture of mandible
d. Infra orbital rim fracture

Ans. b

350. The encircled number in the given instrument formula represents 10 - 80 - 6 - 12: *(COMEDK 14)*

a. Width of the blade
b. Length of the blade
c. Angulation of the blade to the long axis
d. Angulation of the cutting edge of blade to the long axis

Ans. d

351. The control for mastication is normally exercised by: *(COMEDK 14)*

a. Pontine centres
b. Sub cortical centres
c. Cerebellar centres
d. Medulla centres

Ans. b

352. Inflammation of the periapical tissue is sustained by which of the following: *(COMEDK 14)*

a. Stagnant tissue fluid
b. Necrotic tissue
c. Microorganisms
d. Pus cells

Ans. c

353. Perel pontic is: *(COMEDK 14)*

a. Ovate
b. Conical
c. Hygienic
d. Modified sanitary

Ans. d

354. Long acting Local anesthetic agent: *(COMEDK 14)*

a. Lidocaine
b. Prilocaine
c. Bupivacine
d. Procaine

Ans. c

355. "PERICISION" is the sectioning of the: *(COMEDK 14)*

a. Transeptal gingival fibers
b. Horizontal fibers
c. Oblique fibers
d. Apical fibers

Ans. a

356. All of the following are true about H- files except: *(COMEDK 14)*

a. They have good cutting efficiency
b. They are fragile and tend to break easily
c. They are used in torqueing action
d. They have more positive rake angle

Ans. c

A 70-year-old male complains of ulceration on lower lip since 1 month. Patient has history of tobacco chewing since 30 years 6-7 times per day, patient also complains of loss of weight since 2 months and change in voice since one month.

357. A reliable clinical condition to consider for the diagnosis as malignancy is: *(COMEDK 14)*

a. An ulcerative lesion
b. An ulcerative amd painful lesion
c. Ulceration and fixation of the lymph node
d. Bilateral involvement of lymph node

Ans. c

358. In this condition the lymph node enlargement maybe due to: *(COMEDK 14)*

a. Infection of the malignant lesion
b. Reactive hyperplasia secondary to infection
c. Infiltration of lymph node by bacteria or virus
d. Infiltration of lymph node by tumor cell

Ans. d

359. The patient is complaining of change in voice, which nerve could be affected? *(COMEDK 14)*

a. Recurrent laryngeal
b. Internal laryngeal
c. External laryngeal
d. Superficial laryngeal

Ans. a

A 16-years-old female patient reported with chief complaint of small ulcers on the cheek and tongue since one week, Mild rise in temperature was noted on general examination. On oral examination, multiple ulcers were noted on the buccal and labial mucosa. She also reported that she is having her board examination in a week.

360. The likely diagnosis is: *(COMEDK 14)*

a. Bullous permphigoid
b. Minor aphthous ulcers
c. Traumatic ulcer
d. Tuberculoid ulcer

Ans. b

361. The probable etiology is: *(COMEDK 14)*

a. Emotional disturbances
b. Vitamin deficiency
c. Hormonal disturbanes
d. Any of the above

Ans. d

362. The management of such a case would be: *(COMEDK 14)*

a. Antibiotics and analgesics
b. Symptomatic treatment, topical steroids and relaxation
c. Anti-fungal medications
d. Systemic steroids

Ans. b

363. The external carotid artery divides at the level of: *(COMEDK 14)*

a. Angle of mandible
b. Neck of mandible
c. Oblique line of thyroid cartilage
d. Lower border of cricoid cartilage

Ans. b

364. The absorption of dietary triglycerides from the gut is mainly as: *(COMEDK 14)*

a. Triglycerides
b. Monoacylglycerol
c. Diacylglycerol
d. Fatty acids and glycerol

Ans. b

365. The most frequent non sporing anaerobic bacilli isolated from clinical specimen is: *(COMEDK 14)*

a. Bacteroides fragilis
b. Clostridium tetani
c. Prevotella melaninogenica
d. Fusobacterium nucleatum

Ans. a

366. The most common benign tumor of the lung is: *(COMEDK 14)*

a. Hamartoma
b. Alveolar adenoma
c. Teratoma
d. Fibroma

Ans. a

367. "The meeting of accumulate dental needs at the time a population group is taken into the program and the detection and correction of new increments of dental disease on a semi annual/other period basis" is: *(COMEDK 14)*

a. Incremental dental care
b. Comprehensive dental care
c. Total dental care
d. Preventive dental care

Ans. b

368. The recommended rubber dam to provide effective retraction of gingival tissue is: *(COMEDK 14)*

a. Thin
b. Extra heavy
c. Heavy
d. Medium

Ans. c

369. Cells occurring in greatest number in pulp are: *(COMEDK 14)*

a. Cementoblasts
b. Fibroblasts

c. Osteoblasts
d. Ameloblasts

Ans. b

370. The monophase elastomeric material can be used as both tray and syringe material because it has: *(COMEDK 14)*

a. A long setting time
b. It is economical
c. Pseudoplastic properties
d. Better recording of tissues

Ans. c

371. Which of the following material used in orthodontics, commonly causes sensitivity? *(COMEDK 14)*

a. Steel
b. Ceramic
c. Nickel
d. Plastic

Ans. c

372. Cartilage differs from bone in that, the cartilage can increase in size by: *(COMEDK 14)*

a. Apposition
b. Interstitial growth
c. Selective resorption
d. Endosteal remodeling

Ans. b

373. Down's syndrome is characterized by: *(COMEDK 14)*

a. Low incidence of periodontal disease and low incidence of caries
b. High incidence of caries and high incidence of periodontal disease
c. Low incidence of caries and high incidence of periodontal disease
d. High incidence of caries and low incidence of periodontal disease

Ans. c

374. A patient who complains of constant radiating gnawing pain intensified by eating spicy or hot foods, metallic foul taste and has excessive amount of "Pasty" saliva, lesions are extremely sensitive to touch could be: *(COMEDK 14)*

a. Chronic gingivitis
b. Chronic periodontitis
c. Necrotizing Ulcerative Gingivitis
d. Herpetic Gingivostomatitis

Ans. c

375. Oral hairy leukoplakia is implicated with: *(COMEDK 14)*

a. Entero viruses
b. Epstein-Barr virus
c. Hepatitis A virus
d. Coxsackie virus A

Ans. b

376. Advocated apical seal for dowel core is: *(COMEDK 14)*

a. 2 mm
b. 5 mm
c. 8 mm
d. 10 mm

Ans. b

377. Hyperbaric Oxygen Therapy is given the treatment of Osteomyelitis of Jaw: *(COMEDK 14)*

a. 100% Oxygen at 2.4 Atm pressure
b. 95% Oxygen at 2.0 Atm pressure
c. 100% Oxygen at 2 Atm pressure
d. 95% Oxygen at 2.4 Atm pressure

Ans. a

378. Absolute indication for open reduction in Condylar Fractures is: *(COMEDK 14)*

a. Medial dislocation of condyle
b. Deviated condyle
c. Undisplaced condyle
d. Lateral fracture dislocation condyle

Ans. d

379. Choose the correct nerve-pharyngeal arch pair: *(COMEDK 14)*

a. 2nd arch—mandibular nerve
b. 4th arch—oculomotor nerve
c. 3rd arch—gloss-pharyngeal nerve
d. 1st arch—facial nerve

Ans. c

380. Anaphylaxis refers to: *(COMEDK 14)*

a. The severe reaction following re-injection of protein solution in a sensitized animal
b. The severe reaction following primary injection of protein solution
c. The state of immunity developed by repeated injections of any foreign substance
d. The severe reaction resulting from sensitivity to common allergens

Ans. a

381. Infection with Helicobacter pylori is associated with: *(COMEDK 14)*

a. Acute gastritis
b. Chronic gastritis
c. Eosinophilic gastritis
d. Recurrent esophagitis

Ans. b

382. The most important factor associated with causation of head and neck carcinoma's is: *(COMEDK 14)*

a. Intravenous drug abuse
b. Exposure to nickel
c. History of syphilis
d. Tobacco use

Ans. d

383. Which of the following is step in case control study? *(COMEDK 14)*

a. Matching
b. Selection
c. Follow-up
d. Analysis

Ans. a

384. The primary principle of treating endodontic periapical lesions is: *(COMEDK 14)*

a. To eradicate irritants in the root canal system
b. To reduce the inflammation in the periapex
c. To maintain the health of the periodontium
d. To relieve the symptoms

Ans. a

385. Sailography of normal salivary glands reveal the ductal architecture as having an appearance of: *(COMEDK 14)*

a. Sausage string
b. Fruitladen tree
c. Leaf less tree
d. Ball in hand

Ans. c

386. Drug of choice in the treatment of localized form of Juveline Periodontitis is: *(COMEDK 14)*

a. Metronidazole
b. Penicillins
c. Tetracyclines
d. Clindamycin

Ans. c

387. Agent responsible for increasing for VIII activity in hemophilia is: *(COMEDK 14)*

a. Epsilon amino caproic acid
b. Tranexamic acid
c. Avitene
d. Deamino D Arginine vasopressin

Ans. d

388. The abnormalities of tooth morphology in cleft lip and palate patients are mostly observed in Primary and permanent: *(COMEDK 14)*

a. Mandibular molars
b. Maxillary incisors
c. Maxillary molars
d. Mandibular incisors

Ans. b

389. Which of the following is not a bilateral landmark on cephalogram? *(COMEDK 14)*

a. Gonion
b. Condylion
c. Gnathion
d. Porion

Ans. c

390. Antibiotic stomatitis is the other name for: *(COMEDK 14)*

a. Acute atrophic Candidiasis
b. Chronic atrophic Candidiasis
c. Chronic hyperplastic Candidiasis
d. Acute pseudomembranous Candidiasis

Ans. a

391. An example of rigid reversible impression material is: *(COMEDK 14)*

a. Agar-agar
b. Impression compound
c. Alginate
d. Impression paste

Ans. b

392. The Hormone inhibiting both resorption and formation of bone: *(COMEDK 14)*

a. Estrogen
b. Vitamin D

c. Glucocorticoids
d. Parathormone

Ans. c

393. Which of the following is generally the longest root canal on the maxillary first molar? *(COMEDK 14)*
a. Mesiobuccal
b. Distorbuccal
c. Palatal
d. Distolingual

Ans. c

394. Periodontal tissue destruction apically and potentially migrating towards the Gingival margin is called: *(COMEDK 14)*
a. Marginal periodontitis
b. Marginal gingivitis
c. Retrograde periodontitis
d. Chronic destructive periodontitis

Ans. c

395. A data collected for specific purpose and used for the same purpose is: *(COMEDK 14)*
a. Original data
b. Primary data
c. Secondary data
d. Specific data

Ans. b

396. The commonest site for impaction of foreign body in the Gastero Intestinal Tract is: *(COMEDK 14)*
a. Ileocaecal junction
b. Pyriform fossa
c. Pyloric sphincter
d. Cricopharynx

Ans. d

397. Direct Coomb's test is positive for: *(COMEDK 14)*
a. IgA
b. IgE
c. IgM
d. IgG

Ans. d

398. Treatment for recurrent ranula is: *(COMEDK 14)*
a. Incision
b. Excision
c. Excision with adjacent glands
d. Marsupializatio

Ans. c

399. The mean denture bearing area of edentulous mandible and maxilla respectively is: *(COMEDK 14)*
a. 14 cm_2 and 24 cm_2
b. 24 cm_2 and 14 cm_2
c. 14 mm_2 and 24 mm_2
d. 24 mm_2 and 14 mm_2

Ans. a

400. Which one of the following is NOT a lichenoid reaction? *(COMEDK 14)*
a. Graft versus Host disease
b. Fixed drug eruption
c. Pemphigus vulgaris
d. Secondary syphilis

Ans. c

401. Dentoalveolar ablations are caused by: *(COMEDK 14)*
a. Decalcification by acid beverages
b. Mechanical wear
c. Forceful frictional actions between oral soft tissues and adjacent hard tissues
d. Occlusal wear from functional contacts of opposing teeth

Ans. c

402. Frequent periodontal abscesses appear to be an important periodontal feature in: *(COMEDK 14)*
a. Nutritional deficiency
b. Diabetes Mellitus
c. Hormonal imbalance
d. Cardiovascular diseases

Ans. b

403. Antibiotic prophylaxis is not recommended in: *(COMEDK 14)*
a. Making of impressions
b. Dental extraction
c. Replantation of a tooth
d. Gingivectomy

Ans. a

404. Center of resistance for maxilla *(COMEDK 14)*
a. Posterosuperior aspect of the zygomaticomaxillary suture
b. Posteroinferior aspect of the zygomaticomaxillary suture
c. Anterosuperior aspect of the zygomaticomaxillary suture
d. Anteroinferior aspect of the zygomaticomaxillary suture

Ans. a

405. The explosive and widespread form of secondary syphilis in immune compromised individual is known as: *(COMEDK 14)*
a. Condylomata lata
b. Mucous patches
c. Lues maligna
d. Lupus vulgaris

Ans. c

406. Which color of articulating paper is used for diagnosis of premature contacts in eccentric relations? *(COMEDK 14)*
a. Green
b. Blue
c. Red
d. Pink

Ans. b

407. Number of developmental lobes in human permanent anterior teeth: *(COMEDK 14)*
a. 1
b. 2

c. 3
d. 4

Ans. d

408. Dentinal sensitivity is attributed for: *(COMEDK 14)*

a. Neural stimulation of dentinal tubules
b. Craze line in dentin
c. Dentinoenamel junction
d. Pain transmission through movements of find in dentinal tubules

Ans. d

409. DOTS is a community based treatment and care strategy for: *(COMEDK 14)*

a. Filaria
b. Leprosy
c. Tuberculosis
d. Malaria

Ans. c

410. Texas Statewide Preventive Dentistry program is also known as: *(COMEDK 14)*

a. Sharp program
b. Tattle tooth program
c. Smile train program
d. Theta program

Ans. b

411. Thrombocytopenia due to increased platelet destruction is seen in: *(COMEDK 14)*

a. Aplastic anemia
b. Cancer chemotherapy
c. Acute leukemia
d. Systemic lupus erythematosus

Ans. d

412. Which of the following is associated with defective apoptosis and increased cell survival? *(COMEDK 14)*

a. Neuro degenerative diseases
b. Auto immune disorders
c. Myocardial infarction
d. Stroke

Ans. b

413. Local anesthetics block nerve conduction by: *(COMEDK 14)*

a. Depolarising the nerve membrane reducing threshold potential
b. Decreasing the membrane permeability to Na+ ions there by stabilizing nerve membrane
c. Increasing the membrane permeability to K+ ions and thereby depolarizing nerve membrane
d. None of the above

Ans. b

414. The most common variety of soft tissue sarcoma is: *(COMEDK 14)*

a. Rhabdomyosarcoma
b. Liposarcoma
c. Malignant fibrous histiocytoma
d. Synovial sarcoma

Ans. c

415. A Dental professional maybe criminally liable if he/she commits tort: *(COMEDK 14)*
   a. Accidentally
   b. Contributory
   c. Intentionally
   d. Unintentionally

Ans. c

416. The Sigmoid notch is also commonly called as: *(COMEDK 14)*
   a. Coronoid notch
   b. Condylar notch
   c. Rami notch
   d. None

Ans. d

417. The surface of ceramic restoration can be etched by: *(COMEDK 14)*
   a. Phosphoric acid
   b. Hydrochloric acid
   c. Pumice
   d. Acidulated phosphate fluride

Ans. d

Read the Passage and Answer Questions No. 418 to 420

A 48-year-old male reported with the chief complaint of ulcer on the gums and on general examination headache, fever and malaise was observed. On oral examination, sharply punched out crater-like erosions of the interdental papillae of sudden onset were noted. The patient also complained of bad breath.

418. Diagnosis is: *(COMEDK 14)*
   a. ANUG
   b. Pericoronitis
   c. Chediak Higashi disease
   d. Desquamative gingivitis

Ans. a

419. In the first visit, this patient should be treated with: *(COMEDK 14)*
   a. Antifungal drugs
   b. Deep scaling and root planing
   c. Superficial scaling, debriment, chlorhexidine mouthwash
   d. Mucogingival surgery

Ans. c

420. This patient's lower anterior marginal gingiva showed comma-shaped defect called: *(COMEDK 14)*
   a. Stillman's cleft
   b. Dehiscence
   c. Fenestration
   d. Cul-de-sac

Ans. a

Read the Passage and Answer Question No. 421 to 423

A 3-year-old child was brought to a physician, his mother was complaining of cranky child who does not eat well and does not sleep well too. On general examination, his teeth were severely decayed and had signs of malnutrition. The doctor referred him to a pedodontist.

421. What child the dentist suspect? *(COMEDK 14)*
   a. Early childhood caries
   b. Radiation caries

c. Primary herpetic gingivostomatitis
d. PFAPA syndrome

Ans. a

422. In the first appointment, the dentist will: *(COMEDK 14)*

a. Start the endodontic treatment of the grossly decayed teeth
b. Examine the teeth and take radiographs
c. Extract the root pieces
d. Start the restoration of decayed teeth

Ans. b

423. Which among these is not the etiology of this condition? *(COMEDK 14)*

a. Bed-time breast feeding
b. Honey coated pacifiers
c. Frequent medication
d. Viral infection

Ans. d

Read the Passage and Answer Question No. 424 to 426

A 32-year-old male patient complains of swelling in left maxillary region with heaviness in the maxillary sinus following tooth extraction of maxillary first molar. Patient gives a history of tooth extraction one week before with Transalveolar type of extraction.

424. Considering the heaviness in the operated site of the maxillary region the use of Mucolytics helps in: *(COMEDK 14)*

a. Reducing the stasis of mucus
b. Reduces the growth of gram negative bacteria
c. Brings about aeration in the maxillary sinus
d. All of the above

Ans. d

425. The average Mocociliary air flow transport in the maxillary sinus is: *(COMEDK 14)*

a. 5 to 20 mm per min
b. 5 to 20 cm per min
c. 5 to 20 km per min
d. 5 to 20 dm per min

Ans. a

426. The most common microbial population found in a infected maxillary sinus are: *(COMEDK 14)*

a. Poly microbial with anaerobic organism
b. Aerobic organism
c. Fungal
d. Viral

Ans. a

Read the passage and Answer Questions No. 427 to 429

You have injected local anaesthesia for a patient for extraction of lower molar using classical inferior alveol nerve block:

427. Which space has the highest chance of infection with this block? *(COMEDK 14)*

a. Lateral pharyngeal space
b. Pterygomandibular space
c. Para pharyngeal space
d. Pretracheal space

Ans. b

428. If patient develops postoperatively trismus the probable cause may be: *(COMEDK 14)*

a. Injury to the inferior alveolar nerve
b. Toxicity of the LA solution
c. Injury to the lateral pterygoid muscles
d. All of the above

Ans. c

429. If the patient is asthmatic what precautions can you take from the following? *(COMEDK 14)*

a. L.A with adrenaline
b. L.A without adrenaline
c. Should not do the procedure
d. Use steroids before the procedure

Ans. d

Read the passage and Answer Questions No. 430 to 432

The parents of an 8-year-old boy complained of frequent severe bleeding on minor trauma.

430. The patient could be suffering from: *(COMEDK 14)*

a. Hemophilia A
b. Anaemia
c. Attention deficit hyperactive disorder
d. Disseminated intravascular coagulation

Ans. a

431. His blood picture will show: *(COMEDK 14)*

a. Bleeding time is prolonged, clotting time is normal
b. Bleeding time is normal, clotting time is normal
c. Bleeding time is normal, clotting time is prolonged
d. None

Ans. c

432. When they consulted a dentist for a decayed tooth, he advised for checking of prothrombin time (PT and plasma thromboplastin time (PTT), which would be as follows: *(COMEDK 14)*

a. PT is normal, PTT is normal
b. PT is prolonged, PTT is prolonged
c. PT is normal, PTT is prolonged
d. PT is prolonged, PTT is normal

Ans. c

Read the passage and Answer Questions No. 433 to 435

A lady in the second trimester underwent a hemogram and her hemoglobin was found to be 6 mg%. The gynaecologist suggested for IV transfusion of packed red cells to improve the level.

433. How much of iron is absorbed by transfusion of 2 units of packed red cells? *(COMEDK 14)*

a. 2 gm
b. 2 mg
c. 1 gm
d. 500 mg

Ans. d

434. The most common oral change due to nutritional anemia is: *(COMEDK 14)*

a. Enlarged tongue
b. Atrophic glossitis
c. Generalized osteolysis
d. Focal marrow expansion

Ans. b

435. Anaemia can manifest as all of the following, except: *(COMEDK 14)*

a. Headache
b. Vertigo
c. Delirium
d. Tinnitus

Ans. c

Read the passage and Answer Questions No. 436 to 438

A 8-year-old boy presented with swelling on both sides of the face, below the ears of 4 days duration. It first started on the left side and then 3 day later on the right side.

436. Possible diagnosis will be: *(COMEDK 14)*

a. Bacterial sialadenitis
b. Sialadenosis
c. Epidemic parotitis
d. Sialadenitis

Ans. c

437. Cause for the disease will be: *(COMEDK 14)*

a. Herpes simplex virus
b. Cytomegalo virus
c. Paramyxo virus
d. Hepatitis C virus

Ans. c

438. Immunization to this disease can be achieved by the following vaccination: *(COMEDK 14)*

a. MMR
b. BCG
c. Hepatitis B
d. Polio

Ans. a

Read the passage and Answer Questions No. 439 to 441

A 60-year-old diabetic female presented with burning sensation to spicy food. Intra oral examination revealed multiple periodontal abscess and keratotic area in a lace pattern with occasional erosive areas inside the lace pattern:

439. Provisional diagnosis for this lady will be: *(COMEDK 14)*

a. Oral hairy leukoplakia
b. Oral lichen planus
c. Oral squamous cell carcinoma
d. Oral pemphigus

Ans. b

440. Syndrome associated with this disease is: *(COMEDK 14)*

a. Down's syndrome
b. Greenspan syndrome
c. Peutz-Jeghers syndrome
d. Sjogren's syndrome

Ans. b

441. Histological feature will be: *(COMEDK 14)*

a. Elongated rete ridges
b. Flattened rete ridges
c. Saw tooth rete ridges
d. Bulbous rete ridges

Ans. c

Read the Passage and Answer Question No. 442 to 444

A 3-years-child was brought to a physician, his mother was complaining of cranky child who does not eat well and does not sleep well too. On general examination, his teeth were severely decayed and had signs of malnutrition. The doctor referred him to a pedodontist.

442. What did the dentist suspect? *(COMEDK 14)*

a. Early childhood caries
b. Radiation caries
c. Primary herpetic gingivostomatitis
d. PFAPA syndrome

Ans. a

443. In the first appointment, the dentist will: *(COMEDK 14)*

a. Start the endodontic treatment of the grossly decayed teeth
b. Examine the teeth and take radiographs
c. Extract the root pieces
d. Start the restoration of decayed teeth

Ans. b

444. Which among these is not the etiology of this condition? *(COMEDK 14)*

a. Bed-time breast feeding
b. Honey coated pacifiers
c. Frequent medication
d. Viral infection

Ans. d

445. Drug of choice in acute bacterial menignitis: *(AIIMS Nov. 14)*

a. Erythromycin
b. Ceftriaxine
c. Sulfisoxazole
d. Cefoparazone

Ans. a

446. A 10-year-old boy with unsusal small mandible: *(AIIMS Nov. 14)*

a. Will catch up growth in puberty and achieve normal occlusion
b. High chance of developing snoring and obstructive sleep apnea
c. Will require surgery after growth is complete
d. Chances of condylar fracture

Ans. b

447. A 10-year-old boy with class 11 div 1 malocclusion and overjet of 5 mm or more: *(AIIMS Nov. 14)*

a. Maxillary anteriors are more prone to truama
b. Throat inflammation
c. Malnourished child
d. Hyperkinetic child

Ans. a

448. Adequate interocclusal rest space required for the comfort of the patient and health of the tissues is: *(COMEDK 14)*

a. 1-8 mm
b. 4-6 mm
c. 5-8 mm
d. 2-4 mm

Ans. d

449. One of the following is used for root bio-modification: *(COMEDK 14)*

a. Metronidazole
b. Ciprofloxacin
c. Pencillin
d. Tetracycline

Ans. d